Comprehensive Group Psychotherapy

SECOND EDITION

Comprehensive Group Psychotherapy

EDITED BY

SECOND EDITION

Harold I. Kaplan, M.D.

Professor of Psychiatry,
New York University School of Medicine;
Attending Psychiatrist,
University Hospital of the New York University Medical Center;
Attending Psychiatrist,
Bellevue Hospital, New York, New York

Benjamin J. Sadock, M.D.

Professor of Psychiatry,
New York University School of Medicine;
Attending Psychiatrist,
University Hospital of the New York University Medical Center;
Attending Psychiatrist,
Bellevue Hospital, New York, New York

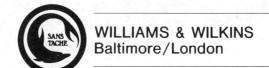

WILLIAMS & WILKINS
Baltimore/London

Library of Congress Cataloging in Publication Data

Main entry under title·

Comprehensive group psychotherapy.

   Includes bibliographies and index.
   1. Group psychotherapy. I. Kaplan, Harold I. II. Sadock, Benjamin J., 1933.
[DNLM: 1. Psychotherapy,   Group.   WM   430   C737]   RC488.C585   1982
616.89′152   82-8369 ISBN 0-683-04521-0   AACR2

Composed and printed at the
Waverly Press, Inc.
Mt. Royal and Guilford Aves.
Baltimore, MD 21202, U.S.A.

Dedicated
to our wives
Nancy Barrett Kaplan
and
Virginia Alcott Sadock

Foreword

At the end of World War II, group psychotherapy was viewed by many members of the psychiatric establishment with a variety of negative feelings ranging from doubt to suspicion to contemptuous rejection. The dyadic relationship and the understanding of the transference neurosis were seen as the essential therapeutic elements of psychotherapy. Many people could not see how the transference neurosis could unfold in a group setting in a manner which would lend itself to analysis, insight, and cure. It can be difficult for someone who did not live through this period to understand the intensity of the conviction with which these beliefs were held. As late as 1960, many fine residency programs in the United States had no teaching of the principles and practice of group psychotherapy. Many fine treatment hospitals relegated it to a secondary role in which groups were usually led for inpatient units by nurses or social workers and only rarely by psychiatrists.

During the last few decades, the use of group has flourished despite these early attitudes. The reasons for its growth and development are multiple. The group approach made it possible for more people to be treated by the same number of therapists. Obviously, this was a highly cost-effective development. The results of group psychotherapy appeared to be satisfactory, and workers in the field reported good results with a variety of patients groups in a variety of settings. It became apparent that the peer pressure of the group could be a useful force for a change even if this force did not reflect traditional concepts of insight. The group therapies also were accepted by a number of nonmedical disciplines, and this extended the cadre of professionals available to offer treatment to a variety of populations.

The reasons for its growth which have been operative are even more powerful in the present. It is obvious, therefore, that the future of group treatment will be even brighter than its recent past history. The desire of more professionals to offer active treatment, combined with the ever-increasing awareness of cost effectiveness, will result in further utilization of these techniques. Perhaps even more importantly, the desire of many individuals to form self-help groups without professional leadership is a movement whose impact is only beginning to be felt. It is always an act of foolishness to prophesize the future, but it seems safe to conclude that these next years will show an increasing popularity and utilization of group techniques.

Not only utilization but the status of the group therapies has changed dramatically. The formal teaching of group techniques is now a requirement for an approved residency training program. Virtually every professional is exposed to group therapy training of one or another type, and virtually every group of people interested in helping themselves with a particular problem has turned to self-help techniques. There is an increasing recognition that there is a method to these activities, and that the method is worthy of scientific study. As is so often the case in the history of science, that which was scorned by one generation is respected by the next. One cannot help but be reminded of Max Born's bitter comment that new ideas are accepted by science only as their opponents die off.

Harold I. Kaplan and Benjamin J. Sadock have combined their diverse and complementary talents once again to produce an outstanding source book for the field. The book is divided into five areas. The first focuses on basic principles, the second on specialized techniques, the third on special categories, the fourth on training and research, and the last on the international scene. They have been successful in obtaining an outstanding group of colleagues to write 58 chapters. They have also appended a glossary for those who are unfamiliar with some of the terminology. It is difficult to imagine that someone interested in an overview of group psychotherapy would require anything beyond this volume. This is an updated edition of a book they first published in 1971, which was very well received by the field. Advances during the intervening years have required a new edition, and the authors have responded to this need in a way that deserves considerable credit. This is an essential volume for any professional interested in the topic, and it is difficult to conceive of a professional who should not be so interested.

Robert Cancro, M.D., Med. D.Sc.

Preface

The first edition of *Comprehensive Group Psychotherapy* appeared over a decade ago. Since then the continued emergence of group psychotherapy constitutes one of the most significant and extraordinary developments in the mental health field.

During this period, alternate views of group therapy as a substitute for individual treatment and as a viable solution to the shortage of trained personnel qualified to care for a growing patient population, the lack of adequate community resources for psychiatric patients, and the high cost of individual treatment have accounted, in part, for the growth of the field. In addition, and more importantly, group therapy has come to be regarded as the treatment of choice for a widening range of patients with highly diverse problems. Concurrently, professionals and laymen alike have evinced a growing interest in the relationship of group therapy to sociocultural processes and systems and to sociological and educational concepts. Predictably, these theoretical developments have been paralleled by the development of myriad therapeutic approaches which vary not only with respect to their underlying philosophy, but also with respect to the planning and conduct of treatment.

The development of an armamentarium of group treatment techniques to meet the diverse therapeutic needs of a varied patient population is commendable in itself, as an indication of the vigor and relevance of group psychotherapy. However, the rapidity with which these techniques have been developed has given rise to serious problems which require prompt resolution if group psychotherapy is to achieve maturity as a scientific discipline. For one, many of the group therapy techniques which are currently utilized, and particularly those which have emerged within the past 5 years, have not been described with sufficient specificity in terms of their goals, the patients for whom such treatment is indicated, and the results they have achieved. Second, there is a dearth of trained professionals qualified to ensure the proper and effective implementation of these techniques.

The organization and orientation of this edition of *Comprehensive Group Psychotherapy* were determined by these considerations. The prescribed aim of this textbook is, of course, to foster professional competence. And, to this end, an attempt has been made to provide a comprehensive survey of the therapeutic techniques which dominate contemporary group practice and the theories and hypotheses on which they are based.

There are no final answers, as yet, to the problems and issues which currently face group psychotherapy and account for the confusion which has permeated this field. But, at the least, the survey presented herein may help to identify these problems and issues and place them in proper perspective.

As noted above, one of the most crucial of these problems is the lack of professionals who must be charged with the responsibility for the future growth and development of group psychotherapy. Thus, a correlative goal of this volume is to underscore the need for adequate—and standardized—training in this discipline, to conform with prescribed professional standards. An attempt has been made in this volume to provide a dynamic and eclectic, but nonetheless structured and systematic, presentation of the body of knowledge currently available in group psychotherapy. Hopefully, the availability of a body of knowledge which can be taught and communicated will stimulate efforts to establish additional programs for training in the skills of group psychotherapy and will enhance existing training programs.

Both editors, in addition to being psychiatric educators, are actively engaged in clinical practice and, in that capacity, have treated patients both individually and in groups. Too often the educator and clinician assume separate functons within our social structure. In fact, this is a false dichotomy, especially when applied to the helping professions. Psychotherapy is an art as well as a science. Consequently, what is taught via the lecture hall or seminar room constitutes just one aspect of the teaching curriculum. Training in psychotherapy must also include clinical exercises performed under the supervision of an experienced clinician who acts as a model for the student.

Authorship

A book written by a single author has certain distinct advantages: It ensures unity and continuity of text and consistency of viewpoint. On the other hand, its scope and dimensions are necessarily limited. The group method of treatment encompasses so many diverse approaches that it would be difficult, if not impossible, for any single individual to discuss them all in sufficient depth and with sufficient objectivity. The editors decided, in light of these considerations, to invite many authors to contribute to this textbook.

The compelling advantage of multiauthorship, in the editors' view, was that each of the group treatment methods covered, as well as those areas in the volume which are concerned with broader theoretical issues, could then be discussed in depth by an expert with special experience or knowledge in a particular phase of theory or practice. Indeed, most of the contributors to this book introduced and developed the group techniques they describe. When the innovators of a particular method were not available for this purpose, their work was summarized by outstanding educators in the field.

At the same time, multiauthorship raises problems with regard to the integration and cohesiveness of material. The editors attempted to deal with these problems by asking our collaborators to follow a specific outline in preparing their contributions. By so doing, we hoped to ensure that each contribution would form an integrated part of the text, without sacrificing each author's unique, creative approach.

Major Modifications in the Second Edition

Although we have retained the basic organization of the first edition of *Comprehensive Group Psychotherapy,* important modifications and changes have been made.

All major psychiatric and emotional disorders discussed in this textbook are in accord with the nosology of the third edition of the American Psychiatric Association's *Diagnostic and Statistical Manual of Mental Disorders* (DSM-III).

In addition, all the sections have been expanded and updated. At least 75 per cent of the material is new, representing significant developments in the field.

Two sections which the editors consider to be classical contributions in group psychotherapy have been retained, although in a somewhat modified form: "Psychoanalysis in Groups" by Alexander Wolf and "Psychodrama" by Zerka Moreno.

Finally, a new and long-overdue innovation is the section on International Group Psychotherapy. This section recognizes the use of the group method of treatment around the world and the original contributions in both theory and technique from investigators working in many different countries.

Acknowledgments

Completing a task of this magnitude required the help of an accomplished and dedicated staff. Nancy Barrett Kaplan and Victoria Sadock provided important aid and assistance throughout the project. We wish to make special mention of Gene Usdin, M.D., and Gail Brenner, M.D., who were especially helpful in advising the editors in the area of international group psychotherapy. Others who helped in the production of this book and who deserve thanks are James W. Sadock, Peter Kaplan, Phillip Kaplan, Jennifer Kaplan, and Judy Drummond.

We wish to offer special thanks to Joan Welsh, head of editorial supervision, for her superb help in the editing of this book. Both her talents and continued friendship are deeply valued. At Williams & Wilkins, James Sangston, Jonathan Pine, Jr., Diana Welsh, and Jacqueline Karkos were of inestimable help. Sara Finnegan, Book Division President of Williams & Wilkins, was also especially helpful.

Virginia A. Sadock, M.D., in addition to writing a number of sections for this book, served as assistant editor and deserves particular mention for her outstanding help in the many editorial discussions and decisions in which she participated.

Finally, the editors wish to thank Robert Cancro, M.D., Professor of Psychiatry and Chairman of the Department of Psychiatry at New York University School of Medicine. He has served as their trusted advisor and collaborator in a variety of psychiatric endeavors including the *Comprehensive Textbook of Psychiatry.* Dr. Cancro heads one of the most important academic and clinical training programs in psychiatry in the United States. The editors have been most pleased to participate and work with the outstanding faculty he has gathered at NYU Medical Center.

H.I.K.
B.J.S.

New York University Medical Center
New York, New York

Contributors

Fern J. Cramer Azima, Ph.D.
Associate Professor, Department of Psychiatry, McGill University Faculty of Medicine; Lecturer, University of Montreal Faculty of Medicine; Co-Director, Therapy Day Center for Emotionally Disturbed Children, and Director, Group Therapy Program, Child and Adolescent Service, Allan Memorial Institute, Montreal, Quebec, Canada

Jerzy W. Aleksandrowicz, M.D.
Associate Professor of Psychiatry, Center for the Treatment of Neuroses, Krakow, Poland

Stanley E. Althof, Ph.D.
Assistant Professor of Psychology, Department of Psychiatry, Case Western Reserve University School of Medicine; Adjunct Clinical Assistant Professor, Department of Psychology, Case Western Reserve University; Staff Psychologist, University Hospital of Cleveland, Cleveland, Ohio

Boris M. Astrachan, M.D.
Professor of Psychiatry, Yale University School of Medicine, and Director, Connecticut Mental Health Center, New Haven, Connecticut

Raymond Battegay, M.D.
Professor and Chairman of Psychiatry, University of Basle; Chief Physician, University Psychiatric Out-Patient Clinic, Basle, Switzerland

C. Christian Beels, M.D., M.S.
Clinical Assistant Professor of Psychiatry, Columbia University College of Physicians and Surgeons; Assistant Attending Psychiatrist, New York State Psychiatric Institute, New York, New York

Michael J. Bennett, M.D.
Instructor in Psychiatry, Harvard Medical School; Staff Psychiatrist, Harvard Community Health Plan; Assistant Psychiatrist, Beth Israel Hospital, Boston, Massachusetts

J. P. Brown, M.B., M.R.C. Psych.
Department of Psychiatry, Hadassah University Hospital, Jerusalem, Israel

Simon H. Budman, Ph.D.
Instructor in Psychiatry (Psychology), Harvard Medical School, and Coordinator of Psychotherapy Research, Harvard Community Health Plan, Boston, Massachusetts

Robert Jean Campbell, M.D.
Clinical Professor of Psychiatry, New York University School of Medicine; Director and Chief of Psychiatry, Gracie Square Hospital; Attending Psychia-

trist, St. Vincent's Hospital and Medical Center, New York, New York

Robert Cancro, M.D., Med. D.Sc.
Professor and Chairman, Department of Psychiatry, New York University School of Medicine; Director, Department of Psychiatry, Bellevue Hospital Center, New York, New York

Wu Chen-I, M.D.
Professor and Chairman, Department of Medical Psychology, Beijing Medical College; Director, Beijing an Ding Hospital, Beijing, People's Republic of China

Stephen A. Cole, M.D.
Assistant Professor of Psychiatry, New York University School of Medicine; and Chief, Family Treatment Unit, New York Veterans Administration Medical Center, New York, New York

Allen H. Collins, M.D., M.P.H.
Assistant Professor of Psychiatry, New York Medical College, Valhalla, New York; Chief of Psychiatry, Lenox Hill Hospital, New York, New York

Donald B. Colson, Ph.D.
Director of Psychology, C. F. Menninger Memorial Hospital; Supervisor, Menninger School of Psychiatry and Menninger Foundation Post-Doctoral Training Program in Clinical Psychology, Topeka, Kansas

Eduardo Luis Cortesão, M.D.
Professor and Director, Department of Psychiatry and Mental Health, Faculty of Medical Sciences, Lisbon; Director of Medical Education and Research, Hospital Miguel Bombarda, Lisbon, Portugal

Atara Kaplan De-Nour, M.D.
Associate Professor of Psychiatry, Department of Psychiatry, Hadassah University, Jerusalem, Israel

John M. Dusay, M.D.
Associate Professor of Psychiatry, University of California School of Medicine, San Francisco; Attending Physician, Langley-Porter Neurological Institute, San Francisco, California

Ahmed Daver Faheem, M.D., D.P.M., M.R.C. Psych. (England)
Assistant Professor of Psychiatry, Department of Psychiatry, University of Missouri-Columbia School of Medicine; Chief, General Psychiatry Section, Harry S. Truman Memorial Veterans Hospital, Columbia, Missouri

Armando R. Favazza, M.D., M.P.H.
Professor of Psychiatry, Department of Psychiatry,

University of Missouri-Columbia School of Medicine, Columbia, Missouri

Guillermo Ferschtut, M.D.
Psychiatrist, Training Analyst and Director of the Institute of Group Techniques; Fellow, Argentine Group Psychotherapy Association, Buenos Aires, Argentina

Jeffrey R. Foster, M.D.
Assistant Clinical Professor of Psychiatry, Mount Sinai School of Medicine; Attending Psychiatrist, The Jewish Home and Hospital for the Aged, New York, New York

RoseMarie Pérez Foster, Ph.D.
Clinical Psychologist, Mount Sinai School of Medicine, New York, New York

Louis A. Gottschalk, M.D., Ph.D.
Professor of Psychiatry and Director, Consultation and Liason Service, Department of Psychiatry and Human Behavior, University of California College of Medicine, Irvine, California; Co-Scientific Director, National Alcohol Research Center, University of California College of Medicine, Irvine, California; Psychiatric Consultant, Veterans Administration Hospital, Long Beach, California

Francis Walter Graham, M.B., B.S., D.P.M., F.R.C. Psych., F.R.A.N.Z.C.P., F.B.Ps.S., F.A.Ps.S.
Honorary Medical Psychoanalyst, Prince Henry's Hospital; Honorary Assistant Psychiatrist, Royal Melbourne Hospital, Melbourne, Victoria, Australia

Jerald Grobman, M.D.
Adjunct Psychiatrist and Consultant in Group Psychotherapy, Lenox Hill Hospital, New York, New York

Martin Grotjahn, M.D.
Professor of Psychiatry, Emeritus, University of Southern California School of Medicine, Department of Psychiatry; Consultant in Gerontology, University of Southern California and University of California at Los Angeles; Training and Supervising Psychoanalyst, Emeritus, Southern California Institute for Psychoanalysis, Beverly Hills, California

Ann Keller Hillman, M.S.W.
Adjunct Faculty Instructor, School of Applied Social Sciences, Case Western Reserve University, Cleveland, Ohio

Leonard Horwitz, Ph.D.
Chief of Clinical Psychology, The Menninger Foundation; Special Consultant, C. F. Menninger Memorial Hospital; Faculty, Topeka Institute for Psychoanalysis, Topeka, Kansas

Edward M. Houser, M.S.W.
Program Coordinator and Field Instructor, Social Work Intern Program, California State University, Long Beach, and University of California, Irvine; Clinical Social Worker, Division of Hematology-Oncology, University of California Irvine Medical Center, Irvine, California

Jarl Jorstad, M.D.
Medical Director, Ulleval Hospital, Psychiatric Department, Oslo, Norway

Mark Kanzer, M.D.
Clinical Professor of Psychiatry, State University of New York, Downstate Medical Center, Brooklyn, New York

Harold I. Kaplan, M.D.
Professor of Psychiatry, New York University School of Medicine; Attending Psychiatrist, University Hospital of the New York University Medical Center; Attending Psychiatrist, Bellevue Hospital, New York, New York

Sigmund Karterud, M.D.
Ulleval Hospital, Psychiatric Department, Oslo, Norway

Howard D. Kibel, M.D.
Assistant Professor of Psychiatry, Cornell University Medical College, New York, New York; Coordinator of Group Psychotherapy, New York Hospital-Cornell Medical Center, Westchester Division, White Plains, New York

Virginia Klein, D.T.R.
Director of Dance Therapy, Payne-Whitney Clinic-New York Hospital, New York, New York

Karl Konig, M.D.
Professor of Psychiatry and Head, Department of Clinical Group Psychotherapy, Center for Psychological Medicine, University of Göttingen, Germany

Irvin A. Kraft, M.D.
Clinical Professor of Mental Health, School of Public Health, University of Texas; Clinical Professor of Psychiatry, Baylor College of Medicine; Senior Consultant, Texas Institute of Family Psychiatry; Attending Psychiatrist, Texas Children's Hospital, Houston, Texas

Irwin L. Kutash, Ph.D.
Clinical Assistant Professor of Psychiatry and Mental Health Science, College of Medicine and Dentistry of New Jersey—New Jersey Medical Center, Newark, New Jersey; Psychological Consultant, Veterans Administration Medical Center, East Orange, New Jersey

Doris J. Lubell, M.A., A.T.R.
Adjunct Professor of Art and Art Therapy, Graduate Art Department, College of New Rochelle, New Rochelle, New York; Art Therapist, Westchester County Medical Center, Valhalla, New York

Joyce H. Lowinson, M.D.
Clinical Professor of Psychiatry and Director, Division of Substance Abuse, Department of Psychiatry, Albert Einstein College of Medicine; Attending Psychiatrist, Hospital of the Albert Einstein College of Medicine, Montefiore Hospital Center, Bronx, New York

Peter A. Martin, M.D.
Clinical Professor of Psychiatry, University of Mich-

igan Medical Center, Ann Arbor, Michigan; Clinical Professor of Psychiatry, Wayne State University Medical School, Detroit, Michigan; Attending Psychiatrist, University Hospital, Ann Arbor, Michigan

James Grier Miller, M.D., Ph.D.
President, Robert Maynard Hutchins Center for the Study of Democratic Institutions and Adjunct Professor of Psychology, University of California at Santa Barbara, Santa Barbara, California; President Emeritus, University of Louisville, Louisville, Kentucky

Jessie L. Miller, M.S.
Santa Barbara, California

Zerka T. Moreno
Director, Moreno Institute, Beacon, New York

Richard L. Munich, M.D.
Associate Clinical Professor of Psychiatry, Yale University School of Medicine, New Haven, Connecticut; Director, Psychiatric Inpatient Services, West Haven Veterans Administration Medical Center, West Haven, Connecticut

Charles P. O'Brien, M.D., Ph.D.
Professor of Psychiatry, University of Pennsylvania School of Medicine; Chief of Psychiatry, Philadelphia Veterans Medical Center, Philadelphia, Pennsylvania

William V. Ofman, Ph.D.
Associate Professor of Counseling Psychology, University of Southern California, Los Angeles, California

John J. O'Hearne, M.D., M.S.
Clinical Professor of Medicine, University of Missouri-Kansas City School of Medicine; Attending Psychiatrist, University of Kansas Medical Center, Kansas City, Missouri

Claude Pigott, M.D.
Consultant Psychiatrist, Institute Claparède, Neuilly, France

Malcolm Pines, M.D., F.R.C.P., F.R.C. Psych., D.P.M.
Consultant Psychotherapist and Former Senior Lecturer in Psychotherapy, University of London; President, International Association of Group Psychotherapy; Vice Chairman, Institute of Group Analysis; Chairman, Training Committee of the Institute of Group Analysis, London, England

Edward L. Pinney, Jr., M.D.
Clinical Associate Professor of Psychiatry, New York University School of Medicine; Assistant Attending Psychiatrist, University Hospital of the New York University Medical Center, New York, New York

William E. Powles, M.D., F.R.C.P.(c)
Professor of Psychiatry, Queen's University; Attending Psychiatrist, Kingston General and Hotel Dieu Hositals, Kingston, Ontario, Canada

A. Venkoba Rao, M.D., Ph.D., D.Sc., D.P.M., F.R.C. Psych., FAMS, FAPA., MRANZ., CP.
Professor and Head, Institute of Psychiatry, Madurai Medical College and Government Rajaji Hospital, Madurai, India

Sheldon D. Rose, Ph.D.
Director, Interpersonal Skill Training and Research Project, School of Social Work, University of Wisconsin, Madison, Wisconsin

Max Rosenbaum, Ph.D.
Clinical Professor of Psychology, Adelphi University, Brooklyn, New York

Bennett E. Roth, Ph.D.
Fellow, American Group Psychotherapy Association; Private Practice, New York, New York

Benjamin J. Sadock, M.D.
Professor of Psychiatry, New York University School of Medicine; Attending Psychiatrist, University Hospital of the New York University Medical Center; Attending Psychiatrist, Bellevue Hospital, New York, New York

Virginia A. Sadock, M.D.
Clinical Associate Professor of Psychiatry and Director, Graduate Education in Human Sexuality, New York University School of Medicine; Associate Attending Psychiatrist, University Hospital of the New York University Medical Center, Bellevue Hospital, New York, New York

Mohammed Shaalan, M.B.B.Ch., D.P.M., N., D.M., M.D. Psychiat.
Professor and Chairman, Department of Neurology and Psychiatry, Faculty of Medicine, Al-Azhar University, Cairo, Egypt

Bo Sigrell, Ph.D.
Assistant Professor of Psychiatry, Psychotherapy Unit, Department of Psychiatry, Saint Göran's Hospital, Stockholm, Sweden

Aaron Stein, M.D.
Clinical Professor of Psychiatry, Mount Sinai School of Medicine of the City University of New York; Attending Psychiatrist and Chief, Group Therapy Division, Department of Psychiatry, The Mount Sinai Medical Center, New York, New York

Norman Sussman, M.D.
Clinical Assistant Professor of Psychiatry, New York University School of Medicine; Assistant Attending Psychiatrist, University Hospital of New York University Medical Center, Bellevue Hospital, New York, New York

Gabor Szonyi, M.D.
Psychiatrist and Psychoanalyst and Leader, Group Psychotherapy Section, Hungarian Society for Psychiatry, Budapest, Hungary

Regin Tischtau-Schroter, M.A.
Research Assistant in Psychology, Center for Psychological Medicine, University of Göttingen, Germany

Teodora Tomcsanyi, Ph.D.
Psychologist and Psychoanalyst and Substitute Leader, Group Psychotherapeutic Section, Hungarian Society for Psychiatry, Budapest, Hungary

Alan B. Wachtel, M.D.
Assistant Professor of Psychiatry, New York University School of Medicine; Director, Medical Behavioral Science Program; Assistant Attending Psychiatrist, University Hospital of the New York University Medical Center, Bellevue Hospital, New York, New York

Myron F. Weiner, M.D.
Professor of Clinical Psychiatry and Vice Chairman, Department of Psychiatry, University of Texas Health Science Center at Dallas, Dallas, Texas

Alexander Wolf, M.D.
Training Psychoanalyst and Senior Supervisor, Postgraduate Center for Mental Health; Attending Psychiatrist, Gracie Square Hospital, New York, New York

Normund Wong, M.D.
Clinical Professor of Psychiatry, University of Kansas College of Health Sciences and Hospital, School of Medicine, Kansas City; Director, Department of Education, Menninger School of Psychiatry, Topeka, Kansas

Contents

AREA A: BASIC PRINCIPLES

AREA B: SPECIALIZED GROUP PSYCHOTHERAPY TECHNIQUES

AREA C: PSYCHOTHERAPY WITH GROUPS IN SPECIAL CATEGORIES

AREA D: TRAINING, RESEARCH, AND SPECIAL AREAS

AREA E: INTERNATIONAL GROUP PSYCHOTHERAPY

AREA A

BASIC PRINCIPLES

A.1 History of Group Psychotherapy

BENJAMIN J. SADOCK, M.D.
HAROLD I. KAPLAN, M.D.

Introduction

In the first edition of this textbook, the importance of studying the origins of the group method of treatment was set forth by Anthony (1971):

The past is conglomerate, complex, confabulatory, and conflictual, but it is incumbent on every worker to resolve these perplexities and complexities for himself and, by so doing, discover his own professional identity and ultimate purpose. Each group psychotherapist must become his own historian and thread his way with open-mindedness and relative impartiality through the shoals of psychobiologically improbable, mythological, mystical, and paralogical ideas of the past and present, asking his own questions and seeking his own answers within the totality of what is known or imagined. He has to undertake this job for himself, since no one can do it for him.

That being so, the very least required of the authors is to point out various landmarks to help Anthony's lonely traveler find his or her way.

Group psychotherapy has been influenced by many persons and philosophies, both American and European, but Americans are usually regarded as the major contributors and innovators in the field. It is especially true today that the major impetus stems from this country. But all along, in this country and Europe, many workers were grappling with similar problems at almost the same time.

American influences

Pratt. The man credited with beginning the practice of group therapy in this country was not a psychiatrist but an internist, Joseph H. Pratt (see Figure A.1-1) In July 1905, Pratt, working in Boston, organized his first group, composed of tuberculosis patients (Hadden, 1975). Most of his patients were severely ill, generally debilitated, and despondent. They were often ostracized from the community, much the same way many mental patients are ostracized today.

Grouped together and often rejected and feared, they seemed ideal subjects for group techniques.

Pratt would meet once or twice a week with 20 to 30 patients at a time. Referring to them as a class, rather than a group, he would lecture about the disease of tuberculosis and the method of cure, and was generally supportive and encouraging about the prognosis. Patients who had responded successfully would present themselves before the group and tell how they had been helped. Difficult patients—those who resisted the method of treatment, which required that they remain at bedrest 8 to 12 hours a day—were seen individually by a nurse, who was known as the "friendly adviser."

Certain techniques used by Pratt are still found in some group methods used today, particularly in homogeneous groups, in which all patients have a common condition. In Alcoholics Anonymous (AA), it is standard practice for the alcoholic to present himself before the group and tell how he achieved the goal of abstinence from alcohol and about the benefits derived therefrom. In both AA and Pratt's group, the process of identification, whereby the sick member takes on qualities and behavioral patterns of the healthy member, is among the therapeutic influences at work.

Marsh. In 1919, L. Cody Marsh, both a minister and a psychiatrist familiar with Pratt's work, began to apply the group method of treatment to institutionalized mental patients. Like Pratt, he referred to the group as a class and to the patients as students. They attended weekly lectures given by Marsh on a variety of topics pertaining to the origins and manifestations of mental illness. Students were expected to take notes during the lectures, and attendance, punctuality, and attentiveness were recorded for each student. Outside reading was assigned, written papers were required, and graded examinations were given. If a student did poorly, he might be required to repeat the course, which was given several times a year. He might also be assigned a tutor to work with him privately.

Marsh arranged discussion groups with all hospital personnel who came into contact with patients—doctors, nurses, social workers, attendants, and so on. He was one of the first psychiatrists to recognize that every encounter a patient had

1

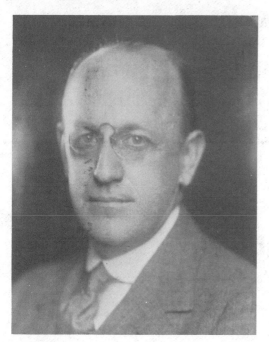

Figure A.1-1 Joseph Pratt. (New York Academy of Medicine.)

within the hospital setting had therapeutic overtones. In this sense, he was a pioneer in the concept of the hospital as a therapeutic community, presaging the work of Maxwell Jones and others in England by many years.

Lazell. At about the same time, another approach to institutionalized patients was used by the psychiatrist E. W. Lazell. His treatment consisted mainly of didactic lectures to schizophrenic patients about their disease. In his lectures, Lazell described the signs and symptoms of the disease and certain aspects of Freudian theory. The results, he felt, were good, and he concluded that patients improved because, in part, their fears were reduced as a result of education. He also believed that the socialization process, defined most simply as patients getting to know one another, accounted for the positive changes he observed. Lazell was one of the first to theorize about the group method of treatment. Pratt tended to view his work more empirically. Lazell was aware that the schizophrenic patient, who might have appeared inaccessible, heard and retained much of the lecture material, and that much of the talking that took place between patients during the lecture was, in fact, the sharing of information, the comparison of symptoms, and the beginning stages of interaction—factors inherent in the process of group psychotherapy that account for therapeutic progress.

Burrow. Lazell and Marsh both worked within institutional settings and with psychotic populations, but at the same time group methods were beginning to be applied to neurotic disorders and to the treatment of emotional illnesses outside of institutions. The main impetus for this parallel movement came from Trigant Burrow (see Figure A.1-2), who also served as a bridge between American and European psychiatry.

Burrow, who received his medical degree at the University of Virginia and studied psychiatry under Adolf Meyer at Johns Hopkins, had met both Freud and Jung in 1909 at Clark University and was analyzed by Jung in Zurich. On returning to this country, he became a vigorous proponent of psychoanalysis and one of the founders of the American Psychoanalytic Association. His interest in the individual's relationship to the social forces of which he is a part soon led to his using the group setting as a vehicle for psychoanalytic treatment.

Burrow called his method group analysis; the term originated with him in 1925. Although he espoused the tenets of psychoanalysis as promulgated by Freud, he was never successful in obtaining Freud's approval of his work to the extent that he would have liked. In group sessions, he encouraged his patients to speak frankly to one another about their thoughts and feelings. He believed there should be no secret about emotional illness or about how persons react to one another. He saw the group member as both the observer and the observed, and he believed strongly that the consensual validation the group as a whole has to offer to the individual member is the main force in effecting greater psychological awareness.

Burrow's continued emphasis on group treatment eventually estranged the growing psychoanalytic community in the United States. In a reorganization of the American Psychoanalytic Association in 1933, he was denied membership in the organization of which he was a founder. Ironically, many years later he was given one of the association's highest honors, the A. A. Brill award, for his scientific contributions.

Wender. Louis Wender regarded the group as a re-creation of the family. He began to use concepts of psychoanalysis in group settings in the early 1930s. Patients viewed the therapist as a symbolic parent figure, and the members of the group reacted to one another as symbolic siblings. Wender encouraged combined treatment, in which the therapist sees the patient individually one or more times a week as well as in regularly scheduled group sessions, a technique that is today growing in popularity. Although Wender's groups were psychoanalytically oriented, his approach was still didactic in that he continued to lecture the patients before each session.

Schilder. Paul Schilder, a psychiatrist better known for his concepts about the body image than for his pioneer efforts in group psychotherapy, began to conduct psychoanalytically oriented groups in the 1930s at New York's Bellevue Hospital. Elaborating on Wender's concept that the group re-creates the family, he also used the technique of free association. He pointed out that thoughts and feelings of one member stimulate associated thoughts and feelings in another. He described, for example, how a patient remembered a sexual assault he made against his sister, with the result that many members of the group recalled similar feelings of sexual attraction to their own siblings. In the group settings, according to Schilder, the patients realized that the thoughts and feelings that seemed to isolate them are, in reality, common to all.

Slavson. During the same decade, Samuel Slavson, originally an engineer by profession, observed that the spontaneous activity of children in certain recreational groups produced behavioral change. He evolved the method of activity group therapy, in which the group leader is permissive and accepting, and the children, who are placed in specially planned groups, are allowed to interact spontaneously. As a result, conflicts are acted out and can be examined. The fact that the children see the therapist as a parental surrogate who permits them to express their hostile or aggressive impulses can be a corrective emotional experience. In a similar way, the withdrawn and fearful child can be encouraged by his peer group and by the therapist to learn new ways of relating.

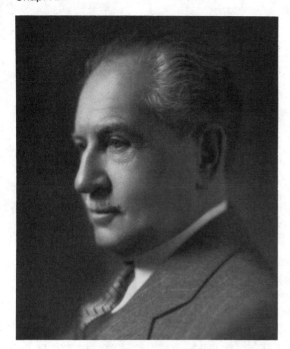

Figure A.1-2   Trigant Burrow. (Courtesy of Hans Syz, M.D.)

Anthony (1971) has described Slavson as having had a major influence on the field. He summarizes his therapeutic stance as follows:

In the therapeutic group, according to Slavson, it is each patient for himself, and the therapist should, therefore, concentrate on the individual rather than on the group as a whole. Slavson recognizes that the individual members affect one another in a variety of ways, including sibling and identification transferences and mutual empathies that make for a collective experience based on the integration of the individual member into the group. The group tends to catalyze the dynamics of the individual patient, accelerating regression, weakening defenses, and at least transiently impairing individuation.

Slavson differentiates between transference and what he calls the basic solidity of the therapeutic relation—what psychoanalysts refer to as the therapeutic alliance. He recognizes that the transference is modified both quantitatively and qualitatively in the group, where he perceives levels of transference.

Slavson played an important role in the group movement as a founder of the American Group Psychotherapy Association in 1948. Composed of psychiatrists, psychologists, and social workers, the organization exists for the dissemination of information among professional group workers. Slavson has also been influential in attempting to ensure adequate and responsible training and leadership in the field.

Wolf. In 1949, the psychiatrist Alexander Wolf published a definitive and now classical work on psychoanalysis in groups that reviewed his experience in group work begun 10 years earlier. Wolf directly applied the principles of psychoanalysis based on Freudian theory to the group setting, and he used the major tools of the psychoanalytic method, such as free association, dream analysis, the elucidation of the transference, and historical development. The therapy group revives the problems the patient had in his original family group. Emphasis is placed on the individual patient and on his relationships to other members of the group and to the therapist.

Wolf originated the alternate session, during which the group members meet regularly without the therapist present. Such a meeting, alternating with a session at which the therapist is present, facilitates more intense interactions between members, and their reactions to the group with and without the therapist present can be compared.

European influences

The temporal association between group work in Europe and group work in this country shows a curious pattern. Pratt, in 1905, was working with groups of tubercular patients. Almost at the same time, Moreno was using group techniques with a variety of patient populations in Vienna. Freud, in 1906, had gathered about him his early followers, who met weekly in study sessions that were as much therapeutic as they were educational. Adler used group approaches in his own work with patients, and, as early as 1918, he formally organized child guidance clinics in Vienna in which group methods were used extensively. Yet there was little, if any, interchange between the old world and the new in that area. Each seemed to evolve independently of the other.

Moreno. Jacob L. Moreno, a psychiatrist, is identified mainly with the technique of psychodrama, which he introduced into the United States in 1925. But he was also one of the European pioneers in group psychotherapy, describing his use of a variety of group approaches as early as 1910. The Theater of Spontaneous Man—the vehicle for psychodrama and role playing—was first set up in Vienna. There, Moreno encouraged the acting out of problem situations to achieve a heightened awareness of the actual conflict and its possible resolution. In his form of group work, the therapist, called the director, encourages the patient, called the subject, to express himself spontaneously by enacting a role out of his past experience or his current life situation. Other members of the group, called the audience, may comment and so be of help, or they may see one of their own problems portrayed and so be helped.

Freud. With the publication of *Group Psychology and Analysis of the Ego* in 1921, Freud directed his attention to group psychology:

Group psychology is concerned with the individual man as a member of a race, of a nation, of a caste, of a profession, of an institution, or as a component part of a crowd of people who have been organized into a group at some particular time for some definite purpose.

Freud differentiated the leaderless group, a mob capable of great excesses, from the leader-centered group, a potential vehicle capable of diminishing anxiety and neurosis. In the group that has a leader, the psychotherapy group members identify with one another and have a common bond to the central figure, who is seen as a parental surrogate. Members react to each other as siblings within the family; as a result, they have mutualities of both love and hate.

Freud's insights into group formation and the transferences that exist between the members, and between the members and the leader, form much of the basis for present-day psychoanalytically oriented group psychotherapy. His influence has been great on those group therapists who use the psychoanalytic model, in that they rely on that theoretical construct as a basic concept underlying their treatment approach.

Freud noted that not only does the leader influence the members of the group, but every individual member acts on every other member. He believed that humans have a herd instinct, as did Trotter, one of Freud's contemporaries. Unlike Trotter, however, Freud did not believe the herd instinct to be primary or indivisible, as he believed the sexual instinct to be, for example. Freud preferred to see a human being as a horde animal—an individual creature in a group led by a chief or leader. With the French sociologist LeBon, another contemporary, Freud believed that large groups or mobs were unruly, capable of excesses, and even dangerous. But he emphasized the crucial role of the leader, and did not think that any group could be understood unless the role of the leader was carefully analyzed. Freud believed that, with appropriate leadership, group therapy was a method that held promise for the alleviation of emotional illness.

Although Freud did not practice group psychotherapy as such, many of his formulations about psychoanalysis and group psychology developed from the study group he organized with his early followers. The study group was composed of about 10 members—including such men as Sandor Ferenczi, Ernest Jones, and Alfred Adler—and met on a weekly basis, beginning in 1906. Freud would elaborate on his various theories as they were being formulated, and they were then explored by the members—psychologists in their own right—through the technique of their sharing together their thoughts, fantasies, and life experiences either to corroborate or to negate the theories as they emerged. Freud apparently participated in this self-exposure to some extent. In addition, Jones, in his biography of Freud, mentioned that, on the ocean crossing to Clark University in the United States in 1909, Freud, Ferenczi, and Jung, shipmates together, shared their dreams and mutually analyzed them.

The study group eventually disbanded as a result of irreconcilable differences in theory that may well have been symptomatic of personality clashes between Freud and some of the members of the group and between some of the members themselves. Kanzer speculated that some formulations set forth in *Totem and Taboo*, particularly the concept of the group's having natural tendencies to attack and destroy the strongest male member, may have evolved from Freud's study group experience, in which he was the object at various times of extremely hostile attacks by some of the participants.

Adler. One of Freud's earliest students, Alfred Adler, was particularly concerned with social and cultural adaptation. Therefore, the relationship of the group to the individual and of the individual to the group were areas he sought to examine. Influenced by certain Marxian concepts, specifically that of the class struggle, he quite naturally began to work with groups and the relationship of the members to the leader, who was, Adler postulated, viewed as a surrogate for many of the oppressive forces operating against the proletariat. Adler's emphasis on the social atmosphere of equality that characterizes the psychotherapy group and on the encouragement, optimism, and support that members offer one another can be considered his major and lasting contribution to group theory. These factors explain important processes that account for the therapeutic influence of group psychotherapy.

Lewin. The trend in group psychotherapy had been to study the individual within the group. Although attempts had been made to examine how the group as a whole functioned, the group was, as Freud put it, simply a collection of individuals gathered together for a particular purpose. It was the social psychology movement, spearheaded by men such as Kurt Lewin, that saw the group as different qualitatively from the simple sum of its parts.

According to Lewin, the group is an entity in its own right, with particular and unique qualities that are different from the individuals of which it is composed. He focused on group dynamics, a term coined by him in 1939, in the same way that Freud focused on individual dynamics. To Lewin, acts of the individual cannot be explained on the basis of an individual's psychodynamics but must be explained on the basis of the nature of the social forces, the field, to which he is exposed. Lewin defined the concept of group pressure, whereby influence is brought to bear on a particular member of the group to the extent that his behavior can be altered. In turn, the individual member influences the group, and together they form a gestalt or whole. Although the group may be composed of heterogeneous elements, it does, nonetheless, function as a unit. Members depend on one another, and each has expectations of the others to the extent that group standards, group ethics, and goals emerge that are unique to a particular group. Lewin's influence on group work has been immense, and the concept of examining the group as a whole must be traced to him.

English school

A number of British psychiatrists and psychologists became interested in group psychotherapy as a result of the need to treat a large number of psychiatric casualties during and after World War II. According to Anthony (1971), the main center for the treatment of the psychiatrically disabled in Britain was at Northfield, and the so-called Northfield experiment provided a rich training ground for a variety of group therapy approaches and theories of group formation. Gathered together at Northfield were analysts whose theoretical contributions remain as important now as they were then.

Bion. Wilfred Bion, now in the United States, is best known for his concept of the group as a whole having a separate mental life, with its own dynamics and hidden structure. Bion (1961) referred to this phenomenon as the basic assumptions, of which there are three. The first basic assumption is that the members of the group are looking for a leader on whom they can depend for spiritual sustenance and protection—the dependent assumption. The second basic assumption is their eventual recognition that such a leader does not exist except in fantasy, that the need for an omnipotent and omniscient figure is irrational, and that they must look to themselves for salvation and survival; in so doing, they form the so-called pairing group and act out the second or pairing assumption. Finally, the group members realize that there may be no one in their midst to fulfill a role that, to their dismay, they realize cannot be filled in any case. They have met for a purpose but have become annoyed and disappointed. Some may choose to stay and fight among themselves or with the leader as to their motives; others may choose to leave and flee from a situation they find unendurable. At this stage, the third basic assumption, the fight-flight assumption, has been realized. Bion did not see the basic assumptions as separate phases in the life of a particular group. All may be operative at the same time, and in varying degrees. The leader must be aware of their existence and, through timely interpretation, enable the group to move to a mature level of functioning, characterized by the individual member's being able to take the final responsibility for decisions and actions.

Foulkes. S. H. Foulkes (1965), one of the main organizers of the group therapy movement in Great Britain, attempted to bridge the theoretical gap between the so-called here-and-now and the there-and-then. He would look at the patient's past life and at its effect on the present; at the same time, he would examine the patient's current modes of interaction, regardless of past experience. He studied the transference situation of the members to the therapist, and was among the first to describe the transference as it also existed between the members themselves and between the members and the group as a whole. Foulkes saw illness in a person as a function of the patient's interaction within a network of other people, and he saw the group as the natural vehicle in which to study psychopathological processes that involve others.

Anthony. E. James Anthony has been and continues to be one of the few psychiatrists able to produce a much-needed and understandable amalgam between clinical phenomena and theoretical constructs about group development. In a classic text, *Group Psychotherapy: The Psychoanalytic Approach* (Foulkes and Anthony, 1957), he dealt with the development of the ego's capacity to create and maintain group relationships. He emphasized the resonance between members of a therapy group, the ability of one member to stimulate related unconscious associations and thought processes in the other, indicating the reactivity of each member to the other. More than any other contemporary authority on group dynamics, Anthony has repeatedly called for a comprehensive system of group psychotherapy. He stated (Anthony, 1971):

> For a scientific purpose, a system of group psychotherapy should demonstrate certain characteristics: It should be impartable to students by the ordinary routines of training, including training therapy, and impartable to colleagues who do not wish to join an esoteric cult to complete their understanding; it should provide a therapeutic model that helps to explain the process of therapy and the process of change; it should carry out periodic research evaluations on the efficacy of its treatment; it should be flexible enough to develop and alter under the impetus of further knowledge and practice; its proponents should remain eternally vigilant with respect to the tightening grip of dogma and fully aware of the limitations as well as the assets of their particular treatment model; and, finally, the system should provide an economic, elegant, and powerfully explanatory theoretical framework linking together group psychology and group psychotherapy in an indivisible whole. There should be special regard paid not only to the individual patient's status and behavior in the current group but also to him as a member of many human groups from infancy on. Group psychology must become developmental if group psychotherapy is to develop further.

Recent developments

The most important developments in recent times are in four areas: short-term group therapy, T-groups, the human potential movement, and self-help groups.

Short-term group psychotherapy. Short-term group therapy is a technique that was first used in the one-to-one setting and was adapted later to the group setting. The number of sessions is limited usually to about 10, and the method is of use for persons in crises who are intelligent and well-motivated to change.

T-groups. The T-group (the "T" stands for training) is an outgrowth of the National Training Laboratories, an organization begun in 1947 by social psychologists, whose goal was to develop ways in which to enrich the educational process. Therefore, the T-group should be composed of normally adjusted people and, in fact, has been called "therapy for normals." The basic goal of the group is not psychotherapy but education, and the individual participant should be healthy enough to learn from the variety of experiences to which the T-group exposes him.

Although T-groups are theoretically not intended to treat mentally ill patients, disturbed people often find their way to the T-group for the treatment of emotional disorders, instead of to traditional forms of psychotherapy. The T-group appeals especially to those people who feel isolated and alienated, who have difficulty in relating to other people, and who lack self-determination. They are attracted to the pragmatic here-and-now approach to human problems, to the promise of emotional enrichment and growth, and—not insignificantly—to the possibility of relieving boredom and adding meaning to their lives.

When not subverted, the training group movement can be—and has been—of great value to countless persons, by virtue of providing sound knowledge about both group dynamics and the structure of organizations.

Human potential movement. The human potential movement is composed of growth centers—loosely organized associations of people who gather together in retreats or rural communities to examine behavior through a variety of group approaches. The growth center has a staff who may or may not reside there, and whose task it is to facilitate the process of personal psychological growth in the participants, who visit for different periods of time—from a few days to several weeks.

The first such community, called Lifewynn, was organized by Trigant Burrow in the 1920s and consisted of about 20 people—students, associates, and patients—who lived and worked together in a summer camp in New York's Adirondack Mountains. In this setting, Burrow attempted to examine the interactions between the members of the community. He was particularly interested in the distortions that exist because people assume facades related to their social roles and professional status. The National Training Laboratories (NTL) today maintains a similar retreat at the Gould Academy in Bethel, Maine. Participants live at the center for several weeks while engaged in the examination of group interaction.

The Esalen Institute at Big Sur, California, founded in 1962 by Michael Murphy, has become the most widely known growth center. Philosophy, psychology, and the meditative aspects of Eastern religions find a forum in the institute's rustic setting. The influence of Gestalt psychologist Fritz Perls (see Figure A.1-3) seems to have been

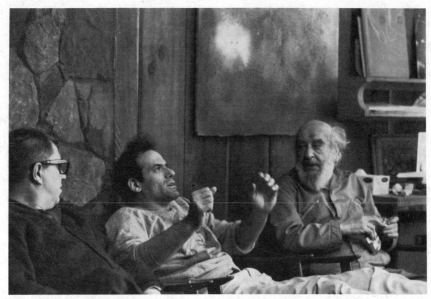

Figure A.1-3   Fritz Perls, *at right*, conducting a group session in which feeling tones are emphasized. (Courtesy of Michael Alexander.)

formidable. Perls believed in shifting levels of awareness, rather than in Freud's topographic theory of conscious and unconscious mental processes. He attempted to integrate a variety of previously defined psychic factors—such as id, ego, and superego—into a unitary whole. Esalen maintains no formal affiliation with other growth centers in the United States, but most centers have been modeled after Esalen's program, which can be considered the prototype.

Self-help groups. Groups in this category are composed of persons who are concerned about coping with a specific problem or life crisis. Usually organized with a particular task in mind, the groups do not attempt to explore individual psychodynamics in great depth, nor do they attempt to change personality functioning significantly. Self-help groups have had a major impact on the emotional health and well-being of a great many people.

A great many different types of self-help groups exist. Members are drawn from highly diversified segments of society, but, regardless of their socioeconomic backgrounds, they are alike in that they are mutually dependent because of their disorder or handicap. Many of the members of self-help groups have joined because the problems from which they suffer have been or are resistant to traditional methods of intervention, or have been ignored by the helping professions for various reasons. The various groups discussed below represent only a small sample of the types prevalent today. Many concern themselves with chronic illness, such as diabetes, renal disease, hemophilia, ileitis and colitis, and, especially, the addictions, such as alcohol and heroin. Special groups are aimed at the handicapped, older women, minority women, battered women, and holocaust survivors.

Alcoholics Anonymous (AA). Founded in 1934 by two alcoholics, one of whom was a physician, AA is the most widely known of the self-help groups. It has developed into a large organization with about a million members, but the basic unit of the small group, composed of alcoholics, re-

mains the agent of change. A rigid credo of total abstinence from alcohol is espoused, and little or no attempt is made to uncover the unconscious psychological antecedents to alcohol abuse. AA has been called repressive-inspirational in nature because great reliance is placed on repeated testimonials by the members about the benefits to be derived from abstinence. Al-Anon is composed of the relatives and spouses of alcoholics, and Al-A-Teen is composed of their children.

Recovery, Inc. Also known as The Association of Nervous and Former Mental Patients. Recovery, Inc., is a self-help after care program organized originally to help maintain the functions of previously hospitalized patients. The organization was founded in 1936 by psychiatrist Abraham A. Low at the Psychiatric Institute of the University of Illinois College of Medicine. Leaders of the small groups are lay people, all of whom are patients or former patients. Meetings are highly structured and inspirational, and they emphasize the conscious control of symptoms and altruism as major factors leading to cure.

Gamblers Anonymous (GA). Founded in 1957, GA is modeled after AA and is composed of compulsive gamblers who seek total abstinence from gambling as the desired goal for its members. When the desire to gamble becomes too great to resist, the tempted member is encouraged to call another member for external control of the impulse, as in AA. Similarly, Gam-Anon is composed of gamblers' spouses, and Gam-A-Teen is composed of their children. With the increased legalization of gambling in this country, GA is expected to assume more and more importance in the future.

Conclusion

Anthony described new developments in group psychotherapy more than a decade ago (1971), and his description still remains relevant to the current state of the field.

Within recent times, a cascade of experimental approaches has inundated the group arena, so that the more conventional procedures have been transiently swamped by fresh waves of novel and largely untried techniques to which the public has oriented itself because of the novelty, the implicit seductiveness, and the promise of quick change. Often there is a pursuit of the unusual for its own sake on the part of the therapist and a craving for new experiences in human relatedness on the part of the patients. It is difficult to say whether the bewildering situation today in the field of group psychotherapy reflects the primitive phase of its development or the disturbing nature of the world. Perhaps both.

If anxiety was the menace to our patients 20 years ago, alienation has emerged as the imperative concern now. The multiple and miasmic urgencies of life today have brought about an impatience with slower historical procedures, and immediate existence in all its calamitous ramifications has become the focus of therapeutic concern. Anything outside the here-and-now is poorly tolerated by the driven inhabitants of this nuclear age. The situation—first postulated by Trigant Burrow many years ago, when he saw therapists and patients in the same predicament—has been incorporated into the existential group movement.

The group therapist is no longer the most psychologically knowledgeable member of the group, the recognized and revered expert in theory and practice; instead, he stands out only by virtue of being the most honest, the most sincere, the most authentic, and the most accepting, both in his commitment to life and to the group. In fulfilling this role, he is obliged to be as open and as honest about himself as he expects the group members to be about themselves. He is offered no special privileges, no diplomatic immunity, no special status. He is a human being among other human beings, a patient among other patients—but perhaps a little more aware of what is implied than are the others in the group.

The development has been a fascinating one. Although it was Freud who first talked of the leaderless group and the deep anxieties that this situation aroused, it was Bion who put these theoretical ideas to the clinical test and examined the panic that ensued at the deepest levels. The group analytical approach, on the other hand, keeps the therapist in the background but sees him as indispensable to the therapeutic life of the group; he does not have to prove his indispensability by defaulting. Today, in some circles, the therapist has become the model of the good patient. He lays on the table not only all his countertransference cards but also his self-recognized human failings, so that he can no longer claim differentiation from his fellow members because of his mental health or superior clinical insights. He is no longer an alarming model of conventional normality. As a consequence, the group can get closer to one another without guilt or shame, since there is apparently no conscience figure to watch over them like the eye of God.

This godlessness has been much exploited by encounter groups. Under the highly emotional impact deliberately fostered by such settings, an exhilarating sense of freedom from prohibitions and inhibitions is rapidly generated. To the uncritical and naive observer, the internal censors seem to have been eradicated or at least put to sleep. Unfortunately, the vacation from conscience is more apparent than real, and more short-lasting than is claimed. The return to conventional circumstances soon reactivates the dormant conscience and may even intensify its more punitive and primitive qualities. Fenichel wrote that the superego is soluble in alcohol; it is also soluble—as Le Bon, McDougall, and Freud pointed out—in the ecstasies occasioned by close group interaction, but there is always a hang-over when reality once again asserts itself. This is, in fact, the oldest lesson in psychotherapy: The internal structures of the mind were not built in a day and cannot be reconstituted over a weekend.

References

Anthony, E. J. Reflections on twenty-five years of group psychotherapy. Int. J. Group Psychother., *18:* 277, 1968.

Anthony, E. J. The history of group psychotherapy. In *Comprehensive Group Psychotherapy*, ed. 1, H. I. Kaplan and B. J. Sadock, editors, p. 4. William & Wilkins, Baltimore, 1971.

Bion, W. R. *Experiences in Groups.* Tavistock Publications, London, 1961.

Burrow, T. *The Social Basis of Consciousness.* Harcourt, Brace & World, New York, 1927.

Ezriel, H. A psycho-analytical approach to group treatment. Br. J. Med. Psychol., *23:* 59, 1950.

Foulkes, S. H., and Anthony, E. J. *Group Psychotherapy, the Psychoanalytic Approach.* Penguin Books, London, 1957.

Freud, S. *Group Psychology and the Analysis of the Ego.* Hogarth Press, London, 1953.

Gottschalk, L. A., and Pattison, E. M. Psychiatric perspectives on T-groups and the laboratory movement. Am. J. Psychiatry. *126:* 823, 1969.

Hadden, S. B. A glimpse of pioneers in group psychotherapy. Int. J. Group Psychother., *25:* 371, 1975.

Le Bon. *The Crowd.* E. Benn, London, 1952.

Lewin, K. *Field Theory in Social Science.* Harper & Brothers, New York, 1951.

Moreno, J. L. *Who Shall Survive?* Beacon House, New York, 1953.

Powdermaker, F., and Frank, J. D. *Group Psychotherapy.* Harvard University Press, Cambridge, 1953.

Pratt, J. H. The principles of class treatment and their application to various chronic diseases. Hosp. Soc. Serv., *6:* 401, 1922.

Schilder, P. The analysis of ideologies as a psychotherapeutic method, especially in group treatment. Am. J. Psychiatry, *93:* 601, 1936.

Slavson, S. R. *A Textbook in Analytic Group Psychotherapy.* International Universities Press, New York, 1964.

Wender, L. Group psychotherapy: a study of its application. Psychiatr. Q., *14:* 708, 1940.

Wolf, A., and Schwartz, E. K. *Psychoanalysis in Groups.* Grune & Stratton, New York, 1962.

Zander, A. The study of group behavior during four decades. J. Appl. Behav. Sci. *15:* 272, 1979.

A.2 Freud: The First Psychoanalytic Group Leader

MARK KANZER, M.D.

Formation of the Group

Therapy for themselves was not the conscious purpose of the members of the first recorded instance of analytic group therapy, but it was a significant instigator and concomitant of their scientific proceedings. This unintended aspect is among the more interesting features, especially as it left a distinct imprint on the development of psychoanalysis itself.

The intimate relationship between the organization of the group and the therapeutic process began when Wilhelm Stekel, who had recently undergone therapy with Freud, proposed regular meetings at which other followers could discuss analysis with the founder of the movement. Thus the Wednesday Evening Society came into being. The exact date of Stekel's treatment is uncertain, but it presumably began in 1901 and may well have continued after the meetings were initiated. In any event, the fantasies now so common among patients—to engage in work with the analyst and ultimately to become an analyst oneself—thus achieved their first gratification.

These fantasies, oedipally motivated, usually extend to the wish to eliminate the analyst and take his place. Such a wish may well have entered into Stekel's constant rebelliousness and ultimate break with the Freudian school. The same constellation was even more marked in the case of Alfred Adler. He also underwent treatment with Freud, a significant fact little noted in the commentaries on their relationship. This information seems to have been divulged only in later years, when it came to light among the posthumous papers of Freud, which were not published until 1960.

The first group was very different from a modern psychoanalytic society. For several decades now, members of psychoanalytic societies have been required to prove their eligibility by completing their own analyses, demonstrating an ability to analyze others, and providing certification as to the soundness of their education. None of these preconditions was possible in the beginning. The early followers were drawn largely from non-medical circles, few possessed therapeutic experience, and none, except Freud himself, had been subjected to more than a modicum of personal analysis. There could be little debate about the principles of the young science. They might be accepted or rejected, but Freud alone had used the necessary investigative tools and was the only authority in the field.

Conduct of the meetings

Certain parallels between the conduct of the meetings, as devised by Freud, and the investigative techniques of psychoanalysis also intensified the therapeutic aspects of the proceedings. Freud's own personality was probably a common factor in both situations—the educational and the therapeutic.

The neutral educator. Freud always presided, so distance was established between himself and his followers. His position as chairman, reinforced by his authority as the foremost analyst, ensured that all remarks were ultimately addressed to him. Correspondingly, he is said to have preferred addressing a particular person, real or fancied, so that, as in analysis, a one-to-one relationship was established despite the group setting.

Free association. An aspect of free association adhered to the peculiar system in force for the regulation of the discussions. After a presentation, each member of the group was called on in turn and obliged to speak when his name was drawn from a Greek urn, which stood in their midst like the embodiment of psychic determinism, if not of fate. The resistance of patients to verbalization under such circumstances found its counterpart in the anxiety experienced by members who were prone to escape on one pretext or another before the drawings began. The imperatives of the urn were to become the targets of more open rebellion as group resistances to Freud mounted.

Topics of discussion. The themes of the unconscious and of sexuality were always in the foreground and in themselves provided natural bridges between the educational and the underlying therapeutic aspects of the discussions. Nunberg describes the tendency of the meetings to drift from the analysis of patients to self-analysis of the members themselves, of their sexual difficulties, memories, fantasies, and personal lives. The conditions for modern group therapy had been created and were to be partly resolved empirically and with scientific insight by Freud and the

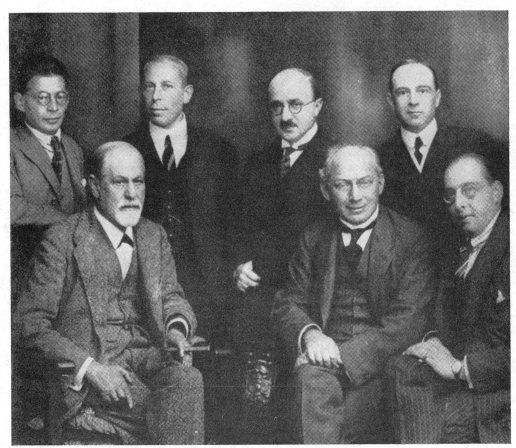

Figure A.2-1 Freud with several of his early collaborators. Top, left to right: Otto Rank, Karl Abraham, Max Eitingon, Ernest Jones; bottom, left to right: Freud, Sandor Ferenczi, and Hanns Sachs. (Courtesy of Louis Linn, M.D.)

other participants. Large areas proved insurmountable through self-analysis, so they required other measures of control.

Interpretations. In the discussions that followed the presentation of a paper, Freud alone had the privilege of intervening at will. The lucidity of his expositions, as impressive in spontaneous utterances as in his writings, lent to a summing-up of the impact of an interpretation. Graf, Wittels, and Reik remember him as always speaking last. Actually, this was by no means the case, and Wittels is probably correct in surmising that, after Freud had spoken, a subject was closed for them.

Working through. Submissive acceptance, the product of awe and relative ignorance, was, of course, countered by ambivalence, negativism, and increasingly informed and independent judgments. The working-through processes, after the interpretations, were diffused through channels of education, therapy, scientific achievement, acting out, dropping out, neurosis, and—in some instances—suicide. Freud naturally became the focal point and mediator among the various strivings that sought expression. When his mediations were successful, he promoted the differentiation of aims and the transformation of instinctual

into neutral energy; when they were unsuccessful, the opposite was the outcome. His own personality was at the center of the entire system.

Freud's personality

Freud's actual personality was revealed to his followers only gradually as it crystallized out from the aura of genius, first encounters, and structured settings for scientific debate. This crystallization was never complete, no matter how long they knew him and no matter how close they came to his inner circle. There is much agreement that central to this inaccessibility was a certain aloofness. Andreas-Salome wrote:

> He enters the class with the appearance of moving to the side. There is in this gesture a will to solitude, a concealment of himself within his own purposes, which by his preference would be no concern of his school or his public.

Similarly, his published self-analyses tell us more of his life than any autobiography has ever revealed, yet one does not really discover in them the inner self of Sigmund Freud.

Only Stekel, according to Ernest Jones, who was not quite accurate, ever dared to address him more familiarly than as "Herr Professor." It is notable that, even after many years, followers were apt to refer to themselves as his pupils or, with a note of deeper reverence, to call him "the Master." Letters addressed to and from his oldest associates were scarcely less formal. Graf spoke of the meetings in terms that compare Freud with a Moses presiding over a religious sect that was sometimes provoking in its insubordination, and Tausk alluded earnestly to psychoanalysis as a "scientific religion."

Yet Freud does seem to have unbent, as far as he was capable, with the group. He appreciated their enrichment of his intellectual and social life after his years of isolation as the first psychoanalyst. He played the part of host, serving coffee and cigars and bringing back gifts from abroad for the "Wednesday gentlemen." The minutes show him engaging in jokes, such as that all cooks were paranoid, especially his own, or crying out unguardedly that a certain patient was an "absolute swine." In contrast to earlier statements, in letters to Fliess, which have been construed as indicating a premature end to his potency, he remarked on November 18, 1908, at the age of 52, that he would write on love when his sex life was extinguished. The human side of Freud and his personal opinions were also revealed when he chided a young colleague, Wittels, for views derogatory to female physicians. Nevertheless, he himself was rather dubious that medicine was a proper field for women, although he joined in welcoming them to the society in 1910.

Still, a deep chasm remained between Freud and his followers. Here one must take cognizance of Freud's unique intellectual qualities, and of an orientation that has been called rigid, but that was probably another manifestation of the same firmness of commitment and adherence to scientific reality testing that had led to the discovery of psychoanalysis and was continued into its development and defense.

In the minutes, illustrations from case histories and dreams follow in unending and fascinating succession as new ideas are constantly adumbrated. A stream of publications bore out the promise of these ideas. Views that his students had laboriously acquired were swept away by the latest bursts of insight. Such a man, as Nunberg pointed out, was an impossible ideal, beyond emulation or identification, and a source of constant frustration to such ambitious followers as Adler and Tausk.

Many felt that he was overly critical in his judgments and intolerant of opposition, yet the minutes rarely bear out this impression. His efforts to teach the correct analytic approach to the inexperienced were, it is true, unremitting, and the contributions that others made did not always seem to him as important or as valid as they were to their exponents. Yet he was mild and scientific in most interchanges, accepted with little challenge and even with admiration the consistent opposition of Adler, and seems to have gained his reputation for severity more because of his role as a superego figure than because of his actual conduct. He was no doubt sincere in his statement in later years that he was disposed to tolerate the shortcomings of his followers in view of their courage in accepting psychoanalysis. Yet these followers seem to have understood and resented this tolerance as well as the conscientious and unremitting efforts to educate them.

Freud's reminiscences, his letters to friends, his fantasies, and his behavior indicate that the tolerance often wore thin and merged into resentment at the unending forms of resistance he encountered. Educational ambition, as well as therapeutic ambition, can be self-defeating to all concerned. Freud's self-image seems to have been that of a patriarch conveying visions of the truth to bickering and unworthy followers, a man for the ages lost among Lilliputians who sought to usurp his accomplishments rather than benefit from them. He inquired of Andreas-Salome why they could not all be like Rank, the dutiful son, although he already sensed the delayed rebellion that would assail him from even that quarter. He was indeed a tormented titan. However, Freud's greatest opponent came from within himself—from the beleaguered ego that sought to be freed from the same patriarchal superego and, still incompletely analyzed, had to be projected through unconscious sympathy into a counteridentification with his own critics in the society.

The Group's Proceedings

The ferments taking place within the group during the educational process may be followed with almost autosymbolic accuracy in the first volume of the *Minutes of the Vienna Psychoanalytic Society*, covering the period from October 1906 to June 1908. This volume opens with a presentation in which Rank dutifully applies the teachings of Freud to a new field, mythology, and closes with a full-fledged challenge to Freudian theories and personal leadership by Adler and his paper on aggression.

From 1906 to 1908, the group showed impressive progress in understanding by the members and in the level of the discussions. On the other hand, emotional attacks on each other increased in frequency and intensity, and a particular charge—plagiarism—became rampant. In the plagiarism charges, there is the appearance of a resistance that had crystallized. Hostilities, displaced from Freud to one another, found intellectualization in the idea that these others sought to deprive them of their claims to originality. These recurrent charges revealed an inner resentment of their own need to borrow from Freud, and their wish to identify with his envied originality. In time, the hostility and the accusations of stealing their ideas were turned against Freud himself.

Group rebellion. With a rising tide of discontent discernible among the disciples toward the end of 1907 and the beginning of 1908—a collective adolescence, one might say, that reflected emergence from antecedent dependency but with a continuing need for Freud's guidance, which was now galling—Freud himself began to show dismay and a longing to pass on the leadership to someone else. Roazen reports that Freud wrote, in a self-analytic mood:

What personal pleasure is to be derived from analysis I obtained during the time when I was alone ... an incurable breach must have come into existence at that time between me and other men.

The growth of a psychoanalytic group in Zurich and the proposal that a first international meeting be held in Salzburg in April 1908 made Freud turn hopefully to Jung on February 18 with the suggestion that Bleuler preside. "My Viennese colleagues would behave better," he predicted.

Two stormy meetings of the Vienna society on February 5 and 12 supply background to Freud's complaints against his own group. At the first of these meetings, Adler brought forward a recommendation that a change be made in the usual methods of conducting the sessions. The urn and its coercive authority came particularly under attack in a transparent displacement from the leader himself. Next, Federn suggested that measures be taken to curb "intellectual communism"—that is, plagiarism. Isidor Sadger, so often the victim, wished the chairman to take more definitive steps to suppress personal invectives and attacks.

With these proposals, the long-standing discontents were finally brought to the surface of group consciousness for discussion. It remained for Graf to go more deeply into the subject and indicate that the proposals "stem from a feeling of uneasiness." Tactfully, he related this feeling to the fact that the group was on the way to becoming a full-fledged organization rather than simply the invited guests of the Herr Professor. Graf suggested that the meetings be transferred from Freud's office to a different site.

Freud responded that he was opposed to using his powers as chairman to suppress any utterances except those conversations that might disturb the speaker. For himself, he waived the right to protect his remarks from plagiarism—a deeply ironic statement. Then, confronting the underlying issues more directly, he expressed the opinion that, if the members could not stand each other or freely express scientific opinions, perhaps the entire enterprise ought to be abandoned. However, he had hopes that deeper psychological understanding might yet appear and assist in overcoming the difficulties. Clearly, he was referring to some advance in self-analytic insight.

Freud's stand, expressed with restraint and dignity, seems entirely correct from both the educational and the therapeutic viewpoints. He took as his baseline an educational situation in which chairman and participants were expected to maintain an alliance directed to promoting the scientific and educational aims that constituted the purpose of the meetings. Self-analysis, promoted by these meetings, should be used to correct divergences from the announced aims.

That Freud would transmute the experiences of this session into scientific and self-analytic terms was to be expected, and the echoes of those experiences are heard in references of later years to

...the uncanny and coercive characteristics of group formation.... The group wishes to be governed by unrestricted force; it has an extreme passion for authority.... The primal father is the group ideal, which governs the ego in the place of the ego ideal.

The destiny of the primal father to be overthrown and replaced by one of the sons was further elaborated in *Totem and Taboo* and was reasserted, despite

better scientific knowledge, in *Moses and Monotheism*. Freud seems to have perpetuated, in his appraisal of group dynamics, unanalyzed fragments of his own family romance.

On February 12, a committee, headed by Adler and appointed to consider the proposals put forward at the last meeting, recommended the abolition of the urn and a widening of the educational process by including book reviews on a more regular basis and brief case presentations by individual members and by giving more notice about longer papers to be presented so that all concerned could be better prepared. The sense of these changes was to formalize the meetings, give the members a greater share of the responsibility, and reduce the overshadowing personal influence of Freud. There was no real solution to the problem of the "ill humor in the empire," as members put it euphemistically, and even the proposal to abolish the urn was blocked, probably out of deference to Freud. However, like the leader, this fetish was stripped of some of its authority. It could still be used to summon members to speak, but they were within their rights if they decided to ignore its call.

Certainly, the meeting at Salzburg in April was not conducive to greater harmony. Freud unmistakably favored Jung and the Zurich group. When he went to America the next year, he took none of the Viennese in his retinue. With his increasing inner and outer withdrawal from the Vienna society, a gap had to be closed.

Transformation of the group

The personal side of the relationship between Freud and Adler was at first obscured behind their polite intellectual discussions, but it figured increasingly in the rifts that grew between them and accompanied a crisis within Freud himself. Adler's boldness in reaching out for intellectual and political dominance of the group was complementary to Freud's increasing withdrawal from the Vienna group and his preference for the Zurich contingency. Freud reasoned that the academic status and Aryan backgrounds of the Swiss offered a greater guarantee for the future of psychoanalysis than did his Viennese colleagues, although it is to be doubted that such rationalizations provided the true motives. As the second International Psycho-Analytical Congress, to be held in Nuremburg on March 30 and 31, 1910, drew nearer, Freud pushed plans to transfer the leadership of the psychoanalytic movement to Jung and its headquarters to Zurich.

Sandor Ferenczi, who had been chosen to convey this message to the Viennese in Nuremberg, succeeded only in uniting the angry delegation behind Adler and Stekel. Freud then decided to resign from the presidency of the Viennese group and to recommend that Adler succeed him. That he should select the man who was the greatest threat to analysis as his successor, even if he regarded him as the most able member of the society, seems to require explanations that have not been forthcoming. Perhaps, as Adler indicated, the choice was not Freud's alone to make. A hint of deeper psychological motives appears in a letter to Ferenczi on April 3, in which Freud refers to himself as a "dissatisfied and unwanted old man." An inner bond with the rebel against the father and the paternalistic aspects of psychoanalysis seems to have been present.

The stage was set for a remarkable group confrontation on April 6, 1910, after the return to Vienna. With the contemplated transition in power from one leader to the other on the agenda, the group meeting was a veritable occasion for a totem meal involving Freud and his "primal horde." Before the assembled group, Freud undertook to carry through his intentions of politely ceding the leadership to Adler, who would have none of this evasion. He criticized Freud for his behavior at Nuremburg and spoke—almost in the language of *Totem and Taboo*, published 2 years later—of the banding together of the group against the founding father of psychoanalysis. Adler then offered a program that clearly promised to replace Freud's administrative and intellectual leadership with his own. The membership was to be widened, as it soon was to admit more of Adler's friends; the society would remove from Freud's office; it would publish a journal, which in time Adler and Stekel edited; and Freud himself, while retaining leadership, would be relieved of administrative duties. Later, Adler used publications of the society and introduced courses to make psychoanalysis a cover for his own views.

Stekel, as first commentator, could not imagine how the group would exist without Freud, whom he nevertheless accused of harboring a deep hatred against Vienna. He suggested that Freud remain as president, Adler be made vice-president with administrative duties, and the forthcoming publication be used to prove, despite the leader's apparent doubts, that Vienna and not Zurich held the key to the future of psychoanalysis. Others joined in the discussion in much the same vein. A note of sadness dominated, not the bitterness and readiness to sweep aside Freud that Adler alone had sounded. Local patriotism emerged repeatedly in the feeling that Freud had mistakenly prized the Zurich analysts as offering a better soil than the Viennese for the future. Wittels commented that his countrymen possessed, as the Swiss did not, "a neurosis which is necessary for entry into Freud's teachings."

Sadger added—in graceful enough fashion for once—that, although Freud had been fed up with the Viennese for two years, they were still ahead of the Zurich group because of his "steady leadership, instruction and advice." A solution was found when, in response to vigorous demands that he at least accept an honorary presidency, Freud agreed to retain a scientific chairmanship while the presidency went to Adler.

At the next meeting, April 13, the transition was sealed symbolically with the total abolition of the urn and the agreement to move the meeting place from Freud's office. The transformation of the Wednesday Evening Society of guests invited to discuss psycho-

analysis with the professor into the Viennese Psychoanalytic Society was complete.

Although the occasion had its melancholy aspects for both Freud and the group, it actually marked the successful completion of a phase in which their mutual purposes had been achieved. Psychoanalysis was no longer a one-man discipline, and, although Freud would remain the intellectual leader throughout his life, the society had become a congregation of scientists with varying views and degrees of competence; it was no longer an assemblage of students who sat at the feet of a master. His faults could now be discerned, tolerated, and understood, just like their own. The children had grown up. The former students, like former analysands, had become sufficiently detached to form new object relationships that still left Freud realistically a teacher and prophet.

What lay ahead for Freud himself at this point was a relapse into temporary isolation and inner scrutiny, from which he emerged strengthened, the guilt for primal parricide shifted from himself to his successor, and freed to rid himself and the movement of a truly incompatible element. It is scarcely a coincidence that the topic chosen for his own presentation at the Nuremburg congress dealt with the problem of countertransference. Throughout 1910, this subject was on his mind. In October, after some months of rest and a period of travel with Ferenczi, he wrote this latest favored disciple and former analysand (whose future revolt was already discernible), conveying some of the thoughts that had been distilled from the experiences and temporary setback with the group: "I am not the psychoanalytical superman that you constructed in your imagination, nor have I overcome the countertransference."

Ferenczi had evidently been engaged in reversing the analytic procedure and exploring the psychology of Freud himself. The master confessed to difficulty in revealing his secrets and acknowledged that his disciple was correct in attributing this difficulty to a permanent incapacity to reach out to others, which was a residue of the traumatic termination of his relationship with Fliess. Freud's disposition to terminate close relationships traumatically went back much further, however. He diagnosed himself, in this letter to Ferenczi, as having regressed to healthy narcissism rather than to paranoia.

As for Adler, once the reins of power were in his hands, he abandoned caution and quickly gave scope to views that carried him increasingly away from the Freudian school. The members of the society, educated by Freud and chastened by their guilt toward the rightful leader, found this departure intolerable, and Adler was forced to resign after a few months in office. This act, too, was part of the group's progress in becoming an educational organization, confident of its own purposes and judgment. When Freud turned toward the group again after a period of self-scrutiny, it received him gladly.

On the personal side, Freud, like Adler, had an ambivalent relationship with an older "brother"—his nephew John, who was a year older than Freud—and guilty memories of a younger brother, Julius, for whose death he felt responsible. With John, he liked to take turns in playing Julius Caesar and Brutus, thus alternating in the murder and revival of a "brother." Adler himself emphasized in his clinical studies the importance of birth order in a family, and his ambivalence with respect to his own brother may well have complemented Freud's. In accepting the opportunity to be Caesar, Adler seems to have opened the way to Freud's long pent-up desire to enact Brutus.

The educational aspects of these meetings promoted an ultimate dominance over the therapeutic, but they also seem to have fostered the emergence of repressed transferences long hidden beneath the cool intellectual exchanges between Freud and Adler. Observers like Graf and Wittels supply pictures of Freud and Adler sitting side by side at the meetings, puffing furiously at cigars. In 1911, the year of the break between them, Freud described, in an addendum to the Schreber case which helped to precipitate their estrangement, a commentary on the myth that the eagle (Adler) establishes its lineage by looking into the sun without blinking. If it does not, the father casts it out of the eyrie. One eagle apparently failed the test. Adler found a similar image and told Freud that he did not propose to stand in his shadow forever. But Bottome relates that Adler confessed, toward the end of his life, that he had not, after all, caught up with his older brother.

The Trial of Adler and Freud

The appearance of the third volume of the *Minutes* in 1974 sheds new light on the transformation of the group, specifically on the "trial" and "expulsion" of Alfred Adler and his followers. This trial was drawn out over a period of nearly a year (1910–1911), and might also have been designated as the dissolution of the original group of Freud and the followers who assembled weekly in his office, ostensibly to learn about psychoanalysis from its founder and only practitioner.

By the end, psychoanalysis had become a world-wide movement with societies in many countries. Representatives of official journals and sympathizers visited the Vienna meetings as though attending a shrine and went forth to stimulate new growth. Yet within this shrine, the leader had been reduced in rank and significance. Adler and Stekel of the original group sat above him as chairman and vice-chairman, and their followers were increasing in proportion to Freud's. His comments were becoming fewer and were becoming paraphrased in the terms of his rivals at every meeting. The situation could not endure, for Freud had formed the group to further psychoanalysis and had no other motive for remaining with it.

Fritz Wittels, who had resigned from the Vienna Psychoanalytic Society for personal reasons in 1910, published in 1924 the best-known account of the deposition of Adler and Stekel, which then became drawn upon by others prior to the publication of the minutes. His information was supplied by Wilhelm Stekel, with whom he was closely associated. How biased and inaccurate it was emerges only with the full

record now available. He depicts Adler as confronted by Freudian "adepts," i.e., followers, in the spring of 1911 (actually the fall of 1910). When Adler responded to demands that he present a connected exposition of his ideas, Wittels asserts he did so to bring about a lasting peace with his teacher. There is little evidence of this motive in his continued aggressive presentation of his own ideas and his diminution of his former teacher's.

Wittels further states that Adler was allotted three evenings for his expositions, and at a discussion on the fourth evening, Freudians "made a mass attack ... almost unexampled in its ferocity." On the fifth evening, Adler was invited to leave the society, which he did with nine followers. Perhaps it tells its own story that Wittels, after penning these lines, sent a copy to Freud and applied for readmission to the Vienna Psychoanalytic Society. Freud replied, mildly deprecated the incorrectness of Wittel's "unauthorized biography," and concurred in the readmission of his ambivalent follower, who thereafter remained a loyal member of the "adepts."

One value of an authentic portrayal of the dissolution of the original group is in order to trace the interrelation of the therapeutic, educational, and finally political aspects of the complicated motivations involved. The fall of 1910 had witnessed the reconvening of the society with the same internecine warfare continuing. On October 26, Freud presented one of the most important of his theoretical papers, *On the Two Principles of Psychic Happenings*, subsequently published in 1911. Actually, it involved an introduction to the reality principle and might have served as a bridge to Adler's "practical" psychology. Adler, however, was cool and would discuss the paper only in terms of his own concepts of organ inferiority as contrasted with Freud's orientation toward the sexual development of the individual. The latter thanked him ironically for the biological and genetic "supplementations" of his paper—code words to call attention to the fact that psychoanalytic considerations, as the basis for debate, were being ignored.

There was no common language—merely a rough sea of conceptual conflicts ahead. The next two sessions offered more of the same, with Freud silent, while Adler, Stekel, and their followers all but completely dominated the meetings. On November 16, Hitschmann, a follower of Freud, did indeed propose early in the session that Adler be invited to offer a systematic presentation of his theories for debate as to whether they could be reconciled with Freud's or at least the differences clarified. Freud intervened to suggest that the nub of the matter might be considered Adler's "masculine protest" in contrast to his own doctrine of repression, which his rival ignored. The entire group voted affirmatively in the matter. No time limit was set, and Adler agreed to proceed on this basis. There was no atmosphere of coercion, and in fact, the major discussion on the masculine protest did not take place until February 22, 1911, 3 months later.

On February 1, however, he had pronounced such bulwarks of Freudian sexual symbolism as dreams of flying, climbing ladders or stairs, and standing on the roof of a house as desires to be important. So-called libidinal tendencies were seen as merely safeguards against being debased by a woman. Similarly, incestuous desires for the mother were interpreted as chiefly the wish to be above her. Freud responded that it was not so much Adler's differing view of various subjects that bothered him as much as it was his tendency to rename Freud's ideas so that discussion became impossible. Thus, bisexuality was renamed psychic hermaphroditism, and masculine protest was described as if it included repression, which was not the case. What Adler sought, he declared, was to eliminate in particular the terms most associated with psychoanalysis. Adler denied any such thing, and Stekel agreed with him. The task of defining the differences was finding rough going.

When, on February 22, Stekel again asserted that he could find no contradiction between the views of Freud and of Adler, Freud observed tersely that he and Adler both did. A comment by Steiner broke through the surface of polite discussions about theory and moved toward depth interpretations; Steiner remarked that the subject matter of the arguments really touched on deep complexes in the speakers. Freud was open to the reproach that he had kept his affects bottled up too long. Adler had deviated more and more from Freud's doctrines and tried to obliterate the essence of his views. If Adler had his way, the ostensible purpose of the association, which was to learn Freud's doctrines, would have to be renounced and the name changed.

Adler, as usual, denied this construction but, at a committee meeting afterward, resigned as chairman because of the now acknowledged incompatibility of his scientific attitude with his position in the society. Stekel resigned as vice-chairman in sympathy. Again, the account of Wittels is manifestly mistaken. Both men continued to attend sessions, as did their followers, and apparently joined in electing Freud to the vacated chairmanship by acclamation. Instead of a mass expulsion, the followers of both men thanked Adler and Stekel for their services and also passed a resolution that the views of Freud and Adler were not incompatible. Only Freud objected to the resolution, and he was unanimously overruled. The notion of a powerful political machine manipulated against the Adlerians simply does not hold up.

During the next 3 months, the proceedings of the society were not less harmonious than usual. On May 24, 1911, after a lengthy silence, Adler made a speech in which he viewed the Oedipus complex and penis envy as simply manifestations of the masculine protest. The summer recess lay ahead, and at the first of the fall sessions, October 11, 1911, it was announced that Adler and 3 of his followers had resigned. Freud then for the first time took a stern stand and stated that remaining members who were close to Adler should resign also—they could not belong simultaneously to his group and to Adler's. Presumably, he did not wish to be spied on and further sabotaged. The 5 remaining Adlerians reminded the society of the resolution that no incompatibility was involved. The issue was put to a vote, and 11 Freudians united against the others, who then left to join Adler's newly formed Society for Free Psychoanalytic Investigation. Its very title, as Steiner suggested, was a challenge and its subsequent course increasingly anti-Freudian.

Thus, where disciples had joined Freud to learn analysis from him, two competing teachers had grown up among them in the last years. Adler and Stekel were forming their own circles of adherents and issuing their own statements through independent publications. Shall the educational or therapeutic proc-esses be judged as unsuccessful for these reasons? Probably not. To the extent that former followers have matured personally and in their outlooks, or even come to form and express divergent reactions, the group process has had its elements of success.

Similarly, in family circles or in colonies that are ready for independence, differentiation is an inherent aspect of maturation. In the end, the three leaders were competing for political control over a group that bore little resemblance to the few respectful followers of Freud who had met in his office to seek instruction scarcely a decade earlier. It was integration under one roof and one leader that was no longer possible, and when Freud announced that the time for termination had come, he was simply recognizing reality in inviting his own followers to remain and the others to leave.

Conclusion

The group that gathered about Freud for instruction in psychoanalysis had multiple functions to perform. It provided a means for continuing his self-analysis and initiating him into group dynamics. It also seems to have provided an impenetrable haven for some resistances. The ostensible educational aims of the other members were all but swallowed up at times by therapeutic needs, aspirations for a career, and a climate that made them into propagandists or antagonists of a revolutionary new concept of the human mind. The triumphs and failures of the group found dramatic expression in the intertwined and opposing personalities and ideas of Sigmund Freud and Alfred Adler.

References

Andreas-Salome, L. *The Freud Journal.* Basic Books, New York, 1964.

Bottome, P. *Alfred Adler.* Vanguard Press, New York, 1957.

Brill, A. A. *The Basic Writings of Sigmund Freud.* Random House, New York, 1938.

Freud, S. *The Origins of Psychoanalysis.* Basic Books, New York, 1954.

Freud, S. On the history of the psychoanalytic movement. In *Standard Edition of the Complete Psychological Works of Sigmund Freud,* vol. 14, p. 7. Hogarth Press, London, 1957.

Freud, S. Group psychology and the analysis of the ego. In *Standard Edition of the Complete Psychological Works of Sigmund Freud,* vol. 18, p. 57. Hogarth Press, London, 1957.

Freud, S. Formulations on the two principles of mental functioning. In *Standard Edition of the Complete Psychological Works of Sigmund Freud,* vol. 12, p. 213. Hogarth Press, London, 1958.

Freud, S. *Letters of Sigmund Freud.* Basic Books, New York, 1960.

Graf, M. Reminiscences of Professor Sigmund Freud. Psychoanal. Qt., *11:* 465, 1942.

Jones, E. *The Life and Work of Sigmund Freud,* 3 vols. Basic Books, New York, 1953–1957.

Nunberg, H., and Federn, E. *Minutes of the Vienna Psychoanalytic Society,* 3 vols. Basic Books, New York, 1962, 1967, and 1974.

Reik, T. *From Thirty Years with Freud.* Hogarth Press, London, 1942.

Roazen, P. *Freud: Political and Social Thought.* Alfred A. Knopf, New York, 1968.

Sachs, H. *Freud, Master and Friend.* Imago, London, 1945.

Wittels, F. *Sigmund Freud.* Dodd, Mead, New York, 1924.

A.3 Group Dynamics

RICHARD L. MUNICH, M.D.
BORIS ASTRACHAN, M.D.

Introduction

The term "group dynamics" refers to the intrinsic nature of groups, the ways in which the group and its individual members affect each other, and the relationship of this interaction to issues of group development, structure, and goals. Part of what makes group dynamics a difficult and complex field is that much that has been said and written about it comes from three separate intellectual traditions: individual psychology, social psychology, and sociology. Each of these traditions has its own theoretical assumptions and distinctive language.

In his effort to understand group life, the psychologist examines the individual, the sociologist focuses on the cultural or structural aspects of the group, and the social psychologist studies the boundary between the social and the psychological, and between members themselves. Insofar as the group consists of individuals with their distinct personality systems, the language and assumptions of individual psychology are relevant. But insofar as behavior in groups is determined by properties of group structure, then that language and those assumptions are inadequate; the traditions of social psychology and sociology become crucial. On the other hand, an exclusive focus on the group itself ignores the experiences of individual members and also, in part, ignores their interactions with other members. The disparity between these languages and the tension between points of view reflect the historical and theoretical roots of the study of group dynamics.

This chapter examines aspects of group life that are active to a greater or lesser extent, irrespective of the structure or the work of any specific group. The emphasis of this examination will be on these processes in smaller, face-to-face groups encountered in most therapeutic contexts. An understanding and appreciation of these processes may help facilitate an awareness of the complex phenomena present in groups so that a group leader can function at an increased level of sensitivity, competence, and effectiveness. These issues will be examined historically, from the point of view of the psychology in the group, the sociology of the group, and the group as a social psychological entity.

History

Sigmund Freud and Emil Durkheim, both born in 1856, made major organizing contributions to their respective fields, psychology and sociology. Freud published *Studies on Hysteria* in 1895, only 2 years before Durkheim's *Suicide.* Their work was undertaken in a rapidly industrializing age, in an intellectual climate characterized by a reaction to the systematic individualism (Locke) and the scientific and political materialism (Hobbes) of the 18th-century Enlightenment, and by the desire to understand subsurface phenomena. In this context, Freud insisted on a relentlessly observational methodology which moved from the concrete word—parapraxis, dream, or joke—to a systematic latent content, and Durkheim was the first sociologist to apply statistical analysis to derive categories of suicide. The bitter battle between Rousseau and Diderot throughout the middle part of the 18th century about which had priority—society or the individual—must also be considered a precursor to the intellectual reaction in which Freud and Durkheim wrote.

Until Freud's paper *Group Psychology and the Analysis of the Ego* (1921), there was little conception of the group except as a mob or collectivity in which one might observe the playing out of individual dynamics. Early group therapy reflected this emphasis on the individual and his dynamics and virtually ignored those relevant aspects of member-to-member interaction and the group process itself. From the point of view of the individual in the group, the importance of the group itself began to be highlighted as an implication of the work of the object relations theorists. In 1932, Melanie Klein published the *Psychoanalysis of Children,* refocusing the analytic inquiry almost exclusively on earlier, pregenital modes of infantile sexuality and the death instinct (aggression). Her formulation pushed the major dynamics of ego and superego development back to the first year of life. Freud had insisted that these structures crystallized with the resolution of the Oedipus complex around age 5, a resolution accompanied by an identification with the same-sexed parent. Klein, however, wrote that reality and real objects affected the child's anxiety situations from the very earliest stages of its existence. Owing to the interaction of the mechanisms of introjection and projection, which make these objects alternately part and not part of the self, external factors come to influence the formation of the personality. That is, parts of these objects might be split off from the self, projected out, and then seen as either loving or hostile. This leads first to a paranoid-schizoid position and then to a depressive position vis-à-vis the world and hence, for our purposes, the group. The more traditionally Freudian contribution to group dynamics, then, had much more to do with efforts of group members to identify with the leader, while the object relations contribution had more to do with group members singly or in various subunits taking on and reflecting various aspects of the personality system.

Influenced by the work of Durkheim, Pareto, and Max Webber, Talcott Parsons published *The Structure of Social Actions* in 1937, and ushered in a sociological line of inquiry involving value orientation, cultural expectations, and behavior patterns. Under the tutelage of Parsons, this second line of relevance for group dynamics came to fruition in the late 1940s and early 1950s at the Harvard University Department of Social Relations, and especially with Robert Bales's idea of the group as a miniature social system. To summarize this conception: A group consists of a system of interaction, the parts of which are interdependent and acting to adapt to the realities of the immediate situation, to accomplish the group's goal, to keep the group intact, and to gratify individual members (Mills, 1967; Edelson, 1970). This point of view led to a rapid increase in research on group process and had a major influence on social psychology. In fact, these sociologists had already been influenced by the work of William McDougall (1920), an early social psychologist, who had formulated various principles for raising collective mental life to a higher level. He alluded to the necessity of a degree of continuity to the group's existence of an idea of the group in the minds of its members, of the need for boundaries and structures in which differentiation and specialization of function could occur, and of the importance of customs and habits developing so that member-to-member relations could be fixed and defined.

Social psychology, the third important line in the development of an understanding of group dynamics, focused in large part on the various interactions between individuals within groups as an effort to illuminate the study of individual motivation and behavior by consideration of social forces. The origin of social psychology has been attributed to August Comte, a French positivist who wrote in the mid-19th century and whose influence was first noticed in the work of LeBon on the crowd and Tarde on imitation. The earliest social psychologists bridged two rapidly evolving disciplines and assisted each in enriching the other. These early investigations include George Simmel's works on group affiliations, Charles Cooley's on the affinity between person and group which originates in the family, W. I. Thomas's on the stabilizing influence of the group, F. H. Allport's social facilitation, Frederic Thrasher's on the gang, George Mead's on symbolic interaction, Elton Mayo's on industrial psychology, M. Sherif's on the development of social norms, and J. L. Moreno's graphic and mathematical sociometry. Along with Durkheim's emphasis on the importance of group ties in the operation of both social and personal control, this body of work moved toward an elucidation of the impact of group life on individuals' emotions, performance, and social and communicational interaction. A more scientific social-psychological approach to group dynamics was ushered in by Kurt Lewin. In several works during the 1940s, he insisted on a strictly observational approach to the derivation of the lawfulness inherent in group life. Creating and manipulating various factors in groups such as leadership, communication networks, group characteristics, competition, and cooperation, Lewin and his followers began to delineate aspects of the group's effect on a single member. Lewin's field theory—which was concerned with group cohesiveness and member interdependence, factors which influence members to remain in the group—represented the culminating point for the contribution of social psychology to group dynamics. Many consider Kurt Lewin the father of group dynamics.

Finally, an empirical and experiential method, that of groups studying themselves—self-analytic groups, T-groups—was developed in the 1950s and became a rich source of data for the rapid, personal, and graphic study of group dynamics. Albeit somewhat artificial, this method illuminated many of the psychological, social psychological, and sociological aspects of group life that are relevant for understanding the trends operative in groups of all types.

Individual Psychology in the Group

The individual entering into a new group moves into a situation in which anxiety is stimulated, personal boundaries are threatened, and various needs are rapidly mobilized and rendered visible. Among these needs are the wish to maintain a sense of autonomy, as well as the strong wish to belong. Some of these needs are satisfied by the establishment of roles, an ordering of relationships between members, group cohesiveness (including a boundary around the group), and a common culture within the group. Other needs, however, are not, particularly insofar as a fundamental source of anxiety for individuals is that engendered in the course of their ambivalent relation to an authority which they both need and fear. In a group without a designated leader, role differentiation and status consensus push certain individuals toward taking on leadership roles in various sectors of the group's functioning (e.g., in task performance, emotional support, expression, or guidance). In a group with a leader, however, the assumption of these leadership roles is always mitigated by the presence of the leader, and other issues come into focus.

Authority and leadership

Freud, trying to understand what he considered the essentially mindless and infantile behavior of groups, invoked the concept of identification. Freud had developed the idea of identification several years earlier, and it was known to psychoanalysis as the earliest expression of an emotional tie with another person. The process of identification was initiated by someone when he took into himself qualities perceived to be held in common with another person. Identification, Freud further hypothesized, not only was the basis for mutual ties between members of a group but was influential in the tie with the leader. This tie with the leader, based on infantile processes and needs, altered the individual's psychological structures, specifically the ego and the ego ideal and their boundaries, in a way that explained the uncanny, coercive, regressive, and mindless characteristics of group formations. As he wrote: "The leader of the group is still the dreaded primal father; the group still wishes to be governed by unrestricted forces; it has an extreme passion for authority; in LeBon's phrase, it has a thirst for obedience." It is important to note, however, that Freud was well known for his insistence on the individual's ambivalence toward authority, as demonstrated in his formulation of the Oedipus complex.

It was the seminal work of Wilfred Bion (1961) that highlighted these processes of ambivalence of individuals toward others and toward the leader in groups. His work is detailed in this section of the chapter because he does not postulate a herd instinct, or group mind; rather, Bion believes that ideas of this sort which develop in groups are the products of regression within individuals, which occurs when people are threatened with a loss of their individual distinctiveness (Rioch, 1970). But this work on group process is also included here because the phenomena Bion described take place very much with respect to the leader of the group. He noticed that groups in his presence invariably seemed to be assembled for two purposes: to function as a work group or as a basic assumption group—the first more or less related to something conscious and designated, the second less obvious but routinely present. In this latter category, three distinct processes were inferred. First, members in the group acted as if the leader was there to give protection and provide security for the members. The group appeared as if its aim was dependency, to be taken care of by an omnipotent, omniscient leader who is idealized to an almost religious level. Passivity in thought and action is the primary mode of being until it becomes clear the leader cannot really fill this role, at least in the way group members had in mind. Disappointment, hostility, and further dependent efforts, even to the point of actual symptomatology, arise within individuals in the group. Efforts to feel and act more responsibly often take the form of a search for a new and more effective leader, one who ultimately suffers the same fate as the original. Predominant emotions expressed in the dependency basic assumption are guilt over the greed for nurturance, anger, jealousy, rivalry, resentment, and inadequacy.

The second process inferred in the basic assumption group is that of fight-flight. Obviously a function whose primary mode is action, the aim of this process is preservation of the group at all costs. As he is viewed as the most courageous and clever of all group members, the leader is called upon to mobilize the group, as if for attack or flight. Whereas the individual predisposition for participation in the dependent basic assumption is an obsessional personality organization, the most receptive valency in the fight-flight group is in those members who facilitate expression or who have a paranoid personality. As fight-flight implies, the mode of the group is avoidance. Predominant emotions in the fight-flight basic assumption are rage, sacrifice, and martyrdom.

The third basic assumption group is pairing. Hysterical personalities are most likely to have the valency for this assumption in this situation. In the pairing basic assumption, the aim of the group is to reproduce itself, the leader is thought to be unborn, and it is as if the future were all that counted. The predominant emotions expressed in a group in this mode are hopefulness, optimism about the future, and sexual embarrassment. Pairing is the antidote to that aspect of a group's development that is concerned with separation and termination.

Basic assumption life rarely, if ever, exists in pure culture. It is never oriented to the adaptive or task priorities of the group; rather, it is a reflection of the fantasy life of individuals within the group, is held anonymously, and is ready to intrude into group life if other group activities—including work in the service of task accomplishment—do not gratify individual needs. The basic assumption life of a group can be used to enhance task performance, particularly if it supports the group's goal, as in a hospital (dependency) or army (fight-flight). Basic assumption life is also a source of energy for a group, a reprieve from the struggles of the task, and an opportunity for individuals to replenish the loneliness associated with role differentiation and goal orientation. The presence of basic assumption life in a group is, for Bion, graphic evidence of the ambivalent conflict between the individual's need for autonomy and his yearning to be a part of the group. The situation of ambivalence leads to considerable distress, efforts to split that distress off from the self, and to relocate it by the process of projections onto—and projective identifications from—another group member, either outside the group or in the leader. There is a great reluctance to allow good and bad to be brought together. Bion argued that the ambivalence and its consequent distress could only be tolerated by the operation of a "group mentality" in which all members collude in the creation of a "culture" reflecting a collective compromise formation. In this group mentality or culture, some individuals are allowed to act, others remain anonymous, responsibility is obfuscated, and guilt and responsibility are dispersed into anonymity (Gibbard et al., 1976). In this context, Turquet has suggested an additional basic assumption, that of fusion. In this basic assumption, the group has no past, no future, and no leader. Activity exists only for the present, and its only aim is gratification and the avoidance of ambivalence.

Peer relations

A parallel to the social-psychological study of member-to-member interaction in groups is Phillip Slater's (1966) important book *Microcosm*. Working from the data generated from a longitudinal study of groups, he examines the elementary social phenomena in the evolution of primitive religious structures. The first part of the book is primarily a clinical exposition of the issues in group development. Of importance for our purposes, Slater, as did Bion before him, begins his discussion of the group process from the point of view of the abstinent leader:

Whereas in macroscopic myth-making it is the perpetual silence of deities which somehow must be explained (or denied), in the training group or therapy group for that matter, it is the more immediate and concrete silence of the group leader. For it is the silence which activates the entire process.

Group members begin by experiencing the leader's silence as an acute deprivation, not only in terms of authoritative direction and personality cues but also with respect to fundamental needs for nurturance. Their fearful response to this deprivation facilitates transference responses that mold from early parental anlage a fantasy of an omniscient and omnipotent protector who will make order from the chaos of their experience. This rapidly develops into a group-level phenomenon and becomes a shared experience.

But the deification fails, and almost inevitably the group moves to some stage of revolution. During the second stage, in which the group revolts, themes of group murder emerge: The leader must die in order for the group to live. In this context, a sense of unanimity is generated, not only by the generalization of the murderous rage but also through the process of scapegoating—that is, by directing hostility generally toward an individual, one whose loyalty to the group revolt may be seen as problematic. But when the leader is the one to be attacked in this manner, a good deal of psychic energy is available for the development of intragroup solidarity. Following the revolt, the theme of cannibalism usually emerges. This theme corresponds to Freud's idea of identification, in that members attempt to incorporate desired attributes of the deposed leader by devouring their possessor. Gradually, the group members take into themselves the skills of the leader, leaving only a remnant of him behind. This remnant is exemplified in the group process by the theme of the sacred king and manifested by perceiving the group as strong and able, and symbolizing the deposed leader as superior.

The third stage of group development deals with the impact of the group revolt on member-to-member relationships with the setting aside of the leader. In this stage, members have a heightened sexual interest in one another, and there are frequent reproduction fantasies, as well as fantasies of the group in some ways reproducing itself. This theme of sexual liberation, in conjunction with incorporation of an identification with the leader during the group revolt, gives rise to the idea that group members will become parents (teachers, leaders) themselves. Unlike the passive, withdrawn role of women postulated by Freud in *Totem and Taboo*, Slater's data identify women as actively encouraging the revolt and the sexuality of the men.

Slater calls the final stage of the group "the new order," a formulation that is quite similar to Bion's conception of the work group. Within this "work group function," the leader is no longer deified, and his skills can be replicated by others. Since the authority and power of the leader have been dispersed throughout the group and into symbols of leadership, individual members' capacity for autonomy is enhanced, and differentiation and individuation begin to take place within members of the group. At the same time, the group has become united around a set of principles, similar to what the social psychologists call a common culture.

The Sociology of Groups

In distinction to psychological and social psychological studies, sociological theory views group dynamics from a perspective that is external to the group. Its focus is much less on the membership and its interactions, than on the group as a system of interaction. Sociologists focus upon those processes and structures which are dependent upon varying group tasks, boundaries, cultural contexts, and forms of leadership. In work on groups, the efforts of sociologists are directed toward the creation of useful models which account for these processes and structures. These models then help order data into an organized and heuristically relevant form.

Models of group

Mills (1967) summarizes six different models of groups. These include the quasimechanical, the organismic, the conflict, the equilibrium, the cybernetic-growth, and the structural-functional models. The specific form of most of these models can be inferred from its name; however, the structural-functional model derived from the work of Parsons, Shils, and Bales encompasses major aspects of most of the others: the systematic ordering of acts and functions of the quasimechanical, the need for member protection and self-fulfillment of the organismic, resolution of serial conflict in the conflict model, the effort to maintain and integrate change into the status quo in the equilibrium model, and the goal seeking and system consciousness feedback loops of the cybernetic-growth model. As such, this model is most useful for our purposes.

The structural-functional model (Parsons et al., 1953) holds that, unless the group simultaneously develops the means to meet its goals, maintain its boundaries, and gratify its members' needs, it will cease to function and be threatened with disintegration. Four interdependent and interacting structures or areas serve to articulate the demands of these functions within the group. Although these areas are not so clearly separable and their names are somewhat artificial, the tasks and work which each represent are relevant for understanding group process.

Adaptation. This area describes the processes by which the group coordinates its resources with the demands of the environment surrounding it. Action in this area involves finding new resources and techniques or molding existing ones for the solution of problems.

Goal attainment. This area is a critical one for obtaining and sustaining member satisfaction and involves the orientation and mobilization of members' efforts to accomplish their collective task. Action in this function involves the expression of positive and negative emotion, especially in relation to the leader or other groups.

Integration. This area monitors and regulates relationships within the group. Action here serves to coordinate and bring harmony to various aspects of and functions within the group, bridging differences and providing symbols for unity.

Pattern maintenance. This group function upholds and represents what the group stands for and the ways in which it will be done. It is an area in which the beliefs, values, and rules of the group combine to form a common culture.

In addition to the separation of group function into these four areas, proponents of the structural-functional model assume the emergence of, or presence in the group of leader-like figures. Leaders monitor the group's progress and take appropriate actions reinforcing and supporting positive movement and redirecting and counteracting negative movement in the areas of adaptation, goal attainment, integration, and pattern maintenance. In addition, leaders introduce new learning into the group's culture in ways that facilitate a balance and interplay among the various goals of the group. This role suggests the critical regulating function of leadership in which not only must the boundary between group and environment be defined, but also determinations must be made as to whether movement in the service of the task is taking place (Astrachan, 1970).

General systems theory, the structural-functional model, and value orientation

The notion of balance and interplay within a social system or group of any sort has been markedly enhanced by the development of general systems theory. This theory defines a system as a set of objects together with the relationships between the objects and their attributes. General systems theory derives from the structural correspondence of systems and is concerned with general system laws applying to any system of a certain type, independent of or unrelated to the specific units within the system (Edelson, 1970).

Using general systems theory and modifications of Parsons's theory of action, Marshall Edelson (1970) postulated a theory of group dynamics which advances the structural-functional model. Edelson's theory outlines the object relations within each function and identifies the manner in which action within a system is ultimately dependent upon the framework of values that group members share:

> ... internalization of a value in a person has occurred when commitment to it exists and does not depend for maintenance upon external sanctions. ... Institutionalization of a value in a group has occurred to the extent that the value has been internalized by the members of the group ... a system of institutionalized values is the essential characteristic of a group, as opposed to an individual entity.

In this model, then, group dynamics are a function of the interaction, the conflict, and the resolution between and among the demands of the four group functions and the value alternative each represents. Although these demands are generated from within the group, as well as from without, each area contributes output to the other areas and receives input from each. In the move from group process to individual member, from the institutionalization of values to the individual's internalization of values, Edelson essentially ignores member-to-member interactions. And, unlike the formulation of the structural-functional model, Edelson does not directly address the issue of leadership or leadership roles in the group. Rather, his formulation assumes that leadership accrues to those persons in the group most representative of specific value alternatives at any given moment.

Group process and the executive role

Drawing from the various models of groups, Mills (1967) suggests 5 interrelated levels of group process through which a newcomer to a group might progress:

overt behavior, group emotions, governing norms, goals, and values.

According to Mills, the newcomer functions "one level after the other until he assumes responsibility for the group as a whole and, in that capacity, operates on all 5 levels simultaneously." Rather than a model of group development, this might be construed as a sociological view of the process of individual development within an established group. Assuming the leadership or executive role involves responsibility for the definition of the group: What would be desirable for it to become? As the hypothetical newcomer to the group progresses through the 5 levels, he experiences new demands, repeated modification of his role, an increase in the complexity of his feedback processes, and an expansion in the range of his options for movement within the group. Although exposing him to more risks, this progression naturally increases the member's effectiveness and value to the group.

An important way, then, in which Mills's model adds to previous ones is in its more specific outline for the functioning of the leadership role. The 4 features of this role include: giving up responsibility for specific parts of the group in favor of the group as a whole, directing interventions to patterns of responses as a way of influencing what the group will become, decommitting himself from previously assumed roles, and standing on the boundary of the group and relating its development to the environment. Two major dilemmas confront the executive role: first, determining which of the plethora of data available to him is relevant, while at the same time becoming aware of as much of that data as possible; and second, determining when he knows enough to act strategically, while at the same time respecting the functional role differentiation and collective development of the group as a whole. As a way of coping with the complexity of the executive role, Mills proposes a paradigm for groups based on the 5 levels of group process. Borrowing from Deutsch, he suggests that the purposes underlying the formation and operation of groups could be classified into five orders: (1) obtaining immediate gratification; (2) sustaining conditions permitting gratification; (3) pursuit of a collective goal; (4) self-determination; and (5) growth. The executive employs this paradigm in the service of remaining equidistant from personality, group, and contextual elements in momentary situations. His strategy of action, therefore, is less governed by the demands of the moment than it is by whether these demands coincide or not with the progressive development outlined in the paradigm.

The five orders of Mills's paradigm are compatible with both the structural-functional model and Edelson's theory of groups. Although Mills repeatedly asserts that each level and each order is interrelated, his paradigm is essentially a progressive one, implying that later steps are impossible without the prior ones. The structural-functional model, particularly the Edelsonian model, has the advantage of not assigning any priority to the functions; rather, each contributes to and receives from the other in a way that more equitably legitimizes the function. On the other hand, it can be argued that these models are too conservative, in the sense that learning can only occur in the context of stability, with radical or revolutionary change being seen as potentially maladaptive.

The Group as a Social Psychological Entity

In its effort to bridge individual behavior and group process, social psychology addresses such issues as group development, role differentiation, member satisfaction, the effect of group size, time perspectives, and group work. The social psychology of groups focuses as well on member-to-member interactions, more so than on the individual member's relation to the group or vice versa.

Group development

At least three models have been proposed to describe and account for the developmental sequence in small groups: the linear-progressive model, the life-cycle model, and the recurring-cycle model (Gibbard et al., 1976).

The linear-progressive model was first proposed by Tuckman after reviewing 50 articles on the stages of group development over time in therapy groups, T-groups, and natural and laboratory groups. It is consistent with the work of Bennis and Shepard and of Kaplan and Roman (1963) and has been given further validation by Runkel *et al.* (1971) in a subsequent study. Tuckman's scheme has 2 essential dimensions: a temporal one and a structural one. In the first stage temporally, the group is forming. From the point of view of the development of group structure, members are testing each other and making efforts to establish dependent relations with other members and the leaders. From the perspective of task activity development, members appear to be orienting themselves to the task. The second stage in the developmental sequence is ushered in by a storming reaction. Group members are experiencing intragroup conflict; an observer might record an emotional response to the task demand. The third stage, known as norming, involves the development of group cohesion as a structural aspect and is represented in task activity as a more open exchange. In the fourth stage, the group is performing. This is characterized by a functional role relatedness in terms of group structure and as experienced by group members. From the point of view of task activity development, one notes the emergence of solutions and insights. Strain occurs in a group when group structure development and task activity development are incongruent. The progression that one notices in Tuckman's scheme is one that moves from an initial testing dependency through conflict to a sense of group cohesiveness and, finally, to the stage of task accomplishment.

Life-cycle models of group development are essentially linear models, with a separation or terminal phase added (Mills, 1964; Mann, 1966; Slater, 1966). An important issue for group dynamics is addressed in the pendular or recurring-cycle model; that is, not only is the linear move toward cohesiveness and intimacy in a group reversed in the process of termination, but interpersonal forces in the group eschew

closeness in order to protect against personal fragmentation and identity diffusion; as group structures develop and the boundary forms around the group, individuals often feel threatened with a loss of self and boundary definition. This might lead to a reversal or pendular movement in the group's development and has led some writers to suggest a more oscillating model (Slater, 1966). Hartman and Gibbard used the pendular notion to conceptualize group development, based on an accommodation to introjective and projective (individual) or inclusive and exclusive (group) processes in the formation and maintenance of boundaries. Borrowing heavily on object relations theory, these processes are conceived of as continuous throughout the life of the group, bringing together aspects of the intrapsychic life of individuals within the group, as well as the evolution of boundaries within those individuals and around the collectivity. Although many social psychologists who write about group development compare the evolution of a group to individual development, rather than a one-to-one correspondence, the processes are parallel.

Role differentiation and member satisfaction

Cartwright and Zander (1953) proposed that a group can be considered to be structured when it has acquired a degree of stability in the arrangement of relationships among its members. While the process of group development contributes to this stability in a general sense, a great deal has been written about more specific member-to-member interaction leading to the development of group structure. In this context, a critical construct for group dynamics is that of role. Role is conceived of as a dynamic structure within an individual (based, therefore, on needs, cognitions, and values), which usually comes to life under the influence of social (interactional, group, or situational) stimuli or defined positions. It includes the individual's expectations of himself in the situation, his expectation of others' reaction to him, and the way he might act in that situation (Edelson, 1970). Thus, each individual has available a repertoire of roles. It differs from the concept of identity and also multiple roles in that, action is involved in fulfilling a role. An important aspect of the arrangement of relationships in a group is that roles within the group become differentiated from each other. As groups develop, expectations emerge from one member to another at various moments in the group's life.

Bales and Slater measured the development of these expectations, the differentiation of roles, and were able to demonstrate the earliest recognizable differentiations within a system: what might be involved, for example, in the action of one person and the reaction of the other. When time of interaction, members interacting, and quality and type of activity were examined, aspects of social differentiation became manifest. The resulting entity is ultimately identified as a social interaction system, a system which itself stimulates the growth of role expectations and role fulfillments. For Bales and Slater, primitive forms of differentiation in the system can be seen as various members give positive reaction, ask questions, attempt to solve problems, and give negative reactions. Some of the processes referred to in the section on group development tend to evoke specialization in the quality and authorship of these activities. In conjunction with certain functions that must be fulfilled if the group is to survive, this specialization leads to the establishing of various roles in the group. For example, a common role which seems to develop in small leaderless groups is that of idea specialist, whose main functions seem to center around the task of the group. This role is usually in interaction with another, which might be called the social specialist, whose functioning exists primarily in the realm of group harmony and support of members. Another dyad which often exists in the small group might include the role of the guidance specialist or the keeper of the group's common culture and his opposite, the emotional specialist, whose task it is to facilitate expressiveness in the group. As these dyads interact within and between themselves, the group gradually builds a common culture, which includes the consolidation of roles, the evolution of a means by which its activity is symbolized, and the construction of a symbol system common to each of the participants. As the common culture grows, roles become increasingly differentiated, in large part because the culture includes the expectations that have developed as to how each person will behave. Although individuals within the group may well have very different opinions about who is best performing various roles, a common culture includes agreement as to the nature of each role and the criteria for its fulfillment.

Important conclusions can be drawn about groups in which there is a high or low consensus about the relative status of all group members. Status consensus and members' perception of progress toward group goals and freedom to participate are the cornerstones of member satisfaction in small groups (Heslin and Dunphy, 1964). As summarized by these authors, when the degree of status consensus is high, especially about the status of the task leader, then member satisfaction tends to be high; that is, there is a preponderance of positive over negative reactions, less factionalism and clique formation, and less competition for leadership. Notably, the converse was also true. Furthermore, status consensus was found to be most prominent when a special kind of group member emerged, one who participated actively in the role of task leader and social-emotional leader. High status consensus could also be achieved if a pair collaborated well in these roles. Finally, high status consensus was generally reported if group members perceived the task specialist as competent. Factors that tended to decrease status consensus were situations of great competitiveness, the absence of a special leader, the imposition of an inappropriate formal leader, and perception of the leader's incompetence.

Further studies reported by Heslin and Dunphy showed that another significant dimension in the assessment of member satisfaction was their perception of the progress toward group goals. Experimentally controlled groups in which goals were not attained (insoluble problems) or where goal attainment was blocked, led to increased factionalism, intermember aggression, and signs of disorganization. Similarly, when the individual needs of members were strong and in conflict with the goals of the group, then member satisfaction and goal attainment were reduced. Deutsch (1949) showed that cooperatively

organized groups were more successful than competitively organized groups in the speed and quality of their productivity. In his study, the high congruence of individual goals with group goals was noted in the cooperatively organized group. An additional factor relating to goal attainment and member satisfaction is that satisfaction with a group can lead to a reinforcement of the behavior conductive to goal attainment.

The third dimension of member satisfaction is the perceived freedom to participate. Much of the data to support this dimension come from communication net and earlier field theory experiments. These studies show that, although all persons in a group do not have an equal need to participate, those groups with a more equally distributed participation—or with members who experienced a felt freedom to fulfill their expectations about participation—experienced higher member satisfaction.

Group size, time perspective and work

Group size, even in the small group, is an important variable in group dynamics. Thomas and Fink divided studies on the effort of group size into two categories: effects for the group as a whole and effects on member behavior. As for the effect for the group as a whole, group performance and group productivity were shown to be enhanced on most measures when group size increases. Speed and efficiency, however, tended to be diminished in the larger group. The reduction in opportunity to speak in groups larger than the sizes that are addressed in this chapter (6 to 14 members) was not accompanied by decreasing participation, particularly in those who already ranked high in this dimension. On the other hand, in groups ranging from two to seven there seemed to be inhibiting factors which prevented the expression of dissatisfaction and disagreement. At the same time, these smaller groups tended to give individuals more opportunity to interact and to exhibit leadership behavior. Finally, the studies reviewed indicated that increases in size led to decreases in group cohesiveness and a subsequent division of labor and clique formation.

Research on the effects of group size on individual member behavior and performance is even more confounded by the nature of the task than that for the group as a whole. General problem solving and individual productivity tend to decrease with larger size, but the quality of solutions to human relations problems tends to increase. No general statements about conformity or consensus can be made, but member satisfaction, as previously noted, decreases with larger groups.

The spacing of group events over time has an impact on the group, but studies are unfortunately confined to a few time-limited self-analytic groups (Harrow et al., 1971). Comparing study groups and T-groups, these authors found that first meetings seem to combine both storming and norming phenomena and that the second meeting was relatively quiet. They also showed that study groups were more concerned with termination than T-groups. Much other information on time and the manner in which time interacts with other issues (e.g., group size, stage of development) is mostly anecdotal. For example, efforts to correlate intensity of experience with duration of group, as in a marathon group, have not been nearly as well demonstrated as the impact of leadership style, i.e., the importance of the charismatic all-knowing leader and potential member disaster in such events. Ziller (1965) reports the group's diminished capacity to accept new members and its heightened implementation of group decisions, particularly in open as opposed to closed groups. He hypothesizes a time perspective as one aspect of this alteration. Members in open groups maintain a continual awareness of the transitory nature of their relationships.

Newton and Levinson (1973) developed a theoretical framework for the analysis of the small work group within the organization. This sociopsychological perspective involves the interrelationship between task, social structure, social processes, and culture both within the small group and in its social environment. The understanding of a group's dynamics must take all four points of view into account, then relate each to its organizational and social context and to its individual members. In this way, these authors provide a synthesis of the individual psychological, sociological, and sociopsychological traditions. Although the concept of task appears self-evident, the clarification of a group's task and maintaining consensus in the group about the group's priorities are critical and difficult aspects of group life. Social structure involves the division of labor and the division of authority within the group. This, of course, corresponds to the concepts of role, status consensus, and the lines of authority that have been discussed earlier. The work group also tends to develop a culture which includes shared values, assumptions, and beliefs that provide a framework for group development and action. As in the case of each of the dimensions, the group's culture is strongly influenced by the culture of the organization in which it exists. Social process refers to not only how a group works in a general way and how it achieves group ends, but also how it works counter to the group's task, culture, and social structure. Social process is the expressive domain, the area involved with member satisfaction and dissatisfaction.

The synthesis provided by Newton and Levinson corresponds in some ways to the sociological model of group proposed by Mills, but it includes most of the concepts discussed in this chapter. As an analytic tool between the social system and individual members but with connections to both of these levels, it is a useful perspective. Nevertheless, the sought-for models which organize experience in and of group dynamics should be thought of more as aids to conceptualizing process, rather than as prescriptions for action. Humankind's irrepressible need for group life is itself a complex phenomenon and, as such, takes a variety of forms. Although there are identifiable patterns, the formation of groups and their resultant dynamics reflect this complexity.

Conclusion

The group therapist leads the group's work. As regulator of the external boundaries of the therapy group and in the managerial role in conducting group treatment, the group therapist needs to be aware of the interactions between the individual psychology in the group and the sociology of the group, as well as the group as a sociopsychological entity. These three contributions to group dynamics combine to exert powerful influences upon group members. The conflict between autonomy and group membership mobilizes anxiety within individual members and leads to a heightened transference readiness, an exacerbation of characteristic role-related and pathological behavior, and a regressive potential, the vicissitudes of which have been documented in this chapter. Member-to-member relationships mirror patterns and conflicts that individuals experience outside of the group. Moreover, as Frank points out, "each person constructs his assumptive world through interactions with others and has a strong need to check the validity of his perceptions and feelings against theirs." Group development and the emergence of a common culture provide a meaningful context and a set of norms by which individuals and the group itself can be measured. The group's boundary provides the safety necessary for the loosening, exposure, and exploration of personal boundaries. In short, the more cohesive a group is, the more likely it is to influence its members.

Kelman describes 3 processes by which influence can be conveyed and accepted in a group: compliance, identification, and internalization. These three processes coincide, respectively, with the social effect of a member's behavior, with the social rootedness of his behavior, and with the value congruence of his behavior. These have obvious connections with the concepts of role differentiation, status consensus, relations to authority, emotional reactions, and group development as outlined in the psychological, sociological, and sociopsychological contributions to dynamics within groups.

References

Astrachan, B. Towards a social systems model of therapeutic groups. Soc. Psychiatry, 5: 110, 1970.
Bion, W. *Experiences in Groups.* Basic Books, New York, 1961.
Bradford, L. P., Gibb, J. R., and Benne, K. D. *T-Group Theory and Laboratory Methods.* John Wiley & Sons, New York, 1964.
Cartwright, D., and Zander, A., eds. *Group Dynamics.* Row and Peterson, Evanston, IL, 1953.
Deutsch, M. An experimental study of the effects of cooperation and competition upon group process. Hum. Relations, 2: 129, 1949.
Edelson, M. *Sociotherapy and Psychotherapy.* University of Chicago Press, Chicago, 1970.
Frank, J. D., Persuasion and Healing: A Comparative Study of Psychotherapy, Baltimore: Johns Hopkins Press, 1961.
Gibbard, G. S., Hartman, J. J., and Mann, R. D. *Analysis of Groups.* Jossey-Bass, San Francisco, 1976.
Harrow, M., Astrachan, B., Tucker, G., Klein, E. G., and Miller, J. The T-group and study group laboratory experiences. J. Soc. Psychol., 85: 225, 1971.
Heslin, R., and Dunphy, D. Three dimensions of member satisfaction in small groups. Hum. Relations, 17: 99, 1964.

Kaplan, S. R., and Roman, M. Characteristic responses in adult therapy groups to the introduction of new members: A reflection on group processes. Int. J. Group Psychother., *13:* 10, 1963.

Kelman,, H. C., The Role of the Group in the Introduction of Therapeutic Change. International Journal of Group Psychotherapy, Vol. 13, pp. 399–432, 1963.

Lebon, G. *The Crowd: A Study of the Popular Mind.* Benn Press, London, 1947.

Lewin, K. Frontiers in group dynamics. Hum. Relations, *1:* 5, 1947.

McDougall, W. *The Group Mind.* Cambridge University Press, London, 1920.

Mann, R. D. The development of the member-trainer relationship in self-analytic groups. Hum. Relations, *19:* 85, 1966.

Mayo, E. *The Human Problems of an Industrial Civilization.* Macmillan, New York, 1933.

Mills, T. *Group Transformation.* Prentice-Hall, Engelwood Cliffs, NJ, 1964.

Mills, T. *The Sociology of Small Groups.* Prentice-Hall, Engelwood Cliffs, NJ, 1967.

Newton, P. M., and Levinson, D. J. The work group within the organization: A sociopsychological approach. Psychiatry, *36:* 115, 1973.

Parsons, T. The Structure of Social Action Free Press, New York, 1937.

Parsons, T., Shils, E., and Bales, R. *Working Papers in the Theory of Action.* Free Press, New York, 1953.

Rioch, M. The work of Wilfred Bion on groups. Psychiatry, *33:* 56, 1970.

Runkel, P. J., Lawrence, M., Oldfield, S., Rider, M., and Clark, C. Stages of group development: An empirical test of Tuckman's hypothesis. J. Appl. Behav. Sci., *7:* 180, 1971.

Schein, E. H., and Bennis, G. (eds.) *Personal and Organizational Change through Group Methods.* John Wiley & Sons, New York, 1965.

Slater, P. E. *Microcosm: Structural, Psychological and Religious Evolution in Groups.* John Wiley & Sons, New York, 1966.

Ziller, R. C. Toward a theory of open and closed groups. Psychol. Bull., *64:* 164, 1965.

A.4   Preparation, Selection of Patients, and Organization of the Group

BENJAMIN J. SADOCK, M.D.

Introduction

When the group concept is used as the psychotherapeutic vehicle for change in personality functioning, careful selection and preparation of patients and careful group organization are essential clinical responsibilities. Group psychotherapy cannot be applied as a blanket form of psychiatric treatment for all types of emotional disorders, even though a great variety of patient populations have been exposed to the method.

Clinical experience shows that patients who have done poorly in group psychotherapy may go on to do well in individual psychotherapy. The reverse is also true; patients who have not made gains in individual treatment have done so in group treatment. As a result, it is often difficult to predict with accuracy which patient will do well in which form of therapy, although certain guidelines can be enunciated.

Preparation

It is important to prepare the patient for the group therapy experience. The preparatory session consists of explaining the processes to which the patient will be exposed, making him aware of the need to be open and honest with his co-patients, and, finally, alerting him to the possibility that he may not like all of the other members, nor they him; but by examining the interaction that evolves, he will learn about himself, in the process developing his own way of thinking, feeling, and behaving—which is, after all, what psychotherapy is all about.

Prospective group therapy patients who are given a preparatory session have a more positive feeling about being in a group than those patients who do not have such a session. Moreover, there is a lower dropout rate, more communication, and a greater sense of cohesiveness among those who are so prepared.

Selection

To determine a patient's suitability for group psychotherapy, the therapist needs a great deal of information that can be gathered only in individual sessions. In the screening interview, the psychiatrist should take a careful psychiatric history and perform a mental status examination so that he has certain dynamic, behavioral, and diagnostic factors in hand.

Dynamic factor

The dynamics of the patient, including commonly used defense mechanisms, are important to determine proper selection. Relationship to peers and to authority figures, current and past, should also be assessed.

Authority anxiety. Those patients whose primary problem centers on their relationship to authority and who are extremely anxious in the presence of authority figures often do better in the group setting than in the dyadic or one-to-one setting. They gain support from the peer group and are thus aided in dealing with the therapist more realistically. Able to identify with others in the group who may have less difficulty in that area, they are eventually better able to perceive the therapist as less punitive or authoritarian than they had believed him to be.

Adolescents generally manifest authority anxiety, and for that reason many workers see group psychotherapy as the treatment of choice for that age group. For the adolescent who has not had a peer group experience, a normal stage in adolescent development, such a choice is especially apt. Therefore, the screening interview should include a careful history not only of attitudes toward parents, teachers, and other adults but, equally important, of the patient's participation in clubs and gangs. One of the most clear-cut indications for group psychotherapy is a history of an isolated, withdrawn adolescence in which the patient has had no exposure to peers. Patients with a great deal of authority anxiety may be blocked, anxious, resistant, and unwilling to verbalize thoughts and feelings in the individual setting, generally for fear of censure or disapproval from the therapist. They may welcome the suggestion of group psychotherapy so as to avoid the scrutiny of the dyadic situation. Conversely, if the patient reacts negatively to the suggestion of group psychotherapy or is openly resistant to the idea, the therapist should consider the possibility of a high degree of peer anxiety.

Peer anxiety. The patient who has destructive relationships with his peer group or who has been extremely isolated from peer group contact, such as a schizoid personality, generally reacts negatively or with increased anxiety when placed in a group setting. For example, some patients whose early development was characterized by a great deal of sibling rivalry and whose hostilities toward or from their siblings were overwhelmingly intense may be unable to tolerate a group and may leave it. For those patients whose nuclear problem is rooted in the sibling relationship, the group can provide the corrective emotional experience necessary for cure; but the psychiatrist must determine the patient's ability to tolerate the degree of discomfort that will be produced. Those patients act out their feelings toward the other members; if properly handled by the therapist, those feelings are subject to analysis and objective understanding. The reality of having other patients with whom they can interact often leads to more insight than does a verbal reconstruction in individual psychotherapy.

For the child who was raised without siblings, the group may produce anxiety because his central position is jeopardized—perhaps for the first time if he has organized his adult life style so as to remain the center of attention. Within the group, those patients demand to have their narcissistic needs gratified by the therapist. But the group setting demands that sharing occur, and such a setting may represent the first time the only child has been in such a position, a position he may be unable to tolerate.

On occasion, the only child may see the group as providing the sibling experience always denied him. The central position that some only children cherish may be anathema to others who were deprived of peer interaction within the family unit as they were growing up. That reaction is especially common if the parents were harsh and punitive and the overwhelmed child longed for allies from whom he could derive support.

In either case—for the only child who is unwilling to share or the only child who longs to share—the group setting rather quickly causes those dynamics to unfold and be subject to examination and ultimate resolution.

Defense mechanisms

Defense mechanisms are mental processes that a person used to protect himself from consciously experiencing anxiety; they enable him to cope with a variety of internal and external stresses. The more knowledgeable the therapist is about the array of defense mechanisms used by a prospective group member, the more helpful he can be in working with the patient within the group. In all forms of psychotherapy, the defensive maneuvers, varied as they may be, are analyzed; but the defenses discussed below lend themselves particularly well to the group method of treatment.

Projection. One of the positive indications for group psychotherapy is the finding that a patient uses the defense mechanism of projection, in which he attributes to others impulses that he finds unacceptable in himself. Such patients persistently blame others for their own inadequacies and failures and distort the realities of the outside world. They are reluctant to talk about their own motives and avoid introspection that may lead to an uncovering of their own unwanted, shameful, and guilt-ridden thoughts. In the one-to-one setting these patients may be unable to establish a working relationship with the therapist because of their tendency to project onto him thoughts and feelings, generally negative ones, that interfere with and are not available for reality testing.

This particular defense mechanism can be effectively dealt with in the group setting by the other group members, who constantly confront such a patient with his distortions as they are directed toward them or the therapist. Such group processes force introspective analysis to occur, and the projective mechanism is thereby eroded. One of the problems to be faced by the therapist is that often the patient using that defense mechanism makes accurate observations about others, since he may be especially sensitive to finding in them the same faults as he himself possesses. Thus, his observations about others may be accurate. Accordingly, the therapist cannot assume that the patient's observations are incorrect; but he must make sure that the projecting member takes responsibility for the same character trait in himself that he notes in others.

Certain techniques have been developed to facilitate that task, such as insisting, at an appropriate stage of treatment, that the member in question begin all his comments with the personal pronoun "I"—"I feel" or "I think"—thus encouraging the introspective mode; rather than the confrontative mode. Regardless of technique, however, the mechanisms of projection, as used by a particular member, must be clearly defined within the group.

Repression, denial, and suppression. These defenses are among the most common. They are characterized by the person's eliminating from consciousness all thoughts, feelings, memories, strivings, impulses, and other mental experiences that constitute a threat to his self-image and the image he wishes others to have of him or her. Repression is similar to denial except that, in denial, it is external reality, rather than internal reality, that is transformed so as not to be painful. Suppression—not to be confused with repression, which occurs outside of the person's awareness—is a conscious attempt to withhold painful material.

Repression, denial, and suppression are particularly well suited for examination in group psychotherapy. When those defenses are delineated in the screening interview, the clinician should consider the advantages of group treatment. It was Schilder who was first impressed with the fact that, when one member recalled an event, other members recalled repressed material, a process that is inherent in every psychotherapy group that has, as one of its goals, an evocation of historical data. The enemy of repression is the stimulation afforded by one member's being able to break through the repressive barrier and to ventilate highly charged material—memories, life events, impulses. However, that breakthrough is not without its potential hazards, and the therapist must be constantly aware of them. Should the repressed material enter consciousness before it can be assimilated effectively, the patient may be overwhelmed with intolerable anxiety. Aware of that potential, the leader, by his skillful management of the group, can evoke the repressed material with the most salutary effects and lead the members to a heightened psychological awareness.

One of the most painful of human conditions is the harboring of a personal secret that produces feelings of sin or guilt. Suppression—the conscious withholding of information about oneself because of fear, anxiety, guilt, shame, or embarrassment—is one of the mental processes attended to by the well-functioning psychotherapy group. In the group, patients may reveal their most hidden secret only to realize that others harbor a similar thought, feeling, or life event. For example, if anger is the suppressed feeling, the group not only examines how and why the mechanism developed but also provides a setting in which resolution can occur and the patient can test new modes of adaptation. When denial is the major mental mechanism used by the patient who finds an aspect of his external life situation too painful to see realistically, the group not only is able to correct the distortion but is capable of helping the patient examine a variety of ways in which he can cope with the situation more effectively. The well-organized group has within it a diverse membership capable of providing role models that enable each to learn from the other. When the denial of mental illness is the major problem, feedback from others in the group may be the first step in getting the patient to recognize that emotional disturbance does exist.

Transference reactions. One of the characteristics of all in-depth psychotherapies, particularly those that are psychoanalytically oriented, is a close examination of the distortions that exist in the feelings of the patient toward the therapist. Such transference examination rests on the premise that the patient reacts to the therapist in the same way that he reacted to significant figures in his past life, and, as this reaction is analyzed, emotional growth and development occur. But sometimes the transference is so intense that it cannot be analyzed in the one-to-one relationship, either because it takes on such negative aspects that the patient can no longer tolerate the feelings and leaves treatment entirely or because it becomes fixed. The fixed transference is static and lacks the more flexible, analyzable characteristics prevalent in the anxiety disorders, for example. The fixed transference is not always negative, however; it can be positive to the extent that it becomes an erotic fixation on the therapist, a condition which may be equally resistant to interpretation and change.

Patients who are likely to develop a fixed or delusional transferential reaction to the therapist, either positive or negative, are best placed in a group in addition to or in place of individual therapy. If the transference is negative, the patient has the opportunity to observe his or her co-patients' distinctly different reactions to the therapist. That observation aids the patient's reality testing, because it becomes difficult to maintain irrational negative attitudes when most, if not all, of the group members have a different perceptual framework. If the transference is positive, the group setting provides the opportunity for certain elements of the transference to be diluted into other members. It also does not allow the patient to harbor the fantasy, common in that condition, that he or she is the therapist's only patient. The fact that the therapist directs his attention to other patients in the group is an inherent reality-testing function built into the group situation.

Predicting how transference will proceed in the course of treatment is one of the most difficult and most important aspects of the initial interview. Examining the patient's reactions to significant persons in his past life helps the clinician make that prediction. At times, the patient's previous therapeutic experiences, whether real or fancied, also provide guidelines, as the following case illustrates.

The patient, a 32-year-old nurse, reported in the initial interview, not without a great deal of embarrassment, that she had had sexual relations with her previous therapist during the last 2 years of her individual psychotherapy. Although she recognized the impropriety of that situation and realized that she needed professional help in alleviating a severe personality disorder, she was aware of her attempts to destroy the therapeutic alliance by repeatedly attempting to seduce the therapist. She welcomed the opportunity to enter a group, which offered her protection from both her own impulses and the expected response of any new therapist she would consult. As treatment in the group progressed, she was able to analyze the use of her sexuality to achieve and maintain intimacy and to protect her from recognizing her deep-seated feelings of unworthiness. It is unlikely that she would have been able to achieve a working alliance in another dyadic situation, since she feared that, if she verbalized her sexual feelings for the therapist, actual seduction would follow.

Isolation. Isolation is the mental mechanism that sets apart an idea from the attached and appropriate feeling tone. The patient may have thoughts that the normal person would find frightening or upsetting, such as wanting to harm himself or someone else. But, when isolation is at work, no affect is attached to the imagery or idea, and the patient shows little or no sign of emotion. Members of a therapy group are usually quite adept at observing the mechanism when it occurs and are able to confront one another with the apparent lack of feeling. When so confronted, the group member in question eventually becomes aware of the defense, and therapeutic reconstruction may begin. In a successful outcome, the defense becomes ego-alien, the ideas and the attached feeling tones coalesce, and insight and behavioral change begin to occur.

Diagnostic factors

The diagnosis of the patient's disorder is important in determining the best therapeutic approach and in evaluating his motivation for treatment, his capacity for change, and the strengths and weaknesses of his personality structure.

Group psychotherapy has been conducted with patients in practically every diagnostic category. The results, both successful and unsuccessful, of treating such a diverse group of patients make it difficult to state with a high degree of accuracy that certain specific mental illnesses are better suited to another form of therapy. Nonetheless, certain guidelines can be set forth about what one may expect in certain major diagnostic categories.

Diagnosis is more than nosological pigeonholing. Those workers who suggest that diagnosis is unimportant in group therapy take too simplistic a view of the diagnostic process, which routinely includes an extensive examination of the patient's chief complaint, along with a detailed evaluation of his past developmental history, including a review of the levels of functioning in various life areas—vocational, familial, social, marital, sexual. The mental status examination provides clues to the psychopathological processes at work currently, in the past, and under

stress, and it also helps predict the patient's characteristic response to stress. Diagnosis includes a variety of postulates about the psychodynamics and defense mechanisms involved, the causes of the patient's emotional disorder, and the desired goals to be achieved. The clinician should be able to make certain inferences about the patient from the diagnosis assigned.

The diagnostic examination must include data about the patient's physical health. No patient should be placed in psychotherapy for an emotional disorder without a physical examination to rule out the presence of an organic disease that may account for some if not all of the patient's symptoms.

Schizophrenia. This large category includes a group of disorders characterized by disturbances of thinking, mood, and behavior that may have the associated symptoms of hallucination, illusion, and delusion. The schizophrenic generally has a history of severe emotional deprivation and may be in poor control of his impulses and in a chronic state of anxiety and agitation. The fear of a loss of reality testing can be omnipresent. Most schizophrenics mistrust others and lead an isolated, socially withdrawn existence.

The group experience can provide the schizophrenic patient with a therapeutic atmosphere that supports reality orientation and encourages him to relate to others so as to combat his feelings of fear and distrust. The emphasis on reality testing diminishes the opportunity to explore unconscious material, which one can attempt with neurotic disorders. The group setting is geared to be socially supportive, and outside group contact has been advocated by some workers because, for many schizophrenic patients, the group provides their only socialization experience in an otherwise bleak and dreary existence.

If group treatment of schizophrenic patients is difficult, it is because of certain technical procedures, rather than because of the group modality. Other patients in the group may interact and interpret in ways that threaten a particular patient's defense system. Skillful handling by the therapist is necessary to overcome that difficulty, although there is some safety in the fact that the schizophrenic in a group is much more leader oriented than peer oriented and is susceptible to interpretations offered by the leader.

If the treatment of a schizophrenic group is conducted by a nonmedical therapist, the services of a physician who can administer appropriate medication should always be made available.

Affective disorders. Patients in this category show disturbances of mood, as in the bipolar affective disorders (manic-depressive illness). When depression is the major symptom and suicide represents a real risk, hospitalization is preferable to outpatient treatment of any kind. Placing the severely depressed patient, who requires a high degree of emotional support and nurturance, in a group as the first therapeutic intervention may aggravate his symptoms, since he is unable to receive sufficient nurturance from the leader. The patient whose depressive illness occurs after he has already been integrated into a group can gain a great deal of emotional gratification from the group experience, but the severely depressed, suicidal patient should not be placed in a new group on an outpatient basis without first having established a strong, positive relationship with the therapist and, if indicated, having received antidepressant medication.

Manic patients, who do not necessarily suffer from conscious suicidal ideas, are particularly difficult patients to manage in the group setting. They tend to display excessive elation, talkativeness, and irritability—traits that often antagonize both the group members and the leader—and they are given to accelerated speech and motor activity, which the group is often unable to control. After the mania has been brought under control psychopharmacologically, those patients do well, however.

Paranoid states. This category includes patients who have delusional manifestations, usually of a persecutory nature. Such patients usually resist most forms of psychotherapy. When there is a risk that the patient will incorporate the group into his paranoid delusion, it is unlikely that effective reality testing will be possible. But when the illness is less severe—as in the paranoid personality, who is still capable of being influenced by the consensual validation of the group—group therapy may be quite effective and, in fact, superior to the one-to-one therapeutic situation. The paranoid tends to be suspicious and jealous and to direct blame at others, behavior that results from his using the defense mechanism of projection. As mentioned earlier, this defense mechanism lends itself to accurate and effective interpretation by the group as a whole. These patients often cannot relate well to other people, and they can use the group as a laboratory in which feedback from peers helps them learn new adaptive patterns that contribute to improved social relationships and to an understanding of the life stresses that caused the paranoid pattern to develop.

Neuroses. Neurotic patients are usually aware of their difficulties, which are mainly manifested by anxiety, and they are generally well motivated to obtain relief from their symptoms. Most group psychotherapy approaches, as well as individual psychotherapy approaches, have been attempted with neurotics, and every category of neurosis has been treated with some degree of success. Psychoanalytically oriented group psychotherapy has been used with the majority of neurotic conditions, but recently phobic disorders have been treated with increasing success by means of behavioral group therapy using operant conditioning and desensitization procedures. Patients who suffer from agoraphobia, who are frightened to go out alone, often can be helped by group members who accompany the patient as he carries out his daily tasks until the condition is ameliorated.

Personality disorders. The patient with a personality disorder may be totally unaware of his lifelong patterns of maladaptive behavior. He usually complains of vague feelings of dissatisfaction with his life, at the same time denying or rationalizing his maladaptive behavior. Group psychotherapy is ideal for these patients because, when they display their characteristic behavioral patterns in the group, the members reflect back to the patient the effects of those patterns on his interpersonal relationships, which are usually either chaotic or nonexistent. Those vigorous confrontations force the patient to examine his behavior. Once he recognizes that it is pathological, he is able to gain some insight into its development and ways to change it. However, certain modifications in technique or frank contraindications to group treatment exist in the following subgroups classified as personality disorders.

Schizotypal personality. Patients with this type of personality disorder are generally shy and oversensitive and avoid close or competitive relationships with others. They experience feelings of rejection without any apparent cause and tend to remain silent about those feelings. The therapist must be able to recognize those emotions, to draw such patients into the group, and to encourage them to participate. A well-functioning group—depending on its composition, the stage of its development, and the therapeutic techniques of its leader—often recognizes the withdrawal pattern in one of its members. But there is a risk that more verbal, healthier patients will overshadow the withdrawn member. Accordingly, specific techniques, such as the go-round, may have to be used to engage his active participation in the group. Patients with a schizotypal personality require a supportive group milieu, and there is no doubt as to the efficacy of the group experience for those patients.

Borderline personality. Borderline personalities are fragile emotionally, with a tendency to mood swings, ambivalent feelings, and loss of empathy with others. Accordingly, they often arouse reactively hostile feelings from other members or, conversely, maintain a fixed emotional pattern within the group of hostility, indifference, or lability of mood. The fixed transferential psychoses mentioned earlier are most often found within this diagnostic category. These patients do not tolerate ambivalence and tend to categorize and stereotype others. In the group they have friends and enemies, and shift fellow group members from one camp to the other with ease. The therapist must be prepared to provide individual sessions for borderline patients who are treated in groups. Reality testing can be helped thereby as the patient attempts to sort out his complex and poorly understood feelings toward the other members of the group.

Schizoid personality. Patients with schizoid personality disorder are lonely people with few if any friends. Superficially, they may appear to be similar to schizotypal personalities, but they are easier to manage in the group because they lack the oddities of thinking, feeling, and perception of the schizotype. Group therapy is particularly useful for schizoids, who are provided with a social network in which they have the opportunity to overcome fears of closeness and feelings of isolation. They learn, in the supportive milieu of the group, to communicate their thoughts and feelings directly to others and, by so doing, move toward more normal behavioral patterns.

Passive-aggressive personality. This personality disorder is characterized by either passivity or aggressiveness. In the passive pattern, the patient is unable to assert himself and assumes a role of chronic submissiveness and compliance. But beneath the unassuming facade may be a great deal of hostility and resentment. The group setting is especially favorable in the treatment of the passive patient on a number of levels. It exposes the passivity to analysis by allowing the patient to become consciously aware of what he may have denied and rationalized previously. Group members confront him whenever he behaves too passively, and he is thus encouraged to become more outgoing and to react more spontaneously with a true expression of feelings. And, in the properly organized group, the passive member can identify with effective role models and so learn new and better-adapted ways in which to make his needs known.

In an alternate pattern of this personality disorder, the patient expresses angry feelings covertly by being stubborn, obstructionistic, or intentionally inefficient. The group usually reacts hostilely to those disguised expressions of anger, thus communicating to the patient the effects of his passive-aggressive behavior on others. Although a group generally disapproves of and refuses to tolerate the persistent pouting, procrastination, and stubbornness of such patients, the group members try to be of help, rather than overtly rejecting the patient, as usually happens outside the group.

Dependent personality. The patient with a dependent personality usually has deep dependency needs that are not being gratified by the external environment, thus leading to disappointment and resentment. The multiple relationships established within the group provide substitute dependency objects and tend eventually to diminish anxiety and the need for the maladaptive behavior pattern. As group therapy progresses the excessive dependency striving can be uncovered. But it is first necessary to examine the patient's character structure, which can be done more successfully in the group than in the one-to-one situation. In the group setting, one or more of the other members may give the patient the support he needs while the removal of his character armor takes place. These patients also dislike being alone, and groups that permit members to contact one another outside of regularly scheduled meetings are desirable, so that a patient can call on a group member when he feels anxious or depressed.

Avoidant personality. The avoidant person is anxious and fearful, and he avoids new or stressed situations. He is needy, and in a group he usually taxes the resources of the healthier members, who complain that they give much to the avoidant personality but receive little in return. In spite of that, however, these patients benefit from the interaction with other people and learn to master their fears and deal with their feelings of loneliness and rejection. Behavioral group therapy approaches have been particularly successful in treating these patients with assertive training methods. Techniques that reinforce the expression of appropriately assertive behavior are used, and the group becomes the testing ground for the changes brought about.

Antisocial personality. Antisocial persons are irresponsible and incapable of significant loyalty to individuals or groups. Their behavior patterns often result in legal or social offenses. Unable to learn from experience, they are resistant to all forms of psychotherapy, and may be particularly unsuited for group psychotherapy, since they do not constructively assimilate the interpretations made by other group members or by the therapist. Because of their inability to adhere to group standards, they are unable to maintain the confidentiality of the group, and for that reason they may have to be excluded from group treatment.

Although attempts have been made, with some success, to work with the antisocial personality in a group setting, those groups have usually been formed in penal institutions, where there is marked external pressure to attend and participate. In a group composed solely of antisocial patients, the group members' massive confrontation techniques toward one another may be sufficient at times to mobilize introspective attempts on the part of some participants.

Disorders of impulse control. Patients who have explosive outbursts of physical and verbal aggressiveness may represent a physical risk to the other group members, for whom the therapist is responsible. If there is a real danger that a patient will act out his aggressive impulses, for example, he should not be included in a therapy group.

The emotional interaction in groups is often heightened, and the control of aggressive impulses is a necessary prerequisite for group membership. Explosive patients need to develop internal control of their tendency to act out. Some of these patients may be able to adhere to external controls established by either the therapist or the group, but they are generally unable to curb their excitability.

The current popularity of encounter groups points up the importance of accurately assessing a patient's ability to control impulses—to verbalize them, rather than act on them. Some compulsive personalities who are excessively concerned with conformity and adherence to standards of conscience may benefit from the acting out of impulses encouraged by encounter groups. But encounter techniques applied indiscriminately to those whose real need is to develop controls are antitherapeutic for the patient unable to control impulses and potentially dangerous for the group as a whole.

Patients who suffer from substance abuse disorders, pathological gambling, or other impulse disorders are usually treated in homogeneous groups. They find mutual support within the group and learn from one another what precipitates the impulse and how it can be controlled.

Adolescent disorders. The adolescent characteristically shows fluidity of behavior in his attempts to consolidate his identity, which is in crisis, as Erikson postulated, during this stage of development. Psychopathology in an adolescent may take a variety of forms—irritability, withdrawal, depression, brooding, shyness, anxiety, and delinquency, among others. In addition, he often has a fear of authority. The group setting allows the adolescent to explore attitudes toward authority more effectively than does the one-to-one situation because in the group he has the support of his peers. Many therapists believe group therapy to be the treatment of choice for most adolescent disorders because it provides a peer experience that the disturbed adolescent may have been denied. Sullivan postulated that, unless such a peer experience occurs during adolescence, there is a risk of overt schizophrenia developing. In that sense, group treatment for this age group may also be a preventive procedure.

Other disorders. A great variety of other disorders and patients with special problems have been worked with in group psychotherapy: homosexual conflict disorders, transvestitism and gender identity problems, alcoholism and other substance abuse disorders, heart disease, and juvenile delinquency. There has been increased interest in the use of group therapy with the aged and those with terminal illness. Petty, Berland, and Puggi described the support to be found in the group setting by the aged who must cope with being alone, and Abrams examined the beneficial effects of sharing fears about death and dying in patients with terminal cancer. The list of special types of problems and specific categories of illness to which the group method of treatment has been applied over the years is practically endless and is as varied and diverse as the range of human behavior.

Structural Organization

Once having decided that a particular patient is suitable for group psychotherapy, the therapist must place him in a group where he can freely communicate with others, including the therapist. The proper organization of the group is crucial if a therapeutic atmosphere conducive to personality change is to occur for all the participants. Therefore, a number of parameters must be considered, which are discussed below.

Size

Group therapy has been successful with as few as three members and as many as 15, but most therapists consider 8 to 10 members optimal. With fewer members there may be too little interaction, unless they are especially verbal. With a larger group the interaction may be too great for the members or the therapist to follow. The number of patients that a particular group therapist can observe adequately also varies. With experience, the range of emotional interaction the therapist can integrate adequately increases to its optimum. And depending on the variables of leadership style and theoretical orientation, the size of the group may also vary.

At times, the composition of the group may determine its size. If, for example, a group contains an extremely verbal, aggressive, dominating member, it may be necessary to increase the size to provide counterforces to offset the monopolist. Similarly, a group composed primarily of withdrawn, schizoid members may require additional members to heighten the level of interaction. Ideally, the group should maintain a constancy, and, within a relatively limited range, the personality make-up of the individual members should be able to provide checks and balances to produce effective interaction.

Frequency of sessions

Most group psychotherapists conduct group sessions once weekly, although Wolf and Schwartz, adhering to a more classical psychoanalytic procedure, have conducted three to five group sessions a week. It is important to maintain continuity in sessions so that themes from a previous session may be carried over, as necessary, to the next without too great a time lag between. Sadock and Kaplan consider group psychotherapy inefficient if sessions are dropped for any reason whatsoever. Thus, they advocate that summer sessions meet even when the therapist is on vacation. When alternate sessions are used, the group meets twice a week, once with the therapist and once without him.

At times, it may be necessay to increase the frequency of sessions during a particular period. But that increase should be done for specific reasons. A member of the group may be undergoing a life stress of sufficient magnitude that he requires the more frequent meeting of the group to provide him with necessary support. Or, the group as a whole may be in crisis—a member may have died, for example—such that only more frequent meetings provide sufficient opportunity for the crisis to be worked through. Certainly, increased frequency should be not capricious but based on a sound appraisal of the needs of a particular member of the group or of the group as a whole.

One of the advantages of co-therapists is that of assuring continuity of sessions. If one member of the co-therapy team is absent, the other can carry the group. When a single therapist conducts the group, the members may be encouraged to meet even when circumstances prevent the leader from attending a particular session.

Length of sessions

In general, group sessions last anywhere from 1 to 2 hours, with the average length being 1½ hours. However, the time limit set should be constant. The limit allows the group to become aware of patterns that may be of significance—such as a particular member's always bringing up a topic meaningful to him just before the group's ending or the group's reacting in a similar manner. If the group session is too short, there may be insufficient time for necessary emotional interaction to develop. Conversely, if the session is too long, the level of emotional interaction may be too heightened to be assimilated cognitively by either the members or the therapist.

The fixed time limit to the session also has the practical advantage of allowing both the patients and the leaders to adhere to the commitments of their everyday lives. It places an optimum value on the necessity to use the time available for group work as effectively as possible. For certain patients, such as those who have difficulty in controlling impulses, the fixed length of the session serves as a model for the setting of limits. And the time limit can be reassuring for those patients who fear a loss of control.

In 1963, Bach and Stoller introduced the concept of time-extended therapy, in which the group meets continuously for 12 to 72 hours. They called the process "accelerated interaction" because the participants are pushed to a heightened level of emotional interaction by virtue of their enforced proximity for an extended period of time.

Enforced interactional proximity and, during the longer time-extended sessions, sleep deprivation, produce a breakdown in certain ego defenses, release affective processes, and promote a less guarded type of communication. However, time-extended groups—marathons, as they have come to be called—are not without their dangers. Careful selection procedures are necessary to determine the capacity of the participants to deal with the increased affective tone of those groups and their ability to maintain cognitive thinking, which normally disintegrates when one is deprived of sleep. Such an assessment is needed to eliminate patients who may suffer untoward psychological effects.

Attempts have been made to integrate marathon experiences within the structure of an ongoing therapeutic group in which the members have already formed a cohesive unit and the therapist is well aware of the interactional potential and ego strengths of the members. Those efforts have been successful in certain instances, especially when a particular group had reached a therapeutic impasse and spontaneous interaction was blocked. In general, however, the causes of group resistance shoud be examined in the regular weekly meetings before time-extended therapy is used. And when it is used, the marathon experience should adhere to the definition of group therapy—the therapist must be especially careful about selection and group organization. Unless those parameters are adhered to, the marathon experience is potentially hazardous.

Homogeneous versus heterogeneous groups

There has been some controversy as to whether the therapy group should be homogeneous or heterogeneous—that is, composed of patients of one sex, age, race, socioeconomic level, symptom, or category of illness, or composed of patients in which those factors vary. In general, most therapists support the view that the group should be as heterogeneous as possible to ensure maximum interaction. Thus, the group should be composed of members from different categories of illness and with varied behavioral patterns; from all races, social levels, and educational backgrounds; and of varying ages and both sexes.

In the heterogeneous group each member receives greater stimulation than in the homogeneous group and is forced to examine and understand what is different about his fellow group members. There is a tacit group agreement to accept what is different, and the adaptive capacity of the individual patient to tolerate difference is tested and reinforced. In addition, the heterogeneous group provides greater opportunities for more effective reality testing, since malfunctioning in one area of living by a particular member may be offset by another member's effective functioning in that same area.

Even homogeneous groups—for example, groups geared to adolescent adjustment problems, personality disorders, and certain sexual disorders—are heterogeneous to some degree. The causes of the disorder, the genetic and dynamic factors, and the patients' life styles vary considerably within any diagnostic category.

The heterogeneous group cannot be organized haphazardly. Certain other factors listed below must be considered for proper group organization.

Diagnostic factors. Some schizophrenic patients can be placed in groups with nonschizophrenic patients. The schizophrenic, who is highly vulnerable to the evocation of unconscious processes, can provide the neurotic patient with the necessary stimulation to break through repressive barriers, which are more intact in neurotics than in schizophrenics. Conversely, the neurotic can provide a high degree of reality testing and support for those ego defenses that have become weakened in the schizophrenic.

Although it is not advisable to place the schizophrenic who suffers from overt delusions or hallucinations in a group made up of neurotics, such schizophrenic patients can be treated in group therapy. Delusional and hallucinating patients can help one another within the group setting. The delusional patient is able to provide effective reality testing for the hallucinating patient and vice versa. And patients with differing delusions challenge one another.

In a group composed of schizophrenic patients, a 41-year-old man complained that he was being followed by a variety of persecutors, who were spying on him constantly. As he was attempting to convince the group of the injustices he suffered as a result, a woman interrupted his story, telling him that he was crazy to harbor such ideas. Others in the group supported her position. The woman in question believed that she was the Virgin Mary. But her delusional system, at variance with the man's, enabled her to mobilize the group and provide reality testing for him. She, in turn, was subject to the same group process when she attempted to convince the group of her false beliefs. Had the group been composed of patients with similar beliefs, that group process could not have occurred, since each patient would have confirmed the delusion of the others. Such collective delusional systems are not uncommon when the organization of the group is not carefully thought out beforehand.

Dynamic factors. When the therapist has a sound understanding of the psychodynamics of a variety of patients, he can organize a group most efficaciously.

For example, if the oedipal conflict is used as a basis of organization, a broad range of effective interactional potentials can be considered. A patient who is competitive with his father can be placed in a group with a patient who competes with his son. A patient who was subject to an overprotective or seductive mother can be placed in a group with such a close-binding mother. The varieties of group organization revolving about this dynamic constellation are almost endless. But each patient should be the mirror image of another; the patients should be complementary with regard to the oedipal conflict. Regardless of the theoretical dynamic construct to which the therapist adheres, he should be able to predict with a fair degree of accuracy how patients will interact within the group.

When the therapist considers the dynamic organization of the group, diagnosis may be misleading. For example, depression in one patient can be the result of a real loss, such as the death of a loved one. In another patient, depression can result from a threatened loss, such as an impending divorce. And in a third patient, it can result from an imagined loss, such as the fear that a loved one has left. A mixture of those various psychodynamic formulations would be desirable in a group; they would add to the potential interactions among the members. The therapist needs a high degree of clinical sophistication to define symptoms psychodynamically.

Behavioral factors. An examination of the patients' life styles and behavioral patterns can also help the therapist organize a group effectively. In so doing, the therapist should choose members with a variety of patterns. The patient whose life style is marked by isolation, withdrawal, and a fear of close relationships is ideally suited for group therapy. Such a patient should be exposed to a member whose life style is marked by an extrovertive or pathologically outgoing personality organization. The patient who is helpless, indecisive, and overly dependent should be matched with one who is impulsive, quick to make decisions—however wrong they may be—and overly independent. In such a group, patients are exposed to new patterns of behavior, and each can learn from the other.

Similarly, life experiences in conflict or in the process of resolution can be a basis on which to organize the group. For example, a patient dealing with the problems of leaving his parents' home can benefit from contact with one who is contemplating or who has successfully negotiated such a move. Patients who have experienced divorce or marriage can help others who are anxious about such life decisions. As life styles and behavioral patterns vary, so do the combinations of patients along those parameters, and the therapist must keep the concept of complementary patterning in mind.

Sexual factors. Most patients who present themselves for psychotherapy suffer from some kind of sexual disorder as part of their psychopathology, regardless of diagnosis and regardless of whether the sexual disorder is the primary complaint. Many sexual conflicts stem not only from psychological conflict but also from educational deficiencies. The interrelationship between the two is exceedingly complex, and the group setting provides a unique opportunity for the patients and the therapist to learn whether a problem is the result of faulty education or psychological problems or a combination of both. Psychological inhibition is suggested when education does not ease the problem, when accurate sex information cannot be assimilated.

For example, many people know intellectually that masturbation is normal, but the typical patient still suffers from some degree of guilt. That guilt is often culturally induced; it may also be the result of traumas associated with masturbatory activity or disturbing masturbatory fantasies. Regardless of the causes, talking about masturbatory experiences can have an almost immediate guilt-reducing effect. The same can be said about other varieties of sexual experience, both normal and abnormal. A member who feels that a particular sexual act is pathological, often discovers that others in the group view it with equanimity. And there is a great difference between being reassured by the therapist in the one-to-one situation that a particular sexual experience is no cause for alarm and hearing others in one's group take a similar position. In the dyadic situation, the patient may see the reassurance being offered as a therapeutic maneuver; group members who openly share accounts of their sexual activities are more reassuring. Furthermore, the sharing of experience has an educational effect.

In certain situations, such as homosexuality, the group may be organized unisexually. Advocates of that approach point out that the homosexual's anxiety about discussing and examining the dynamics of his situation may be too great, especially in view of societal pressures that still exist against that form of behavior, if the other members of the group do not have a similar orientation. The therapeutic goal—whether adaptation to heterosexuality or better adaptation to homosexuality—also plays a part in determining whether to place the homosexual in a mixed group. In general, most heterosexually oriented groups are tolerant of various sexual behavior patterns but tend to pressure the homosexual person to change his orientation. If that pressure is consonant with the person's goal—that is, if the homosexuality is ego-dystonic—placement in a mixed group may be indicated. But the therapist must be aware that such group pressure may be premature or ill timed and serve only to raise the patient's anxiety level. In the case of the person interested in improving his adaptation to homosexuality, rather than changing his sexual orientation, the therapist must be sure the group is willing to work toward that end. There is greater social acceptance of homosexuality today than in the past, and this trend should make it easier to find heterosexual groups able to help the homosexual work out his commitment to homosexuality.

Although there is no firm contraindication to placing a homosexual in a mixed group, those pitfalls should be kept in mind. Or the therapist could begin the treatment of the homosexual in a homogeneous group and later, depending on the patient's progress, consider a transfer to a mixed group.

Socioeconomic factors. Patients from different socioeconomic levels can be integrated into the same group with salutary effects. Juxtapositions of different social and economic factors can heighten the psychological awareness of the members involved. If, for example, a patient who has achieved financial success but who is anxious about not having earned a college degree is placed in a group with a patient who is anxious about his limited financial means but who does have a college degree, one can predict the potential value of their interaction, which would have been lost had a college degree been a prerequisite for group membership.

Racial, religious, and ethnic variations in group composition can also be used effectively. When that is done, it is desirable to include more than one member from any given background; two members with similar backgrounds provide mutual support and identification and so enable each to tolerate the minority position. That suggestion applies whether one is working with blacks in a predominately white group or with whites in a predominately black group, for example. And, early on, the therapist should make a statement of policy to the effect that one of the group standards is to respect the differences between members. Such a statement by a leader with prestige is an important prerequisite for modifying attitudes toward minority ethnic groups.

Of particular relevance is group work with the poor conducted by a middle-class therapist. Poor patients may feel the therapist cannot understand their situation, and sometimes that is so. The group setting is particularly advantageous with such patients. In a one-to-one situation the therapist may not be able to distinguish between psychological stress and real stress produced by adverse socioeconomic factors. The mutual support and understanding among group members helps to close that cultural gap and aids the therapist in making distinctions.

Age. Adults can be treated in groups with an extremely broad age range. Patients between 20 and 50 can be effectively integrated into the same group. Age differences aid in the development of parent-child and brother-sister models. Patients have the opportunity to relieve and rectify interpersonal difficulties that may have appeared insurmountable, as illustrated by the following.

A 22-year-old man was included in a group with a man of 49. The older patient had adopted a stern, authoritarian position with his son over the length of his hair and other aspects of his life style that resulted in their complete alienation. The younger patient had not spoken to his father in 3 years because of a similar family situation. Both group members were able to work through feelings toward their own son and father, respectively, by means of their interaction, which was, as expected, stormy at times.

In organizing the adult group, the therapist should be careful not to have only one member representative of the extreme age group. It is likely, for example,

that a woman of 50 in a group of other adults between 20 and 30 would be subject to a variety of transferential mother surrogate reactions on the part of the younger members. Although that situation can be tolerable and therapeutic for all concerned, it may be intolerable and antitherapeutic if all the younger patients had mothers whom they despised.

Both the child and the adolescent are best treated in groups composed of patients in their own age group. Some adolescent patients are quite capable of assimilating the material of the adult group, regardless of content, but they should not be deprived of a constructive peer experience that they might otherwise not have. In addition, adolescents often have severe authority problems, which would increase their anxiety level in an adult group. With peers they are better able to express feelings toward the authority figure represented by the therapist and to find support from their co-patients. That is not to exclude all adolescents from adult groups; but, before placement, the therapist should assess the adolescent's prior peer experience. If that experience was deficient, the patient should not be denied adolescent group placement.

Conclusion

Even when the most careful thought has been given to its organization, each group develops a unique ambiance that cannot be replicated. As each individual person is unique, so is each group. The challenge of proper group organization is for the therapist to be as aware as possible of the potential varieties of interaction that may unfold.

The better the clinician's ability to postulate a hypothesis about the interaction between patient A and patient B and the constructive potential in that interaction, the more assured he can be about his having organized the group properly. The gratification in group work is to be able to help the participants achieve emotional growth and development as a result of their collective interaction.

References

Bernardez, T., and Stein, T. S. Separating the sexes in group therapy: An experiment with men's and women's groups. Int. J. Group Psychother., *29*: 493, 1979.
Bieber, T. B. Combined individual and group psychotherapy. In *Comprehensive Group Psychotherapy,* H. I. Kaplan and B. J. Sadock, editors, p. 153. Wiliams & Wilkins, Baltimore, 1971.
Borriello, J. Acting out character disorders. Am. J. Psychother., *27*: 4, 1973.
Burke, J. D., White, H. J., and Havens, L. L. Which short-term therapy. Arch. Gen. Psychiatry, *36*: 177, 1979.
Cunningham, J., Strassberg, D., and Roback, H. Group psychotherapy for medical patients. Compr. Psychiatry, *19*: 135, 1978.
Grotjahn, M. Learning from dropout patients: A clinical view of patients who discontinued group psychotherapy. Int. J. Group Psychother., *23*: 346, 1973.
Leopold, H. Selection of patients for group psychotherapy. Am. J. Psychother., *11*: 634, 1957.
MacLennan, B. W. The personalities of group leaders: Implications for selection and training. Int. J. Group Psychother., *25*: 177, 1975.
Wong, N. Clinical considerations in group treatment of narcissistic disorders. Int. J. Group Psychother., *29*: 317, 1979.

A.5 General Living Systems Theory and Small Groups

JAMES GRIER MILLER, M.D., Ph.D
JESSIE L. MILLER, M.S.

Introduction

Group psychotherapy, like other psychiatric techniques and like the mental health sciences in general, cannot depend for its conceptual integration on a body of generally accepted and empirically established fact, as many medical specialities can depend upon biochemistry and cellular biology. The necessary basic research findings are not, as yet, available. While Freud outlined a group psychology that is still of fundamental importance to group psychotherapists, he did not develop group therapy to the extent that he did the psychology of the individual person (Anthony, 1972). Some experimental findings from the field of group dynamics have provided important insights into many aspects of group processes, but no generally accepted theory of groups has developed from this work. Currently, it is believed that general living systems theory can provide a useful conceptual integration for the understanding of groups, including therapy groups (Anthony, 1972). While it does not offer a new system of therapy, the theory offers a novel conceptual context in which all of the factors involved in a group situation can be interrelated and brought to bear on the therapeutic process.

Basic Concepts

General living systems theory regards groups as part of the set of living systems that includes all life on earth. The living systems are included in a larger set of concrete (real or veridical) systems, living or nonliving, into which the entire physical universe is organized. General living systems theory is, therefore, the part of general systems theory that is concerned with living systems.

Systems

Not all material things are systems. A system must have parts (or units or components); these parts must have some common properties, be interdependent, and interact within the system. These are the minimum requirements for any sort of system. In addition to these, living systems of all sorts must have certain other attributes that allow them to carry out life processes.

Random arrangements of matter-energy that have no common properties are not interdependent and do not interact in systematic ways. For example, the local landfill or a pile of unrelated spare parts—are not systems.

These requirements also restrict the definition of a group to exclude a collection of people randomly assembled on a corner or in a waiting room, although any such gathering of people can become a system and, therefore, a group, as Freud recognized (Miller, 1978).

The living systems are aggregates of matter-energy—like the nonliving objects around them—but are more complex in structure and organization. They form a hierarchy in which each more advanced level is made up of systems at lower levels. Systems at any given level are more like each other in many ways than like systems at other levels. They have similar components—that is, systems at the level below. Although they may vary in size, they are larger, on the average, than systems at the level below them and smaller than those at the level above. Seven such levels can be readily identified: (1) cells, with nonliving molecular components; (2) organs, composed of cells aggregated into tissues; (3) organisms, composed or organs; (4) groups, with organism and smaller group components; (5) organizations, usually made up of groups, although large ones may have smaller organization components, and small ones may have some individual organisms as components; (6) societies, composed of organizations, groups, and individuals; and (7) supranational systems, with societies and organizations as their components.

The increase in complexity seen in levels of living systems from cells to supranational systems is a result of the evolutionary process by which the higher levels developed from the lower. The more complex, higher level systems are not, however, simply aggregations of lower level systems. A description of systems at a higher level only in terms used for those at the level below is necessarily incomplete. Systems at each level have emergent characteristics (characteristics that are made possible by the new forms of system organization as they develop) not found at the level below. This fact is expressed in the saying that "the whole is greater than the sum of its parts."

The most important way in which living systems differ from nonliving is their ability to combat entropy for varying periods of time—that is, to maintain themselves, to grow and repair damage instead of undergoing steady—if sometimes slow—disintegration from the moment they form, as nonliving systems do.

Living systems do this by taking in, processing, and putting out matter-energy and information. Information is order, formal patterning, or complexity as opposed to randomness and disorder. The shape of an artifact, the nature of the train of pulses along a neuron, the sequence of dots and dashes in Morse code, and the arrangement of words in a message are all information.

Information is carried across system boundaries from the environment and is transmitted within systems on markers. A marker is a form of matter-energy such as electromagnetic waves, neural pulses, sound waves, or molecules of a great variety of chemical substances. The information conveyed by a transmission of markers affects processes of the receiving system. Information flows coordinate all subsystem processes and make it possible for living systems to maintain their relationships with their environments and suprasystems.

Money and other monetary exchanges like checks and credit cards are special forms of information that transmit economic meaning to human systems. Monetary information is carried through social systems on wampum, paper, metal, or electronic markers.

Information is not the same thing as meaning, which is the immediate or delayed effect of information input to a system. An input has meaning if future processes of a system are different than would be predicted if it had not been received. For example, a cell that binds a particular type of molecule will start or stop production of a specific protein after receiving an input, or a man will change his plans after receiving a message.

Structures and process

Systems have two sorts of parts: components, which are structurally discrete, separate organizations of matter-energy; and subsystems, which are single components or groups of components that carry out a particular process in the system. Components may or may not be systems. Subsystems are always systems at a lower level than the reference system.

At any given moment in time, the parts of a system are arranged in space in a specific pattern. This is the system's structure. Possible structural relationships among subsystems and components include their position relative to one another, order along a spatial dimension, direction along a spatial coordinate, their density in the system, the size of the area over which they are distributed, and containment of one subsystem or component by another (Miller, 1978). The number of subsystems and components in the system is an important structural characteristic, since interrelationships among subsystems and components increase as a direct function of their number.

Process is change over time. It includes the ongoing function of a system, with actions, some essentially reversible, succeeding one another from moment to moment. It also includes history, which is less readily

reversed, or irreversible change. Birth, growth, death, and their equivalents at levels above the organism are examples of historical changes. Temporal relationships like duration, temporal order, and pattern in time of processes and spatiotemporal relationships—like pattern of action, direction of action, and entering or leaving containment of one subsystem or component by another—are examples of process relationships (Miller, 1978).

Each subsystem of a living system processes matter-energy and information in varying amounts and proportions to provide an essential process for the system. Every subsystem keeps particular system variables in steady state by means of adjustment processes among its components. The system as a whole maintains system-wide variables in steady state by adjusting the processes of its subsystems.

Each type of system and subsystem has characteristic adjustment processes which start and stop processes or which adjust rates of flow of matter-energy and information within subsystems or system wide. These keep the variables controlled by one or more subsystems from changing beyond a particular range that is normal (although not necessarily desirable) for the particular system. Fluctuations within this range in response to variations in matter-energy and information flows occur in steady states. When historical change occurs, the normal values of some variables change. When one member of a family group goes away to college, for example, the others adjust their rates of interaction to compensate for the loss, and a new steady state is created.

It is important to establish normal values for the variables of a given type of system and to develop measures or indicators for each. This has been accomplished for many physiological and some psychological variables of human organisms. Much less is known about normal structure and function at levels above the organism. Without such established values, it is difficult to know what is pathological in these systems. It is also important to know which adjustment processes are normal for a particular type of system, which indicate extreme values of variables and a lack of optimal steady states.

Many adjustment processes of living systems are activated by feedback from other parts of the system itself or from outside the system. In feedback, a part of the output from a system is returned as input and affects subsequent processes. Negative feedback cancels deviations or corrects errors so steady state is maintained. Positive feedback intensifies an ongoing activity so the feedback information increases the rate or other aspect of the activity. Such change can be useful to the system if it is self-limiting, but it can also be disruptive because it alters variables and changes steady states to produce structural or functional change in the system. When such change is rapid and not limited, it can be explosive. A disagreement that escalates into violence is an example of an explosive outcome of positive feedback.

The use of "structure" in general living systems

theory is quite straightforward, referring always to the distribution of matter-energy in space. For example, the "structure of personality" would not be referred to. "Personality" is a term that describes behavior and is, for that reason, a process term. It includes, among other things, characteristic adjustment processes and interpersonal style. Personality theories are sets of concepts which are usually based on traits—that is, on repeated similar responses of a system, as recognized by an observer. "Id," "ego," and "superego" are thus considered to be hypothetical constructs rather than structures, although the behaviors they refer to, like other behavior, have their correlates in processes of information-processing subsystems—that is, in structures of the central nervous system.

At all levels, all living systems must perform—or have performed for them—certain essential subsystem processes in order to remain alive and to continue the system type or species from generation to generation. Nineteen essential subsystem processes have been identified, although alternative conceptualizations are possible. Two of these subsystems are concerned with both matter-energy and information in significant amounts, while the others process primarily matter-energy or primarily information.

Since each of these processes is essential to the life of the system (with the exception of one, the reproducer, which is essential for the continuation of the species or type of system), a system lacking structure for a particular subsystem process may depend for that process upon the larger system of which it is a part (its suprasystem), upon another system similar to itself, or upon systems at a lower level. Such a system is dispersed. While some deciding processes may be dispersed, a system cannot remain a system if all its decider processes are dispensed to other systems.

Groups as Systems

Human groups, like other systems, exist to carry out some activity or serve some purpose in their suprasystems. Families, work groups, psychotherapy groups, social groups, teams, and committees are all examples of groups, each of which processes matter-energy and information in differing amounts and proportions in order to achieve the purposes for which it was formed.

Living systems, including groups and the individual persons in them, also have internal long-term purposes, which are preferred steady-state values of particular variables. These are derived from the genetic endowment of human organisms, from the purpose for which a group was formed, and from the learned values a system develops through reinforcement or lack of it from within or outside the system.

Living systems also have short-term internal goals which, if attained, will achieve the purposes for which they strive. A pioneer family, for example, may have the purpose of surviving through a long, cold winter. To achieve this end, they work toward the goal of storing firewood and food, making warm clothing, and securing their cabin against the weather. Values, purposes, and goals may, of course, be concerned with information processing, as well as with matter-energy processing. Social, intellectual, philosophical, and moral purposes and goals are related to steady states of variables of information-processing subsystems.

A system's values are not always congruent with the values of its suprasystem, nor do its internal purposes necessarily coincide with its suprasystem's purposes. As a result, it may have divergent goals. When a system and suprasystem conflict in this way, however, the system is often regarded by the suprasystem as deviant or pathological.

Structure

The components of a human group are individual persons or smaller subgroups. When a group is assembled, its members are usually close enough so that face-to-face interaction between any two people is possible. Ordinarily, members can see and hear each other, and each can, at least potentially, communicate directly with any of the others.

The smallest number of members a group can have is, by definition, two. A therapist-patient dyad is, therefore, a group, but their interaction does not constitute group therapy. The lower limit of number in a therapy group is three—two patients and a therapist.

The upper limit of number of group members is indefinite. A childless married couple and a couple with 22 children are both groups. An organized group of protesters may be very large. The next higher level of living system, the organization, is distinguished from a group not by the number of people in it but by the presence of two or more echelons in its decider subsystem. Upper limits are set for particular sorts of groups for convenience or other reasons, as the limits for psychotherapy groups are set by the exigencies of the therapeutic process.

The number of members a group has significantly affects its processes. Triads are unlike dyads, for instance, because each member of a three-person group intervenes between the other two and because, in addition to the dyadic relationship between each member and every other, there is an indirect relationship between each dyad and the third member. A therapist who sees married couples together is well aware of these interrelationships. Research on the effects of the number of members on group processes has produced some conflicting findings but shows that many-membered groups differ significantly in many ways from groups with fewer members. Five appears to be the most satisfactory number for problem-solving groups, since each person in a group of this size can express feelings and actively work for solutions, while still regarding the feelings and needs of the others. With more members, groups necessarily limit the amount of talk-time for each; at the same time, all members must maintain more relationships.

As a result, fewer opinions are expressed, while more information is offered and more suggestions are given. There is less consensus. Showing solidarity increases, and in some studies, more dissatisfaction is expressed. Strains, however, are less in groups with more members, possibly because it is easier for a member to avoid deep involvement. Individual variability is greater in the large-number groups.

The arrangement of group members in space is also significant in the processes of some sorts of groups. Position in the group, for example, affects the probability that a member will exert leadership. The pattern of leadership proved to differ in six-, seven-, and eight-member groups. Seating position also determined what seats were preferred. At a rectangular table, a designated leader usually sat in the end position. Preferred seats in this seating pattern are those next to her or him. In other patterns, preferred seats may be opposite the leader, or no seats may be preferred. Position in a circle in discussion groups affected the probability that one member would directly follow the other in speaking. Those seated opposite the speaker were more likely to speak next. The most usual pattern of seating in therapy groups is a circle, and, of course, it is significant if one or more members of the group sit outside the circle, turn their backs, or choose to retreat under a table.

Subsystems

The subsystems of groups are composed of group members in varying combinations. A subsystem process may be assigned to a single member or to a subgroup, or all the members may participate in it. It is important to note that a subgroup—like a clique or friendship cluster—is a subsystem only if it is the structure for one of the essential subsystem processes.

Since the number of members is often fewer than the number of subsystems whose processes must be performed, each member must ordinarily take part in processes of more than one subsystem. There is no one-to-one relationship between components and subsystems.

Living systems often have inclusions within their boundaries. These are parts of the environment that are enclosed by the system and are not a part of the system's living structure.

Some of these are artifacts used as nonliving components to carry out or assist in a subsystem process. These include the artifacts that replace missing parts of a living system, such as robots in a factory work group, and the materials brought into a system to be used in subsystem processes, like the table and chairs in a group therapy room. Other inclusions have no part in subsystem processes or may be harmful to the system.

Living systems can also be inclusions in other living systems. Other inclusions are a consultant who enters a group to assist in some process, patients in a hospital, the audience in a theater, and refugees in a detention center maintained by a society. Lepers, typhoid carriers in a hospital ward, and a violent psychotic intruding into a therapy group are potentially harmful inclusions.

Groups often lack structure for one or several subsystems and must depend upon the organization of which they are components or upon some other system to provide that process for them. Groups (like rural families or exploring parties) that live or work far from supportive organizations must make provision for more subsystem processes than groups that meet for brief periods. Social clubs, therapy groups, experimental groups, and many work groups often lack significant matter-energy-processing capabilities. Members do not usually live together in these groups. They depend upon other systems—such as their families, a hospital, or other organizations in the community—for many essential processes. These groups primarily process information and usually have most or all of the information-processing subsystems represented in their structure.

A description of the structure and processes of each of the 19 subsystems of groups is presented below. The names given to the subsystems were chosen to be as appropriate as possible for all seven levels of living systems. It is impossible to find general terms that are in ordinary technical use at all levels. Consequently, some subsystem names are used that are not in common use in psychiatry or in the group field. These terms are, however, all ordinary English words and are easily understood by both scientific and professional people.

Indeed, the following discussion seems relevant to both individual and group psychotherapy because it contributes to the holistic understanding of the many sorts of group activity in which people engage. Such understanding is useful whether a group, like a family, is the system being treated by a psychotherapist, or, like a therapy group, is a tool in the therapy of its members.

Subsystems Which Process Both Matter-Energy and Information

REPRODUCER

A reproducer is the subsystem which is capable of giving rise to other groups similar to the one it is in.

Structure

Groups are reproduced by those individual persons, other groups, or higher level systems that produce an implicit or explicit charter for a new group and select, recruit, or bring together its members.

Process

Reproduction of a group is not the same as the biological reproduction of the individual organism members of the group. The object of group reproduction is the formation of new groups. In this process, the charter is analogous to the genetic material of organisms. Both act as templates or blueprints that specify the structure and processes of new systems.

A group's charter can be a formal legal document, such as a marriage contract; it can be the directions given to a newly formed work group by their organization superiors; or it can be an informal agreement among people who intend to form a group or who recognize that they are already a group. The contract that is the basis of the therapeutic relationship in transactional therapy is an agreement between a patient and a therapist that they will enter into a dyadic relationship to work toward a stated goal, such as holding a job for a certain period. It is an explicit charter for that patient-therapist dyad.

The reproducer of groups is often dispersed to another system, such as an organization or large group, or to an individual.

Groups and systems at levels above the group do not reproduce themselves as cells and organisms do, but they accomplish a comparable achievement. They unite components of matter-energy (persons) into an operating system. This is true even of families, since, when parents procreate children, they are not reproducing groups but producing organisms that will be components of the existing family and other groups. The reproducer of families includes the dyad that comes together to mate and any other organizations or people that may be involved in the legal, institutional, or familial processes that are prescribed in all societies when new families are founded.

The reproducer in other sorts of groups may be the organization that establishes a new group or committee, a person who brings a group together for some purpose, a group that divides into two or more smaller groups, or a number of people who choose to come together into a group. The reproducer of a therapy group includes such components as a hospital or other organization that determines that a group will be formed, whoever is responsible for selecting group members, and a therapist who meets with members to establish a group and gets the group started.

BOUNDARY

A boundary is the subsystem at the perimeter of a group that holds together the components of the system, protects them from environmental stresses, and excludes or permits entry to various sorts of matter-energy and information.

The boundaries of groups, as of other living systems, are regions of increased density which can inhibit matter-energy or information transmissions into or out of the system. Since all living systems are open systems, there must be regions in their boundaries through which matter-energy and information can pass.

Structure

Because of the physical separateness and independent mobility of the component organisms, boundaries of groups and systems at higher levels lack the physical continuity that characterizes the membranes, capsules, skins, and exoskeletons that form the boundaries of systems at levels below the group. For the same reason, boundaries of systems above the organism are often capable of rapid change in shape. This dissimilarity between the boundaries of cells, organs, and organisms, on the one hand, and groups and higher levels of social systems, on the other, may hide the essential similarity of their processes. The boundaries of separate groups can also interpenetrate as their members move about. The boundary components that process matter and energy in some groups are different from those that process information.

A distinction must be made between the boundary of a group and the borders of the territory which the group occupies or claims as its own. The territorial borders are geographical limits, like the outer limits of a family's farm, the walls of the room in which a committee meets, or the part of a forest defended by a primitive band. These borders are often marked and protected by artifacts like fences or walls.

The matter-energy boundary of the living group system is composed of some or all group members. Members at the periphery are boundary components. Other boundary components include the group members assigned to maintain buildings, fences, or other artifacts at the territorial border; those acting as guards or door-keepers; and those who determine what matter-energy can cross the boundary into or out of the system.

The information boundary subsystem of a group includes all group members so long as they are able to communicate with one another or are coordinated by stored information. If communication is totally disrupted and no coordinating information has been stored, the information boundary disappears, and, until it can be restored, group members must act separately as individual organism systems. Special boundary components are those persons who determine what information may enter or leave the system.

Boundary processes of several kinds may be dispersed to other systems, most commonly to organizations. The building and room in which a group meets are often maintained by an organization, such as a hospital or office building or apartment management. Home owners are more and more commonly protected by security systems operated by organizations that install and respond to alarm signals. Police and fire departments also have boundary maintenance and protective functions for groups in the community.

Divergence can be found among system theorists in their use of the boundary concept as it relates to the boundaries of the organism members of groups. In the theory being presented here, a boundary is always a continuous or discontinuous material structure which carries out processes appropriate to the level of living system in which it is found. An organism's boundary is its skin or other outer covering. The boundaries of the organ subsystems of organisms are the membranes that surround organ components, like the liver or stomach, as well as the less readily identifiable structural separations between functional parts of nervous systems.

In the system being presented here, therefore, there is no talk of the "boundary of the self." Here, the self is regarded as an abstracted construct used to represent a set of subjective experiences and observable verbal and other behaviors, rather than as a separate entity represented by a specific set of neural components.

For similar reasons, introjection and projection are conceptualized not as transactions at the boundary of the self but, rather, as adjustment processes that take place within and among information-processing subsystems within the endocrine and nervous systems, although the verbal or behavioral evidence of such processes is indeed output over the organism's boundary.

Process

Boundaries carry out three separate but related processes: (1) they are barriers to flows of matter-energy (including people) and information into and out of systems; (2) they filter certain sorts of matter-energy and information, allowing some kinds to cross into or out of the system but not others; and (3) they maintain a steady-state differential between the interior of the system and its environment, making it more likely that a given sort of matter-energy or information will be on one side of the boundary or the other.

In general, inputs not needed or wanted by the system, harmful or excessive inputs, or inputs of inappropriate size, shape, chemical structure, or information content are excluded from entering, while their opposites are admitted. Some sorts of matter-energy and information are retained inside the system and prevented from passing the boundary into the environment.

The rooms or buildings that enclose a group's territory act as barriers to unwanted matter-energy and information and protect the group from harmful inputs. Doors are open only to people a group wants inside. Windows are closed against rain and cold air.

Two sorts of information can flow across group boundaries. The first consists of patterned inputs carried in speech, writing, and other sorts of communications. The second is monetary information. Money is information because a marker of metal or paper carries the message that it can be exchanged for a certain value in goods, services, or other money, depending on current prices.

Flows of certain sorts of communication information into or out of the system are restricted by many sorts of groups. Families often prevent magazines and television shows they consider unsuitable from entering the home. Therapy groups commonly agree that group discussions will not be reported outside the group. Some group therapists limit the sorts of information that members can bring into the group. Early childhood memories are usually acceptable inputs from a group member, but some therapists restrict the subject matter of the group to the immediate group situation, excluding past history and experiences of group members.

The nature of the information boundaries of groups allows them to remain systems even when members are not face to face. A group of soldiers in the field remains coordinated and within the group information boundary by the use of radio. A child away at school can participate in family group processes and thus remain within the group, using long-distance telephone. Such communication channels need not be open at all times, but they must be available. Families that are separated by war or disaster and cannot find each other lose their system boundaries. Members become parts of other groups or live separately.

Coordination by stored information can maintain a group's information boundary so that a group that meets for a limited time is able to remain a system between meetings. Members store information about the place and time of the next meeting, come together as planned, and continue the group process, perhaps having carried out agreed-upon activities in the meanwhile.

Subsystems Which Process Matter-Energy

INGESTOR

An ingestor is the subsystem which brings matter-energy across the group boundary from the environment.

Structure

The subgroups or single members that bring into a group whatever matter and energy are needed for its processes are ingestor components. Ingestor components include members of families who shop for the things required for the family and its home or who harvest home gardens, and refreshment committees of social clubs and members of work groups who bring in materials needed for a job. New members of groups, except members born to a family, are matter-energy inputs. They are brought in by ingestor components who invite or recruit them, as, for example, in the case of a therapist who adds a patient to an existing group.

No components for this subsystem are regularly parts of some sorts of groups, either because they process information and meet for short sessions or because the process is dispersed to another system. Groups that meet in buildings maintained by an organization, for example, receive heat, cool air, and illumination as services provided by that organization. Therapy groups with fixed membership need make no provisions for ingesting, the exception being those whose marathon sessions extend for many hours or even for several days.

Process

Division of the labor of the ingesting process according to sex has been traditional in families and social groups and is often carried over into other sorts of groups as well. However, these traditional assignments can no longer be taken for granted. It is important to observe how families in treatment carry out this essential ingesting process.

DISTRIBUTOR

A distributor is the subsystem which carries input from outside the group or input from its subsystems around the group to each member.

Structure

A subgroup or single member may be the component responsible for assuring that matter-energy of various sorts is appropriately distributed to group members in accordance with their needs and the subsystem processes they perform. Components of this subsystem are often lacking in therapy groups.

Process

In most families, the parents are responsible for distribution among family members of the matter-energy that is both appropriate for them and necessary for their health and comfort. In some, however, the process of food distribution is so informal that even very young children take what they want from cupboards or refrigerators, whether or not such food is appropriate.

Some work groups depend upon an artifact, e.g., an assembly line, for distribution of material to members of the group. This subsystem is often made up of all group members who take the materials they need from a supply.

CONVERTER

A converter is the subsystem which changes certain inputs to the group into forms more useful for the special processes of that particular group.

Structure

Families ordinarily have this subsystem. Work groups that prepare materials for use in making a product do also, but converter structure is frequently trivial or lacking in social groups, therapy groups, or others which process information.

All members of families can be converter components except the very young and the helpless. Choppers of wood, grinders of corn, and seamstresses who cut cloth for clothing are all components. Similar components can be found in many work groups.

The converter of groups is often dispersed to organizations that provide materials ready for processing. Many modern families, for example, buy their meat from organizations in the form of neatly packaged chicken pieces or hamburger already ground, instead of having to butcher animals themselves.

PRODUCER

A producer is the subsystem which forms stable associations that endure for significant periods among matter-energy inputs to the group or outputs from its converter. The material synthesized is for growth, damage repair, or replacement of components of the system, or for providing energy for moving or constituting the group's outputs of products or information markers to its suprasystem.

Structure

This subsystem is always present in families, but some other sorts of groups disperse the producer to other systems. Parents who, by procreating, add new members to the family group are members of this subsystem, since they produce basic components that make up the system. The process of production is reproduction at the organism level. Family members who cook, build furniture or other artifacts, or create art objects for the home are components of a different sort. Any family member who takes care of or nurses other members is a producer component because the people who receive care participate more fully in the systems process.

Many producing processes are upwardly dispersed to organizations. This is true of much health care of group members.

Process

Care of the physical health of group members is a producing process, but what about mental health, which is the concern of group psychotherapy? Is the therapist a producer component of the therapy group?

Psychotherapy is directed toward altering patients' thought processes and behavior by what is fundamentally a learning or relearning process. Learning is a change in the associator, an information-processing subsystem that makes associations among items of information. Group psychotherapists are, therefore, a part of the associator, rather than the producer, subsystem of the group.

If drugs are used as adjuncts to therapy, associations take place at the cellular level between neurons and molecules of the drug. The abundant research on stress and on psychosomatic medicine shows that changes in matter-energy processes can occur with emotional disturbance and that some of these can be reversed by psychotherapy. It is reasonable, then, to consider a psychotherapist a producer component, as well as an associator component of the therapy group. He is also a producer component of one or more organizations, since he is a member of the health delivery systems of the city in which he practices and the state which licenses him.

MATTER-ENERGY STORAGE

Matter-energy storage is the subsystem which retains in the group, for different periods of time, deposits of various sorts of matter-energy.

Structure

Components of this subsystem are the members of subgroups responsible for keeping supplies of materials and making them available when needed. This subsystem is usually found in familes, which keep supplies of clothing, food, and many other sorts of things on hand. It is of particular importance to groups that must be self-sufficient for some reason, like parties of explorers, space travelers, or families on remote farms. Groups that meet for short periods to process information may need no components for this subsystem, since the members may be supplied by other groups or organizations. In some groups, the subsystem is limited to someone who keeps supplies of such things as writing materials, coffee, or soft drinks for the group.

Many groups disperse important parts of this subsystem upward to their suprasystem organizations, which store materials for the group's processes, or to organizations like shops and other businesses, which make long-term storage of larger quantities unnecessary by keeping stocks of matter-energy available. The subsystem is often dispersed to individual members who bring their own supplies of needed materials.

Process

The process of storing matter-energy by groups and other living systems involves three separate activities: (1) putting into storage; (2) maintaining in storage over time; and (3) retrieving from storage.

EXTRUDER

An extruder is the subsystem which transmits matter-energy out of the group in the forms of products or wastes.

Structure

A group member who carries waste materials out of a group's meeting place to a trash can, members of a group who decide to terminate the membership of one or more people in it, a therapist who eliminates a patient from a group because that patient no longer needs treatment (in which case the patient is a group product) or because the patient is unable to benefit from therapy, a member who takes a group's product to market, and even a member who opens the window to let cigarette smoke out, are all components of this subsystem.

The extruder is often upwardly dispersed to an organization whose employees pick up the waste materials for a work group, clear away a seminar's discarded paper, or remove a group's product from the work area.

Process

Removal of products and wastes from a group's territory is either continuous, as it is when finished products are moved away from a work group on an assembly line, or episodic, if it takes place at regular intervals or only when a group finds it necessary.

An accumulation of products or wastes in a group's territory can impede group processes. The rate of removal of such substances must be related to the rate at which they accumulate. If, for example, carbon dioxide expired by group members cannot be replaced by fresh air at a sufficient rate, the group's efficiency declines in direct relationship to the severity of the oxygen lack.

MOTOR

A motor is the subsystem which moves the group or parts of it in relationship to part or all of its environment or moves components of its environment in relation to each other.

Structure

Systems at the group level and above, composed as they are of independently mobile separate systems, lack the sort of motor subsystems found in systems whose components are held together within skins or membranes. Movement of a group is dispersed to the separate members, each of whom uses her or his own motor subsystem, or the group moves with the use of artifacts like station wagons, buses, or elevators. Two or more members often work together to move something that impedes a group's progress, like a large rock or a dead tree from a family's yard.

Process

Group movement takes place when the whole group moves from place to place, when members move in relationship to one another in the group's activities, or when artifacts or environmental objects are moved by group action.

Many sorts of groups perform complex movements which require a high degree of coordination among components. This is true of basketball teams, dancers, and work groups of many sorts. Often, two or more group members combine their individual motor subsystems to do work that a single member could not do alone, like pushing a car out of a snowbank. There are, of course, groups in which movement plays little or no part in the system activities.

SUPPORTER

A supporter is the subsystem which maintains the proper spatial relationships among members of the group so that they can interact without weighting each other down or crowding each other.

Structure

Living systems at the level of the group and above do not have internal structural supporters. They make use of buildings, furniture, or specialized apparatus to support their human components in the spatial relationships conducive to the group's processes. In some groups, members support other members, like a parent holding an infant to feed it, or acrobats forming living pyramids.

Process

The subsystem provides firm or rigid support so there is little action to describe.

Subsystems Which Process Information

INPUT TRANSDUCER

An input transducer is the sensory subsystem which brings markers bearing information into the group, changing them to other matter-energy forms suitable for transmission within it.

A transducer brings the markers on which information is carried into the system and changes them while retaining essential characteristics of the signal being transmitted. An organism's eyes, for example, transduce information from a marker of visible light to neural pulses that can be transmitted over the optic nerve to the central nervous system. A radio transduces information from electromagnetic waves to light and sound waves.

Structure

The components of input transducers at this level are those group members who bring information into the group either directly from the environment or from their own memories of past input. Single members or subgroups, like committees, form this subsystem. Each person is an input-output system who receives, processes, and outputs information to a group. Multiple transductions may take place within an organism system, but the final transduction is from neural pulses to some form of movement which transmits signals that can be perceived by other group members. Speech, written reports, gestures, and body language are examples.

All members of therapy groups are ordinarily parts of this subsystem. Artifacts like radios, television sets, and telephones are used in some sorts of groups to augment the human transducers.

Process

The input transducers of living systems can be described in terms used for mechanical and electromagnetic transducers, although no great degree of precision of description has yet been achieved at levels above the organism. For example, each transducer component has characteristic processing times, distortions, and channel capacities.

Processing times are very long for stored information when, for example, early childhood memories are recalled and recounted to a group. Distortions are caused by malfunction of an organism's eyes, other input transducer components, or the characteristics of a person's internal processing of information. Mistakes, personal bias, psychoneurosis, and lies are some of the causes of distortions. Channel capacity is the maximum amount of information a component (a channel) can process in a given time. The channel capacity of a group input transducer can be increased for some sorts of transductions by having more than one member report the same event and combining all their reports.

INTERNAL TRANSDUCERS

An internal transducer is the sensory subsystem which receives, from subsystems or components within the group, markers bearing information about significant alterations in these subsystems or components, and which changes them to other matter-energy forms of a sort which can be transmitted within it.

Structure

Informal groups and groups with few members usually include all members in this subsystem. Larger or more formal groups sometimes delegate certain members to perform this subsystem process. A committee to determine the attitudes of members and report them to the group is an example.

Communications transduced by this subsystem may be about tasks carried out by group members or feelings and attitudes of members. The transductions are from sensory inputs to the organisms that constitute the subsystem to neural codes to muscular outputs, just as in the input transducer. Information is drawn from experience and from memories and is subject to processing time constraints, distortions, and limited channel capacity in the same way.

The two sorts of communications transduced by the internal transducer are called "work" and "emotionality" by Thelen (1954), "internal" and "external" systems of the group by Homans (1950), and "task-related" or "socioemotional" acts by Bales (1950).

Some groups plan time for discussing the group process, criticizing the group's work, and expressing feelings and attitudes. In others, the process is informal or may take place only when members become disturbed.

CHANNEL AND NET

A channel and net is the subsystem composed of a single route in physical space or multiple interconnected routes, by which markers bearing information are transmitted to all parts of the group.

Structure

Communication takes place when a message passes from a transmitter to a receiver over a channel. Channels include the air through which sound waves and electromagnetic energy are propagated, telephone wire, physical contact, or other media. All the channels that connect components of a system form a net which, in the case of systems like a human organism or a large organization, can be exceedingly complex. Many channels are two-way, but some are one-way only. Every member of a group is, at least occasionally, connected into the net by a minimum of one two-way channel, or one on which he can send and another one on which he can receive messages.

Auditory and visual channels are most commonly used in assembled groups, although some work groups use communications equipment like walkie-talkies or conference telephones. Bodily contact is important as a form of communication among members of some families. When groups have dispersed, members may communicate over suprasystem channels, such as telephones.

The structure of group communication nets—that is, who communicates with whom—can vary greatly, even in groups with the same number of members and similar processes. If all members are connected by open two-way channels, the net is totally connected. Nets can be constrained in various ways so that certain channels are closed. A group in which all communication must flow to or from a particular person is an example.

Process

The structure of the communication net of a group exerts a major influence upon its processes. Experiments with artificially constrained group nets have shown a totally connected group, in which anyone can talk to anyone else, to be satisfying to its members. But many such groups found it necessary to develop their own constraints in order to get their tasks done. Parliamentary rules in a board meeting, or agreement to allow each member of a group to speak in turn, are net constraints imposed for the sake of orderly process in some groups.

A form of constraint that has been used in some therapy groups requires all communications to be addressed to the therapist. More commonly, however, members may speak to the group as a whole or to any other member, as well as to the therapist.

As members of a group interact, its communication net develops its own characteristics. Some channels are used frequently, others rarely. Subgroups of people who communicate with each other to the exclusion of others may form, often with one member as spokesman for the whole group. Cliques that exclude other members of a group from participating in discussions or other critical processes are causes of dissatisfaction and disruption in some groups.

DECODER

A decoder is the subsystem which alters the code of information into a private code that can be used internally by the group.

A code is an ensemble of markers that convey meaning to a living system. This is a very broad definition that covers, in addition to the symbolic codes usually referred to in information theory, the sort of coding that a chemical molecule must have if it is to act as a signal in cellular processes, and the codes used by neurons, pattern recognition, and perception of the environment by organisms.

It is useful to distinguish three types of codes, increasing in complexity, which are used in encoding and decoding by living systems: (1) An alpha code is one in which the ensemble of markers is composed of different patterns or spatial arrangements of physical artifacts, like door keys, chemical molecules, or some sorts of environmental events. Hormones are complex organic molecules which are made up of various groupings of carbon, hydrogen, and other atoms. The message a hormone carries is coded in the spatial arrangement of its atomic components. It signals cells to start, stop, or alter the rate of specific processes. Perceptual events are decoded similarly as "a square" or "a funnel cloud" because of their physical characteristics such as shape, color, or type of movement. (2) A beta code is based on variations of process, such as different temporal patterns of signals or different patterns of intensity of signals. Beta codes are used in nervous systems of animals and human beings. Some perceptual coding is beta-coded. A sound increasing in intensity is frequently decoded as approaching. (3) A gamma code is an ensemble of symbols taken from a language of some sort, such as hand signals, words, mathematical symbols, or the dots and dashes of Morse code.

Human groups ordinarily use gamma codes in communication with other systems. Almost any repeatable sequence of acts, arrangements of matter-energy, marks on stone or paper, or pulses of energy can be given symbolic meaning by agreement between senders and receivers. When a baseball manager scratches his nose, it can mean "bunt" to a batter; a red light means "stop"; a pile of rocks marks a path; and a distinctive sign warns of atomic energy in use. Both Chinese ideographs and Western alphabets function efficiently to express ideas.

Structure

All group members are ordinarily part of this subsystem because they individually decode information input to the group. Specialized components are translators, interpreters, and members who explain the meaning of a communication or event to the others.

Many sorts of groups have private codes that convey meaning to them but are not understood by people outside the particular group or particular type of group. Families frequently use special words and descriptive terms. Work groups use technical terms and slang not commonly understood by other members of the organization which is their suprasystem. Therapy groups use specialized terms that members learn and use within the group. "Games," "parent," "child," "script," and many others have specialized meanings in transactional therapy, just as the terminology of psychoanalysis does in psychoanalytic groups.

Process

An interpreter who makes it possible for a person who speaks a foreign language to take part in the conversation of a social group is decoding the foreign language for the benefit of the group. A member of a work group who can read the output from a computer and explain it to the other members is also decoding.

One of the major activities of therapeutic groups is interpreting (decoding) behavior or statements of patients. The therapist is the only one who does this in some sorts of groups, but in others, members may offer interpretations of their own and others' output.

Decoding patients' gamma-coded output is only a part of the decoding that goes on in therapy. Body language, which is decoded in all sorts of interpersonal situations, is of particular importance when a patient is unable to put his feelings in words or his behavior contradicts his statements. When a trembling patient says, "I'm not afraid," group members decode both words and behavior and may decide that he is afraid.

Behavior—like absence from group sessions, selection of a particular chair, or sitting at some distance from other members—can also be decoded in therapy. Some therapists also decode a patient's dreams or offer alternative explanations of past events.

ASSOCIATOR

An associator is the subsystem which carries out the first stage of the learning process, forming enduring associations among items of information in the group.

Structure

At the levels of the group and above, the association of items of information must be done by one or more organism components, since learning (associating plus storing in memory) takes place within the nervous systems of members. Ordinarily, all members of groups are associator components, but, for group learning to take place, it is not necessary for every group member to make all associations. Individual members and subgroups can be specialized components of this subsystem.

Process

Group learning, like individual learning, is made evident by changed behavior. If one member makes a critical association and directs the others in such a way that the behavior of the group is altered, or if each member makes the association separately, with the same result, group learning has occurred.

Neither organisms nor groups learn without feedback in the form of knowledge of results or error correction. Group learning, like organism learning, is facilitated by reward and inhibited by punishment, either of which can come from within the group or from the suprasystem and environment.

Groups that interact over time associate words and ideas and form concepts that establish the code, or private language, used within the group. Each group member also learns his part in the group processes and the role he will play in group interactions. These individual associations result in the characteristic interaction patterns of the group. Successful groups learn behaviors that facilitate group processes, produce high morale, and make the group attractive to its members. Interactions that result in poor performance, dissension, dissatisfaction, low morale, and group termination also occur. Altering the pattern of learned pathological interpersonal interactions is a common goal of family therapy.

Dance groups, marching bands, gymnasts, and many sorts of work groups, among others, learn coordinated skills, such as patterns of movement or a flow of work that is most efficient for that group. A member of a string quartet hears his own instrument and also the other three. A distinctive group sound and style is produced as a result of these feedbacks which blend each individual performance into a group output.

Research on group learning has used simplified situations such as learning lists of nonsense syllables, but some of the results may apply to group learning of other sorts. With multiple nervous systems working together, each member needs to process less information, and each has different prior experience to contribute. Members correct one another's errors, so that groups have more opportunity to profit from error feedback. Also, information input to the group may receive more attention when several people are receiving it.

MEMORY

A memory is the subsystem which carries out the second stage of the learning process, storing various sorts of information in the group for different periods of time.

Structure

This subsystem usually includes all group members, each of whom stores information in his own nervous system. In addition, specialized components also exist. Secretaries and people with specialized training are examples.

Artifacts are important in group memory. Correspondence files, financial records, minutes of previous meetings, photographs, and tape recordings are all used in preserving information in groups. This subsystem may store money for a group, or another system, like a bank, may do it.

Process

Information storage, or memory, involves four separate processes: (1) reading information into storage; (2) maintaining it in storage; (3) losing or altering it during storage; and (4) retrieving it from storage.

Storage in individual human memories is, of course, the fundamental form of group information storage. Crucial aspects of the culture of preliterate groups—such as language, songs, dances, art forms, religion, and history—are stored only in this way. Each generation passes this information to the next. In these groups, certain members—older people, people who are especially talented, or people who are deemed worthy of being the repositories of important secrets—play an important role in this essential function.

All storage in human memory is subject to loss from storage as people forget. It is also subject to distortions that result from imperfect understanding, individual intrapsychic processes, or deliberate alteration. It may also not be immediately retrievable, especially if it happened long ago or seemed unimportant when it happened. If several group members store information, their memories can be compared to produce a more accurate memory.

Some group therapists use human recorders, who are not members of the group, to observe and describe behavior and write an account of the verbal exchanges. Others use tape recorders. If these records are used in later activities, they are parts of the group memory.

DECIDER

A decider is the executive subsystem which receives information inputs from all other subsystems and transmits to them information outputs that control the entire group.

Structure

The decider components of groups are those individual members or subgroups who establish the purposes and goals of the group, make operating rules, guide and control group processes, make choices among available alternatives, select means of implementation, and designate which components will implement each decision.

Deciders of groups vary in their procedures, from an extreme authoritarianism, in which a leader or boss makes all the decisions, to complete democracy, in which all members vote on every issue. It is not unusual for decider processes to vary within a single group from one mode of decision to another. A democratic structure, in which all members participate equally, may be considered suitable for some decisions, while some may be made by a committee, and still others by the leader or president.

Decider structure of certain groups is prescribed by the suprasystem. This is true of work groups in which the boss is expected to make all decisions on work-related issues. (For example, the group can decide democratically where to go for lunch.) In such groups, the boss is often part of a complicated echelon structure in the suprasystem organization which makes the decisions through its decider components.

The decider structure of families is culturally determined in societies, although some families deviate from cultural norms.

Group therapists are ordinarily decider components, particularly in initial sessions. Each method of group psychotherapy prescribes its characteristic group decider structure, which is somewhere on a continuum from being extremely authoritarian to being extremely democratic.

Leaders emerge in the course of interaction in certain groups which have no prescribed decider structure. Some are single-issue leaders, but some become authoritarian deciders with the concurrence of other members. Others influence the democratic process by attracting followers and getting their ideas accepted.

Process

Deciding in groups, as in living systems at other levels, appears to follow four stages: (1) establishing purposes and goals; (2) analysis; (3) synthesis; and (4) implementation.

Establishing purposes and goals. The purposes and long-term goals of groups are prescribed by the suprasystem or by the group itself. A psychiatric unit determines that group psychotherapy will be practiced by its staff, with the long-term goals of increasing the number of patients who can receive psychotherapy, improving their psychological health, and providing experience for resident physicians. A club forms with the purpose of benefiting the community and the goal of raising $10,000 annually for charity.

Within these constraints, groups set shorter-term or more specific goals from time to time, as necessary. Each group member also has individual goals, conscious or not. It is possible that some of these individual goals are at variance with group goals. The contract in transactional group psychotherapy is an explicit statement of a goal upon which therapist and patient agree. A major goal of therapeutic groups is to help members achieve their individual goals of improved comfort and function by means of the group interactions.

The purposes and goals of a group represent the hierarchy of values of the group, whether explicit or implicit. The social club that raises money for charity instead of choosing some other activity is expressing a value and so is a work group that sets limits on the daily production of any member. When values conflict, the hierarchy or order of importance of values is reflected in the choice.

Analysis. In this stage of decision making, a group decider confronts a situation or problem, evaluates what sort of adjustment processes are needed to improve or solve it, and discovers what alternatives are available. These may present a binary choice between clear-cut alternatives or may involve the study of many variables. The outcome of alternative choices cannot always be foreseen.

This stage appears in a therapeutic group when a member asks for help in a life situation. Proposed solutions will reflect group and individual values and goals. If the problem is a marital one, values relating to the permanence of the marital bond, the roles of the sexes, and the importance of children are likely to surface.

Each proposed solution carries its own costs in money, time, and personal inconvenience, discomfort, or unhappiness. Each has some probability, high or low, of solving or ameliorating the problem.

Synthesis. This stage involves the actual determination of a strategy for action, allocation of matter-energy or information, or agreement upon a judgment. From the alternatives offered, the decider selects one. Some receive scant consideration, since they appear too costly or unlikely to work. At this stage, influence processes and power relationships among members of a multiple-member decider come into play. An objectively less desirable alternative that is backed by a powerful, influential person often has a better chance than the excellent solution proposed by a weak or unpopular one. Group decisions are not guaranteed to be optimal.

The research on group influence processes is extensive. Male sex, high status, prestige, good social skills, and a greater amount of activity in the group all contribute to a member's being able to influence group decisions in a simulated jury or a real legislative committee.

Implementing. In this stage, if action is to be taken, the group decides how and by which member or members the decision will be carried out.

There is little useful research in the way groups typically implement their decisions, but studies have been made of the effectiveness of group decisions (Miller, 1978). Group productivity was taken as a measure of effectiveness. Productivity was found to increase when a decision was urgently needed, when the group believed that it had sufficient power to implement its decision, when communication among members was adequate, when procedure was orderly, and when all group members felt free to participate. Productivity diminished when members expressed more self-oriented needs. Groups with formal procedures and designated leaders were no more nor less productive than less formal groups.

ENCODER

An encoder is the subsystem which alters the code of information input from a private code used internally by the group into a public code which can be interpreted by other groups in its environment.

Structure

Any member or subgroup that expresses the meaning a group wishes to convey in language suitable for communication outside the system is an encoder component. Communications can be encoded by the whole group working together or by designated members. Clubs often have secretaries who encode messages for them. A family member who writes a letter for the family or who can encode family business into a language not used within the family, like a foreign language or technical terms, is an encoder.

A social worker who fills out forms for a family and a consultant who composes advertising material for a board of directors are dispersed encoder components.

Process

The encoder subsystem, like the decoder, is concerned with meaning. Groups that prepare information for use in the suprasystem must encode their information outputs for transmission into the suprasystem channel and net, changing from one natural language to another or from informal expressions or technical jargon to formal language, or simply agreeing upon what they want to say and putting it into symbolic form. One sort of group uses artistic calligraphy on fine paper; another uses a rude gesture.

Therapy groups have little need to encode messages to other systems. If the need arises, the therapist or another member is delegated to encode the message.

OUTPUT TRANSDUCER

An output transducer is the subsystem which puts out markers bearing information from the group, changing markers within the group into other matter-energy forms that can be transmitted over channels in the group's environment.

Structure

The foreman of a jury who communicates the group's decision to the court, a spokesman for a group of prisoners, and a secretary who transmits phone messages from a group, are all components of this subsystem. The same member or subgroup that acted as encoder is often also the output transducer. This subsystem can be dispersed to another system, such as a messenger who delivers a singing telegram or a spokesman for a labor union who submits a work group's grievances to its employer.

Telephones, telegraph machines, and other artifacts are used in this subsystem.

Process

As in input and internal transducing, one or more human nervous systems transduce information from one marker to another for output from groups. Information from the group encoder is input to the person or subgroup doing the transducing, processed, and output to the suprasystem on a suitable marker. The member or subgroup doing the transducing, types and mails a letter, speaks over a telephone, uses semaphore signals, spells out a team's name on the gym floor, or transmits a signal in some other form into suprasystem channels.

General Living Systems Analysis of Groups

A systems analysis of a group or other living system begins with a review of the structure and processes of each of its subsystems, similar to the systematic procedure used by a physician in a physical examination, and continues with a study of the adjustment processes by which system wide steady states are maintained.

Both the physical examination and the subsystem review are intended to determine whether the variables controlled by each subsystem are within ranges considered normal for the type of system and for the particular system being reviewed. With specific pathological processes identified, the system wide effects of the pathology on structure and process can be understood.

Although the sort of precise tests and measurements available to an examining physician have not been developed for the group level, a group can be compared with other groups of the same sort in similar environments to determine to what extent it deviates from accepted norms. Within any society, for example, laws and customs determine what family structure and processes are typical. A family is considered pathological if it deviates too greatly from these cultural norms. Emotional disturbances of family members, criminal behavior, marital difficulties, and poor relationships to other systems in the environment, such as neighboring families and schools, are often regarded as symptoms of pathology.

No norms exist for therapy groups, but each group therapist learns what sort of processes benefit patients and what sort do not. The critical subsystem processes in these groups are those of the information-processing subsystems. Analysis of these can show when and where intervention in the group process by the psychiatrist would be useful.

Each type of group has characteristic adjustment processes that serve to keep its internal variables and its relationships in the suprasystem and environment in steady state. A work group must satisfy the demands of the organization that employs it and, to that end, must have efficient internal processes that allow the members reasonable satisfaction with their jobs. If the work load is suddenly increased, the group adjusts its rate of processing or in some other way changes its processes to get the job done.

The term "steady state" does not imply a value judgment. An organism can be in a steady state of good health or of chronic illness. A group, similarly, can maintain healthy or pathological steady states. Both normal and pathologial steady states are maintained by adjustment processes.

Adjustment processes reflect a system's values and always carry a price tag. A system that is aware of its options and their probable costs selects the least costly adjustment process available to it. A married couple that valued community opinion and the permanence of marriage, for example, exchanged not a word for several years, a costly adjustment process that made it possible to avoid terminating the marriage.

The most important adjustment processes of therapy groups are made to the meanings conveyed by information flows among group members. Interpersonal communication in these groups allows members to become aware of their own and others' personal dynamics and serves as a tool for effecting change in members' understanding of their own and others' thoughts, feelings, and behavior. If the group process is successful, these insights can be carried over to other groups of which therapy group members are components, such as their families, work groups, and social groups.

Both cognitive and emotional communication among group members alter group adjustment processes. Group members experience intense emotions and learn new modes of interaction as they become aware, through feedback, of others' responses to their own communications, gain insight into their own past experiences and their feelings about themselves, and learn to appreciate the feelings of others.

The group therapist has a special role in the group, particularly in early sessions, since he or she is expected to monitor the group process in such a way that group and personal changes occur. The therapist supports the group in placing limits on certain sorts of behavior; provides factual information, interpretive feedback, and emotional support where necessary; and helps to guide the interactions among members in therapeutic directions. If the group indulges in social conversation, avoiding the less comfortable work they need to do, the therapist must get them back to useful interactions. If they are like a group of good children, depending upon the therapist as an adult, they must learn that is what they are doing. As the group learns, these responsibilities of the therapist may diminish in importance.

Systems Analysis of a Family

A subsystem review based on the theoretical approach presented here was used by members of a clinical seminar conducted by Shafii to analyze a family being treated by staff members. This analysis was used to decide the direction of further treatment. The patient was Jeff S., an adolescent boy under treatment for anorexia nervosa. Both the psychiatrist who was treating him and the social worker who worked with the family were among the participants. Two levels of living systems were of concern in this case: the patient, an organism; and the family, a group. Subsystem reviews were made of both systems.

ORGANISM LEVEL

The physical and neurological examinations of the patient disclosed no structural abnormalities in any subsystem. On admission, however, his heart action was abnormal, and he had not moved his bowels or urinated for an excessively long time. These signs and symptoms disappeared when he began to eat and drink. These distributor and excretor malfunctions, as well as his failure to ingest food or permit storage of matter-energy in the form of fat in his body, were considered secondary to pathological information processing. Other findings in information-processing subsystems were as follows.

Input transducer

Jeff was extremely sensitive to noise, a symptom frequently observed in starving people. Ordinarily, however, the oversensitivity disappears when the matter-energy lacks are corrected. In this patient, it continued after his physical problems had been corrected.

Internal transducer

The patient said he was not hungry or thirsty. He wore several layers of heavy clothing throughout the year and complained of being cold in the steamy summer when others were uncomfortably hot. The conference questioned whether his problem was in the internal transducer or other information-processing subsystems. It appeared probable that the input transducer components that report skin temperature and the internal transducer components that respond to blood temperature and composition were functioning normally, but that Jeff's reported lack of hunger and thirst and his atypical response to what others perceived as excessive heat were evidences of pathological decoder or decider processes. It was suggested that adaptation had occurred in the internal transducers so that they no longer responded to a drop in blood sugar level that would normally have excited them. Such adaptation occurs in normal people who often report less discomfort from hunger after the first few days of a fast. Adaptation may well have been involved also in his unusual response to temperature.

Channel and net

The channel and net of human organisms and of animals with similar nervous systems consists of neural tracts that transmit information throughout the body, as well as the blood vascular system that carries chemically coded information from its source to target organs. No abnormality was found in Jeff's channel and net subsystem.

Decoder

Perception of the environment and of internal states of the system is a decoder process. The abnormal body image of patients with anorexia nervosa is a result of abnormal decoding of information. It was considered possible by conference members that Jeff decoded temperature information aberrantly, with the result that what other people perceived as excessive heat was not experienced in that way by Jeff. They could not decide whether internal transductions of hunger and thirst were transmitted and decoded normally, or whether his report that he was neither hungry nor thirsty was accurate. Either the denial that could result in an inaccurate report of his perceptions or repression that

would keep the sensations from reaching consciousness would be decider rather than decoder processes.

Associator

Jeff was estimated to be somewhat above average in his ability to learn. His A and B grades in school were considered to be the result of overachievement. Psychological tests given in the hospital revealed some difficulty with abstract thinking.

Memory

The patient's memory was excellent.

Decider

No emancipation was permitted by Jeff's authoritarian father, who exercised complete control over all aspects of the lives of his wife and children. Jeff's goals were set for him. He was motivated by reward and punishment, rather than by the sort of internal motivation appropriate for a boy of 16. Money was the usual reward. His father's displeasure, which he showed by yelling, was punishment. There was not a consistent reward system or assignment of responsibilities to Jeff and his siblings.

Neither Jeff nor his family appeared to consider what might be good for him. His behavior was directed toward maintenance of an unthreatening family steady state, rather than toward the desirable steady states of his own physiological and psychological variables.

The unusual direct reward-and-punishment system imposed by Jeff's family produced behavior considered obsessional by the hospital staff. His parents accepted the fact that he did no work without payment. He would continue drawing pictures or writing indefinitely so long as his parents paid for his productions. On the ward, he would draw until aides stopped him.

Jeff lacked the ability to limit his behavior in other areas as well. When he became interested in collecting, he filled his room with objects he had collected until he had to move out.

This characteristic, and probably some glimmering of an adolescent striving for independence, appeared to be involved in his illness. He and his father were both overweight and had undertaken a program of diet and jogging together. Jeff was rewarded for weight loss. He also made it plain in the hospital that he was proud of being a better weight loser than his father. These motivations were much more important to him than the hunger and thirst which he said he did not experience. His psychiatrist was uncertain whether these drives were repressed, suppressed, or denied.

Encoder

Nothing remarkable was found in this process.

Output transducer

Nothing remarkable was found in this process.

GROUP LEVEL

A subsystem review of the family group was done on the basis of the case history presented by the social worker, who saw the parents together and, occasionally, each separately. The four younger children in the family were not included in the therapy.

Jeff's father was a successful professional man who appeared serious and anxious at all times. His personality characteristics included lack of affect, rigid thinking, obsessive defenses, a strong superego, and a somewhat phobic orientation to the world. He feared losing control, which caused him to deny emotions and to limit his sexual activity. He and his wife were never allowed to go out in the evening together or to go on vacation without the children, because of his fears that something would happen. He wanted to keep the family together as much as possible.

Jeff's mother was an attractive housewife who related to others in a passive, dependent way, frequently behaving like a child with her husband. She attempted to meet her needs in indirect ways, avoiding confrontation, and fluctuated between expressing affection and denying all feelings. She did appear to be intelligent and to have good judgment. It also appeared that she was aware of how families usually operate. She said she felt guilty when she expressed anger and frustration at the family's life style.

Structure and processes of several subsystems appeared to be abnormal in this family. The seminar detected pathology in the following subsystems:

Boundary

Mr. S. was the primary boundary component.

The boundary to matter-energy was less permeable than is usual in families of this sort. The family lived in a small house on a very large piece of property, which isolated them from their neighbors. The father's insistence on doing everything together as a family kept the children inside the group boundary to the extent that it was possible with school-age children.

The boundary to information of this family was also pathological, since the father acted as a censor to exclude information he considered harmful. By discouraging friendships, he sought to limit input of information from outside the family.

Distributor

The usual impediments to movement of family members through the family's living space had been removed by Mr. S., who took locks from most of the inside doors, removed some doors, and would not allow anyone but himself to lock the bathroom door. The distributor channels were, therefore, more open than usual. Family members were denied the assurance of privacy they would have preferred.

Supporter

The house was too small for the number of people it held. Jeff's father resisted building the new home the family could well afford. As a result, seven people shared three small bedrooms. This supporter failed to provide adequate separation among components of this system.

Decoder

All information that entered this family was interpreted by Mr. S. in terms of his own fears and suspicions. These distortions could not be corrected by comparisons among family members because that was forbidden. As a result, the children accepted their father's distorted perceptions and ideas as accurate reflections of the world.

Internal transducer

Verbal communication of feelings and attitudes by family members was restricted by Mr. S. Even the mother did not tell her husband how she felt, since he made it clear he did not want to hear such things. She did convey her emotions by pouting and crying when she was unhappy or dissatisfied, but no discussion took place between parents about this behavior.

Channel and net

All members were connected in the channel and net by two-way channels, but the sort of information that could flow in the channels was restricted. The father told everyone what they should do and did not want feedback unless it supported him. At the time the study was made, it was not known whether subgroups in the family, such as the twins or the girls and the mother, had special communication channels that they used in the father's absence.

Decider

This family had an unusually centralized decider, in which the father was the sole effective component. The mother did not control even those aspects of day-to-day life that are usually considered a woman's province, like planning meals. Although three of the children were in their teens, they had no increased participation in family deciding.

This decider was abnormal also in the fact that there was little or no upward flow of suggestions, ideas, or feedback from below. The father made decisions on the basis of his own flawed perceptions, and these controlled even minute aspects of the family life and the personal lives of family members.

It seems clear that the abnormal steady states of this family, as well as Jeff's symptoms, were responses to the pathological decider subsystem, which reflected pathology at the organism level—that is, the subsystem and adjustment processes of Mr. S. The seminar had little hope that the other children would weather adolescence without problems or that the family would improve its interactions without intensive treatment for both the patient and the family group to correct, to whatever extent possible, the pathological processes disclosed in this analysis.

Conclusion

General living systems theory analyzes the structure and processes of living systems at seven levels, their actions in relation to other systems in their environment, and the ways in which systems at each level are like and unlike those at other levels. The insights it provides can increase understanding of the processes with which group psychotherapy is concerned, and, as evidenced in the case material presented above, it can be useful in diagnosis and treatment of individual patients and groups.

References

Anthony, E. J. The history of group psychotherapy. In *Sensitivity through Encounter and Marathon*, H. I. Kaplan and B. J. Sadock, editors, p. 4. E. P. Dutton, New York, 1972.

Bales, R. F. *Interaction Process Analysis: A Method for the Study of Small Groups*. Addison-Wesley, Cambridge, Mass., 1950.

Homans, G. C. *The Human Group*. Harcourt, Brace, New York, 1950.

Miller, J. G. *Living Systems*. McGraw-Hill, New York, 1978.

Thelen, H. A. *Methods for Studying Work and Emotionality in Group Operation*. University of Chicago Press, Chicago, 1954.

Vassiliou, G., and Vassiliou, V. G. On the alternation of group transaction patterns and its therapeutic actualization. Int. J. Group Psychother., 27: 75, 1977.

A.6 Nonverbal Behavior in Groups

JOHN J. O'HEARNE, M.D.

History

Nonverbal behavior was common in healing ceremonies of groups as diverse as American Indians, Africans, and ancient Greeks. All of these cultures used group gatherings with music, song, dance, touch and use of fetishes or symbols such as sand painting, when a person or an entire group needed to be healed. Shamans and other healers frequently touched those who came to be healed. Healing frequently included mind-altering conditions, such as deprivation of sleep or of food and the sound of drums or other musical instruments.

After the Industrial Revolution, when individual privacy became more available, medicine became more scientific, i.e., less based on ritual, myth, and reunion with networks of others. Treatment of the sick became more of an individual matter. Healers still touched, although they relied less upon symbolic means of cure.

As Freud revolutionized much of the Western world with his introduction of dynamic psychotherapy, treatment of emotionally and mentally ill individuals became more individualized. Those who sought psychotherapy came to expect a talking treatment; such talking treatment was taught to new practitioners by having them tell their teachers what the therapist said and what the patient said. Mention was made of what patients seemed to be feeling and what therapists thought was happening. Some teachers asked what therapists felt at the time. New therapists came to depend more and more upon what was said. In so doing, other aspects of communication came to be slighted in comparison with the importance of words. Skilled therapists still paid attention to the totality of the communication process, noting such occurrences as changes in the analysand's productions when the therapist turned her head (O'Hearne, 1981).

Beginning in the 1950's, other models for working with people in non-task groups proliferated. These groups emanated from the field of T-groups and encounter groups of the human potential movement. While psychodynamic group therapists operated primarily from the medical model of an ill person seeking treatment for a diagnosable disease, these new groups had a different philosophy. They emphasized that a person does not need to be sick in order to get better. Leaders in these groups had seldom been trained as vigorously as dynamic group therapists. Many such leaders prized themselves as leading groups on a passionate basis as compared with a more cognitive approach. As Schutz indicated, the purpose of the leader was to do whatever is needed to help the members of the group attain their own growth goals, using whatever seemed to move the group along (Schutz, 1967). Some of these groups had a casualty rate approaching 10%—high enough that if it were a drug, the Food and Drug Administration might not permit its being marketed (Lieberman et al., 1973).

Some group psychotherapists participated in these human potential groups and integrated techniques from them back into more conventional dynamic group psychotherapies (Mintz, 1969; O'Hearne and Glad, 1969). These techniques usually included variations in the duration of group sessions. Virtually all of them included a new interest in nonverbal behavior in group psychotherapy.

Contributions from Social Theory

Linguists and anthropologists have made us aware of the fact that verbal components in conversation carry the smaller part of our total message in most situations in everyday life. Estimates of the social meaning carried by verbal components in conversation range between 7% and 35% (Knapp, 1972). What, then, carries the remainder? If we recognize that all behavior is communication, we have most of the answer to this question. We must also recognize that behavior is influenced greatly by context and that, in all communication, two orders of information are present (Watzlawick and Beavin, 1977). These two orders are the content of the message and the relationship aspect of the message. For example, the simple question to a friend, "How much are beans worth today?" may elicit a simple answer: "Eighty-nine cents a can." However, if he answers with his back turned, or his eyebrow lifted, or his nose wrinkled, or his voice pitch raised, the responder provides not only the answer; more importantly, he tells the questioner how to interpret the relationship between him and the questioner.

Social theorists who study communication often regard psychotherapy literature as reductionistic. Such literature often hints that what goes on between therapist and patient can be diagrammed in simple cause-effect style, with arrows clearly showing what happened. If the therapist interprets behavior in transference terms, more arrows need only be added. Social theorists are more likely to look with a systems view, finding feedback loops and circles, with each event seeming to cause other events (Scheflen and Scheflen, 1972; Argyle, 1975).

Both theorists, however, are right. A psychotherapy group is a system made up of individuals who are dealing with their own internal processes, constantly interacting with the others in the system, holding the system steady, tending to resist change and also to change the system. To overlook any of these aspects is to oversimplify the problem.

Nonverbal Communication (NVC)

The symbol "NVC" refers to nonverbal communication between two or more individuals. Included here are all aspects of the communication except words. It is not necessary that either person attempt to communicate with the other. It is impossible not to communicate with another human being when in their presence.

It is not necessary to be silent to use NVC. In addition to saying words when we speak, we use prosodic signals of timing, pitch, and stress in our utterances. If our speech were entirely like that of voice-simulating computers, life would not be much fun. Our NVC modify our verbal productions so much that they may entirely cancel their meaning. A complement given with a sneer exemplifies this double-level message. When the non-word aspect of a communication contradicts the word aspect, the effect of the transaction is usually governed by the nonverbal aspect.

Since all behavior has meaning, any list of how we behave nonverbally must remain incomplete. Among these behaviors are: how we look, sound and smell; how and what we move; how closely we place ourselves to others; how we display affect; how we illustrate what we mean in words and special gestures which we use to communicate commonly understood meanings; and whether we arrange ourselves in space so as to indicate interest or disinterest, whether we and our group are open or closed to others, and whether we literally trust others behind our backs.

To those who can interpret them, we give indications of which parent-pleasing behaviors we still live out in highly predictable ways (Kahler and Capers, 1974).

The lay press has popularized some of the research on NVC, selling books which purport to tell people what various postures and gestures mean. For instance, folded arms are said to indicate that people are "closed." They are not told that large-shouldered men may be looking for a place to rest their heavy arms and shoulders, or that women may simply be keeping themselves warm when they cross their arms.

As the grammar employed in our use of words can not be learned from one simple book, neither can the grammar of our nonverbal language be learned from one simple book. Just as good native-born speakers of a language are only marginally aware of the rules they follow as they speak, so do those who readily express themselves remain only marginally aware of the usually unwritten rules they follow. In fact, fluent speakers are often especially uncomfortable when joining a psychotherapy group, partly because they know that they are more likely to reveal themselves inadvertently in nonverbal than in verbal fashion. They may also have an awareness that our bodies change when we feel emotion, and that these changes reveal not only something of what we are feeling but what we wish or fear others would do about our feeling. They may intuitively recognize that most of our major emotional expressions could be interpreted in any culture around the world, with no words being exchanged (Ekman and Friesen, 1975).

There is a story attributed to Mark Twain, whose wife strongly objected to his cursing. As the story recites, she decided to cure him of his bad habit. So, one evening while putting the studs in his shirt and tying his tie, she cursed for the entire time. When she had finished, he smiled, kissed her on the cheek and said, "Well, Hon, you got the words. But you ain't got the music yet."

To separate words from "music," the following experiment may be found useful. Watch and listen to a televised drama until you understand the program. Then adjust the sound so that you can no longer hear. Watch for a time and predict what will be happening when you again increase the volume so that you can hear.

Since there are at least a thousand gestures and since the face is capable of over 200,000 different expressions, the therapist who decides to increase his attention to NVC in therapy sessions may find it easier to focus attention at first on only several aspects of NVC, such as head nodding, color of lips, breathing, or wheather the person moves his vertical body axis while speaking.

If the therapist only notes the distribution of the patient's body mass, he will learn somthing. If he notes that the patient looks "top heavy," he will be especially alert for this patient's feeling that he cannot stand on his own, cannot support himself. Or, if a patient has a small upper body and his lower belly is much larger, we may expect to find that this person will never feel filled. He is likely to need a very strict treatment contract in order to be clear about what can and cannot be accomplished in therapy. If the patient has a large chest which moves little as he exhales, we may anticipate that he will keep his heart literally and figuratively protected in its almost rigid case. He will likely live with a stringent set of rules for his own conduct and wish others would do the same. We can predict that at some point in therapy he will be able to cry deeply and loudly, releasing years of grief, and showing us the hurt child within him.

Kurtz and Prestera (1976) believe that every disturbed person has disturbed respiration. Many of the "body therapies" focus intensively upon breathing (Lowen, 1975). So do some forms of yoga. Any therapist can learn a great deal about a patient's resistances simply by watching carefully to see when the patient suddenly stops breathing.

For instance, an asthmatic patient stopped breathing whenever she talked about her mother, her sister, her home city, and how frightened she was when she was without a complete survival plan in a strange city. Calling her attention to this resulted in a smile and a resumption of her talking. Asking her to breathe when she talked again of similar matters resulted in her feeling less frightened. When asked to continue to talk about them and to breathe out deeply as she completed each topic, she first felt anger, then started to cry softly. When the therapist said that she cried like a child who wanted no one to hear her, she said, "I knew early in life that I couldn't trust my mother. I didn't want her to hear me cry." When the therapist said, "Of course. She can't breathe your air for you," she was startled. She said her former therapist helped her be angry at her mother at similar points. When the therapist said, "Right now, do you want to be angry at your mother or breathe your own air?" She smiled, shook her shoulders with relief, threw her head back and took a deep breath, exhaling fully.

Smell

While only a few patients actually smell bad, there are more who overuse perfume or cologne, or who are afraid to come to a group meeting without using a breath freshener. As this behavior is noted, it is material for analysis just as is any other communication.

Sound

Since most middle-aged people have a decrease in their ability to hear higher notes, the therapist and other group participants may note difficulty in hearing those who speak in low volume but with high-pitched voices. They will have special difficulty in hearing sibilant sounds such as *f, v, c.*

Many group members repeatedly became angry with the young adult woman who kept her head tucked low while she spoke. She repeatedly aimed her voice and eyes at the center of the floor. Her baby-like voice was not congruent with her considerable ability both at tennis and in business. Repeated confrontations were not effective in changing this "split." She was asked to speak just softly enough that the therapist could almost hear her. The group laughed at this paradoxical direction (Watzlawick et al., 1974). As she complied, she laughed. When she was asked to now roar in a whisper, she laughed again and did so. Then she softly began to cry while telling of wanting to win her father's love by being quietest of all the children while he slept during the days. The therapist asked if she ever won the prize of being favored first by her father. She had not. Then she was asked if her father would now love her if she remained his good little girl. She nodded no. The therapist placed an empty chair immediately in front of her and asked her to pretend her father was sleeping in that chair and to softly tell him that she was being quiet so she would not wake him and that he would then love her. When she did, she was asked, "Is he still asleep?" When she nodded yes, the therapist moved the chair to the other end of the room and asked her to take three deep breaths and now wake him up to tell him. The entire group joined in her laughter as she roared "Wake up and pay attention to me."

Movement

Absence of movement in a therapy group is as much a matter for analysis as is absence of speech. What patients do not move is at least as important as what they do move. The person who sits motionless, expressionless, in a group is certainly presenting an Iron Man mask to the group. And, the tighter the mask, the more we must respect his need for it in the first place.

One of the first ways we note an individual's movement is in his postures and gestures. Lowen (1975) gives a particularly clear account of hang-ups which people demonstrate in their postures. He illustrates how some people look like they have a coat hanger between their shoulders, while others have a pronounced widow's hump in the form of a pronounced lump of fatty tissue over the seventh cervical vertebra. The coat hanger look is associated with individuals who are constantly frightened or ready to be; the widow's hump is associated with individuals who are ready to be instantly angry. He says that schizoid characters may demonstrate a posture similar to what would happen if a noose were placed around their neck, while some borderline individuals may have a posture resembling that of a crucified man. People who have thus frozen their bodies can seldom discharge the motion in their emotion. (The Latin root of emotion means to move away.)

Lowen emphatically believes that people with hang-ups do not have their feet planted firmly upon the ground, ready to support themselves. He and other followers of Wilhelm Reich emphasize grounding as the opposite of hang-ups and as a prerequisite for the effective expression of emotional tension.

The face

If therapists could only see the faces of their patients, they would still have access to huge amounts of information. By careful observation of facial movements, therapists can discern whether people are depressed, excited, happy, or sad without hearing a word of what they say. Patients with a long history of treatment in individual psychotherapy sometimes find this aspect of group psychotherapy bothersome. They say, truthfully, that there is no place to hide in a group.

Absolute symmetry in faces does not exist. The Christ nature in Albrecht Dürer's portrait of Christ was gained by making the two sides symmetrical. The split in facial symmetry is usually vertical. The two eyes are seldom identical in appearance. Kurtz and Prestera (1976) list information which may be gained from looking at each eye separately. They believe that the right eye indicates qualities of activity, maleness, doing, and relationship with one's father, while the left eye indicates the opposite of these.

It is usually simple to assure patients that no face is symmetrical, that we can learn much from looking at each side separately and integrating what we see. This is done most easily by using videotape playback, utilizing a close-up lens and marking off portions of the screen. Since Gestalt techniques focus so sharply on splits and reintegration, they are very useful here. The patient can be asked to speak as though first one side and then the other is his totality, and then to integrate the split.

When therapists realize that some people use their eyes for purposes other than seeing, they have important avenues open for clarifying such uses. They include using eyes to pin the other person down, look daggers at others, act as vacuum cleaners to suck others dry of emotion or attention. They may certainly be used to make sexual invitations.

People who frequently raise their eyes and eyebrows repeatedly, nod with their chins ending near their chest, commonly use tentative words, like "You know?", are also often found to make declarative sentences but to end them as though they were questions. This "please me" sequence, along with four other compulsively driven behaviors, has been chronicled by Kahler and Capers (1974). Those who master his simple system of markers and use them on a second-by-second basis can usually describe adaptation patterns and major interpersonal tendencies within a maximum of several minutes' interaction. This can be done with minimal attention to content of the patient's history.

The central portion of the forehead has been referred to as the wisdom spot or third eye, for instance, in kundalini yoga. To demonstrate how chronic tension in this area limits our view, our choice of emotional responses, and what we invite back from others, the following exercise is suggested. It may also be found useful in sensitizing patients with chronic frowns to what they do to themselves.

While looking into a mirror, imitate a state of anger or worry. As the forehead and areas around the eyes tense, it will be noted that the full field of view is constricted. Tension usually is felt down into the shoulders. Does this look invite others to relax and be friendly with you? Could it lead to a tension headache?

People with chronic muscular tension around the eyes usually have tension also at the junction of the muscles of the neck and the posterior portion of the skull. Headaches often originate in this area. Sometimes, all the psychotherapy in the world does not alone produce relief from this tension. Sometimes medications are necessary; sometimes massage helps. Sometimes Rolfing, Feldenkrais, or Alexander methods help.

A man began psychotherapy because of increased conflict between himself, his wife, his parents, and some of his business colleagues. He drove himself to excellence and worked long hours. He seemed friendly; his eyes were bright. He sat almost rigidly frozen in the group. Analysis of this freezing of motion and feeling did nothing for his chronic pain and tension around his eyes and at the back of his skull. He did not want to stare; he could not refrain from it. Of course, his efforts to stop made his condition worse (Watzlawick et al., 1974). Analysis of his smiling at his troubles was satisfactory; reduction of his "be strong" compulsion was more resistant (Kahler and Capers, 1974).

In one group session, he attempted to smile bravely through his headache which centered around his eyes, which he kept fixed upon the therapist. When a group member said that he acted like he had forgotten that he did not need to smile so bravely, nor try so hard, his eyes moistened with tears and he said, "I can't let go." The therapist asked if he would sit on the floor between the therapist's knees. He did. The therapist pressed firmly upon the muscles of his neck where they joined his skull. When the patient let his head relax and fall forward, the therapist then massaged this area. As he relaxed more, the therapist massaged the mastoid region at the insertion of the sternocleidomastoid muscle. To increase tension on this muscle, he put the patient's chin in his hand to turn his head. The patient jerked his head upright and only relaxed it when the therapist said, "You've tried long enough. Let me hold your head up." As he relaxed and the therapist continued the massage while talking to other group members, the patient cried softly at first, then

sobbed, "I'm so tired. I've tried so hard." When he said this, the therapist pressed firmly with his thumbs into the back muscles near the seventh cervical vertebra. At first, the patient resisted, then bowed his head and began to cry. He sighed, "I'm tired." The therapist said rather loudly, "I can't hear you." The patient said, slightly louder, "I'm tired." Now very loudly, the therapist said, "I can't hear you." The patient straightened up and angrily yelled, "I'm so damn tired of carrying you all on my back." He was instructed to stand, to throw his shoulders back each time he repeated this loudly. After venting his anger, he then told how he had felt responsible for his father's business, his mother's happiness, his family's welfare. While talking, he began to slump his shoulders and a group member said, "You look like you are picking them all up again." The therapist said, "It's your turn now." He straightened up, took a deep breath, and smiled. His original decision was now analyzed, and he understood how he had kept waiting for approval from both his parents and that he could never get this in the way that he wanted it.

In subsequent group sessions, he was monitored on what he did for his own pleasure while he worked through his anger and grief at never being able to get the approval and love for which he had worked for so many years (O'Hearne, 1981).

The mouth and nose are frequently used together to express such emotions as varying degrees of anger, nausea, disgust, surprise. For instance, patients who claim to be disgusted but who do not show slight elevations of nose and lip on at least one side are probably inaccurate or nonauthentic in naming their emotions. Similarly, the person who says she is emotionally repulsed and who then lightly licks her lip is probably non-authentic.

Masseter tension

The strongest muscles in the body for their mass are the masseters, whose chief function is to close the jaws and hold the rear teeth together. Sustained tension here is most likely to be due to dental malocclusion or to the "bite of resentment." People with dental malocclusion are often misdiagnosed as having psychological problems. A simple test is to insert a flat toothpick between the rear teeth on each jaw separately and have the patient close his jaws gently. If this simple test provides some tension relief, he needs dental consultation.

The patient who "bites off his words" is frequently using only the front of his mouth for his oral aggression. He underuses his rear teeth and is likely not to "hang on" to a project or problem until it is finished. Patients with the chronic bite of resentment are likely to "hang on" to resentment so that their therapy is prolonged. If they have a good working relationship, the therapist may ask both of these patients to slowly bite on a roll, such as a folded small towel or roll of facial tissue. (This should not be done if the patient has dental bridges because of the risk of fracturing these expensive bridges.) The first patient is usually reluctant to "get his teeth into biting" (Perls et al., 1951). Biting exercises can be prescribed for him. If he has been demonstrating resentment, the second patient is especially reluctant to let go. If the therapist playfully growls as if playing with a dog, the patient is likely to growl back and to hold on. The therapist can then attend to others in the group, allowing the resenter to decide when to let go. The duration of his holding on is important to analyze (Perls et al., 1951).

The shoulders and chest are so important that only brief mention can be made of them. People who are afraid of their emotions literally do not breathe easily. The patient who barely moves chest, neck, or head literally acts like a frightened rabbit. By so doing, he further increases his fear. Here, the James-Lange theory of emotion has at least as much relevance as the Gestalt theory of fear leading to inhibited breathing, leading to hypoxia, producing more anxiety. When the therapist notices a patient whose shoulders are bent forward and rounded, he can feel the effect of this posture upon emotional expression by imitating the patient's position and breathing. Similarly, imitation of the patient who squares his shoulders or throws them back or who keeps his chest full of air will quickly enlighten the therapist about some of the patient's defenses. Such quiet, non-ridiculing imitation of a patient's posture will often provide the therapist with his own visual and kinesthetic cues as to how the posture defends the patient, helps him cope, and prevents him from releasing his emotions in a safe, appropriate, ethical fashion.

This is especially easy to do with the hands. Imitation of the hand picking often done by agitating obsessive-compulsive people will help the therapist see that the patient keeps a closed circle, picks on himself, aims at precision, keeps his power within himself, and injures himself slightly. Hurried drumming of the fingers, especially while others are talking, provides awareness of the demand these people place upon themselves and others relative to time, and of their impatience with how others use time. Parental pointing of the index finger is sometimes done from the Parent ego state, sometimes as a child imitating a parent.

Many books omit the foot as a nonverbal indicator. There is one foot motion which is especially important to watch: the "put-on-the-brakes" position in which the toes are dorsiflexed as if the person has just put on the brakes in an automobile. We are especially likely to see it if a person is about to confront another and is uneasy about this, or if he is about to discuss a subject with whose presentation he is uneasy. Analyzing the resistance here may be more important than the content.

Some therapists deliberately provide both individual and joint seating arrangements for group psychotherapy sessions. Here, patients can sit alone or can experiment with physical closeness to others. Seldom does a new patient voluntarily occupy the middle of a three-cushion sofa. Whoever occupies that position must decide how closely they will sit comfortably near somebody else and whether they will touch or not. Not touching is as much a matter of communication as is hand holding or compulsive comforting of those who cry. This is especially easy to do in those who initiate a touch but stop it in midair.

Inhibition of natural touching behavior is common in new patients in group psychotherapy until they determine the culture of the group relative to touching and until they have learned that there are many reasons and ways to touch other than sexual. The author believes that sexual acting out is less likely to occur in psychotherapy groups where touching occurs than in those where it is rigidly proscribed.

Subgroups identify themselves by turning at least parts of their bodies toward each other and extending parts of their bodies, such as elbows or feet, to mark that they are set apart. They do this also by identifying themselves as "withs" by sitting close together, looking primarily at each other, and waiting for one person to speak for the subgroup (Scheflen and Scheflen, 1972).

Those individuals who are less comfortable with closeness will literally set themselves apart by increasing distance between themselves and others. If they have paranoid or sociopathic trends, they will usually sit so they can see everyone else and take special care that the space behind them is not occupied. More schizoid and phobic individuals tend to sit near the door.

By studying expert therapists, Bandler and Grinder (1975) have noted that people represent their conceptions of the universe in four modalities: visual, kinesthetic, auditory, and olfactory-gustatory. They note that the individual reveals his ways of contacting the universe by various patterns of eye movement and by choices of words appropriate to their dominant modes. Skill in these areas helps the therapist meet the patient "where he is," rather than demanding that the patient accept the therapist's mode of representing and contacting "reality." For instance, if a person is highly auditory, talking alone may suffice for most of his therapy. If the patient is highly kinesthetic, movement plus analysis and new learning is much more likely to facilitate his changing. If he is highly visual, we can use visual predicates, such as clear picture, sharp focus, or new view, in talking with him, and our rapport very quickly will improve.

The studies of these authors and their followers buttress related studies explicating the utility and rationale of touch and movement in psychotherapy groups (Mintz, 1969; O'Hearne, 1972, 1976).

Those individuals who represent the world kinesthetically are especially likely to benefit from movement and touch in treatment. Those who are more visual may profit from seeing conflict worked out rather than talked out. In addition, groups may often benefit from nonverbal activities. Since no one can predict their exact outcome, they are referred to as experiments rather than exercises.

To do these safely and most productively, the therapist himself should have had some personal experience with them. The therapist should prevent injuries by setting limits, by not using a nonverbal experiment without a clearly defined purpose, and by the almost universal need for discussion and working through of what happens. The therapist should also inquire about cardiovascular and musculoskeletal and other systems if pertinent, as in those activities requiring physical endurance or strain or contact.

Discussion of such exercises without paying tribute to modern Gestalt practice would be like reinventing the wheel, since all of them are designed to clarify, confront, and experiment with inefficient Gestalten (Polster and Polster, 1973; Hatcher and Himelstein, 1976). One of the major deficiences in Gestalt technique is the absence of working through; the principles of analytic therapy are highly useful for this part of the work, as well as for analyzing resistances to such experiments. A few of these are listed below.

Sculpting a traumatic scene with group members as stand-ins for those originally present and having the concerned patient view it from the side clarifies the trauma and provides an opportunity to discuss it. The therapist may elect to have the patient then move the various "statues" to make the outcome as he would like to have it.

At those times when the group is very quiet and not

highly resistant, the therapist has several experiments he can suggest. He can have people center themselves in the room if they believe they are heavily involved in the group or more peripherally if emotionally distant from the group's activity. He can have them sit or lie comfortably where he leads them on a guided fantasy or can play recorded music, such as Debussy's La Mer, while they make their own fantasy. He can have them focus attention on their breathing, then subvocally call themselves by their favorite names, using part of the sound with inspiration, the remainder with expiration.

Starting new groups is facilitated by having members pair up, stand at two arms' length from each other, then one arm's length, then blur their vision by putting their faces less than 5 inches apart. Or, they may be asked to mill around the room at first without looking at each other; gradually look up and choose a partner; sit down, wordlessly; look closely at each other until they can remember each other's face with their eyes shut; look again, squint at partner, close eyes and remember someone from their own past who has some similarity to the partner; discuss with partner. As with all role playing, they must be sure that they have "removed" the face they "put on" the partner. This exercise is especially good for teaching patients about transference distortions.

The issue of sharing in groups can be demonstrated by having each pair share one piece of paper, each person having a different colored crayon, taking turns making marks on the paper. This inevitably elicits discussion concerning cooperation and competition—"my space, your space."

Where a newcomer is convinced he cannot make his way into a preexisting group, the group may be asked to stand, link elbows, and exclude the newcomer, whose task is now to make his way into the group. This is a very rapid way of integrating a newcomer.

When a non-paranoid person finds trust difficult, this dilemma may be dramatized by asking him to pick someone to catch him as he stands with stiff knees, back to the catcher, and falls backward into the arms of the catcher. Initially, the therapist should probably be at the side of the catcher. The entire group can be involved in this by standing, the individual in the center, the group encircling him. He falls backward and is slowly passed around or across the circle while he keeps his knees stiff. (If music is desired for this, Ravel's Bolero is excellent.) Many women with orgasmic dysfunction find this a difficult exercise. When cured, they do not.

Reaction formations against rage can often be demonstrated and provide good working-through material by having the person kneel in front of a well-padded surface, link his hands above his head, arch his back backward, then come forward and hit the padded surface repeatedly. They frequently scare themselves and must often be urged to continue, later making noises as they exhale. Frequently, they begin to curse and yell. At the conclusion, have them repeat the movement, but this time very slowly and gently. Frequently, they caress the surface and cry at this point. This latter is important to demonstrate to them that they still have control over their rage. A tennis racket can be used with even less risk to the hands in this exercise.

A gentler exercise for working with aggression is to have participants pair up, put the palms of their hands together without talking, and have their hands successively get acquainted, dance, argue or fight, "make up," and part. Then discuss.

Patients who are convinced they are helpless or that their anger will hurt someone may be asked to lie on the floor,

belly down, and arm wrestle with someone else. The elbows must be touching to minimize injury. They are instructed to go slowly and not to suddenly throw the other person. They are asked if they will abide by this agreement. If so, a signal is given for them to begin. With elbows together, a very small woman can arm wrestle with a much larger, more heavily muscled man. She is usually amazed at her strength.

There are many Gestalt techniques for "going around," such as having the hyperindependent person stand in front of each person in the group and say, "I don't need anything from you." If this experiment is timed for an instance when his reaction formation is most strained, he can seldom go all the way around the group without changing his mind.

If the therapist wants the group to work in the area of oral-dependent strivings, he can ask them all to lie comfortably on the floor, let the floor support them while they relax with knees bent. Then have them put their hands straight up, breathe deeply for a while, then begin to say "Mama" at whatever sound level they want. They usually begin quietly and end loudly.

If the group is in a state of low energy and activity, some of Lowen's (1975) grounding exercises may help a great deal. Since the head is low in some of these exercises, the implicit message is that the group need not always do everything head first with great intellectualizing.

If the group approaches sexual conflicts only peripherally, they might all be asked to stand, close their eyes, move their hips in unison with recorded music, and thrust their hips forward when certain motifs occur. Many modern songs are useful for such work. Closure of the eyes reduces possible embarrassment. This experiment usually ends with great laughter and facilitates discussion of sexuality.

The question usually arises: Does the therapist's touching the patient complicate treatment? Any behavior of the therapist can complicate treatment, including both touch and rigid non-touch, laughter and rigid avoidance of laughter. Some therapists comfortably hug patients of either sex when the patient has made a "break through" in his treatment or at the successful termination of therapy. These therapists are confident they can differentiate between provocative hugs, clingingly dependent hugs, and hugs of celebration. Other therapists violently eschew them.

The above are samples of some nonverbal experiments. Each therapist's creation of his own experiments, designed for specific moments, will be part of his own joy in making therapy more creative and, hopefully, more helpful, more rapidly. The working-through process is often helped by having seen, heard, and felt the conflict differently than talk alone can produce.

References

Argyle, M. *Bodily Communication.* International Universities Press, New York, 1975.

Bandler, R., and Grinder, J. *The Structure of Magic,* vol. 1. Science & Behavior Books, Palo Alto, CA, 1975.

Ekman, P., and Friesen, W. V. *Unmasking the Face.* Prentice-Hall, Englewood Cliffs, NJ, 1975.

Hatcher, C., and Himelstein, P., eds. *The Handbook of Gestalt Therapy.* Jason Aronson, New York, 1976.

Kahler, T., and Capers, H. The miniscript. Transct. Anal. J., *4:* 26, 1974.

Knapp, M. L. *Non-Verbal Communication in Human Interaction.* Holt, Rinehart and Winston, New York, 1972.

Kurtz, R., and Prestera, H. *The Body Reveals.* Harper & Row, New York, 1976.

Lieberman, M. A., Yalom, I. D., and Miles, M. B. *Encounter Groups:*

First Facts. Basic Books, New York, 1973.

Lowen, A. *Bioenergetics.* Penguin Books, New York, 1975.

Mintz, E. Touch and the psychoanalytic tradition. Psychoanal. Rev., *56:* 3, 1969.

O'Hearne, J. J. How can we reach patients most effectively. Int. J. Group Psychother., *22:* 446, 1972.

O'Hearne, J. J. How and why do transactional-Gestalt therapists work as they do. Int. J. Group Psychother. *26:* 163, 1976.

O'Hearne, J. J. Good grief. Transact. Anal. J., *11:* 85, 1981.

O'Hearne, J. J., and Glad, D. D. The case for interaction. Int. J. Group Psychother., *19:* 268, 1969.

Perls, F., Hefferline, R. F., and Goodman, P. *Gestalt Therapy.* Dell, New York, 1951.

Polster, E., and Polster, M. *Gestalt Therapy Integrated.* Brunner/

Mazel, New York, 1973.

Saretsky, T. *Active Techniques in Group Psychotherapy.* Jason Aronson, New York, 1977.

Scheflen, A. E., and Scheflen, A. *Body Language and Social Order.* Prentice-Hall, Englewood Cliffs, NJ, 1972.

Schutz, W. C. *Joy: Expanding Human Awareness.* Grove Press, New York, 1967.

Watzlawick, P., and Beavin, J. Some formal aspects of communication. In *The Interactional View,* P. Watzlawick and J. H. Weakland, editors, p. 56, W. W. Norton, New York, 1977.

Watzlawick, P., Wakeland, J., and Fish, R. *Change: Principles of Problem Formation and Problem Resolution.* W. W. Norton, New York, 1974.

A.7 The Role of the Leader in Group Psychotherapy

MYRON F. WEINER, M.D.

Introduction

Leading a psychotherapy group is a far more complex undertaking than conducting individual psychotherapy. The group psychotherapist has many more stimuli to deal with, has less ability to attune himself to individual intrapsychic processes, and is more exposed to his patients or clients than the individual psychotherapist. Consequently, he has less control over the process with which he is dealing, has much less information about it, and is more vulnerable to manipulation than the individual psychotherapist.

Group therapists seem generally more comfortable with self-display than therapists who prefer to work one-to-one. The relative looseness of the group therapist's hold on the therapeutic reins may facilitate acting out and use of the group for ordinary social gratifications by the leader and the group members. It also enhances the potential of the group for doing damage to vulnerable members.

The leader's responsibilities, his tools for working with the group, and the impact of styles of leadership and the attributes of the leader on the functioning of the group must all be considered. The leader and the group are in a process of constant change and interchange, with the role of the leader changing as the needs of the group change, but with the leader generally supplying the group's direction. Although he has a wide variety of roles available to him, the leader can never become fully a member of the group without losing his position of leadership and his therapeutic leverage. It is a lonely business for the therapist, perhaps more lonely than individual therapy because

he witnesses the formation of emotional ties without being able to partake of them. In this sense, group therapy may be a greater strain on the interpersonally hungry therapist than individual therapy (Grotjahn, 1975).

The Leader's Responsibilities

The leader's responsibilities begin before his first meeting with a group. He must make certain tentative decisions, including the goals for the group, the therapeutic means, the optimal style of leadership, the most appropriate type and number of group members, and the group rules. If he or she works in an institutional setting, the leader must establish an atmosphere conducive to the conduct of groups and to the referral of potential candidates for group therapy. This requires an intimate acquaintance with the power hierarchy of the institution (Berne, 1966) and considerable groundwork in acquainting the staff with the therapeutic potential of groups. An effective group therapy program can be undertaken only after institutional resistances have been dealt with (Kadis et al., 1974).

When starting a new group, the therapist ideally spends time with each potential member to screen for suitability, to develop a feel for each person as an individual, to establish a therapeutic contract, to work through resistances to entering the group, and to establish a positive emotional tie.

If a new leader enters an established group, he needs preliminary information about the previous goals for the group, the level at which the group has operated, the nature and number of participants in the group, the former leader's style, and the contractual aspects of the group.

SETTING GOALS

Setting goals requires that the leader have a therapeutic frame of reference and requires that he formulate goals which can be understood and consensually validated by group members. A shared cognitive framework facilitates emotional learning in groups. As the leader attempts to formulate goals for the group he wishes to undertake, he must concomitantly identify the prospective members of his group and assess their ability to reach these goals.

In setting goals, the therapist must also take into account his level of training and expertise in four areas: his ability to teach principles of psychologically healthy functioning, his sophistication about psychopathology, his mastery of psychological interventions, and his self-awareness. A good teacher with little sophistication about psychopathology and little formal awareness of group techniques can often conduct a repressive group well. A leader who teaches well, who has sophistication about psychopathology, and who is technically well equipped can conduct ego-supportive groups well, even if he lacks significant awareness of his own unconscious processes. By contrast, the leader of an evocative group need not be a talented teacher, because his therapeutic medium is confrontation and interpretation, not explanation or modeling. However, he must understand psychopathology well, must be able to employ group process to facilitate the emergence of material from the unconscious, and must be sufficiently self-aware to help him guide the group interactions without stimulating acting out.

In addition, setting goals requires that the therapist know the support available should the group members require additional help through medication or hospitalization.

ESTABLISHING THERAPEUTIC MEANS

The therapeutic means includes the level at which the group operates as well as the types of intervention employed by the therapist. The basic levels of group psychotherapy are: repressive (behavioral, guidance, didactic), ego-supportive (counseling, interactional), and evocative (psychoanalytic group psychotherapy) (Kadis et al., 1974). Repressive groups are classes in which the leader teaches means to deal with conscious attitudes and concrete reality problems. Ego-supportive groups focus on conscious attitudes and also on the effects of preconscious attitudes on interpersonal relationships in the here and now of the group and in everyday life. Evocative groups allow emergence of material from the unconscious through group members' reactive associations and the development of transferences within the group (Wolf and Schwartz, 1962).

The level at which the group operates determines the basic types of intervention appropriate for that group (Weiner, 1970). Appropriate interventions in a repressive group deal with problems in the here and now through practical suggestions by the leader and other group members. Patients in such groups are frequently taught about their psychodynamics and psychological vulnerabilities.

Mr. Q., a self-educated man who functioned as an engineer, had achieved significantly greater self-esteem through group therapy and had become a more effective manager and employee through his increased ability to assert himself and to stand his own ground. Nevertheless, he still experienced episodes of depression that could not be attributed to work, family, or intrapsychic pressures. Part of Mr. Q.'s group treatment was teaching him to recognize depression and to differentiate it from actual failure on the job or in his interpersonal relationships, thereby enabling him to turn more quickly to antidepressant medication instead of suffering needlessly for months at a time.

The therapist may tell a group member directly that he or she is very sensitive to interpersonal losses and encourage the building of a supportive interpersonal network to help in the event of losing any single source of support. Material which emerges from the unconscious is actively suppressed in these groups.

The basic interventions in ego-supportive groups deal with the dynamics of behavior in the here and now and the preconscious attitudes and emotions, such as fear of authority or unexpressed anger, which motivate the behavior. The vehicles for therapeutic progress are direct feedback about self-defeating behaviors in and outside of the group and identification of the group members with healthy behaviors modeled by others. The leader supplies an intellectual underpinning by pointing out that behavior is determined by feelings of which people are often unaware and is motivated by certain unfinished emotional business or by the unconscious wish for a psychological payoff (Berne, 1964).

Mrs. A.N. sought therapy because she felt she had no personality of her own, that she only reacted to the demands of her husband and job and expressed little of her own needs and desires, with which she felt greatly out of touch. Because she did not know what she wanted for herself, she had become a puppet for others to manipulate.

The reaction of the group to Mrs. A.N. was warm and positive. In the group, she was initially quiet and inhibited, a problem that was compounded by the fact that she cried each time she dealt with an emotionally significant issue. As therapy progressed, she told of her feeling that she and her father had been crushed by her mother. She, for example, was a gifted musician but had meekly accepted her mother's profession of nursing.

As she became comfortable in alternate sessions, the group noticed a difference in her behavior in the absence of the leader. She expressed herself well, interacted well, and did not cry. Over time, it became evident that she had transferred aspects of her relationship with her mother to the therapist but was still unable to alter her behavior in spite of understanding it.

The therapist dealt with her by gently playing out the uncaring aspect of her mother's relationship with her. He stopped responding to her occasional requests for advice and, instead, turned them back on her, sometimes shrugging his shoulders and saying that he did not know what to do either. The other group members had little difficulty understanding the therapist's tactic, but were nevertheless angered by his failure to respond to her requests. As the other group members expressed their anger on her behalf, supported the expression of her anger, and praised her when she began demanding what she felt entitled to, her behavior changed. She was at first troubled by her bitchiness but later became proud of having developed definite likes and dislikes and having become aware of her needs and willing to seek their satisfaction in appropriate ways.

In contrast to the education and advice giving in repressive therapies, which suppress unconscious material, and feedback in ego-supportive therapies, which calls attention to preconscious attitudes and feelings, the therapist of the evocative group uses interpretation to bring to consciousness the unconscious roots of attitudes and behavior and to tie them to each member's primary object relations: a genetic reconstruction.

Mr. B. was a man in his late twenties who operated a manufacturing business. He had been a chronic stutterer and an academic failure at college. In addition, he had great difficulty making sales calls or business trips because of anxiety-provoked diarrhea.

Mr. B. had made significant headway in reducing his symptoms through group therapy. His stuttering had diminished markedly. He had returned to college and was doing well, and his nervous diarrhea was abating.

He stormed into group angrily one day, after having been severely chastised by his father, who officed in the same building with him, and periodically dropped in to give unsolicited, unwanted advice. Mr. B. announced angrily that he was going to quit his job and let his father run the business. The therapist reminded him that the business was his, not his father's and that, if he quit, there would be no business. He was startled and pleased by the therapist's remark, because it was his first significant positive awareness of his separateness from his father, which he had expressed previously through negative means, such as failing in college and refusing to work in his father's business.

Later, after working on material from dreams of shooting policeman and being held captive by strangers, Mr. B. was also able to deal with his wish to be dominated by his father and his need to pay the price of humiliation.

Anxiety-reducing repressive interventions are employed at times when high anxiety would be detrimental to the members of any group, whether repressive, ego supportive, or evocative. Because evocative techniques raise anxiety, they are best reserved for groups in which the members are psychologically well integrated and in which there is adequate support for a member who becomes temporarily overwhelmed.

CONTRACT MAKING

In psychotherapy, a contract between a therapist and a potential patient is an explicit, noncoercive, mutually agreed-upon statement of the tasks each is to perform, and the ends to which those tasks are a means.

Contract making is important in psychotherapy as a corrective emotional experience, as defined by Al-

exander and French (1946) and as described by Strupp (1977). The patient learns cooperation and mutuality instead of negativism, passive aggression, or manipulation as a means to deal with others. Contract making acknowledges the patient's influence in the therapeutic process, encourages the patient to assume part of the responsibility for the treatment, and also allows for changes in methods and goals of treatment based on periodic reevaluation of the progress of treatment by therapist and patient alike.

An evaluation contract is the first contract made between a group therapist and his prospective group member. It is an agreement that the prospective patient will reveal enough about himself to enable his prospective therapist to evaluate him for treatment. When the therapist concludes that the referred patient is a good candidate for one of his groups, he offers a therapeutic contract for negotiation.

In the ideal therapeutic contract, the therapist shares enough of his ideas about the patient's problems and the means by which he hopes that he and the patient will address these problems that the patient can make a rational decision to cooperate, to suggest alterations in the method, or to seek help elsewhere.

An appropriate therapeutic contract includes a description of the group and its members (without breaking confidences) and may include an orientation to the issues with which the group is currently dealing. It always includes the group rules. Most therapists of outpatient groups indicate that information which arises within the group will be held in confidence by all of its members.

In outpatient groups, the leader usually makes some provision in the contract about outside contact between group members. The majority of therapists who conduct outpatient groups suggest that outside contacts with other group members be reported and discussed within the group as a means to maximize the therapeutic value of the group. In repressive groups, outside contact and mutual support between group members is frequently encouraged.

Also included in the contract for group members are the time and place of group meetings, the fee arrangement, and fees for missed sessions. Failure to clarify those aspects of the group may point to significant countertransference.

The therapeutic contract also calls for each group member to use his share of the group's time. Failure to use his share of the group's time is dealt with as a resistance at a level appropriate to the group and the individual members.

Proscription of physical contact or violence by one group member toward others is part of the contract with groups of patients with poor impulse control, such as institutionalized delinquents or adults who have committed violent acts.

It may also be useful to build an agreement termination into the therapeutic contract. The leader may explain that group therapy is often uncomfortable at first and that new members often think strongly about quitting during the first few months and may ask each potential group member to discuss a decision to leave in a certain number of group sessions before actually quitting.

Alternate sessions also need to be discussed if a patient is to enter a group in which alternate sessions have begun.

A process of renegotiation begins once the group convenes. At the beginning of the group, the leader reviews the therapeutic contract with each member, helps the members to achieve an appropriate degree of cohesion, and establishes the area of discussion and the psychological level at which events will be discussed.

Once assembled as a group, the members help determine the goals for the group and the means by which they will be reached, including the role of the leader, the structure of the group, the length and frequency of meetings, and alternate sessions.

SELECTING MEMBERS

The selection of patients for a group is a complex process that depends largely on the psychological fit between the candidate, the group leader, and the group for which the candidate is being considered.

In considering a candidate for his group, the leader must ask himself if he can establish sufficient rapport, and if he can tolerate the demands likely to be made. The leader must also be aware of his emotional reactions to new patients and try to screen out those persons with whom he will interact poorly because of his personality or his present life situation. Indications of potentially interfering emotional reactions include the offering of contracts that are much more liberal or stringent than the therapist's ordinary contracts, and intense emotional reactions to the candidate which stimulate dreams and fantasies (Langs, 1973).

The evaluation of a candidate for group psychotherapy begins with an assessment of ego strength. Ego strength varies from time to time in relation to social, psychological, and biological factors. Changes in a member's ego strength may call for different interventions by the group leader or transfer from one group to another or from group therapy to another type of therapy.

Ego strength is determined by evaluating a person's history and his present behavior in life, by formal examination, and by assessing the quality of his interaction with the therapist. Three basic qualities are searched for: the ability to constructively alter one's environment, the assumption of appropriate responsibility for one's self and others, and the

assumption of different roles toward one's self and others as needed to meet the present demands of life (Weiner, 1982). These qualities encompass impulse control, including the ability to tolerate emotional tension and to delay gratification. They are evidenced by a history of success in endeavors which require concentration and assumption of personal responsibility, such as school and work, and the establishment and maintenance of positive, cooperative, and intimate relationships as boss, underling, child, friend, lover, spouse, or parent.

A candidate's compatibility with the group must also be considered. A highly functioning neurotic would probably be quite uncomfortable in a group of marginally coping people, just as a chronic schizophrenic would feel ill at ease in a group of highly interactive, socially skilled persons. The interaction of personalities, level of intelligence, psychological-mindedness, and cultural variables must also be considered.

The third aspect of patient selection for groups is how well the candidate will be able to work in the group at the time he is available to enter the group. The nature of the group and the events in the life of the group are relevant here. If a new member enters as rage is building toward the group leader, it may be displaced onto the new member. If he enters too soon after the departure of an important group member, the group may be too involved in grieving or in denying the loss to be able to accept a new member.

DEVELOPING STRUCTURE

The therapist establishes the communicational structure of the group (Kadis et al., 1963) (see Figure A.7-1).

Professionally led repressive and ego-supportive groups often have vertical or triangular communication. In these groups, interaction with the leader is the most important therapeutic element; the interaction with other group members is of less importance. As a consequence, the strongest bond is to the leader. Although group members develop skills in coping, leadership does not emerge from within the group. This type of leadership is generally adopted by an authoritarian or charismatic leader. Virtually all therapy groups begin with vertical or triangular communication and revert to this type of communication in

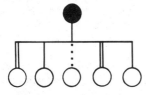

1. Vertical Communication,
   Leader-centered Group

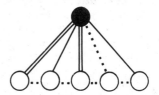

2. Triangular Communication,
   Leader-centered Group

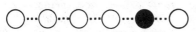

3. Horizontal Communication,
   Authority-denying Group

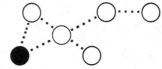

4. Unstructured Communication,
   Authority-denying Group

Figure A.7-1   Types of group communication.

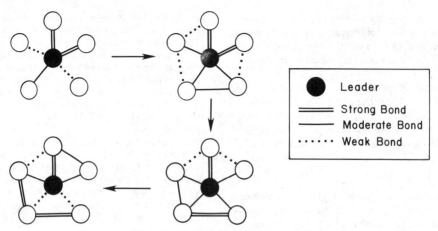

Figure A.7-2   Evolution of bonding in group-centered group with circular communication.

times of stress or at times when the leader feels that his control of the group is threatened.

Horizontal communication is typical of unorganized groups or groups in which the designated leader is unable to assume the leadership role and no leadership has emerged from within the group. Bion's (1961) basic assumption group is an example of this type of group interaction. Status-denying leaders also tend to stimulate this type of interaction (Robertiello, 1972).

Many different types of groups have circular communication. Repressive, ego-supportive, and evocative groups may all employ circular communication to encourage interaction and interdependence of group members. The therapist may foster circular communication by taking a back seat after establishing a group norm of member interaction or may implement it by actively encouraging members to react to each other. Circular communication can be used to hold the group at any psychological level from advice giving to free association.

Circular communication stimulates strong emotional ties and emotional reactions between group members (see Figure A.7-2). This means that multiple transferences may occur, that social relationships are prone to develop, and that the ties of group members to one another may become stronger than their ties to the leader. This type of group interaction may be difficult for the leader who feels that he must occupy the central position in the group or be in charge of the group interaction at all times, because group members will temporarily emerge as leaders as they become more comfortable with their assertiveness, and the group will begin to challenge the leader who allows his group members to unite. The advantage of circular group communication is its stimulation of the members to depend on themselves and each other.

MANAGING G-RESPONSES

The therapist must anticipate and deal with G-responses, the ubiquitous reactions of groups which can obstruct or augment the therapeutic process.

All groups tend toward homeostasis, an empathic consensus between group members which establishes the least anxiety-provoking manner in which they can operate together. Homeostasis is allowed to develop when group tensions are running too high and is actively opposed by the therapist when the group's comfort seeking interferes with its work. Group climate refers to the type of homeostasis at which the group arrives or to the predominant mood or activity of the group over the course of a few sessions. A group can develop an intellectualizing climate as the result of the leader's emphasis on cognitive understanding, or it can develop a climate in which emotions are readily experienced or acted upon. The group can develop hostile or friendly climates or climates of uninvolvement or intense emotional interdependence. Group homeostasis and climate are constantly modified by the interaction of the leader with the group and also change in reaction to the material with which the group deals.

Cohesion is the group members' sense of belonging, their loyalty to each other, and their willingness to work together and assume responsibility for one another in pursuit of their common goals. Group cohesion can block or facilitate change. The group can unite against the leader, or it can establish emotional bonds between members that block appropriate feedback. The leader attempts to stimulate cohesion at the beginning of group and at times when the intactness of the group is threatened; he does so by pointing out concerns and attitudes common to many group members.

Displacement of aggression may take the form of intense attacks on the therapist or on other group members. This displacement occurs when the object of several group members' hostility cannot be dealt with directly, because group members fear losing that person's approval or fear that they will destroy him or her. The group's anger is displaced onto a less-valued member who symbolizes some aspect of the person or situation that stimulates the hostility. It is the responsibility of the leader to detect such displacements when they occur and to decide whether to allow the displacement to continue or to interrupt it by clarification, confrontation, or interpretation.

Group members of low status who are disliked by others in the group frequently bear the brunt of hostility whose original aim was the leader or a more valued or influential group member. It is the leader's task to see that the group's anger is directed properly and in such a way that it serves a constructive purpose. Unfortunately, many people who suffer as scapegoats actively volunteer for the role by encouraging hostile or demeaning attitudes toward them. In these instances, the leader must also recognize the behavior of the scapegoat as a provocateur. At times, the leader must actively interfere with the group's expression of anger toward a scapegoated member or come between the group and the provocateur whose active masochism conceals his passive sadism toward other group members.

Plateauing is the tendency of the group to advance rapidly and then stall for a period of time, as though each breakthrough is followed by heightened resistance at the new level of function. Plateauing may be a function of resistance or may be a new level of homeostasis for the group. It is the leader's job to distinguish between the two and to react accordingly.

DEALING WITH RESISTANCES

A resistance is anything that slows or subverts the therapeutic process. The group resistances found in the therapeutic groups are group silence, social conversation, advice giving, labeling, and subgrouping. Resistances shared in common with individual therapy are transference and acting out.

Group silences are best managed by asking direct questions of group members and by then asking other group members to respond to the answers given. When the leader begins questioning a group member during a period of silence, he may pick a neutral topic, such as an account of recent events in the member's life, or may ask how he or she reacts to the silence in the group.

Social conversations in a group can be managed by gently changing the subject to one more appropriate for the group.

Advice giving and labeling of certain behaviors as games with payoffs are useful aspects of group treatment which can become resistances to deeper penetration into intrapsychic and interpersonal issues. When they become resistances, the leader points out that the group members can deal best with the emotional issues by allowing themselves to react emotionally to what is happening in the group, instead of giving advice or labeling each other's behavior. Advice giving and labeling can also be minimized by encouraging group members to associate to events in the group or to fantasize about other group members.

Subgrouping may be a subtle resistance, and the group leader may not become aware of the formation of a subgroup until after it has become deeply entrenched. Subgrouping is disruptive to the therapeutic process because the relationship between several members of the group goes on out of the view of the group as a whole and, therefore, cannot be dealt with. Subgrouping is dealt with by identifying the special relationship between several of the group members. Whether or not a special tie is acknowledged, the subgrouping members are reminded of one of the basic group rules—that all communication between group members outside the group is important and needs to be brought up in the group.

Transference is a source of significant resistance in groups. Depending on his approach, the leader may reinforce, circumvent, explain, interpret, or ignore transferences. Generally speaking, transferences are left alone as long as they facilitate progress. Thus, the transference expectation that the therapist will help and the transference-based perception of the therapist as accepting and understanding are usually uninterpreted. When the transference leads a group member to expect that the group and the therapist will accept any kind of behavior, it must be dealt with. Generally speaking, the therapist reinforces the positive transference and minimizes negative transferences in repressive and ego-supportive therapies, while the entire range of transferences may be challenged in an evocative group. Transferences occur to the leader and to all the other members of the group, with varying degrees of intensity. The leader has an additional therapeutic tool for dealing with transference in group therapy; the reactions of other group members who can serve distorted perceptions and overdetermined emotional reactions.

Acting out is a compulsive, repetitive behavior based on transference and on impulses stirred up in treatment (Langs, 1973). There is much more potential for acting out in group therapy because of emotional contagion, because of multiple transferences and identifications with other group members, and because members of a therapeutic group are not under as close scrutiny as patients seen individually. Acting out differs from taking advantage of a group as a social or sexual outlet. Acting out is based on unconscious resistance. As such, it cannot be dealt with solely through establishing a therapeutic contract forbidding certain kinds of behavior. Acting out can only be dealt with by psychological means if group members have sufficient ego strength and impulse control to integrate the relevant information. The rapidity with which transferences and acting out develop is an important clue about group members' ego strength; the more rapidly they develop, the less strong the person's ego, unless the therapist is actively promoting their development. For example, sexual activity between therapist and patient is more often a function of the therapist's interpersonal vulnerability than the patient's seductiveness (Dahlberg, 1970). Acting out should be suspected when group members' behavior together is unreported, concealed, or violates some aspect of the group contract.

When the leader detects antitherapeutic activity in repressive groups, he explains that it is antitherapeutic and curtails it if possible. In ego-supportive groups, its compulsive quality and interpersonal significance are made the issue. In an evocative group, the behavior is dealt with through clarification, confrontation, and, finally, by interpretation of its genetic significance.

DEALING WITH EVENTS IN THE GROUP'S LIFE

Ongoing groups develop a group life, and the events in the life of the group, such as changes in status of the group members and the addition and loss of members, become part of the group process.

The leader bears the primary responsibility for integrating new members into the group and for helping to avoid premature termination. To minimize dropouts, adequate support should be available during the period of introduction into the group. In some cases, it is useful to introduce two new members at once as a means to reduce their sense of isolation. Other group members will require individual sessions to help them acculturate.

The therapist should allow the group time to reintegrate following periods of crisis and should avoid introducing new members at times of high group tension. If this cannot be avoided, it may be useful to orient a potential new member to the problem with which the group is struggling before he enters the group.

The Leader's Problems

The leader's problems include awareness and use of his own personality and style of leadership, dealing with crises in the life of the group, managing G-responses in such a way that the group task is facilitated, dealing with transference and countertransference issues, and dealing with his own personal needs as they are stimulated by outside events or events in the life of the group.

STYLE

Style refers to the quality of the therapist's behavior in the group and the quality of interaction he stimulates or allows. Usually, the therapist's style is more strongly related to his personality and his personal needs than his theoretical orientation (Yalom, 1975). Narcissistic or interpersonally needy therapists find means to become the center of attention of their groups and have difficulty tolerating alternate sessions. One such therapist encouraged alternate sessions which were to be held in his office but forgot to unlock the door for 3 consecutive weeks. Dependent therapists turn to the group for support of their decisions. Authoritarian therapists impose their judgments and formulations on their groups.

Co-therapists can help to keep therapy on the right track. Interpersonally needy therapists may use co-therapists to diminish the effects of their social hunger on the group. Authoritarian persons can use co-therapists to mitigate the force of their personalities. New therapists can use co-therapists to help them develop expertise and also to help

become aware of their interpersonal and intrapsychic blind spots.

Group therapists are more prone to adopt a self-disclosing style than individual psychotherapists. This is in some measure due to the differences in personality of therapists who are drawn toward group psychotherapy, who may have greater interpersonal needs and greater exhibitionistic tendencies than individual therapists and may worry less about therapeutic exactness. Feeling much kinship with his group, feeling need for others, and being less occupied with transference-countertransference issues, the group therapist tends to more readily lower the therapeutic barrier (Tarachow, 1963).

The pertinent issues with regard to self-disclosure are not how much or how little but what kind and under what circumstances. Leader disclosingness in therapy groups does not enhance disclosure by group members (Weiner et al., 1974). Appropriately timed self-disclosures of the leader's reactions to group members in the here and now seem to have positive value, as do occasional personal disclosures by the leader which convey respect and trust to group members and which help augment their reality testing (Weiner, 1978). Therapists of adolescents and adolescent groups also report that a modicum of personal openness about one's own feelings in the group and during one's own adolescence are useful in facilitating positive identification and enhancing trust (Weiner and King, 1971).

Much attention has been paid to the triad of therapist-offered conditions of accurate empathy, nonpossessive warmth, and genuineness as the *sine qua non* of successful psychotherapy (Truax and Mitchell, 1971). In a recent reappraisal, Mitchell et al. (1977) found that the accumulated data neither support nor reject the overriding influence of these three variables. They undoubtedly contribute positively in many cases, but their potency and generalizability are not as great as once thought.

Whitehorn and Betz (1954) proposed an A-B variable that distinguished therapists who were successful in the psychotherapy of schizophrenic patients from therapists who were unsuccessful with schizophrenics. Type A therapists were willing to become involved at a personal level with their patients and responded to them as people, while Type B therapists held themselves aloof and responded in a detached impersonal fashion. Further research indicates that there are real A-B differences in therapists; A's are more socially marginal and more comfortable with verbal modalities, and B's deal better with language as a set of formal logical symbols and probably seek and enjoy cognitively complex activity, but the A-B variable does not predict any important process or outcome parameters in therapy (Razin, 1977).

At present, more is probably known about ineffective and damaging styles than about helpful styles. Sexual intimacy with patients is often damaging (Dahlberg, 1970); group leaders' failure to recognize people in their groups as individuals is highly frustrating and generally nonproductive; and studies of encounter groups show that group leaders who are highly intrusive, who offer little emotional support or cognitive framework, and who are controlling and highly idiosyncratic in their approach to persons in the group often damage people with little self-esteem, few coping skills, and high expectations of the group. Studies of other aspects of leadership style are offered by Gurman and Razin (1977).

DEALING WITH CHANGES IN STATUS

Changes in a member's status through marriage, divorce, bereavement, birth of a child, graduation from school, or gain or loss of a job, all affect the homeostasis and climate of the group.

Changes in status that are valued by other group members stimulate envy, competitive feelings, and hope. Losses in status of group members through being fired or laid off arouse fear of similar losses in other group members and may temporarily create a climate of hopelessness and helplessness in the group.

DEALING WITH REACTIONS TO SEPARATION AND LOSS

The group offers multiple opportunities to deal with other separations and losses in addition to the loss of the therapist. Anxiety over separation at vacation time or other absences of the therapist occurs in groups as in individual therapy but is cushioned by other group members' availability during this time. This separation anxiety is usually most marked at the time of the group's first scheduled absence from the leader.

If disruptive tension arises in relation to the group's first vacation from the leader, the leader can reduce the tension by explaining to the members that their uneasiness is a normal result of memories and feelings associated with significant past losses that everyone has experienced. If the group is able to tolerate the tensions generated, the leader can ask group members to discuss their feelings about the impending separation and their past experiences with separations and can ask group members to project themselves into the future and imagine themselves during the period of time in which the therapist will be gone and the group will be adjourned.

The leader also needs to anticipate the premature terminations that frequently occur in reaction to vacations and other separations. For this reason, many group therapists build a 4-week notification period into the therapeutic contract.

The loss of a group member, whether expected or unexpected, has wide repercussions in a group. If a member graduates, envy is stimulated, as well as fear of discharge from the group before sufficient independence has been achieved. If a member leaves without having made significant headway, group members wonder about the therapist's potency and can put the group leader on the defensive about his therapeutic abilities. It also tarnishes group members' omnipotent fantasies about the leader. Again, there is a significant tendency to avoid issues raised by the loss of the member who prematurely quits. At the time of a premature loss of a group member, it is imperative that the group leader deal with its effects

by helping the members to discuss their own thoughts about staying or leaving.

The most traumatic losses are due to death, especially death of a group member by suicide. Kibel (1973) suggests that the therapist deal with this type of crisis by sharing his grief, by increased activity, by structuring the group more highly, and by offering individual sessions as needed.

Other Factors

There are a number of therapeutic factors which give the group therapist extra leverage in dealing with his patients: group pressure, multiple interaction, feedback, multiple identification, multiple transference, reactive association, and carom.

It has long been known and is well objectified (Asch, 1955) that group pressure can strongly modify group members' behavior and judgment, depending on the attractiveness of group members to one another, the extent to which they value each other's approval, and the pressures the group members can bring to bear on one another. The therapist can bring group pressures to bear by simply encouraging the interaction of group members. When working in schools, prisons, or hospitals, the therapist must be aware that certain group norms will interfere with the progress of the group, and he may have to develop a core of group members whose norms differ significantly from the prevailing norms in the institution before much headway can be made.

Multiple interaction brings each member's characteristic interpersonal behavior into the group. As each member becomes himself in a social sense, there is opportunity for feedback by other group members about the effect of each member's behavior on the others in the group. Promoting this type of awareness is extremely important in dealing with character pathology and with the secondary gain of neurotic symptoms.

As a consequence of multiple interaction, multiple identifications and multiple transferences develop. Identifications and transferences which are positive and which can be well integrated are unchallenged. Those which are defensive or destructive are challenged. Group therapy offers multiple objects for identification and transference development in the therapeutic situation, thus broadening the opportunity for emotional growth and for conflict resolutions.

The leader may press for reactive associations when emotionally loaded subjects arise in groups. The reactive associations of other group members illuminate the problems of all other members of the group, as well as the protagonist of the moment. When an emotionally hot subject arises, he asks each member's reactions at a level appropriate for that group at that point in time. The leader must also stay alert for caroms, in which comments or behavior of one person in the group have an impact on a member who was not part of the interaction. The vicarious therapeutic or harmful experience can go unnoticed unless the leader pays careful attention to the nonverbal behavior of group members, including posture, facial expression, and alterations of the seating arrangement.

The Therapist's Management of Himself

The therapist as a person impinges significantly on the therapeutic process. The therapist's reactions and interventions are colored by his values, his personality, and his personal needs. The therapist is also affected by the emotional pushing and pulling of his patients. These difficulties are compounded in groups, because of the sheer number of interpersonal stimuli, the effect of group pressures on the leader, and the relatively exposed position of the group leader.

Through experiences as a group and individual therapist, life experiences, supervision, and personal therapy, group leaders become aware of their personalities and the impact of their personalities on others. The best information about the impact of the leader's personality on groups and the impact of groups on his personality comes from direct observation of his interaction in groups by a more senior co-leader or by a supervisor reviewing videotapes of the leader conducting a group. All therapists evolve a style of interaction with certain kinds of patients and certain kinds of groups. As a group leader in training becomes aware of his style, he develops a means for detecting unusual amounts of emotional pressure in the therapeutic situation. Departure from one's usual style of dealing with certain types of people and situations indicates to the leader that he must search himself and his interaction with the patient carefully to detect the source of the emotional pressure (or lack of pressure) and to ascertain if his change of style is therapeutic, antitherapeutic, or irrelevant. In addition to changes in therapeutic style, there are other indications of unusual types or degrees of involvement by the therapist, such as preoccupation with or indifference toward certain group members and recurrent dreams about them. In this situation, the therapist's mental checklist should be: (1) What is the nature of my reaction? (2) What am I reacting to in the patient or group? (3) What am I reacting to in me? Personal values? Personal need? Countertransference? (4) Does my behavior need to be altered? (5) If it needs to be altered, in what way?

As the therapist grows professionally, he becomes aware of his vulnerabilities and attempts to deal with them or compensate for them, sometimes by using a co-therapist, sometimes by referring patients to other therapists, sometimes by seeking personal treatment in supervision.

One category of patients, the borderline personality, invariably creates emotional storms in their groups and their therapists as they project unacceptable parts of themselves onto others and then react against these disowned, projected attributes. An emotional storm in the therapist can be a valuable clue to the presence of a borderline patient in his group. Other sensitivities occur because of events in the therapist's personal life. However, there are many times at which emotional reaction of the therapist to the patient is an appropriate response to the material he is presented.

The therapist must also be aware of the ways in which his group members conform or fail to conform to his cherished values, whether they be education, upward motility, or interest in automobiles or athletics.

Finally, the therapist must develop sufficient tools for self-exploration that he can recognize countertransference, the stirring up of his own unconscious conflicts by members of a group. The source of countertransference reactions can be sought in his dreams, the quality of his behaviors and feelings toward the person(s) in question, the therapist's associations, and the types of fantasy the therapist can produce in relation to him or them.

If the therapist's countertransference feelings do not alter his behavior with the patient(s) in group in question, nothing needs to be done for the sake of the patient. The therapist, on the other hand, may wish to satisfy his curiosity or alleviate his own discomfort, which he can do by introspection, by discussing his feelings with a colleague, or by seeking supervision or personal therapy.

If the therapist is behaving in a way which he regards as nontherapeutic and cannot alter his behavior, he has many routes of action. He can call his behavior to the group members' attention and ask for their reaction as a means to help him understand. He can videotape and review his session with the group, by himself, with peers, or with a supervisor. He can acquire a co-leader. He can seek supervision or personal therapy; or, if all else fails, he can transfer the patient or group to another therapist.

The therapist owes himself and his patients a satisfying life for himself outside of the office. Otherwise, he is overly vulnerable to his own needs and to the transference expectations of his group.

Conclusion

There are enormous technical and emotional complexities in leading therapeutic groups. Before undertaking the treatment of groups, prospective group leaders should have a grasp of individual psychopathology, the pathology of interpersonal relationships, and some knowledge of normal psychological and interpersonal development.

To be an effective group therapist, a prospective group leader must develop an appreciation of normal behavior in social and work groups and of levels of intervention as they relate to ego strength and dynamic or descriptive diagnosis. He must also learn how to deal with events in group life in such a way as to further the progress of his group at an appropriate psychological level.

Mature self-awareness is another important asset of the group leader, and includes awareness of one's strengths and liabilities, and a willingness to seek a co-leader, consultation, supervision, or personal therapy when needed. The active cultivation of non-work-related interests is also of benefit to therapist and group members alike. It ensures a balanced view of the group and of life by the therapist, and thereby promotes a balanced treatment in which the treatment needs of the group members and the personal needs of the therapists do not become confused.

References

Alexander, F., and French, T. M. *Psychoanalytic Therapy: Principles and Application.* Ronald Press, New York, 1946.

Asch, S. E. Opinions and social pressure. Sci. Am., *193:* 31, 1955.

Berne, E. *Games People Play.* Grove Press, New York, 1964.

Berne, E. *Principles of Group Treatment.* Oxford University Press, New York, 1966.

Bion, W. R. *Experiences in Groups.* Basic Books, New York, 1961.

Dahlberg, C. C. Sexual contact between patient and therapist. J. Contemp. Psychoanal. *6:* 107, 1970.

Grotjahn, M. Growth experience in the leader. In *The Leader in the Group,* Z. Liff, editor, p. 146. Jason Aronson, New York, 1975.

Gurman, A. S., and Razin, A. M., editors. *Effective Psychotherapy: A Handbook of Research,* Pergamon Press, New York, 1977.

Kadis, A. L., Krasner, J., Weiner, M. F., and Winick, C. *Practicum of Group Psychotherapy.* Harper & Row, New York, 1974.

Kadis, A. L., Krasner, J. D., Winick, C., and Foulkes, S. H. *Practicum of Group Psychotherapy.* Harper & Row, New York, 1963.

Kibel, H. D. A group member's suicide: Treating collective trauma. Int. J. Group Psychother., *22:* 42, 1973.

Langs, R. J. *The Technique of Psychoanalytic Psychotherapy,* vol. 1. Jason Aronson, New York, 1973.

Mitchell, K. M., Bozarth, J. D., and Krauft, C. C. A reappraisal of the therapeutic effectiveness of accurate empathy, nonpossessive warmth, and genuineness. In *Effective Psychotherapy: A Handbook of Research,* A. S. Gurman and A. M. Razin, editors, p. 482. Pergamon Press, New York, 1977.

Razin, A. M. The A-B variable: Still promising after twenty years? In *Effective Psychotherapy: A Handbook of Research,* A. S. Gurman and A. M. Razin, editors, p. 291. Pergamon Press, New York, 1977.

Robertiello, R. C. The leader in a "leaderless" group. Psychother. Theory Res. Prac., *9:* 259, 1972.

Strupp, H. A reformation of the dynamics of the therapist's contribution. In *Effective Psychotherapy: A Handbook of Research,* A. S. Gurman and A. M. Razin, editors, p. 3. Pergamon Press, New York, 1977.

Tarachow, S. *Introduction to Psychotherapy.* International Universities Press, New York, 1963.

Truax, C. B., and Mitchell, K. M. Research in certain therapist skills in relation to process and outcome. In *Handbook of Psychotherapy and Behavior Change,* A. E. Bergin and S. L. Garfield, editors, p. 299. John Wiley & Sons, New York, 1971.

Weiner, M. F. Levels of intervention in group psychotherapy. Group Process, *3:* 67, 1970.

Weiner, M. F. *The Psychotherapeutic Impasse.* Free Press, New York, 1982.

Weiner, M. F., Cody, V. F., and Rosson, B. Studies of patient and therapist affective self-disclosure. Group Process, *6:* 27, 1974.

Weiner, M. F., and King, J. S. Self-disclosure by the therapist to the adolescent patient. In *Adolescent Psychiatry,* P. Giovacchini and S. Feinstein, editors, p. 499. Basic Books, New York, 1971.

Whitehorn, J. C., and Betz, B. A study of psychotherapeutic relationships between physicians and schizophrenic patients. Am. J. Psychiatry, *3:* 321, 1954.

Wolf, A., and Schwartz, E. K. *Psychoanalysis in Groups.* Grune & Stratton, New York, 1962.

Yalom, I. D. *The Theory and Practice of Group Psychotherapy,* ed. 2. Basic Books, New York, 1975.

A.8 Indigenous Healing Groups

ARMANDO R. FAVAZZA, M.D.
AHMED DAVER FAHEEM, M.D.

Introduction

Since physical and mental disorders are found in every culture, it is not surprising that efforts to heal these disorders are also ubiquitous. In technologically advanced societies, many persons with severe disorders seek a cure or relief from symptoms by engaging in a dyadic relationship with a health professional who utilizes a scientific approach (such as a physician, nurse, or psychologist), although the services of pseudoscientists (such as chiropractors) may also be utilized. Persons with less serious "disorders" sometimes may seek help from folk, religious, or "pop" healers; some utilize purely supernaturalistic approaches, some practice a mixture of scientific and supernaturalistic approaches, and others practice unorthodox, sometimes bizarre healing methods, often under the rubric of "humanism" or "holistic health" (Gaviria and Wintrob, 1979).

In cultures where the Western, scientific outlook prevails, diagnosis and treatment are usually a private, individual matter between the patient and the health professional. The paradigm is exemplified at its most extreme by a few rigid psychoanalysts who refuse to speak with anyone other than the patient. In Western cultures, a group setting is usually considered inappropriate for purposes of diagnosis but may be utilized for treatment, e.g., mental health professionals may bring strangers together for group therapy. Network therapy involving "natural" groups holds great promise for the future. Self-help groups where persons with similar conditions share experiences and provide support and advice are quite popular; most were formed either by health professionals or by patients in consultation with a health professional, and most have written principles and guidelines.

In cultures where Western science is not paramount, both diagnosis and treatment are often a public, group matter involving not only the patient and healer but also the patient's family, social network members, and his entire community. The origins of indigenous healing groups are usually obscure, and rarely, if ever, do these groups have any written materials.

Three indigenous healing groups in disparate cultures will be described in this chapter: the Guardian Spirit ceremonial of the Coast Salish (North America); the dream groups of the Senoi (Malaysia); and the zar cults (Ethiopia, the Nile Valley, and Iran). These groups have been selected because, together, they demonstrate a wide range of healing practices.

The Guardian Spirit Ceremonial of the Salish Indians

For years, Native Americans have been subjected to an unwelcome challenge to their traditional ways by the white man. They have been forced to adopt alien ways under the name of progress and to give up their long-held beliefs and traditions, sometimes under the threat of legal punishment. This has frequently led the native population to confusion and identity crises, with resulting emotional difficulties such as depression, alcoholism, anxiety, and criminal and aggressive behavior.

After years of oppression and turmoil, Native Americans have started to revive their old traditions, to reestablish their old identity, and to use indigenous methods of dealing with their emotional problems. The Salish Winter Dance is one such revived Indian tradition which has been transformed in modern times. The ceremonial uses group dynamics to heal troubled tribal members. By symbolically experiencing death and rebirth, each dancer undergoes a process of personality depatterning and reorientation and emerges with a new and healthy identity. The Salish are natives of the upper Frazer Valley of British Columbia. The group under consideration here numbers about 2,000 persons who live in the upper Stalo region.

THE TRADITION OF THE SALISH WINTER DANCE

The Guardian Spirit Complex is an ancient phenomenon of considerable cultural and psychological significance for the many Native American societies. The winter spirit dance was the major ritual involving the Guardian Spirit Complex of the Salish-speaking people and was considered to strengthen the vitality of the people. Winter was considered the most appropriate time for ceremonies concerning the guardian spirits who arrive and depart with the cold season.

Spirit dancing was outlawed in Washington Territory by decree of the Superintendent of Indian Affairs in 1871 under the threat of prosecution, disgrace, and punishment. The ceremonial was considered a vestige of a bygone age of barbarism.

The following discussion is based on Jilek's excellent monograph (1974).

Revival of spirit dancing

The resurgence of spirit dancing on the Indian reserves of the upper Stalo region started in 1967–1968. There have been many changes in the original ceremony and its organization. English has been substituted for the original Salish language for important communications. Fundamental to the North American Guardian Spirit Complex is the vision experience as a means of obtaining and controlling supernatural power. The vision experience is obtained by producing an altered state of consciousness. Obtaining this altered state of consciousness is very much dependent upon the subject's motivation, as well as by situational and sociocultural factors, but may be facilitated by certain conditions and techniques effecting temporary changes of brain function.

Conditions playing a major role in the production of altered states of consciousness in the traditional Salish Guardian Spirit quest are: social isolation associated with prolonged nocturnal vigilence, expectant alertness, and monotony; motor hyperactivity and mental excitation associated with prolonged fear and emotional stress and followed by exhaustion and fatigue; sleep deprivation; hypoglycemia induced by fasting; dehydration due to fasting, sweating, purgation, and forced vomiting; hypoxemia due to hyperventilation from prolonged diving; exposure to extreme temperatures from bathing in ice cold water; and self-inflicted painful stimuli.

Spirit illness

The advent of the winter dance season is heralded by the sickening of those who have acquired dancing power. They become anorectic, insomnic, distraught, weak, and emaciated. Several therapeutic measures are prescribed for the cure of winter illness. The patient must sponsor a spirit dance during which the therapist summons the patient's guardian spirit. The patient then demonstrates his spirit's powers by singing, dancing, and ritual acts. Subsequent winter illnesses are diagnosed by the patient himself and require public exhibition of the spirit power by its owner in the dance ceremony.

In examining the symptomatology of contemporary spirit illness, Jilek (1974) introduced the concept of anomic depression, defined as "a chronic dysphoric state, characterized by feelings of existential frustration, discouragement, defeat, lowered self esteem and sometimes moral disorientation." He indicated that this state is often the basis of the specific psychic and psychophysiological symptoms manifested by contemporary sufferers of spirit illness.

The symptomatology of contemporary spirit illness resembles that of neurotic depression. It includes anorexia, insomnia, apathy alternating with restlessness, dysphoric moods with crying spells and nostalgic despondency, somatizations (usually pain), and sometimes also conversion reactions (paralysis and fainting spells). In the foreground of the syndrome is the melancholic aspect of spirit illness. The depressive reaction appears often to be triggered or aggravated by mourning for deceased ancestors and for the golden age of the Indian past. Nostalgic and melancholic ruminations of this type preoccupy the patient's mind more and more as the spirit illness progresses.

Symptoms peculiar to spirit illness as manifested today are: singing and hollering during sleep; hallucinations or illusional perceptions with a culture-specific content, e.g., visions of guardian spirits, deceased dancers, ceremonial paraphernalia and acts, or hearing of spirit songs; and dyspnea with sighing respiration (a culture-specific explanation for this symptom is the supernaturally caused lack of air around the patient).

Spirit illness is generally considered to be potentially contagious and can be contracted through close contact with a powerful spirit dancer.

THE THERAPEUTIC PROCESS OF CONTEMPORARY SPIRIT DANCE INITIATION

Death-and-rebirth is the central theme of the spirit dance initiation, expressed through the professed purpose of the initiate "finding his song and dance." The initiator is a healer who, by the power of a Guardian Spirit, symbolically "clubs to death" the initiate's faulty and diseased self in order to awaken in him the potential for total change and to guide him on the path of Indian tradition. The initiate is named and treated as a baby who is fed, dressed, constantly attended, and guarded by "babysitters." In this state of complete infantile dependency, in the quasiuterine shelter of the dark long house cubicle, the initiate hatches his power and prepares to grow with it into a more rewarding existence.

In the process of initiation, three major therapeutic approaches are used: (1) personality depatterning through alternating sensory overload and deprivation, (2) physical training, and (3) indoctrination.

Personality depatterning and reorientation

The candidate is kept in the long house, and is secluded in a dark cubicle usually for a period of 10 days. The length of this seclusion (which, after 4 days of passive endurance, is interrupted by frequent strenuous exercises) varies with candidates and ritualists. It seems to depend mainly on the novice's motivation and his—unconscious or conscious—cooperation in "finding his song and dance."

Personality depatterning starts with an initial shock treatment known as "clubbing," "grabbing," or "doctoring up" of the candidate and is aimed at rapid induction of an altered state of consciousness. Often there is a temporary loss of consciousness. Various methods used to facilitate this include sudden bodily seizures, immobilization by physical restraint, blindfolding, various forms of tactile and kinetic stimulation (such as hitting, biting, and tickling the initiate while he is simultaneously uplifted, lowered, swayed, and whirled about), and auditory stimulation by loud drumming, singing, and howling in the initiate's ears. This treatment is administered by teams of eight workers under the supervision of the initiator who signals orders by shaking his ceremonial staff. This "grabbing" procedure is repeated at least four times. Each time the workers complete four circles around the long house hall with their candidate, whose moaning cries become progressively weaker until he appears lifeless, pale, and rigid when finally bedded in the cubicle.

When the black-painted ceremonial workers seize him, the candidate is touched or "marked" with a ceremonial staff wielded by the initiator or his assistant. Although this is not more than a gesture, merely imitating the "clubbing to death" of a victim, some candidates immediately fall into motionless rigidity. It appears that these candidates had previously showed signs of very severe spirit illness and that they derived a certain prestige from their instant initiation. They usually sing and dance as soon as they wake up from this "death."

Through the 4 days of the depatterning phase, the initiate is blindfolded; he has to lie still and is forbidden to talk or to move even in sleep or when sweating under his heavy covers on the fringes of which sit the "babysitters" or "watchmen." He is starved, and his fluid intake is restricted; at the same time he is "teased" and "tested" with tasty salmon bits held close to his mouth. Every day he is again exposed to the initial shock of the "grabbing" procedure in order to make him "die" again. These maneuvers aim at bringing forth the novice's song.

This strict regime is continued until the initiate "gets his song straight"—usually within 4 days. He is then duly invested with the traditional uniform, hat, and stick in sign of his rebirth. The Guardian Spirit itself appears in a dream to the novice in the smokehouse cubicle, or in a visionary experience during the training which follows the initiate's investiture.

Physical training

The phase of physical training is associated with intense indoctrination and is supposed to "make the newborn baby strong." It lasts for at least 1 week and consists of daily runs around the smokehouse hall or outside, often barefoot in snow; daily swimming in ice cold water; and frequent rounds of dancing to exhaustion in the smokehouse.

The initiates feel their newly acquired power when their song bursts forth from them and the leaping steps of their first dance carry them through the long house, spurred on by the drums and the chanting and clapping of the crowd.

Didactic aspects of spirit dance

The theoretical indoctrination of spirit dancing includes the direct teaching of the rules and sanctions of the Guardian Spirit, the recounting of spirit lore, presenting examples of the works of the spirits, and presentation of cultural propaganda.

Ceremonial speakers display considerable skill in suggestive psychotherapy. When teaching the new dances, the ritualists speak with ancestoral spiritual authority, instilling in the initiate a sense of personal responsibility toward his elders and his people. The new dancer must maintain the secrecy of the ceremony and faithfully observe the ceremonial by attending as many dances as he can. Of utmost therapeutic importance is the prohibition of alcohol intake, and also of smoking and of taking illicit drugs.

Observance of general and individual ceremonial rules is enforced by both social and supernatural sanctions. During the initiation period, the "babysitters" or "watchmen" supervise the novice's behavior and also protect him. Group pressure is probably even more important. A novice who reneges by leaving the ceremony and by breaking the rules is not only inviting supernatural retaliation but also rejection by his group; all kinds of social troubles—which he invariably gets into—are expected. If a young dancer continues to misbehave, his sponsors warn him they are going to invite people to *Potlach*, where prominent leaders will elaborate on his wrongdoings and "preach" to him, which is felt to be a public shame.

The initiation process ends with a disrobing ceremony. The new dancer dresses in his initiation garb until the end of the season during which he was "grabbed." The therapeutic implication of this ceremony is that it documents the candidate's successful cure from spirit illness. Together with his uniform, the initiate sheds the last vestiges of his old personality. The new dancer is presented to the public as yet another example of the healing and regenerating power of the Guardian Spirits. Not until 4 years after initiation does a person become fully established and considered capable of assuming important roles in the initiation procedures.

Volunteers with or without spirit illness are considered as candidates, as are all those who show apparent symptoms of spirit illness. Antisocial acting out, alcohol or drug abuse, and mistreatment of one's spouse are behavioral problems which may be considered indications for initiation. Mockery of the ceremony or its participants is also felt to be an indication, as is being the spouse of a participant, especially if other indications are present.

In spite of the stressful procedures to which the novices are subjected, no serious accidents during the initiation procedures were described by Jilek.

ANNUAL WINTER THERAPY

The holding of spirit dances throughout the winter is valuable for the active dancers and also benefits the entire local population. Active participation is expected from the audience, drawing them into the therapeutic enterprise. Winter is a time of high unemployment, increased family and marital conflict, and increased alcohol and drug abuse. This results in increased demand for medical attention. The winter spirit dance incorporates the techniques of group psychotherapy, cathartic abreaction, psychodrama, direct ego support, and physical exercise.

Several observers have underlined the psychotherapeutic role of spirit dancing. There is unanimous group support for the participants, who often manifest a violent expression of anguish and despair.

The principles of group therapy are operant in spirit dancing in that it provides the participant with support, protection, acceptance, and stimulation. The participant is turned from egocentric preoccupations to collective concerns and the pursuit of collective goals. Group solidarity is stressed in speeches during ceremonial gatherings. Nondancing participants are involved in organizing the dances, making uniforms, providing meals, and tending the fires. Many drum, sing, shield the dancers from the fire, or help them back to their seats. Those in the audience clap hands or beat sticks in time with the dancer's chant. They all share in the responsibility of satisfying the Guardian Spirit.

Cathartic abreaction occurs as the dancer enters an altered state of consciousness and relives the coming of his song, which then breaks forth from him in a tremendous affective and motor discharge. The dancers may tremble, sob, moan, and perform various gestures in the course of their abreaction, with the active support of an interested and helpful audience. This helps the dancer learn to accept his emotions and, at the same time, to control them.

Dramatic acting out of affect through the personification of supernatural beings who are culturally available has been utilized for psychotherapeutic purpose in many cultures. The choreographic drama of the spirit dance is a form of therapeutic psychodrama by virtue of its combination with a cathartic abreaction in an appropriate group setting.

The positive attention which the ritual leaders and the people focus on the active dancers provides direct ego support. There is increased public recognition and acceptance of the dancers, and a subjective sense of pride and well-being as the spirit powers afford the owner protection, good luck, and success. The belief that the spirits can easily be offended by neglect or infringement of the ceremonial rules results in a genuine interest in preventing such behavior, and implies a personal responsibility towards one's group.

Physical exercise is offered by the rigorous training the active spirit dancers go through from fall to spring every year. This helps produce a subjective sense of physical and mental well-being.

THERAPEUTIC EFFECTIVENESS

Jilek concluded that for an Indian clientele the indigenous therapeutic procedures of the spirit dance are superior to Western methods in the management of two symptom complexes: (1) conditions of ill health with prominent psychoneurotic and psychophysiological components—these patients figure in Indian lore as miraculous cures after having been "in and out of hospitals, given up by doctors"; and (2) antisocial and aggressive behavior—this is often associated with alcohol or drug abuse and is emotionally or physically destructive to self and kin.

Spirit dancing also seems more helpful in treating Indians with alcohol problems than is Western medical and psychiatric treatment. The leading ritualists and some prominent participants are total abstainers, and most of the active spirit dancers abstain throughout the ceremonial season. All new dancers keep sobriety during the season of their initiation.

Inebriated persons are not permitted to attend ceremonials, even if they are not active dancers. This has generally discouraged Indian drinking in the upper Stalo region during wintertime. In addition, the culture propaganda associated with the winter spirit dance suggests involvement in off-season festivals, during the summer months. However, the majority of spirit dancers continue to consume liquor outside the ceremonial season. Most feel free to do so after their first year of participation in the ceremonial is over, although they generally reduce their intake compared to before their initiation. Indian Alcoholics Anonymous groups recognize the value of spirit dancing, and some senior participants recommend continued active participation for those with serious alcohol problems. Although some participants return to drinking and drug abuse, the spirit ceremonial provides most active dancers with sobriety for at least 5 months each year and reduces the risk of alcohol abuse in other participants.

At a time when the Indian population is in a state of disarray and depression, ceremonials like Salish spirit dancing take great importance in personality development and sociocultural identity formation, from which are derived feelings of social and emotional security. The Indian youth's quest for a Guardian Spirit, therefore, is a quest for his identity and meaning in life. Initiation is no longer only for the cure of a ritualized pathomorphic state, but helps to overcome sickness and faulty behaviors contracted by exposure to an alien culture through rebirth as a true Indian. This is the ritualist's message at the names-giving ceremony—part of the initiation process—in which the revival of ancestral names is solemnly proclaimed and witnessed.

What in the past was a ritual with psychohygienic aspects is now an organized Indian effort at culture-congenial psychotherapy. There appears to be a current general renaissance in group rituals as tribal leaders struggle with ways to counteract the widespread demoralization and poor health of Native Americans (Jilek, 1978).

Senoi Dream Groups

The Senoi are a tribe of about 12,000 persons who live in relative isolation in the central mountain range of the Malay Peninsula. They are thought to constitute the most tolerant and nonviolent society in the world with practically no crime or destructive conflicts (Dentan, 1968). The Senoi are also thought, from anecdotal reports, to have a low prevalence of chronic physical or mental disorders. Living in long community houses constructed of bamboo, rattan, and thatch, they guide their affairs on the principles of contract, agreement, and democratic consensus. All this is achieved by group interactions that produce high degrees of psychological integration, emotional maturity, social skills, and attitudes that promote creative, rather than destructive, interpersonal relations. The Senoi reportedly have no jails, no police force, and no hospitals or facilities for mental disturbed persons. They have no written language.

Senoi psychology is remarkable for its unique reliance on group dream interpretation and on dream expression in a cooperative reverie. The Senoi consider dreaming to be an adaptive process; every dream is thought to be a mental image of the external world and is a visual representation of a person's inner psychological concerns. Sometimes these images conflict with each other or with the basic psychosocial orientation of the dreamer. Once internalized, these conflictual, hostile images turn man against himself and against his fellows as manifested by physical, psychological, and social malfunctioning. Through the process of dream interpretation, however, the dreamer is able to confront his hostile images in a therapeutic manner.

Each morning, children are invited to recount the previous night's dreams to their parents, and adults discuss their own dreams with peers: " ... every dream symbol and situation is discussed ... every member of the group freely expresses his opinion as to its meaning ... and those who come to consensus act on the meaning of the dream which they accept in effecting some sort of group project" (Stewart, 1953). Thus, if a person dreams of a new type of hunting trap, the group members will help him to build it. Or, if he dreams of a song or poem, he is encouraged to express it to the group.

When a dream is interrupted because of anxiety, the Senoi believe that the dreamer must resolve his underlying fear, anger, or sexual desires. If a child, for example, is frightened into wakefulness by a dream about death or falling or travel, he is instructed to complete his dream in order to overcome his fears. Since all dreams have a purpose, the dreamer is instructed to relax and to enjoy himself, even if the dream is fearful. A dream of falling, for example, allows the dreamer to travel to the source of the spirit that has caused the fall. Upon encountering the falling spirit, the dreamer is expected to relax and to remain asleep, even though frightened, so that he may receive the spirit's power. A dream of dying is explained as an attempt by the dreamer's spirit to receive the powers of the other world. Thus, with this type of advice, praise, criticism, and social interaction, dreams of anxiety and terror become enjoyable experiences, and the fear of falling is transformed into the joy of flying.

If a person dreams of harming another person, then he must give a gift to that person while awake; conversely, if he is injured by another person in a dream, that person is expected to give the dreamer a gift. If he dreams of fighting a monster, he is instructed to dream of conquering the monster and to call upon his friends for assistance in the dream. The Senoi teach that a dreamer should always advance and attack when confronted by danger. The defeated monster then becomes a helpful spirit in later dreams.

Telling dreams to close friends, to casual acquaintances, or to persons who appear in the dreams is like giving a gift to them. Even when a dream places another person in a bad light, the person is usually happy to know about it and interacts with the dreamer in a positive way.

Some of the most significant dreams for the group are those dreamed by recognized leaders of ceremonial trance dances. These leaders invite dream characters to visit them during the trance dances and to provide guidance for personal and community actions. In the "cooperative reverie," a rite of passage from adolescence to adulthood, the young dreamer achieves the ability to accept dream characters. Often the dream characters will agree to appear only after the dreamer agrees to engage in some act that benefits the community as a whole.

The social and psychological processes involved in Senoi dream interpretations have been outlined by Stewart as follows:

1. Children receive social recognition and esteem for discovering and then publically relating their inner fears as manifested in dreams. As long as the child follows this procedure, he will be accepted by his peers, parents, and other adults, no matter how terrifying the dream content that he expresses.

2. The workings of the mind are rational rather than mysterious; this rationality is maintained during sleep as well as during wakefulness. Thus, a person should make decisions and arrive at resolutions in his nighttime thinking as well as in daytime.

3. The forces that are experienced in a dream can be controlled and directed if the dreamer relaxes and adopts an appropriate mental set. The person who publically reveals his dreams for the group to interpret is better able to control his life than is the person who conceals or represses his dreams.

4. Since dreams give rise to imaginative thinking and

creative activity, it is important to uncover and to eliminate any anxiety that interrupts the dream process.

Thus, the Senoi model of a good citizen is that of a person who maintains good will toward others and who communicates his waking thoughts and his dreaming thoughts to them for approval and for criticism. The Senoi dream group allows for open, verbal discussion of potentially conflictual thoughts and feelings. What results is a high degree of interpersonal cooperation and an apparent minimum of rivalry and strife.

Nubian Zar Groups

Zar refers to healing ceremony and to a class of spirits prevalent in Ethiopia, the Nile Valley, and some areas of Southern Iran (Kennedy, 1967; Saunders, 1977). Although there are geographic variations, the following account of Nubian zar ceremonies can be considered characteristic.

The purpose of zar ceremonies is to cure or to alleviate the symptoms of mental illness by dealing with the causative zar spirits which inhabit the patient. Most commonly, participants in zar ceremonies are women who, in Western terminology, are suffering from anxiety, somatoform disorders, mild depression, and chronic schizophrenia. Patients participate in zar ceremonies as a last resort. When the usual curing methods have failed, it is assumed that the patient's illness has a supernatural cause. The evil eye of envy, the breaking of taboos, and sorcery are all thought to produce mental illness associated with zar possession. Once it is determined that zar spirits are causing a disorder, the patient becomes inextricably associated with these spirits for the rest of her life and assumes a perpetual responsibility to satisfy her spirits by attending ceremonies for others and by participating in a special zar performance at least once a year.

A patient who suspects that she is possessed by zar spirits will consult a sheikh (male) or sheikha (female) who interrogates her and arrives at a presumptive diagnosis. If there is a general consensus that the patient's symptoms are most likely caused by zar possession, a zar ceremony is performed. A full ceremony lasts for 7 days, although shortened ceremonies may be held if the patient is unable to afford a full one or if her illness is mild or if she recovers quickly.

The zar ceremony is held in a large room or special enclosed arena. Although the leader, his assistants, and the musicians are usually men the ceremony is attended by current women patients, along with their female relatives and friends; by women who have been cured in the past and who are present to satisfy their spirits and to support the new patients; and by women who simply enjoy the ritual spectacle or who hope to receive answers to pressing personal questions.

There is a central stage area for the sheikh and his helpers. Doors and windows are closed, and the only light comes from lanterns. The room temperature is high to stimulate the spirits. The patient is dressed like a bride in new white clothes and jewelry. The room is filled with perfume and the smoky fragrance of incense.

Music and dancing are important elements of the Nubian zar ceremony. The sheikh begins the ceremony with songs and with drumming; each special song is associated with a particular zar spirit. Thus, members of the cult shake, dance, and often go into a trance when the song associated with their particular zar spirit is played. The sheikh goes into a trance during which his zar questions the patient's zar in order to certify an accurate diagnosis and to learn the name of the possessing zar. On behalf of the patient (who is also in a trance), the sheikh's zar demands that possessing zar leave the patient in peace and no longer cause her to be ill. Before her zar leaves, however, it usually demands special favors, such as new clothes, jewelry, and expensive foods. It is the duty of the patient's family to gather round the prostrate woman and to pacify her zar by granting its demands. Sometimes the patient gets to keep the goods demanded by her zar, although she may have to return some or all of them to her family and friends. She may lie on the floor for a brief time, as if dead, until a special song by the sheikh brings her back to consciousness. In addition to treating the patient(s), the sheikh also prescribes cures for audience members and tells their fortunes during the ceremony.

The zar ceremony ends with a ritual animal sacrifice. The animal's blood is rubbed on the patient's face and body; some blood is mixed with spices, henna, and water in a potion that the patient drinks. The animal is cooked for a feast, and then the patient leads the other possessed participants of the zar to the Nile River, where they all bathe.

Zar ceremonies fulfill many of the psychological and social needs of the participants. They serve as a socially sanctioned safety valve and are an accepted method for wish fulfillment. The demands of the patient's zar represent items that the patient's husband has not provided and that he normally would not give to her.

The zar ceremony results in neither insight nor verbalization of social-psychological problems nor working-through of conflicts. Rather, emotions are aroused and intensified through the dramatization of a dangerous confrontation with evil spirits. The special ceremonial atmosphere, the rituals, and the wearing of new clothes heighten the drama. The ceremony is so emotionally charged that various therapeutic activities become easily possible as normal social rules are temporarily suspended and the forces of evil are in evidence.

The success of the ceremony depends upon constant group support. Group members pay a great deal of attention to the patient, help her to gratify her wishes, and, by attributing the patient's difficulties to supernatural powers, absolve her from responsibility for her illness.

The many symbols and rituals used in the ceremony—the bride's clothing, animal sacrifice, the smearing and drinking of blood, the purifying bath— all contribute to the evocation of deep emotions and help to intensify the patient's faith in the process and her awareness of group support; the guiltless patient is encouraged to give vent to her repressed and suppressed emotions in a joyful yet mysterious atmosphere of singing and dancing. In fact, Kennedy (1967) compared the zar experience to a "culturally staged dream," where superego controls are dissolved and the patient's repressed wishes are allowed free expression.

Summary

Examples of indigenous healing groups from three different cultures have been presented. None of these groups is scientific in the Western sense, although, through trial and error and through cumulative practical experience, they appear to benefit group members.

One commonality among the groups is the linkage of the healing experience with an alteration in consciousness, although this linkage differs somewhat for each group. Prince's review (1980) examines psychotherapy as the mobilization of endogenous healing mechanisms. He notes:

What does a suffering person do on his own? He may go to sleep, or take a rest, he may withdraw and try to puzzle out the reason for his suffering, he may socialize or go on a drinking spree, he may buy himself a new horse or, less commonly, he may deprive or otherwise punish himself or commit suicide. On the other hand, involuntary coping mechanisms may come into play. He may dream, or have a religious experience, or go crazy. Suffering individuals, when they have exhausted their own resources, often turn to a specialized healer or healing institution. We will argue here that most of the treatments that the healers offer are simply an exaggeration or extra development of the above named endogenous mechanisms.

If Prince is correct, then perhaps an alteration in consciousness may be regarded as a gateway for the release of endogenous healing mechanisms; the Senoi utilize their dreams; the Salish utilize a religious-like experience, as well as dreams; and the zar cult participants utilize a culturally staged dream.

In the Salish ceremonial, the experience of altered consciousness serves several purposes: (1) it metaphorically symbolizes the "death" of the old, troubled self; (2) it psychophysiologically renders the initiate more amenable to persuasion; (3) it provides an opportunity for cathartic abreaction; and (4) it facilitates the emergence of new identity as the initiate receives the Guardian Spirit in a dream and discovers his song.

Sleep is, of course, the most commonly experienced altered state of consciousness. Sleep cures for mental illness have a long history in Europe. Yoruba (Nigeria) healers sometimes induce prolonged sleep in psychotic patients by using Rauwolfia drugs.

With a few notable exceptions, the therapeutic use of dreams is uncommon. Temple incubation, the process of receiving healing advice or of being cured while dreaming in a sacred temple, was practiced in Babylon, Egypt, Greece, and Rome. Many case histories of this healing technique as practiced by Asclepian cults have been collected. The Iroquois Indians believed that the fulfillment of wishes revealed in dreams preserved good health and cured illness. Psychoanalysts use dream interpretation to get at the workings of the unconscious mind, as do the dream doctors of the Digueno Indians of Southern California.

The Senoi's reliance on dream expression and interpretation is truly remarkable. The process appears to be therapeutic not only for the individual but also for the entire community. By encouraging the open discussion of dreams, the Senoi avoid interpersonal and intrapersonal conflict. They recognize that dreams contain potentially disruptive wishes but, by shared interpretation of these dreams, they are able to preserve the peace. Although the dreamer is not responsible for the content of his dreams, he is responsible (with the group's help) for the resolution of troublesome dreams. There is an interesting anecdotal literature on attempts by a few group psychotherapists to establish Senoi-type dream groups with American patients (Goodall, 1972; Greenlief, 1973).

In zar cult practices, the therapist and the patients undergo an altered state of consciousness for both diagnostic and healing purposes. While in a trance, the patient is allowed to speak words and to express emotions that otherwise might remain repressed and suppressed. While the patient is in a trance, everything she says and does is ascribed to the zar spirits, therefore relieving her of responsibility.

A second commonality among the three healing groups is their ongoing nature. None of the groups is time limited, and group members are invited to participate for the rest of their lives. The continuous availability of group participation is a common feature of healing groups in many cultures and prompted Harwood (1977) to note:

One must begin to question why psychiatric therapy has tended to stress independence from the therapeutic relationship as a goal rather than the cross-culturally more common practice of rehabilitating and socializing the sufferer into a long-term mental aid group.

In Western cultures, many self-groups, such as Alcoholics Anonymous and Recovery, Inc., could be called long-term mental aid groups. Most therapy groups conducted by mental health professionals, however, have some type of time limitation, although long-term chronic care clinics that combine individual therapy with group participation have been written about (Favazza, 1975).

A third commonality among the groups is their large size. No attempts are made to limit the number of participants; anyone who desires to join the group and who fulfills certain criteria is invited to attend. In fact, the large size may increase the therapeutic efficacy of the group, e.g., the ritual processes appear more magnificent when done on a large scale, desirable effects such as trance states and emotional abreaction are facilitated by contagion, and group support for participation is enhanced.

A fourth commonality among the groups is their public nature. Healing is accomplished not in private but, rather, in public open view. In fact, group members include not only identified patients or troubled persons but also family, friends, community members, and cult devotees. By the public appearance of the patient and by the public involvement of so many other persons, not only is the stigma associated with mental illness dissipated, but also societal approval for attempts at remediation is clearly expressed. Indigenous healing groups recognize the interconnectedness of the patient with his social network and with the community at large and of public health with private health.

Conclusion

Group therapy is a common and ancient treatment modality found in cultures throughout the world. Although there is little hard data on the efficacy of indigenous group therapeutic practices, it is probable that they do serve a useful purpose. The commonalities described here among healing groups in three disparate cultures—their large size, their ongoing and public nature, and their linkage of healing with an altered state of consciousness—provide a basis for scientific study. While it may not be possible or even advisable to adapt some indigenous group healing practices to Western-style group psychotherapy, we should not summarily dismiss these practices without further investigation.

References

Dentan, R. K. *The Senoi—A Nonviolent People of Malay*. Holt, Rinehart and Winston, New York, 1968.

Favazza, A. Outpatient treatment of the chronically ill. *Curr. Psychiatr. Ther., 15:* 263, 1975.

Gaviria, M., Wintrob, R. Spiritist or psychiatrist. J. Oper. Psychiatry, *10:* 40, 1979.

Goodall, K. Dream and tell for the fuller life. Psychol. Today, *6:* 32, 1972.

Greenlief, E. Senoi dream groups. Psychotherapy, *10:* 218, 1973.

Harwood, A. *Spiritist As Needed*. John Wiley & Sons, New York, 1977.

Jilek, W. G. *Salish Indian Mental Health and Culture Change*. Holt, Rinehart and Winston, Toronto, 1974.

Jilek, W. G. A quest for identity: Therapeutic aspects of the Salish Indian Guardian Spirit ceremonial. J. Oper. Psychiatry, *8:* 46, 1977.

Jilek, W. G. Native renaissance: The survival and revival of indigenous therapeutic ceremonial among North American Indians. Transcult. Psychiatr. Res. Rev. *15:* 117, 1978.

Kennedy, J. G. Nubian zar ceremonies as psychotherapy. Hum. Organ. *4:* 185, 1967.

Mann, L. Cross-cultural studies of small groups. In *Handbook of Cross-cultural Psychology*, H. C. Triandis and A. Heron, editors, vol. 5, p. 155. Allyn and Bacon, Boston, 1981.

Prince, R. H. Variations in psychotherapeutic procedures. In *Handbook of Cross-cultural Psychology*, H. C. Triadis and J. G. Draguns, editors, vol. 6, p. 307. Allyn and Bacon, Boston, 1980.

Saunders, L. W. Variants in zar experience in an Egyptian village. In *Case Studies In Spirit Possession*. V., Crapanzano, and V. Garrison, editors, p. 177. John Wiley & Sons, New York, 1977.

Stewart, K. Culture and personality in two primitive groups. Complex, *9:* 3, 1953.

AREA B

SPECIALIZED GROUP PSYCHOTHERAPY TECHNIQUES

B.1 An Overview of Group Methods

WILLIAM E. POWLES, M.D.

Definition

Marshaling a field as complex and changing as that of the group therapies is a daunting task. Fortunately, the total number of modes of group psychotherapy appears to be rather finite.

Slavson (1960) divided the whole field of the psychotherapies into three broad bands: counseling, guidance, and psychotherapy proper.

Counseling is the process of assisting a patient or client with finding the solution for a relatively immediate, circumscribed problem or personal decision. Groups, Slavson argues, are not a good modality for counseling because of the relative acuteness, reality orientation, and concreteness of both problems and agenda, and because it is essentially impossible to keep a group of people focused tightly on problem discussion and solution.

Guidance Slavson defined as pursuing the ramifications of defined problems beyond their concrete issues into matters of attitudes, using a freer pathway toward ultimate problem resolution. Slavson argues that guidance can be very well undertaken in groups.

Psychotherapy, Slavson suggests, has no other agenda than the free expression and exploration of human experiences. Such a definition implies that a focus on problem solution is a resistance in the psychotherapy process, although, naturally, successful therapy has as an ultimate goal the solution to the problems of the patient or client in his ongoing life outside therapy. Psychotherapy proper, he argues, is also particularly well undertaken in the group setting.

This initial, very broad comparison defines counseling in a way which excludes it from the field of group psychotherapy. Included are two broad types of therapy: guidance, which explores reality problems in depth, and psychotherapy, which maintains its principal focus on spontaneous (free-associational) personal communication.

Powles (1964) suggested some rules or yardsticks for defining the group psychotherapies—what shall be included and what excluded. They might be paraphrased as follows:

(1) A group of troubled people is assembled and meets regularly for the purpose of improving the personal well-being and effectiveness of its members. (2) A leader or therapist is involved, whose personal well-being and effectiveness, including his professional expertise, is recognized as superior to that of the patients or clients. (3) Group process or dynamics is somewhat explicitly and purposefully exploited as an instrument of therapy.

By these rules, some helping groups can be conceptually excluded from the field of group psychotherapy—for example, recreational or educational groups whose aims are to improve specific skills rather than general well-being and effectiveness, and which do not capitalize clearly on group processes, or self-help groups such as Alcoholics Anonymous or Weight Watchers, in which either a therapist is not recognized or group process is not explicitly utilized.

Some further practical boundaries need to be drawn. For example, how large is a group before it stops being a group? When therapy is done with a group large enough that it cannot be in intimate face-to-face contact, or large enough that all its members cannot regularly be together for meetings, such large-group therapy will be excluded from our comparisons. This leaves within the boundaries of group psychotherapy, the face-to-face, family-sized group of up to a dozen persons. Again, a further boundary: included are only face-to-face groups who form, or become intimately acquainted, over some months; groups which meet only for a weekend or a few meetings do not develop a structure and process which can be utilized as an instrument for therapy. Again, are couple and family therapy to be defined as within or without? It seems they should be placed outside the boundaries of group psychotherapy on two grounds: (1) They involve in one case a tiny specialized group, the couple, and in both cases a group which has been formed and closed over a considerable length of time, unlike the groups of strangers assembled in group psychotherapy proper. (2) There is probably more heterogeneity of theory and more disagreement about what constitutes couple and family therapy than even within the field of group psychotherapy proper.

Therefore, large-group therapy, therapy with brief, short-lived groups, and couple and family therapy will be considered cousins, outside the immediate group psychotherapy family, i.e., members of an extended family who require serious consideration as collaterals.

Overview

The group therapies may be classified by combining these six dimensions:
1. Locus of responsibility: Therapist- versus group-centered
2. Composition by problems: Homogeneous versus heterogeneous
3. Principal approach: Supportive versus confronting
4. Focus of attention: Problem- versus person-centered
5. Modality used: Actional versus communicational
6. Chief emphasis: Conceptual versus experiential

Fortunately, in the real world, the huge numbers of possible permutations of these dimensions do not exist; rather, the main types of group therapy boil down to a rather finite number of clusters:

Cluster A

This type is somewhat therapist centered, homogeneous as to problem, supportive, problem centered, and actional—group guidance (Slavson, 1960) for a variety of problems, from alcoholism to sexual difficulties. This is perhaps the most common type of group therapy practiced in clinics and agencies (e.g., Hadden, in Rabin and Rosenbaum, 1976; Rice et al., 1981).

Cluster B

This type is group centered to various degrees, heterogeneous as to problems, supportive and confronting by turns, person centered, communicational, and conceptual—the psychoanalytic and cognate group psychotherapies. This is perhaps the most common type in private practice of group psychotherapy (e.g., Rosenbaum's and Whitaker's chapters in Rabin and Rosenbaum, 1976).

Cluster C

This type is therapist centered, heterogeneous, confronting, person centered, actional, and experiential—classical psychodrama.

Cluster D

This type is therapist centered, confronting, problem and person centered, actional, and experiential—the newer eclectic and integrative group psychotherapies using transactional analysis, psychodrama, gestalt, nonverbal and body exercises. This type is characterized in the work of Knobloch and Knobloch

(1979), Sacks (Rabin and Rosenbaum, 1976), and many others.

Differences

The most difficult problem in classifying the group psychotherapies is that of discerning and conceptualizing the real differences in therapeutic process and outcome among (and within) these various clusters and modes. Research in the complex variables of group psychotherapy is probably in its infancy. One must, therefore, make guesses and assumptions about what kind of group accomplishes just what. Such assumptions, or guesses, relate to differences in patients enrolled in various groups—for example, we can hardly call the members of certain groups patients at all, while in other groups distress and disability are high; differences in therapist style and conviction—autocratic, permissive, intellectual, intuitive, warm and supporting, cool and confronting, etc; differences in group climate—group as locus of authority, cohesiveness, experiential versus conceptual culture, length of life of the group and its culture, etc. In turn, outcome areas include such variables as symptomatic recovery from distress; degrees of increased personal effectiveness, with or without conceptual insight; different kinds of persisting insight into the self, into other people, into the dynamics of group life; and the durability, or otherwise, of such changes.

Group Composition

A rather small number of explicit discussions of indications and contraindications for the group psychotherapies have been published. There are more discussions concerning selection and rejection of patients for the group and group composition. These range from rather metapsychological and abstract to practical and clinical; they leave the impression, probably quite correctly, that we are only generally aware of indications and contraindications, and that putting people together in groups is still partly a matter of guesswork and luck. It is much like issuing invitations to a party—a very practical matter of who will get along with whom and what collection of guests will make a good party. Indeed, composing a group is often anchored by the stern reality of a very limited pool of patients or referrals from which to choose.

If a patient's ego functions and controls are relatively intact and his life situation stable, he can be directed toward a formal, contracted psychotherapy plan or at least a contracted trial of psychotherapy. But if the patient's ego functions, controls, and communication ability are impaired and his life situation is unstable, the patient is assisted with hospitalization, milieu therapy, pharmacological and physical therapy, social casework, and environmental manipulation. This patient may well be considered, following stabilizing action, for formal psychotherapy.

A patient whose problems will be early manifest in a group setting, who is either at an oedipal level of development or in marked dependence on the family, and who is socialized sufficiently to gain something from group effort, should be directed toward some form of group psychotherapy. On the other hand, a patient whose problems cannot easily be demonstrated or visualized in the group setting but must be inferred and conceptualized by an expert, whose individual therapy is floundering, and who is unsocialized in a late pregenital position, should have a form of psychotherapy other than group—for example, analytic psychotherapy, psychoanalysis, behavior therapy, couple therapy, family therapy. Such a patient might well be referred later for group psychotherapy.

Skynner conceptualized a "sandwich" distribution of patients suitable for group psychotherapy in a way which seems to combine some practical findings of others. Skynner posits that certain very immature persons, with poor individuation (early pregenital fixation) can relate to a group as a mass, with therapeutic benefit. Persons with somewhat better individuation and autonomy (late pregenital fixation) do not do well in groups, while those with still more mature organization (oedipal level) will also do well in groups, relating to the group members as clearly defined objects. In practical terms, certain chronic schizophrenics, or patients suffering a schizophrenic defect state, may be able to utilize group psychotherapy for mutual support and problem solving, probably in the form of group guidance, in a homogeneous, problem-shared group. The same would go for various types of stabilized, very dependent personalities. But marked compulsive and hysteroid personalities or patients suffering from disabling neuroses probably fall under the late pregenital contraindication.

Conclusion

Group psychotherapy is a general mode of psychotherapy oriented to the social nature of man and characterized by the exploitation of group relationships and processes by a trained expert; for our purposes, this means the use of a face-to-face group of around eight people, who meet for a long enough course to form into a tight-knit working instrument. Generally, group psychotherapy polarizes between an open-ended, free-floating, nondirective discussion method and a problem-focused, behaviorally oriented, therapist-directed method. As yet, little of certainty is known regarding what patient should be most cost effectively offered what type of group. However, in addition to the general indications for psychotherapy, there are a number of precepts which are worth taking seriously—if only to test them in research—and which offer something midway between total guesswork and clinical certainty in weighing the merits of different group modalities for one's patients.

References

Heath, E. S., and Bacal, H. A. A method of group psychotherapy at the Tavistock Clinic. Int. J. Group Psychother., *18:* 21, 1968.

Knobloch, F., and Knobloch, J. *Integrated Psychotherapy.* Jason Aronson, New York, 1979.

Powles, W. E. Varieties and uses of group psychotherapy. Can. Psychiatr. Assoc. J., *9:* 196, 1964.

Rabin, H. M., and Rosenbaum, M., editors. *How to Begin a Psychotherapy Group: Six Approaches.* Gordon and Breach, London, 1976.

Rice, C. A., Day, M., et al. Topical papers: Aspects of psychoanalytic group therapy. Am. J. Psychiatry, *138:* 63, 1981.

Skynner, A. C. R. *Systems of Family and Marital Psychotherapy.* Brunner-Mazel, New York, 1976.

Slavson, S. R. When is a "therapy group" not a therapy group? An outline of the principles and practices of counseling, guidance, and psychotherapy. Int. J. Group Psychother., *10:* 3, 1960.

B.2 Combined Individual and Group Psychotherapy

NORMUND WONG, M.D.

Introduction

The use of a combined individual and group approach appears to have arisen out of practical necessity, creative innovation, a desire to amalgamate the best features of individual and group treatment, and sheer frustration when individual or group therapists simply did not know what next to try in order to help a patient. The first paper on combined therapy was written in 1949 by Wender and Stein. A large number of articles on the subject followed in the 1950's and 1960's, with fewer publications appearing in the 1970's and early 1980's.

For the most part, this treatment modality was started by individual therapists, who began to experiment with groups and to supplement individual sessions with group therapy when they discovered the unique advantages of the group. Various arrangements have emerged, ranging from the use of one group session to complement an individual analysis conducted on a five-times-a-week basis to the employment of an occasional individual meeting with patients who may be seen two or three times weekly in a psychotherapy group. When a patient is in concurrent intermediate or long-term dyadic and group psychotherapy with the same therapist, the process is referred to as combined psychotherapy. If two or more therapists treat the patient concurrently, but one therapist provides the individual treatment while the other one or two render group psychotherapy, the process is termed conjoint therapy.

Within this accepted definition of combined treatment, a number of variations can be found. Sager (1960) prefers the term "concurrent therapy," instead of combined psychotherapy, to stress the equal importance of both therapies in the patient's treatment. He advocates that the patient be engaged in continuous and simultaneous treatment in group and individual sessions with the same therapist. The number of individual sessions is not changed once the patient enters combined treatment. Kadis and Markowitz (1958) classify combined treatment into three categories: (1) therapist-centered; (2) therapist-group-centered; and (3) group-centered combined treatment. In the therapist-centered approach, the therapist uses the group as an adjunct to the individual therapy, in order to elicit interaction phenomena to be worked through in subsequent individual sessions with the patient. In the therapist-group-centered combined treatment, the therapist uses the group to modify the transference phenomena. Here, the individual and group sessions are manipulated by the therapist in order to relieve the pressure of transference and countertransference feelings. In group-centered combined treatment, the therapist lays great stress on the inherent curative and maturational properties of the group and places himself in the role of an expert group participant. Individual sessions are kept to a minimum, as they are viewed as an expression of resistance on the part of the patient to the group process, to the therapist, or to both.

Fried (1955) believes that the two different modalities of treatment should be used not in parallel fashion but combined into a larger unit of treatment. Each form of therapy enables the patient to take better advantage of the other. She stresses that the benefits of combined treatment come from the cross-fertilization between individual and group therapy. Most practitioners of combined therapy believe that this approach provides the best features of individual and group treatment. In 1955, Hulse found that the results of combined treatment approached the depth and intensity of the reactions of intensive psychoanalytic therapy. In his opinion, combined therapy stood somewhere between psychoanalysis and the use of individual or group psychotherapy alone.

A review of the literature reveals a variety of opinions regarding the purported advantages of combined treatment over either individual or group psychotherapy. Green (1953) feels that the combined approach affords greater opportunities for working issues through. With this method, it is possible to pick up on material expressed in a group which frequently cannot be followed up because of pressing issues and concerns from other members and the lack of available time. Fried reports that combined treatment shortens the withdrawal periods of orally frustrated individuals and increases their productivity. Papanek (1954) finds that combined treatment has stimulating effects on both therapists and patients alike. Hulse (1955) reports that combined therapy is particularly effective in reinforcing interpretations made by the therapist, deepening insights, and strengthening reality testing. Material can be brought up first in individual sessions to be tested out and then brought to the group. He also notes that there is increased productivity during the early stages of treatment and a more intensified working-through process in the later stages. Catharsis is stimulated,

and conflictual material arises more freely. Insights are reinforced, and greater over-all reality testing results from the use of the combined approach. Lipschutz (1957), a pioneer in this method, finds that combined treatment reduces the stress resulting from the group setting by modifying tension from transference and countertransference manifestations. He feels the combined approach offers the therapist a better awareness of the current conflicts in the patient's life and helps prevent untoward reactions of the patient in the group.

Sager states that concurrent or combined treatment provides the patient with a better means of understanding and of working through problems. In the group setting, the patient is able to reenact the conflicts surrounding the dyadic and triangular relationships and the familial and social constellations. It is especially potent in dealing with the patient's ego defenses and ways of coping. In the individual sessions, the patient is provided the opportunity to more thoroughly work through historical material relating to oedipal and preoedipal problems. In contrast to other authors who write about combined therapy, Sager emphasizes that group psychotherapy is not to be used to help individual therapy in overcoming resistances or by providing material for the individual sessions. Nor is the patient's individual analysis to be considered ancillary to the group psychotherapy. He stresses that, in conducting the patient's individual analysis, the analyst should function in his customary way. There should be no major departure from the therapist's role either as an individual or group therapist. However, he recognizes that the two forms of therapy do provide material for each other which can be traced through the latent content.

In 1964, Cappon stressed that combined treatment was more effective in exploratory and integrative work with patients than either individual or group therapies separately. Battegay (1972), although critical of combined treatment, feels that it offers a deepening of insight and social learning processes. Sakles (1972) concludes that each of the treatment modalities in combined treatment draws from and complements the other. In their comprehensive overview, Scheidlinger and Porter (1980) state that character reconstruction does occur with great alacrity and depth with combined treatment.

A number of other advantages can be enumerated. Patients who tend to terminate treatment prematurely if placed in individual or group psychotherapy alone, often do well with a combined approach. The excessive anxiety and stresses created by group therapy, or the too intense transference reactions in dyadic treatment, can be alleviated in combined treatment. Patients are better able to accept interpretations and confrontations when these are presented in both the individual and group sessions. There is greater acceptance of interventions, which eventually lead to improved insight and reality testing. Patients may become more amenable to intense reconstructive therapy with the combined approach. Often, time and financial constraints prevent individuals from entering an individual psychoanalysis. Combined therapy can be a very satisfactory substitute which enables them to attain the same therapeutic goals. In combined treatment, problems on various developmental and psychological levels can be intensively worked through and an understanding of the patient's personality defenses and sources of anxiety can be obtained. This approach also makes it possible to understand the cultural and familial factors which contributed to the individual's personality. There are advantages for the therapist as well, for he can observe the patient's behaviors in vivo, and blind spots of either the patient or the therapist may be verified more easily. There is a greater interpersonal and intrapsychic understanding of the patients with this comprehensive treatment approach.

Indications for Combined Treatment

Combined therapy has been employed in a number of clinical situations. In 1955, Hulse reported that the use of combined treatment was fully justified with patients showing character disorders of long standing. Schecter (1959) feels that patients who tend to relate predominantly in a rather exclusive or incestuous manner or who show great difficulty communicating in pairing and sibling situations would benefit from this approach. Durkin (1964) and Tabachnick (1965) both believe that patients who have problems with isolation should be treated with combined therapy. According to these investigators, such patients have a fear of interpersonal contacts, cannot communicate easily with others, and show a general inhibition of instinctual drive derivatives. Wilder (1974) recommends the use of combined treatment for those individuals who have been in analysis for a long time and are showing difficulty with the resolution of their transference neuroses. Combined treatment has also been used by many clinicians when they feel that patients are at a treatment impasse, manifest stubborn or long-standing resistances, have been unable to apply the insights gained from either group or individual therapy, are close to termination in dyadic treatment and may benefit from a group experience, and when they believe some patients would gain from intensive psychotherapy but because of time and financial considerations cannot afford analysis. An attenuated version of combined treatment is practiced with psychiatric inpatients in many institutions as described by Green (1953) and Beran (1961). Most clinicians who work with hospitalized patients employ a combination of individual and group approaches. But because of the lack of intensity and limited duration of the treatment, with a few exceptions, these approaches would not meet the definition of combined treatment. When patients are hospitalized for a lengthy period, a combined approach may be very helpful in order to provide the working through of specific issues, manage distorted and dangerous fantasies, and reduce excessive anxiety.

Wolf (1974) feels that individuals showing fairly intact egos, the oldest or nearly the oldest siblings in a large family who were prematurely forced to assume surrogate parental roles, patients who experience sudden panic or severe depression, those who are unable to verbalize basic problems, silent members, severe sadomasochists, acting-out patients, and patients plateaued in treatment are amenable to combined treatment. Brende (1981) reports that combined therapy can often be effective for Vietnam veterans.

A number of authors urge that combined treatment be used with great care and only for specific indications, because this approach may confuse and complicate the transference in both modalities, resulting in increased resistance and causing therapeutic difficulties. This reservation has been supported by Fried (1954), Jackson and Grotjahn (1958), Papanek (1956), and Stein (1964). Some patients falling into specific diagnostic categories are believed to be good candidates for combined therapy. Fried (1955) recommends the use of this technique for passive-narcissistic patients with the rationale that they would be forced to deal with reality. Such patients could partially gratify their dependency needs in the private sessions, where they would also have the opportunity to analyze the search for their unrealistic ego ideals. With the aid of the group, they would ultimately experience the devaluation of their unattainable ego ideals and sustain the necessary disappointments to enable them to form more of a self-identity. She also advises the use of combined therapy for orally frustrated individuals with paranoid character trends.

Wong (1979, 1980) pointed out the advantages of combined treatment for borderline and narcissistic patients. With this approach, patients have the opportunity to form idealizing and mirroring transferences in dyadic treatment in unimpeded fashion, are provided transitional objects in the group to reduce their fears of engulfment and retaliation which are frequently projected onto the therapist, and are afforded a chance to redress the fixations which occurred during the separation-individuation stage. The group experience is especially valuable for narcissistic patients in helping them work through the issues of grandiosity and aggression and in easing the therapist's countertransference burden. In the group, borderline patients can find a variety of role models to "try on for size" as they work through feelings of separation and abandonment en route to the establishment of a mature integrated self. The individual therapy fosters and maintains the therapeutic alliance, nurtures the development of idealizing and mirror transferences, and helps attenuate the often fantastic fantasies stirred up in a group setting.

Wolberg (1960) also favors the use of combined treatment for borderline patients; however, she carefully points out that the patient should not become a member of a therapeutic group until the patient's defenses of detachment have been penetrated and the fears of close relationships with other people are being overcome. The patient should have expressed a desire to join a group or have shown some effort to be a functioning part of a group which is not necessarily a therapy group. Stein states that borderline patients with character and ego defects and certain patients with oral-narcissistic traits can benefit from combined treatment.

Both Mintz (1966) and Bieber (1974) discuss the advantages of combined treatment for homosexual men. Mintz advocates placing these patients in heterosexual groups whose members have a heterosexual orientation. Mintz finds that combined therapy offers these patients an opportunity to dissolve rationalizations about homosexuality, develop a stronger sense of personal identity through contact with women and heterosexual men, draw out unconscious anxieties related to heterosexual drives, and provide corrective emotional experiences which increase their self-esteem. Bieber also feels that combined treatment is helpful in the treatment of male homosexual patients. In contrast to Mintz, however, Bieber employs an all-male homosexual group. Patients for this treatment are evaluated on an individual basis. Bieber concludes that the combined approach is contraindicated for those individuals who cannot discuss their condition with other patients, are unable to tolerate the multiple relationships formed in a group, and need the continuity and intensity of a one-to-one treatment situation. Homosexuals with underlying psychotic states and individuals whose hostilities, distortions, and anxieties would interfere with the group process are considered unsuitable candidates for combined treatment.

Rosenbaum (1960) recommends the use of combined psychotherapy for the treatment of passive-dependent and hostile-dependent personalities who are extremely oral and demanding. Wolff and Solomon (1973) suggest that withdrawn schizoid personalities are candidates for this approach. In the dyadic therapy, they can experience a relationship with the therapist which corresponds to the early infant-mother situation, while, in a group setting, they are able to learn how to share the parent therapist with others. Conflicts involving multiple and varied types of relationships can be worked through which are similar to family childhood experiences and the interaction present in a wider social network. Heigl-Evans and Heigl (1974) support the use of combined treatment for schizoid patients, pointing out the need of these individuals for an individual therapist and the stimulus afforded by the group which helps them relate to other human beings. They also suggest the application of this modality for hysterical patients, because they would benefit from the group feedback. Individual therapy would sustain and protect these patients, while in the group they could learn to appreciate the consequences of their erratic, impulsive behavior and of their blind spots.

In summary, the indications for combined treatment can be grouped under specific conflicts, diagnostic categories, and a few selected situations. They are illustrated in Table B.2-1.

Contraindications for Combined Treatment

There is relatively little in the literature about contraindications for the use of combined therapy. Because he feels that hysterical personalities do not profit from a group experience, are incapable of utilizing group feedback, and exploit the group for their own exhibitionistic purposes, Battegay (1972) believes combined treatment is contraindicated for these patients. Wolf describes the following patients who should not be treated with this approach. They include individuals who are classified as borderline psychotics, patients who wish to control and to seduce the therapist or to isolate him from the rest of the

Table B.2-1
Indications for Combined Therapy

Patients with specific conflicts
    Have "incestuous" manner of relating to others
    Show difficulty in pairing and sibling situations
    Exhibit problems dealing with isolation
    Cannot tolerate intense dyadic treatment relationship
    Are oldest siblings who were forced to assume family responsibilities prematurely
    Tend to act out
    Are very silent in dyadic treatment
    Are orally frustrated and possess paranoid trends
    Show difficulties from Vietnam military experience
Patients in certain diagnostic categories (DSM-III)
    Narcissistic personality disorders
    Borderline personality disorders
    Male homosexuality (ego-syntonic and ego-dystonic)
    Schizoid personality disorders
    Histrionic personality disorders
    Dependent personality disorders
    Passive-aggressive personality disorders
Other indications
    Patients acceptable for psychoanalysis but lack time, money, or access to psychoanalyst
    Patients in termination phase of psychotherapy

group, and regressed psychotics who manifest pre-oedipal attachments to the prior individual therapist or to the group analyst himself. Scheidlinger and Porter feel that there are only two major clinical contraindications to combined treatment. These include the classic psychoneuroses, which are best treated with intensive individual psychoanalysis, and some borderline psychotic and masochistic patients. Such individuals have extremely fragile ego structures and may respond to the addition of group psychotherapy with enhanced anxiety, regressive behavior, or repression.

Technique

Some therapists may see their patients in individual treatment for a long time, place them in a group with themselves, and then withdraw the individual sessions. Other psychotherapists may begin treatment with patients in a group but later see the patients only in individual treatment. The above two approaches are not what we define as combined treatment. Most practitioners of combined therapy prefer a preparatory phase of individual therapy before adding group psychotherapy to the treatment plan. The length and frequency of the individual therapy vary and appear to be guided by the following principles. Papanek, Schecter, and Sager stress the need first to establish a transference and then work through some of its infantile aspects before placing the patient in combined treatment. According to Scheidlinger and Porter, some clinicians wait until the transference manifestations are established in individual therapy and at least partially understood. The acute situation and symptoms for which the patient originally sought treatment should have subsided, and the patient should be able to tolerate the anxiety and stresses of the group.

Before embarking on a course of combined treatment, the clinician should establish a diagnosis, understand the dynamics of the patient, establish a therapeutic alliance, and educate the patient to the process of therapy. The duration of individual therapy may vary from a few weeks to a few years. Most practitioners of combined treatment tend to place their patients in individual therapy for 1 to 2 years before adding the group modality. If a patient remains in individual treatment too long before entering combined therapy, some clinicians feel that the patient may find it difficult to relinquish the fantasy of being special; once in combined therapy, he or she may show a variety of reactions—excessive frustration, anxiety, rage, withdrawal, resentment, or undue dependency.

Other therapists favor the use of group therapy first and only later add individual sessions. This approach may be helpful for individuals who are psychologically unsophisticated and may learn how to think psychologically when placed in a group which is able to offer support, opportunities for universalization, altruism, ventilation, and catharsis. Scheidlinger and Porter point out that the group-first approach is useful if the transference in the dyadic relationship is viewed as too frightening to a patient. Individuals with previous psychoanalytic experience may be placed in a group before starting combined treatment.

Green (1953) and Beran (1961), who describe the treatment of inpatients, favor the use of group therapy first before starting combined therapy. Beran finds that withdrawn and suspicious persons cannot tolerate individual contacts in the beginning, but in a group their fears and suspiciousness are gradually lost when patients are offered an opportunity to give and take in a friendly group atmosphere.

The decision as to when to place the patient in combined therapy also varies, depending on the therapeutic progress being made by the patient, the time available to the therapist and patient, and financial considerations. In private practice, it may take a long while before the clinician has a sufficient number of patients to employ the use of combined treatment. Some writers start all their patients in combined treatment from the very beginning and do not provide any individual sessions.

Once in combined treatment, patients may be seen in individual therapy for the same or a reduced number of visits or may be gradually withdrawn altogether from individual treatment. The number of individual sessions may range from a minimum of one visit every other week to as many as five meetings weekly. Most practitioners see their patients once or twice weekly in individual sessions and in one or two group sessions, each lasting 1½ hours. Papanek (1956) objects to too-frequent group meetings. She recommends that groups be held not more than once a week and views alternate meetings as being superfluous

and potentially harmful. There is the danger that group life may substitute for real life and a gang culture hostile to the outside environment may develop. Aronson (1964) leaves the responsibility for the frequency of individual meetings with the patient but with the understanding that the therapist may schedule an individual session when it seems indicated.

Objectives of Group Sessions

In combined treatment, the group modality provides the advantages commonly ascribed to therapy groups in general. However, its objectives differ somewhat from the customary practice of group psychotherapy alone, for it is only half of the overall treatment. The impact of individual treatment and the presence of the same therapist in both settings are ever-present undercurrents in the group. In contrast to individual treatment, group therapy provides patients opportunities in a safe environment to interact with others in a setting reflective of society at large, mutual support, different learning situations, a chance to express and benefit from altruism which in itself may be therapeutic, and opportunities for identification and catharsis. It also promotes and encourages free expression of thoughts, behavior, and affects toward other patients and the therapist. In addition, the group provides multiple transference objects, a large number of stimuli in the treatment setting, feedback about the individual's behavior from a variety of perspectives, and an increase in personal awareness of the impact a person makes upon others. The emotional contagion often present in groups may help lift repressions in patients who in individual therapy alone cannot come to grips with their feelings. In the group, patients may feel more comfortable with aggressive feelings and receive help with acting-out behavior because of the reassurance and support offered by other members.

Group therapy differs from individual treatment in a number of ways. It works on a more conscious and less regressed level and tends to be more reality oriented and focuses less on fantasies. In 1953, Sullivan pointed out that the group situation tends to evoke and revive those past attitudes and feelings that are chiefly related to the juvenile and preadolescent eras. This led Schecter to comment that such group-provoked attitudes may inhibit behavior and feelings which are characteristic of and derived from the infantile and childhood eras. Lastly, group therapy depends more on interaction among its members and activity than on free association. Its focus is more on the "here and now" instead of the "there and then."

When combined with individual treatment, group therapy provides some additional functions. These include an outlet for and control of intense, unmanageable transference phenomena which otherwise could disrupt or even destroy treatment; the reduction and resolution of some resistances which are seemingly intractable in individual therapy; opportunities for risk taking to try out new behaviors which have been analyzed and worked through in individual treatment; and the management of excessive dependency needs where the patient learns to share the therapist with others. By watching other members and their reactions to the therapist, through feedback from other group members, and a reduction in the intensity of the transference, patients are afforded increased opportunities to strengthen and develop their observing egos. Confrontations and insights which may not have been effective in individual therapy may assume significance and validity when they are voiced in the group setting. Finally, the group sessions can serve as a catalyst to promote progress in individual therapy.

One of the objectives of the group sessions is to provide the therapist with a chance to see the social facets and interpersonal behaviors of the patient which might otherwise be difficult to evaluate in individual treatment. The therapist can observe the adaptive mechanisms employed by the patient in a different setting and determine to what extent certain issues in individual treatment have been successfully worked through and applied in a group setting. Because most therapists feel that they must be more active and transparent in a group setting, combined treatment affords them a chance to see how adaptive and successful are their behaviors in the two arenas.

Objectives of Individual Sessions

Most therapists practicing combined treatment ascribe to an individual psychoanalytic, uncovering, or exploratory approach. With a few exceptions, treatment will be long term, such as a year or more. The objectives of individual therapy in combined treatment differ from group psychotherapy in several aspects. Regression to an earlier level of development occurs, and dreams, free association, and fantasies are encouraged and explored to a greater extent. More emphasis is placed on a detailed study of intrapsychic rather than interpersonal matters. Intense preoedipal and oedipal transferences are commonly encountered in individual psychotherapy, while in group therapy sibling transference tends to predominate. Overall, the transference phenomenon in individual treatment is usually more intense and regressed than in group therapy. Greater attention is paid to the working through of neurotic structures instead of underlying character defenses. Individual sessions may provide for greater insight and depth of understanding.

When combined with group therapy, the individual sessions serve additional functions. These include the development of sufficient trust and confidence in the therapist to enable the patient to enter group therapy. Because the therapeutic alliance or working relationship must be sufficiently developed to enable the patient to withstand the anxiety and stresses of the group, part of the function of individual therapy is to prepare the patient for a group experience. Resistances and defenses brought out in a group can be

examined and further worked through in the separate sessions. In the group, the therapist and patient share another experience in common which will have an influence on their relationship in the dyadic situation and offer further material for study. In combined treatment, more of the therapist's personality is revealed, and this influences the transference in individual psychotherapy. For patients with relatively weak ego structures, extra attention may have to be paid in individual sessions to supporting the patient and reducing the anxieties arising from the group experience. When the combined treatment format is employed, patients may request fewer or more individual sessions, and the reasons for the request must be explored. New meanings are frequently attributed to the individual meetings. Material from the individual sessions will often be carried over to the group session. Patients seen in group psychotherapy alone may manifest intense rivalry and envy toward those members in combined treatment, and there may be great anger expressed toward the therapist and feelings of rejection by patients who are in group treatment solely.

Table B.2-2 summarizes some of the general characteristics of individual and group therapy when they are used together in combined treatment.

Transference

In the American Psychoanalytic Association's *Glossary of Psychoanalytic Terms and Concepts*, transference is defined as an unconscious process which involves the displacement of patterns of feelings and behavior originally experienced with significant figures from a person's childhood to individuals in one's current relationship. Transferences may be intra- or extra-analytic and positive or negative. Various opinions exist regarding the transferences in combined treatment. Some clinicians believe that the transference becomes diluted and split, contaminated and

Table B.2-2
General Characteristics of Treatment Modalities in Combined Therapy

	Individual Modality	Group Modality
Orientation	Insight oriented, intrapsychic	Reality oriented, interpersonal
Mode of expression	Emphasis on free association, dreams, and fantasies	Emphasis on reality-based, interpersonal behavior and learning
Level of regression	Infantile, stressing feelings from childhood era	Juvenile, stressing feelings from preadolescent era
Major emphasis	Intrapsychic exploration, focusing on neurotic structures	Interpersonal relationships, focusing on character defenses
Feedback	Single source and restricted	Multiple sources and spontaneous
Attitudes	Neutral	Altruistic, mutual support

inhibited in its development, and less intense and made more difficult to manage in combined treatment. Others feel that the transference manifestations are not greatly affected or become more intense and that there may be a reinforcement of positive as well as negative components. The manifestations of transference are also influenced by the actual relationship between the patient and therapist in each of the two treatment settings, the timing of the combined treatment, the patient's personality, the composition of the group, and the style of leadership of the therapist.

Shay (1954), Lipschutz, and Jackson and Grotjahn point out that tension in the transference is reduced in individual sessions with the combined treatment approach. Berger concurred in these findings in his paper of 1960. Fried, Papanek, Schecter, and Sager comment on how the group can be used as a defense against the transference in individual treatment when combined therapy is employed. Stein reported in 1964 that the transference to the leader is split and deflected onto the group members. Tabachnick notes similar findings. In 1972, Sakles stated that transference toward the leader is diluted by the group in combined treatment. Battegay observes that combined treatment creates difficulties in the transference. The intensity of the transference in individual treatment is disturbed, for each patient wishes to be treated as the special beloved child. On the other hand, Slavson (1950) and Spanjaard (1959) conclude that the deflection and inhibition of the transference from the leader to the group lead to increased intergroup tension, which serves as a major dynamic factor within the group.

Other authors such as Lipschutz feel that the transference in the treatment situation is not disturbed; instead, the patient becomes more aware of it. In 1952, Lipschutz observed that the positive transferences with the analyst became strengthened in the group with the combined approach. In 1960, Sager claimed that the intense regressive transference was not interfered with in combined treatment. On the contrary, some authors feel that the transference is intensified with the combined approach, in comparison to the use of group therapy or individual treatment alone. This position was taken by Hulse. Papanek agrees and states that the transference may become more intense, reactivating childhood experiences with the parent. Berger (1960) points out that the negative aspects of the transference can be brought out more fully because the dependency factor is reduced. The intense anxiety associated with relating to the therapist as a transference object in individual treatment can be diminished when, at the same time, the patient is also being treated in the group. Bieber (1964) concludes that the anxiety in the transference can, indeed, be lessened without decreasing the intensity of insight. It may be that there are basic differences in the transference elicited by the combined approach and the issue is not a quantitative measure of the transference but, rather, of qualitative differences of the transference.

It is generally agreed that multiple transferences are elicited when a combined approach is employed, although the transferences may be more transient than those seen in individual therapy. Fried (1954) states that in the group there are a large number of transference objects and a rapidly changing and unstable quality associated with them which allows for quick fluctuations in transference feelings. This view

is supported by and elaborated upon by Berman (1950), Beukenkamp (1955), and Wolf and Schwartz (1962), who concur that in combined treatment the group can provide multiple transference figures which nevertheless lead to very intense reactions. Bieber believes that the basic transference remains unchanged in combined treatment. New transferences may be seen but their basic nature does not change. Stein classifies the differences in the transferences found in combined treatment as follows. The transference in individual treatment tends to be basic, primary, and may be called central or vertical. In the group, the transference may be labeled peripheral, secondary, sibling, or horizontal. Sager comments that the group does not appear to materially affect the transference and its working through, as long as the analyst continues to practice psychoanalysis in the individual sessions. In the group setting, a parental transference occurs which shows manifestations of the presence of other family members, while in the individual sessions, the parental transference is typically reflective of the triangular relationship.

Table B.2-3 describes the transference manifestations usually encountered in combined treatment.

Countertransference

Countertransference refers to attitudes and feelings which may be only partly conscious or unconscious that the therapist harbors toward a patient. They may arise because of the therapist's own unconscious conflicts, and unless the therapist is aware of them, the treatment of the patient may be affected. It has been stated that combined therapy may be indicated for patients whose transference feelings have become too intense or negative toward the therapist in an individual setting and whose treatment is jeopardized. But when the therapist becomes acutely uncomfortable or unable to manage the intensity of the transference feelings, combined treatment is helpful.

The treater should be aware that countertransference manifestations are sometimes operative in the decision to recommend this modality of treatment. In combined treatment, the therapist must realize that therapeutic flexibility is called for. In the group, the therapist's actions are constantly on display, and some therapists are made acutely anxious and uncomfort-

Table B.2-3
Transference Manifestations in Combined Treatment

	Individual Modality	Group Modality
Level of regression	Infantile and early childhood periods	Juvenile and pre-adolescent periods
Types	Generally parental, primary or central	Usually sibling, secondary or peripheral
Intensity	Intense	Diluted
Objects	Usually limited to one at a time	Multiple

able. Analysts who are not accustomed to a vis-à-vis treatment situation or group therapy may have intense reactions to no longer being the sole person or object of the patient's attention, as well as having to share the patient with others. If parental feelings toward patients have not been worked through, the therapist may be too protective of a patient in a group and come to the rescue too often, to the detriment of the latter. "Convoying" phenomena may be observed. Additional manifestations of countertransference reactions are commonly revealed through forgetting what certain patients may say in a group, feelings of boredom or inattention toward certain patients, and irrational, strong emotional responses.

It is possible that a therapist's countertransference feelings may be manifested through boredom, discouragement, or frustration and are the ostensible reasons for placing a patient in combined therapy. However, this is not to state that they are contraindications for the use of this modality. Also, as pointed out by Wolff and Solomon, when a therapist is very invested in group therapy, the group can be idealized, and the therapist may persuade patients to join. Therapists who are unable to confront the hostility about terminating a patient's individual treatment may skirt the issue by referring them for a combined treatment. Battegay comments that a therapist's countertransference feelings may trigger competition among the group members. Wilder reveals how the group situation can often bring out countertransference manifestations in the group more than in the individual treatment situation. But opportunities to analyze countertransference may be increased in the group setting. Countertransference manifestations can arise more frequently when patients criticize the therapist in a group; the therapist generally has less control in that situation than in one-to-one treatment. If the therapist feels exposed and is made uncomfortable and vulnerable, he or she tends to be more self-revealing and feels less adequate in the group setting. Thus, countertransference feelings may arise. Wolf (1974) notes that the analyst who uses combined treatment tends to become more active, questioning the need of total frustration of the patient's archaic needs, less neutral, more challenging, shows a greater appreciation of the patient's family life, and seems to demand less regression in the individual sessions. Lipschutz's observation that combined therapy provided a richer and more stimulating experience for the analyst remains unchallenged even today.

Confidentiality

Most therapists practicing combined therapy inform their patients in advance that material from individual sessions may be brought up in the group session and vice versa. They prefer, however, that the patients do the bridging. Therapists do advise patients that material discussed in individual sessions may be referred to and encourage their patients to bring it into the group if it appears to be helpful and thera-

peutic. Few therapists bind themselves to strict confidentiality by restricting discussion of material within the therapeutic modality in which it was originally brought up. To agree to such an arrangement is to play into a resistance which colludes against change in therapy and may be a reflection of countertransference feelings.

Some authors offer a somewhat different perspective. Greenbaum (1957) stresses that there should be a separation of the material between the two modalities. Sager points out the need for a certain separation between individual and group material, stating that defenses would be raised in individual treatment and productivity stifled. He agrees that information received privately from the patient should rarely be introduced into the group unless the patient himself freely does so. Usually, therapists ask the patient's permission to bring material from the individual session into the group. The therapist should not discuss actions of other members, dynamics, or symptoms in individual sessions, for to do so would violate the confidentiality of patients. It would also be a seduction and convey a message of specialness to a patient, favoring him or her above the others.

Case History

Miss J., a 24-year-old schoolteacher, was referred for psychiatric treatment by her internist because of longstanding somatic symptoms, difficulties with authority figures at work, and her inability to maintain heterosexual relationships. Although she was bright, articulate, and attractive, her relationships with men usually ended in bitter arguments wherein the man was devalued and discarded. Following 2 years of individual therapy, on a twice-a-week basis, her treatment seemed to come to a standstill. She idealized the therapist, who could do no wrong. Her infatuation with him led to constant, provocative behavior and resulted in a series of pseudoemergency phone calls. She refused to analyze her behavior and continued her acting out with supervisors at work. There was obvious splitting occurring. It was mutually agreed that she might make better progress with a change in the therapeutic format, and she consented to combined therapy.

Miss J. became one of eight members in a newly formed close-ended group. All the members were in combined treatment with the same therapist. Two had been in individual treatment less than 1 year; the other six had been in therapy 2 or more years. Four of the members were felt to have borderline personality disorders, and one of these (Miss J.) also manifested pronounced narcissistic pathology. One patient was a narcissistic character but exhibited few borderline features. The remaining three patients had other disorders—one person was diagnosed a hysterical personality, another a phobic individual with severe obsessive-compulsive features, and the third was a chronic depressive character. Two members dropped out of this group after 2 years; the others terminated as a group 4 years later. Another borderline patient joined the group 3 years after its inception and remained with the group until it terminated.

Miss J., who was aggressive and determined to be the leader, quickly took charge. She became the group interpreter and soon established a pattern for the group of letting everything hang out. She also adopted a detective-like, probing attitude. The anticipated defensiveness and animosity created by her approach was counteracted by the personalities of the three nonborderline patients, in particular by the narcissistic patient, who was by profession an entertainer. The group members showed a low level of anxiety and were not susceptible to much guilt. They were themselves aggressive individuals and had been carefully prepared during individual sessions to expect personal confrontations.

Initially, because of her psychological sophistication, Miss J. was perceived by some members as a ringer who had been put into the group to keep them on track and to stimulate them. They considered the group to be a laboratory in which they were to learn about themselves and how they reacted to people. Although the illusion about Miss J. soon faded, the group did not lose sight of the therapeutic goals which were reinforced in the individual sessions. The members gradually saw through Miss J.'s defensive maneuvers and pointed out to her how she protected herself by focusing on others in an aggressive fashion. Eventually, she came to realize that her attacks upon the other patients represented a disavowal of the hated parts of herself which she feared and had to actively control; thus, she projected them onto other people. In turn, she was able to experience how she was used by other borderline patients in a similar manner.

Miss J. shared her job difficulties relating to supervisors with the group members and re-enacted her conflicts within the group. Although never fired from any position, she came perilously close to being dismissed by outraged supervisors at work and of being scapegoated in the group because of her attitudes. A physically attractive person, she wore blouses with plunging necklines and displayed her legs to advantage whenever she dealt with male members. In the group, she flaunted her sexual escapades with prominent men and described how she could easily seduce and humiliate them. Her exhibitionistic actions would intrigue the group and temporarily allay her feeling of loneliness but would be followed by a sense of emptiness and chronic rage.

Although Miss J.'s appearance, behavior, and affect might easily lead one to diagnose her as a hysterical personality, a more malignant underlying disorder existed. She was unable to separate from a cold, very masculine, and controlling mother. Her father had divorced her mother when the patient was very young, and he died during her course of therapy. Her younger sister never knew her father. Miss J. suffered severe somatic symptoms and had marked identity problems. During her treatment, continuing changes occurred in her manner of dress, hair style, makeup, speech mannerisms, and personal opinions. In her own words, she was desperately seeking to find "the real Miss J."

In the group, the members confronted Miss J. with her chameleon attitudes and chronic rage. In the individual therapy, she was afforded the safety and opportunity to work through her identity diffusion and the resolution of her grandiose self. She was able to learn through individual therapy that her acting out in the group and her destructive social relationships on the outside represented at one level, a flight from the oedipal situation and, on a more regressive plane, the need for an idealizing parent who was missing from her life. During the last year of combined therapy, Miss J. was finally able to maintain a healthy relationship with a professional man whom she later married. Over the course of her therapy she had gone through a total of 25 lovers, often with destructive results.

During her participation in combined treatment, Miss J. gained some insight into her narcissistic resistances, which were initially manifested in individual therapy by an over-idealization of the analyst and therapy. For example, she felt that treatment would provide her with techniques which would further her professional success and rid her of the bad

parts of herself. She would learn more about herself and be able to attract a marriage partner befitting a person of her beauty and intelligence. In the individual sessions, she hid her envy and aggressive feelings behind an idealizing, albeit patronizing, attitude toward the therapist, all the while engaging in sadomasochistic love affairs on the outside.

Once combined treatment was begun, a dramatic change occurred in her individual sessions. Expressions of rage and envy toward the group members as well as toward the therapist surfaced. Aggressive themes of wanting to usurp and belittle the analyst in the group aroused feelings of intense anxiety in her individual sessions. As those feelings were worked through, the patient recalled the loss of her once loved but psychologically impotent father who fled the family when the patient was 5 years old. Her father was happily remarried, but he saw the patient infrequently. Her mother often expressed her bitterness and open disappointment that the father's second marriage was so satisfying. The apparent loss of the therapist to the other group members and the realization that he cared about other patients besides her proved narcissistically mortifying but therapeutically useful for Miss J. After being in combined therapy for 2 years, she went through a period of depression, reliving the loss of the idealized father. As her depression lifted, she was able to verbalize her anger and rage over the desertion instead of acting out the conflict.

The transference paradigms were manifested in the group through her relationships with the members and were further dealt with in both her group and individual sessions. Her reactions in the individual sessions often became grist for the group mill. The father transference toward the therapist alternated with that of the good-bad mother transference and eventually carried over to the group, which came to be viewed as the good mother. At varying times, Miss J. reacted to the women in the group as though they were her more attractive sister or mother, while she related to the men like they were her suitors or male supervisors.

The individual sessions were the glue that held these people together, allowing for heated interchange in the group between members, the emergence of projective identification, splitting, and a vast range of intermember and therapist-member transferences. When the group terminated after 6 years, the members regarded one another with affection and respect. In follow-ups, the therapist learned that some kept in touch occasionally by phone or met for lunch.

Criticisms

The practice of combined therapy does not lack for critics. Some therapists who are in the sole practice of individual therapy object to the concurrent use of group on the basis that the transference is not allowed to develop to its fullest, while those practicing primarily group psychotherapy feel that the group anxiety is not resolved in the group setting and even avoided with the use of combined treatment. Most of the criticism protests how group therapy becomes impaired. Slavson (1950) and Foulkes and Anthony (1957) feel that group psychotherapy should not be mixed but used alone. They find the intensive regressive transference fostered in individual treatment incompatible with the diminished or diluted transference which is required for functioning in the group. Other critics believe that the concurrent use of individual sessions dilutes the potency of the group and provides a resistance to group treatment. Such an opinion is voiced by the British school of group psychotherapists who practice group analysis. Rosenbaum (1952) states that in combined treatment the group is merely used as a social setting, while treatment is carried out in the individual setting. He grants that occasionally individual treatment is done in the group, but most of the reactions of the group members and their understanding of dynamics are really resolved in individual treatment. The group is not utilized to its full capacity, and treatment may become overly intellectualized. Transferences are avoided and not dealt with in the groups, dreams are not discussed, and much of the work is shunted to the individual session.

Conclusion

If the therapist consciously or unconsciously stresses the importance of the individual sessions over the group meeting, he or she may contribute to the patient's resistance to the group and undermine its effectiveness. Battegay finds that, in combined treatment, subgroups form between the patients and therapist and the group is rendered impotent. Members not in combined treatment form subgroups within the group, creating difficulties. The group is no longer group but becomes leader oriented. Consequently, freedom in the group is greatly hindered. Sakles contends that in combined treatment there is a withholding and draining off of the group energy which injures the nature flow of group process. The discharge of affect or tension in individual sessions reduces the pressure to express it in the group.

Wolf states that the therapist using combined treatment shows little regard for the therapeutic effectiveness of group therapy. He feels that combined treatment should not be employed routinely; the use of individual sessions may arise from countertransference needs of the therapist. The regular use of individual hours along with group therapy, according to Wolf, leads to increased resistance, blocks reality testing, and prevents vigorous mutual investigation in the group. He fears that in combined treatment the patient may avoid group participation, misuse the group in order to avoid relating to the analyst, create destructive behavior either in the group session or in the individual sessions, and become infantalized. According to Wolf, the occcasional use of individual hours in conjunction with group psychotherapy is permissible when such use is realistically necessary and appropriate. But whenever this occurs, the patient should tell the group what transpired in the individual meeting.

The reader must render his or her own judgment about combined treatment. Those who have employed it seem totally convinced of its efficacy, while others who protest its legitimacy are perhaps too hesitant to attempt it.

References

Aronson, M. L. Technical problems in combined psychotherapy. Int. J. Group Psychother., *14:* 425, 1964.

Battegay, R. Individual psychotherapy and group psychotherapy as single treatment methods and in combination. Acta Psychiatr. Scand., *48:* 43, 1972.

Beran, M. Combined individual and group therapy within a hospital team set-up. Int. J. Group Psychother., *11:* 313, 1961.

Berger, I. L. Modifications of the transferences as observed in combined individual and group psychotherapy. Int. J. Group Psychother., *10:* 456, 1960.

Bieber, T. B. Group and individual psychotherapy with male homosexuals. J. Am. Acad. Psychoanal., *2:* 255, 1974.

Brende, J. O. Combined individual and group therapy for Vietnam veterans. Int. J. Group Psychother., *31:* 367, 1981.

Cappon, D. Discussion. Symposium on combined individual and group psychotherapy. Int. J. Group Psychother., *14:* 438, 1964.

Durkin, H. Discussion of symposium on combined individual and group psychotherapy. Int. J. Group Psychother., *14:* 445, 1964.

Foulkes, S. H., and Anthony, E. J. *Group Psychotherapy: The Psychoanalytic Approach.* Penguin Books, London, 1957.

Fried, E. The effect of combined therapy on the productivity of patients. Int. J. Group Psychother., *4:* 42, 1954.

Fried, E. Combined group and individual therapy with passive narcissistic patients. Int. J. Group Psychother., *5:* 194, 1955.

Green, J. A treatment plan combining group and individual psychotherapeutic procedures in a state mental hospital. Psychiatr. Q., *27:* 245, 1953.

Greenbaum, H. Combined psychoanalytic therapy and negative therapeutic reactions. In *Schizophrenia in Psychoanalytic Office Practice*, A. Rivkin, editor, p. 56. Grune & Stratton, New York, 1957.

Heigl-Evans, A., and Heigl, F. On the combination of psychoanalytic individual and group therapy. Gruppenpsychother. Gruppendyn., *8:* 97, 1974.

Hulse, W. C. Transference, catharsis, insight and reality testing during concomitant individual and group psychotherapy. Int. J. Group Psychother., *5:* 45, 1955.

Jackson, J., and Grotjahn, M. The treatment of oral defenses by combined individual and group psychotherapy. Int. J. Group Psychother., *8:* 373, 1958.

Kadis, A. L. and Markowitz, M. Group psychotherapy. In *Progress in Clinical Psychology*, vol. 3, p. 154. Grune & Stratton, New York, 1958.

Lipschutz, D. M. Combined group and individual psychotherapy. Am. J. Psychother., *11:* 336, 1957.

Mintz, E. E. Overt male homosexuals in combined group and individual treatment. J. Consult. Psychol., *30:* 193, 1966.

Papanek, H. Combined group and individual therapy in the light of Adlerian psychology. Int. J. Group Psychother., *6:* 136, 1956.

Rosenbaum, M. The challenge of group psychoanalysis. Psychoanalysis *1:* 42, 1952.

Rosenbaum, M. What is the place of combined psychotherapy? A comment and critique. Top. Probl. Psychother., *2:* 86, 1960.

Rosenbaum, M. What is the place of combined psychotherapy? A comment and critique. Top. Probl. Psychother., *2:* 86, 1960.

Sager, C. Concurrent individual and group analytic psychotherapy. Am. J. Orthopsychiatry, *30:* 255, 1960.

Sakles, C. J. Role conflict and transference in combined psychodramatic group therapy and individual psychoanalytically oriented psychotherapy. Group Psychother. Psychodrama, *25:* 70, 1972.

Schecter, D. E. Integration of group therapy with individual psychoanalysis. Psychiatry, *22:* 267, 1959.

Scheidlinger, S., and Porter, K. Group therapy combined with individual psychotherapy. In *Specialized Techniques in Individual Psychotherapy*, T. B. Karasu and L. Bellak, editors, p. 426, Brunner-Mazel, New York, 1980.

Shay, J. Differentials in resistance reactions in individual and group psychotherapy. Int. J. Group Psychother., *4:* 253, 1954.

Slavson, S. R. *Analytic Group Psychotherapy.* Columbia University Press, New York, 1950.

Spanjaard, J. Transference neurosis and psychoanalytic group psychotherapy. Int. J. Group Psychother., *9:* 31, 1959.

Stein, A. The nature of transference in combined therapy. Int. J. Group Psychother., *14:* 413, 1964.

Sullivan, H. S. *The Interpersonal Theory of Psychiatry.* H. S. Perry and M. L. Gawel, editors, Norton, New York, 1953.

Tabachnick, N. Isolation, transference-splitting and combined therapy. Compr. Psychiatry, *6:* 336, 1965.

Wilder, J. Group analysis and the insights of the analyst. In *The Challenge for Group Psychotherapy—Present and Future.* S. De Schill, editor, International Universities Press, New York, 1974.

Wolberg, A. The psychoanalytic treatment of the borderline patient in the individual and group setting. Top. Probl. Psychother., *2:* 174, 1960.

Wolf, A. Psychoanalysis in groups. In *The Challenge for Group Psychotherapy: Present and Future*. S. De Schill, editor. International Universities Press, New York, 1974.

Wolff, H. H., and Solomon, E. B. Individual and group psychotherapy: Complementary growth experiences. Int. J. Group Psychother., *23:* 177, 1973.

Wong, N. Clinical considerations in group treatment of narcissistic disorders. Int. J. Group Psychother., *29;* 325, 1979.

Wong, N. Combined group and individual treatment of borderline and narcissistic patients: Heterogeneous versus homogeneous groups. Int. J. Group Psychother., *30:* 389, 1980.

B.3 Structured Interactional Group Psychotherapy

HAROLD I. KAPLAN, M.D.

BENJAMIN J. SADOCK, M.D.

Introduction

It is generally conceded that the human personality does not evolve solely from biological determinants. Nor is the texture of the child's earliest relationship with his mother the sole determinant, however crucial it may be for his later development. Personality can best be understood as the combined product of the child's biological endowment and his psychological experience, which derives in large measure from his interaction with all the key individuals in his social environment—not only with his parents, but also with his siblings, aunts and uncles, friends and teachers, etc. Implicit in this formulation is the etiological proposition that all emotional and mental difficulties that cannot be attributed to constitutional or organic factors must be considered to arise from disturbances in the individual's interpersonal relationships. It follows, then, that if it is to be effective, psychotherapy must provide the patient with a corrective emotional experience, or, more accurately, with a series of corrective interpersonal experiences which in turn will enable him to modify the learned emotional responses which underlie his neurotic behavior patterns. The kind of corrective emotional experience that is a prerequisite for the success of treatment could not be provided within the framework of the one-to-one doctor-patient relationship, since individual psychotherapy seems to create a special situation which, in itself, is an unnatural medium for emotional change and growth.

Individual psychotherapy seeks to illuminate the relationship between the patient's current problems with other people and within himself, on the one hand, and his conflictual feelings toward crucial figures and events in his past, on the other, by exploring his transference responses to the therapist, who is traditionally cast in the parental role. Concomitantly, the therapist, by assuming attitudes toward the patient

which differ significantly from those held by his parents, may produce what Alexander (1950) called "the corrective emotional experience." Apart from the fact that the efficacy of this particular technique is open to question, individual psychotherapy can be criticized on the grounds that it emphasizes one sector of the patient's psychological experience. This is not to say that individual psychotherapy does not permit the patient to act out a variety of roles in his relationship with the therapist. However, by virtue of the fact that the therapist is the sole focus of cathexis, such manifestations are limited to a level of fantasy when they involve a variety of people in the patient's life.

The multiple transference components of the patient's behavior might emerge more clearly in a group situation, where he is given an opportunity to engage in dynamic interaction with a number of individuals. In contrast to individual psychotherapy, group therapy represents reality; and in this setting, the corrective emotional experience acquires new depth and meaning. The patient faces a variety of people who are possible targets for his transferential reactions and responds to them to the extent of his abilities. In the process, he is forced, under pressure from the group, to recognize the distortions in his response to selected members of the group. At the same time, he comes to understand that these inappropriate responses derive from repressed feelings and attitudes which were originally directed toward figures and situations in his past. Finally, the patient is motivated to explore and, ultimately, to modify these inappropriate impulses and attitudes, by his compelling need to be accepted by the group.

From these considerations, it was concluded that an individual approach to psychotherapy was not sufficient in itself, and, in 1953, Kaplan began to treat groups of patients for the first time, using a new directive approach called structured interactional group psychotherapy. At the same time, however, it was realized that group therapy could not supplant individual therapy entirely, particularly when treatment is based on psychoanalytic concepts.

The overriding goal of group therapy is to effect permanent changes in the behavior of the individual patients who comprise the group. But there is not sufficient opportunity in this setting to elicit from each group member the genetic and dynamic data which, according to psychoanalytic theory, are essential to the understanding of human behavior. In fact, the lack of detailed data regarding individual patients constitutes a major source of the criticism which has been leveled at group therapy. Presumably, these data would not be required for experiential-existential group approaches which focus on the "here and now," i.e., on the patient's immediate emotional response, and attach little importance to the origins, meaning, and implications of that response. It is the authors' contention, however, that behavior (and symptoms) cannot be modified without reference to their pathogenesis and content. A detailed anamnesis of each group member would, therefore, be considered a paramount requisite for the success of treatment. Inasmuch as these data can only be obtained in individual session, it was stipulated that all group patients must also see the therapist for individual treatment. From the outset, it was assumed that the combined use of group and individual treatment would enhance the possibility of a successful therapeutic outcome, and the results of these efforts in the years since attest to the validity of this assumption.

Therapeutic Philosophy

Structured interactional group psychotherapy evolved, within this theoretical framework, from two interdependent premises: (1) what is generally referred to as the directive approach to group therapy—that is, the success of treatment can best be assured if the therapist assumes an active role as leader of the group; (2) if the therapist is to function effectively in this capacity, combined individual and group therapy is a mandatory condition of group therapy. Obviously, this is an oversimplified delineation of the components of structured interactional group psychotherapy. The content of the premises on which this treatment approach is based, their underlying rationale, and the nature of their interrelationship all merit further elaboration.

Design

The various methods of group therapy are frequently viewed as a continuum. Those methods which entail a high degree of structuring on the part of the therapist (and have limited therapeutic goals) are placed at one end of the continuum; unstructured methods which entail minimal activity on the part of the therapist (and attempt to fulfill the traditional goals of psychotherapy) are placed at the other end.

Structured interactional group psychotherapy belongs in the middle of this continuum. The therapist structures much of the group's activity; however, his efforts to control and direct group interaction are specifically designed to implement the traditional goals of psychotherapy. Thus, such structuring consists in the application of specialized techniques which enhance the traditional techniques of group therapy

and serve, thereby, to facilitate treatment. More precisely, the therapist structures the group's activities by actively intervening to circumvent the methodological problems which are inherent to this treatment modality. And although some therapists believe that these problems can be ultimately resolved through spontaneous group interaction, it seems that undirected interaction exerts a negative influence on the treatment process which may, in fact, impede their possible eventual solution.

A brief discussion of some of the characteristics of traditional forms of group therapy, as compared to structured interactional group psychotherapy, may serve to clarify the role and function of the therapist in each setting. In traditional groups, each patient achieves catharsis and varying degrees of insight into his difficulties through his own efforts. Concomitantly, the patient's progress will depend, in large measure, on the degree to which intrapsychic and interpersonal factors restrict or foster his participation in the group process. In theory, each patient comes to the fore at various times during a group session, either of his own volition or at the insistence of other group members. In actual fact, however, one or more patients in a traditional group may remain withdrawn and uncommunicative for long periods of time. In structured interactional group psychotherapy, the therapist takes specific steps to correct this imbalance. For example, at each session, group activity focuses on a particular member of the group who has been selected beforehand by the therapist. Through this and other techniques, which are discussed in detail below, the therapist is able to ensure the participation of each patient in the group. Moreover, since participation in group treatment must be properly channeled if it is to yield therapeutic gains, the therapist may intervene, within the framework of structured interactional group psychotherapy, to further enhance the patient's efforts to achieve catharsis and insight into his difficulties. These activities on the part of the therapist are the cornerstone of structured interactional group psychotherapy.

Admittedly, traditional group therapy permits greater spontaneity among group members. On the other hand, the spontaneous emotional interaction which is a paramount feature of traditional group therapy may block or retard therapeutic progress. Emotions such as rage, anger, and distress are infectious. When the intensity of such emotions exceeds the limits of the patient's tolerance, the group situation becomes chaotic. Accordingly, structured interactional group psychotherapy attempts to avoid the perils of the affect-laden group. In his role as group leader, the therapist provides the guidance which is essential if cognitive processes leading to insight are to occur.

INTEGRATION OF PSYCHOANALYSIS AND OPERANT CONDITIONING

Liberman has described operant conditioning in the therapeutic setting as the use of the therapist's overt and covert responses to reinforce the patient's adaptive patterns of behavior and to inhibit his maladaptive patterns. When a group therapist directs attention toward a withdrawn member who has just contributed to group interaction for the first time and when he approves of and accepts the contribution, then he is selectively strengthening and reinforcing that mature behavior. Such reinforcement may also take place between members of the group.

When a particular group member is the focus of attention and interest, the therapist has many opportunities to apply verbal operant conditioning methods. By reinforcing selected behavior of the group members, either collectively or individually, he is able to effect behavioral change.

A passive man who was unable to assert himself was asked by the therapist to make a critical comment about each member of the group—including the therapist—in a go-around. Reluctant to do so at first, he eventually acceded to the request. After completing the task, during which he was able to tell one member that she was obese and another that he was an opportunist, the passive patient received the approval of all the members. Assertiveness was thus reinforced.

As used by the authors, operant conditioning in structured interactional group psychotherapy is adjunctive to the cognitive insights and the corrective emotional experience that psychoanalytic practice affords. The two frames of reference are not mutually exclusive in this treatment method. The working through of a transference distortion—such as seeing the therapist as a stern, punitive father figure—can be effected not only by the leaders and the other members' interpretations within the psychoanalytic frame of reference but also by operant techniques. These techniques reinforce the patient's ventilation of angry feelings consonant with that tranferential reaction—but do not reinforce the fantasied retribution he had come to expect as a result of past experiences. Thus, structured interactional group psychotherapy serves as a bridge between psychoanalysis in groups and behavioral group psychotherapy.

INTEGRATION OF INDIVIDUAL AND GROUP THERAPY

There is general agreement that group therapy is more effective and less troublesome when it is carried out in conjunction with individual treatment. As noted above, the multiple transference components of the patient's behavior emerge with greater clarity in the group setting. However, for obvious reasons, the origins and implications of the patient's transference to the therapist and to other group members can be explored in greater depth in individual sessions. Concomitantly, individual sessions provide the patient with an opportunity to express feelings he is not yet ready to discuss in the group. They may also serve to reassure those in whom the group experience has aroused excessive anxiety, to give overly shy members an opportunity to communicate with the therapist, and, generally, to solidify gains made in the group.

These considerations apply, to varying degrees, to all methods of group therapy. However, the integration of individual and group therapy has a particular significance for structured interactional group psychotherapy. The therapist's detailed knowledge of each member of the group, which can only be acquired in the intimacy of one-to-one treatment setting, and his continued awareness of the emotional status and needs of each patient are crucial to the success of his efforts to direct and control group interaction and group interrelationships. At the same time, the therapist's individual relationship with each patient in the group reinforces his role as leader and removes the taint of authoritarianism from his efforts to structure the treatment process. For, in a sense, the therapist's activities in the group setting are perceived as an extension of his traditional role in individual treatment.

Formation of the Group

Eligibility

As a general rule, those patients who are seen individually by other therapists are not considered suitable for structured interactional group psychotherapy. Structured interactional group psychotherapy can be truly effective only if the group therapist has sufficient genetic and dynamic understanding of each patient in the group; and, as noted earlier, this knowledge can only be acquired in individual treatment. If his eligibility for structured interactional group psychotherapy is not contraindicated on these grounds, the prospective patient is seen by the therapist for diagnostic evaluation in one or more initial interviews before he is accepted for psychotherapy.

Formal diagnosis is based on the criteria set forth in the *Diagnostic and Statistical Manual* (III), issued by the American Psychiatric Association. In the course of these initial interviews, the therapist formulates a comprehensive statement of the fundamental aspects of the patient's life, i.e., somatic, intrapsychic, interpersonal, and cultural. On the basis of this data, the therapist is able to assess the patient's eligibility for psychological treatment in general and for combined individual and group therapy in particular.

Obviously, not all patients who are accepted for individual treatment would, from the outset, be considered suitable candidates for structured interactional group psychotherapy. Individual treatment can help, in such instances, to prepare the patient for the group experience. However, such patients are relatively few in number. Because of its unique features, eligibility for structured interactional group psychotherapy is not subject to the restrictions which necessarily limit participation in more traditional methods of group therapy.

Accordingly, the choice of patients for structured interactional group psychotherapy follows the same lines as for individual psychotherapy. Patients who are inaccessible to individual treatment because of organic or constitutional defects or extreme regressive states must also be excluded from group therapy. With these exceptions, structured interactional group psychotherapy can generally be used successfully to treat patients who suffer from every type of neurosis and personality disorder, including those syndromes which are not generally thought to be amenable to group therapy. By virtue of the fact that it incorporates specific techniques to ensure participation by every member of the group, depressed and withdrawn patients can benefit greatly from this type of treatment. Patients who suffer from conditions variously described as schizotypal, latent, borderline, or prepsychotic states are also considered eligible for structured interactional group psychotherapy. And, once again, this can be attributed, in large measure, to the unique features of this type of group psychotherapy. In his role as group leader, the therapist uses his skills to control the amount of stimulation to which these patients are exposed, to diminish anxiety, and, in general, to assuage the emotional tensions which lead to disorganized behavior.

Composition

As a rule, groups tend to function best when they are heterogeneous, not only with respect to clinical entity but also with respect to such factors as sex, age, social status, and cultural background. Ideally, then, the group will include individuals who demonstrate enough variety in personality and emotional problems to prevent reinforcement and overintensification of their difficulties. To the extent that this is feasible, the group should comprise an equal number of male and female patients. And, finally, heterogeneity—with regard to age, social status, and cultural background—facilitates communication and interstimulation among group members. However, some similarity in these areas may be desirable. To illustrate, although patients from 16 to 60 may benefit from structured interactional group psychotherapy, in a group of young individuals one middle-aged patient might feel isolated and out of touch.

Groups which are heterogeneous with respect to clinical entity are not suitable for all patients. When all the patients in a group have similar difficulties, they share a certain commonality of suffering which may facilitate their participation in treatment. Two types of patients seem to do best in a homogeneous group: Acting-out adolescent patients, particularly those with drug abuse problems, and regressed patients. In any event, heterogeneous groups should not include more than one or two patients in these categories. Because they are so demanding of the time and attention of the therapist and of the other group members, these patients generate a great deal of resentment, which can have no therapeutic value and may block the treatment process.

Patient Orientation

The sooner the patient joins a group, the better his prognosis. The therapist explains to the patient that the cornerstone of his treatment will be individual psychotherapy; group therapy is presented as an additional modality which is available to the patient to supplement individual treatment, in much the same way that a laboratory session serves to supplement a chemistry lecture. Nevertheless, most patients express initial anxiety about the prospect of group therapy which cannot be entirely alleviated by this explanation.

The new group

Introducing different group members to each other upon the formation of a new group or introducing a new member to the members of a pre-existing group involves essentially the same process. Invariably, patients are uncomfortable and anxious at their first group therapy session; therefore, it is the task of the therapist to make this experience as untraumatic as possible.

At the first meeting of a new group, the group leader discusses the procedures and rules of structured interactional group psychotherapy. He then asks each member to talk about himself briefly, i.e., to give his name, age, and martial status and to summarize his educational background, work status, and the major emotional problems that brought him into therapy. Each member is allocated from 5 to 10 minutes for this purpose. However, within this time period, the therapist may supplement the patient's introductory statements with significant details that he feels the group should be aware of, provided, of course, that he has not been placed under any restrictions in this regard by the patient. If a patient does not want to disclose a particular aspect of his life at the first group session, the therapist must not bring it up until the patient's resistance has been worked through. Ultimately, however, the patient should be prepared to talk as candidly in group as he does in individual sessions.

The therapist's intervention may take other forms during these introductory self-summaries. When patients are too verbose, he may have to limit discussion, even though at this early point in treatment the patient may experience the therapist's intervention as a rejection, which will have to be worked through in individual session. Conversely, withdrawn and schizoid members may have to be drawn out and given support. Above all, each member of the group must have an opportunity to talk during this first session. The patient who is unable to participate for one reason or another may feel neglected; and while some patients may feel an immediate sense of relief because they have escaped exposure, this can only delay their integration into the group. In other instances, the patient may perceive this neglect as indifference to his problems on the part of both the therapist and the group, and he may withdraw from treatment altogether.

Once a new group has been formed, it has a life of its own, independent of the admission of new patients from time to time and the equally sporadic discharge of others. This, in turn, is a reflection of the stability and continuity of treatment, as epitomized by the therapist.

The new member in group

In time, each group develops a culture of its own, and the older members transmit the particular standards which have been adopted by the group to new patients when they enter therapy. This is a gradual process, however, and the new member must feel comfortable in the group before it can occur.

During his first group session, the patient is introduced by name, and provides a capsule summary of his background. Each of the regular members then introduces himself in turn; he gives his name, age, and occupation and briefly discusses the problems that brought him to therapy for the edification of the new member. Ten or 15 minutes may be devoted to these introductions. During the remainder of the group session, the new patient is up for discussion, a technique which is discussed in further detail below. The new patient is not told beforehand that he will be the center of the group's attention, lest this prospect evoke excessive anxiety. But this is rarely perceived as a betrayal by the therapist. Once the group is in session, the procedure is explained and its traumatic aspects minimized; the patient is further reassured by the protective presence of the therapist. In theory, the procedure is a relatively simple one. The group members ask the new patient questions about himself. In fact, when the group is more sophisticated and experienced, such questioning is reminiscent of a skilled psychiatric examination. Although it may cause some temporary discomfort, this procedure helps to integrate the newcomer into group psychotherapy more rapidly, inasmuch as both the older members and the new member acquire some knowledge of one another's background and emotional difficulties at the outset.

Treatment Plan

Physical setting

The setting in which group therapy is conducted has received minimum attention in the literature. It has been the authors' experience, however, that specific aspects of this setting may help or hinder group interaction; as such, these routine details merit brief consideration.

Obviously, the room used for group psychotherapy should be large enough to comfortably accommodate all the members of the group; physical discomfort due to overcrowding, however minor, will, in most cases, reinforce the patient's resistance to therapy. Within the consultation room, it may be useful to have the members of the group sit in an unbroken circle; that is, individual patients are not separated from each other or from the group as a whole by physical barriers, e.g., conference tables, etc. The advantages of this circular seating arrangement as a symbol of group unity are self-evident.

Size of the group

The number of patients in the group will depend on the size of the consultation room. Provided that adequate space is available, a group may include as many as 15 or 16 members. Ideally, however, the size of the group will be limited to 10 or 12 patients. It can be speculated that 1 or 2 of the members of any typical group will be withdrawn schizoid patients whose participation will be minimal, and another 1 or 2 members will be absent from any given group therapy session, which means that from 6 to 8 patients will actually participate in each session. Efforts to have every patient participate in every session, at least to some extent, are most likely to be successful in groups of this size. If the group is too small, it may succumb to long periods of inpenetrable silence. And, if the group is too large, not everyone who wishes to

participate can do so within a fixed time period. Under such circumstances, it becomes more difficult to prevent secondary discussions between 2 or 3 members, which lead to group fragmentation.

Length of group therapy sessions

Group therapy sessions may vary in length from 1 to 2 hours. The group requires at least 1 hour to get suitably involved in the problem under discussion. However, no discussion or series of discussions can hold the attention and interest of either the group or the therapist if the session continues for more than 2 hours. (For this reason, among others, the group therapy marathon has always seemed to be of limited value, unless, of course, the therapist has carefully screened each participant beforehand and considers him capable of such sustained interaction and has further established that the patient can tolerate the continued stress which is a concomitant of this innovation.) It has been the authors' experience that, after a certain period of time, patients can no longer assimilate the intense stimulation of group therapy and that the length of the group therapy session must be determined by such psychodynamic variables.

Apart from such considerations, the therapy session should not extend beyond the limits of the therapist's ability to function effectively, and this has particular relevance for structured interactional group psychotherapy. Furthermore, the therapist must assess his clinical capacity at the outset. Due to the misconception—which, unfortunately, is nonetheless prevalent—that psychiatrists sell time (they sell their unique professional skills, not their time), it is important that all the groups treated by the therapist be allocated the same amount of time, and that the same amount of time be allocated to the same group each week. This must be clearly established by the therapist at the first meeting of each new group, and he must insist on strict adherence to this schedule. Varying the time arbitrarily causes patients to feel cheated. But, more important, many patients are reassured by the therapist's ability to control the length of the session, for this is perceived as a manifestation of his ability to control the group. If the therapist cannot control time, how can he be expected to control the group's aggression and hostility?

Frequency

Typically, 1 group session is held each week, so that 4 or 5 group sessions are held a month. It may be useful to increase the frequency of sessions, so that an extra group session may be held on a regular basis. For example, a group which meets regularly every Tuesday may also have an extra session on the first Thursday of the month. In any event, it is essential to establish regular meeting times which should only be changed if the therapy session falls on a holiday or if the therapist is ill or cannot be present for other reasons. Because regularly scheduled group sessions are important to the success of treatment, it is essential that missed group sessions should be made up by scheduling an extra meeting for the preceding or following week; proximity in time to the missed session helps to reinforce the concept of regular meetings. Although the concept of regularity is stressed, it may be necessary to increase the frequency of group meetings temporarily, if the resistance encountered in a group has, in the therapist's opinion, reached critical proportion. This should not be done arbitrarily, but only to overcome certain unique resistances of the group as a whole or of a particular member.

Finally, structured interactional group psychotherapy differs significantly from traditional methods of group therapy in respect to the frequency of group sessions, in that the group meets regularly during the summer month while the therapist is away on vacation. Briefly, during this period, the members meet without the therapist and report to him weekly on the content and procedure of each session. There is no charge for group sessions scheduled while the therapist is on holiday; but the attendance of the patients at these group meetings is mandatory (unless, of course, they are away on vacation themselves); indeed, it is considered as important as attendance at the regular sessions during the year. There is no guarantee that the patient's symptoms will remain in remission or that he would use this period to consolidate his gains; on the contrary, he may lose valuable ground. Consequently, structured interactional group psychotherapy can be maximally effective if it is provided throughout the year.

Financial considerations

The fees for psychotherapeutic services vary from one area of the United States to another and differ according to the background, skill, and reputation of the psychotherapist; in addition, within any given area, they will be determined by the supply and demand for psychiatric specialties.

The financial arrangements for structured interactional group psychotherapy pose important and unique problems which differ significantly from those encountered in individual psychotherapy. To begin with, patients in group therapy must feel confident of their equality in the eyes of the therapist. Therefore, as evidence of the therapist's lack of bias, all patients are charged the same fee for each group session, regardless of their financial resources, which group they have been assigned to, or the length of time they have been in treatment. This approach diminishes rivalry between group members and serves to preclude crises in the doctor-patient relationship which might otherwise arise on this account. In contrast to the uniformity which characterizes fees for group therapy, fees for individual psychotherapy are determined by a variety of factors; the patient's income, the therapist's customary fee at the time the patient begins treatment, frequency of therapy sessions, etc.

Rules and Procedures

Confidentiality

Structured interactional group psychotherapy is based upon a fundamental positive relationship between the patient and therapist and between the patient and other group members. One cornerstone of this dual relationship is the patient's firm conviction that his communications in both the individual and group treatment settings will be regarded as confidential and privileged information. Catharsis can take place only if the patient is secure in this knowledge. Consequently, the abrogation of confidentiality—whether inadvertently, by the therapist, or deliberately, by a member of the group or by a member of another group—may seriously impair treatment and, in extreme cases, precipitate its termination.

Doctor-patient relationship

Before he enters group therapy, the patient is encouraged to be as open with his group members as he is with the therapist in individual session. At the same time, however, he is assured that he will not be compelled to discuss any detail of his life with the group until he is ready to do so. And patients frequently do explore sensitive areas with the therapist in individual session which they cannot bring themselves to raise in group therapy sessions.

However, there are exceptions. In one group, a patient reported that he had an atrophied testicle as a result of a trauma, a fact he had made known to the therapist previously in individual session. At this point, another member of the group reported that he, too, had only one testicle, the result of a congenital anomaly, a fact of which the therapist had not been aware. The patient then explained that he had been too embarrassed to mention this in individual session. Once he found out that someone else had the same affliction, he no longer felt this overwhelming sense of shame, and he was able to talk about this problem.

However, as noted earlier, such situations occur rarely. In the normal course of events, the patient discusses such sensitive areas with his individual therapist first. If he does not want a specific matter brought up in the group, the patient must inform his therapist accordingly, prior to the group session, so that the therapist will not raise the issue himself when he feels it is in the patient's interests to do so. Unless the patient has imposed a specific prohibition, the group leader will automatically assume that any material discussed in individual session may also be discussed before the group. When the patient imposes such a restriction, the therapist should attempt to explore with the patient the various factors which underly his resistance. Although the therapist may agree that a particular subject should not be covered in group, at least for the time being, more often the therapist will attempt to dissuade the patient from avoiding the subject.

Whatever the source of his resistance, if the patient does not wish to discuss a subject, it is incumbent upon the therapist to honor his decision. To be treated in such a manner—that is, to have his wishes respected and honored—is most reassuring to the patient. Conversely, any violation of the patient's confidence would seriously impair the doctor-patient relationship, which, in turn, would have an adverse effect on treatment.

Ethics of group relationships

Similarly, the positive relationships between the patient and other group members, essential if group therapy is to be effective, are based in large measure on adherence to these ethical principles. Accordingly, when he enters group therapy, each patient is informed that the contents of all therapeutic sessions are confidential and must not be discussed with anyone outside the group. When a patient breaks this rule, he is immediately advised by the therapist that he will not be permitted to continue in therapy if he violates it a second time.

Chain reaction phenomenon

Information may also be spread between groups. It is particularly important, for example, that the confidentiality be emphasized when husbands and wives who see the same therapist in individual session have been assigned to different groups. Under such circumstances, one can understand that marital partners will be strongly tempted to gossip about discussions that take place in the respective group sessions, but such gossip is no less dangerous and potentially destructive to therapy.

Friends and other members of a family who are in individual treatment with the same therapist but in different groups are subject to the same temptations. For example, suppose that patient A in group I, patient B in group II, and patient C in group III are close friends socially. Patient A may then be tempted to discuss some particularly interesting item he has learned from a patient in his own group (I) with his friends, who may then pass this information on to their co-patients in groups II and III. While such a chain reaction dissemination of information is usually harmless, it does represent a violation of confidentiality, and, as such, it can present serious problems. Accordingly, while the therapist must expect chain reactions, he must exert every effort to reduce them to a minimum. And, when they do occur, it is his responsibility to confront the persons involved and to make the necessary interpretations.

Extratherapeutic contact

As the group as a whole and his fellow group members as individuals become a emotional focal point for the patient, there is an increased tendency to socialize, i.e., to establish contact with the group outside the treatment setting. However, contact outside the group may be undesirable on several counts. Socializing threatens confidentiality; socializing conduces to sexual acting out, which may constitute a therapeutic crisis; and excessive extratherapeutic contact may impede the patient's growth and development as a social being.

After they had been in therapy for 3 years, the members of one group who had been permitted to socialize had developed few outside relationships. Since their social life revolved around the group, these patients simply had not had an opportunity to test new modes of behavior with others. Only after socializing was prohibited and group members were forced to form relationships in the outside world was there evidence of progress in this area.

Termination of treatment

The patient who terminates therapy by mutual agreement with the therapist is discharged with medical advice; the dropout is discharged against medical advice. After the patient and the therapist have agreed that the patient is ready to terminate treatment, the patient remains in group therapy for a 3-month trial period before this decision is finalized. This permits the patient to withdraw from treatment gradually, and it gives the therapist additional time to carefully evaluate the patient's psychological status. If all goes well, the patient is discharged from treatment with the understanding that he can return to the group whenever he feels the need to do so for any number of follow-up sessions. Research seems to indicate, however, that most patients avail themselves of this privilege only sparingly. More frequently, their relationship with the group tapers off gradually, although they may remain in contact with one or two group members. And, in turn, this is a measure of the success of treatment.

Specialized Techniques

Structured interactional group psychotherapy is based upon the dynamics common to all psychotherapy: relationship, catharsis, insight, ego strengthening, reality testing, and sublimation. The techniques employed are based on the fundamental principles of psychoanalytic theory. Thus, they include exploration of the patient's personal history to facilitate the expression of repressed material and ward off tendencies to act out, the use of free association and the interpretation of dreams, and the analysis of transference phenomena and of resistance.

Structured interactional group psychotherapy is unique, however, in that it also employs specialized therapeutic techniques, geared to this particular treatment modality, which are specifically designed to enhance the traditional procedures delineated above.

The patient is up

The cornerstone of structured interactional group psychotherapy, theoretically and technically, is the procedure whereby a specific patient is up for discussion by the group. Its purpose is to foster participation in treatment. Such participation is essential if the patient is to achieve creative change within himself and in his relationship with others; furthermore, there is a close correlation between the extent to which the patient participates in treatment and the degree of change he is able to achieve. On the whole, the articulate patient rarely presents a problem in this respect. However, the participation of the withdrawn or schizoid patient—who is encountered just as frequently in psychotherapy—becomes an overriding therapeutic goal. "The patient is up" ensures fulfillment of this goal.

In essence, each week, the therapist selects the patient he feels will benefit most from group interaction to be the focus of the therapy session. In a sense, the session belongs to this patient. Typically, he will talk about himself for 15 or 20 minutes; at the conclusion of this monologue, the group will begin a general discussion which will continue to revolve around the patient who is up. The therapist may interject his comments, either in the course of the patient's initial presentation or during the subsequent group discussion, if he feels that certain relevant aspects of the patient's behavior have not been covered or have not received sufficient emphasis. Thus, to a significant extent, the therapist provides the structure, organization, and substance of the group session.

As the center of attention, the patient who is up occupies an enviable position in the group, and patients frequently vie for this opportunity. In fact, many patients keep a rather careful record of which patient is discussed each week in order to make sure that all the members of the group are up for discussion the same number of times each year. Moreover, since the therapist makes the final decision as to who is up for discussion each week, these records serve to ensure equality of treatment. Nevertheless, such equality in frequency of discussion is not always feasible. A patient who is going through a period of crisis may have to be the focus of group attention in two or three sessions out of cycle. Group members tend to accept this without protest; they understand that occasionally a patient may need extra time when he is faced with an emergency. Conversely, they will object if a dominating, grasping patient tries to get more than his fair share of the group's attention; such a patient usually evokes considerable hostility on the part of his co-patients.

As noted above, the therapist's decision with regard to the selection of the patient who is up is based on his evaluation of the needs of the individual members of the group. Thus, the withdrawn schizoid patient, who finds it difficult to relate to others and who will not participate in group discussions voluntarily, will have to be forced to participate in treatment. Group members rarely make an effort on their own to draw these patients out. As a rule, the members of a newly formed group, in particular, will tend to overlook such patients and to direct their attention to the verbal, articulate, and insightful patient. The fact remains, however, that even if the therapist must set the stage for this response, it is extremely beneficial for the withdrawn patient to feel that the group is interested in him and wants to know more about him.

The go-around

Intimately related to the preceding technique, which is designed to ensure participation in treatment, is a procedure referred to as the go-around, which seeks to involve the patient more deeply in therapy by encouraging him to explore and verbalize his emotional problems. When he is the focus of a group session, the patient makes himself available for psychological exploration. Such exploration is facilitated by the go-around, whereby each member of the group is given an opportunity to discuss his personal response to the patient who is up.

In broad outline, after the group members are seated in a circle, as is customary, the therapist decides on the starting point of the go-around. Each patient then proceeds in orderly sequence to evaluate the focal group member and to explore his transferential feelings toward him until all the members of the group have participated in the discussion. Spontaneity is encouraged, and patients may enter the discussion out of turn. Yet the therapist must see to it that such spontaneity is kept within certain bounds. When affective reactions reach chaotic proportions, the group takes on the characteristics of a mob. Psychotherapy cannot proceed unless rational cognitive processes are brought to bear upon affective responses. Contrary to the view held by proponents of the encounter method, the ventilation of affect, in itself, has little psychotherapeutic value. Since the group situation is conducive to this form of expression, group therapy can be effective only if patient interaction is directed and controlled by the therapist, who can then make orderly, constructive interpretations. Finally, at the end of the go-around, the therapist may summarize its content and suggest particular areas of further exploration during the after-session.

The after-session

After the formal group session has been terminated, the group members continue their discussion of the patient who is up at an after-session, which is held outside the therapists's office and without his presence. Attendance at the after-session is mandatory.

Since the after-session may continue for several hours, it is most practical to schedule it in the evening so that patients who work or have other commitments during the day can attend. Most patients can usually manage to attend formal group therapy sessions during the day, since these are less time consuming. As a rule, groups meet with the therapist from 5 to 6:30 P.M. and proceed from there to the after-session, which may last until 11 P.M. or midnight, depending on the patient being discussed, the content of the session, etc.

Practical arrangements for the after-session are made by the members of the group, although they may—and frequently do—consult with the therapist before specific plans are finalized. Most often, the after-session is held at the apartment of a group member who lives in the general vicinity of the therapist's office. If several group members live in the area, their apartments are used in rotation. Obviously, the availability of a member's home for therapy sessions, no matter how ideally located, may be outruled on several grounds. The presence of the patient's mate or children would, for example, constitute a limiting factor.

Whether or not the patient's mate is in therapy himself, he will have definite opinions and feelings about his mate being in treatment. Depending on his personality structure, he may support the therapeutic efforts of his spouse or represent a potentially destructive influence. These attitudes and prejudices will be transmitted to group members if the mate happens to be around during an after-session held at his home and may require subsequent interpretation by the therapist. But, apart from such considerations, complete privacy is a mandatory condition for the after-session because of the highly personal and confidential nature of group therapy. This means that a patient may have to persuade her mate to visit a friend on the evening the group meets, which may not be easy. When children are involved as well, it becomes even more difficult to ensure the group's privacy. Nevertheless, patients do seem to manage somehow, so that arranging for after-sessions does not usually present an insurmountable problem when two or three homes are potentially available to the group for this purpose. But, when it does arise, this problem must be dealt with. The use of a private meeting place is essential for effective group therapy; a restaurant, for example, will not suffice.

There is an added advantage in having the group meet in a patient's home. The group has an opportunity to learn something about the patient's environment. In one instance, the group was particularly appalled by the shabby home of a patient who had been perceived as a natty dresser, a man about town. Indeed, this was the facade he presented to the world. In fact, however, this patient was extremely despondent, and his shabby, depressing surroundings accurately reflected his inner sense of despair.

After-sessions should be distinguished from the alternate sessions which are a frequent component of traditional group therapy approaches. Both are held without the therapist. However, in contrast to the after-session, which represents an extension of the formal group therapy session, the alternate session is held on another night of the week. But the most important difference between them lies in the fact that, in contrast to the after-session, attendance at alternate sessions is usually poor, and they tend to be disjoined and nonproductive.

Summer sessions

As mentioned earlier, the group continues to meet on a weekly basis during the summer month that the therapist is on vacation. Usually, a schedule is prepared the week before the therapist's departure, indicating in which patient's home the sessions will be held. Because patients have more time to travel, these vacation sessions are frequently held at the homes of group members who live in the suburbs. And, as is the case during the rest of the year, the therapist encourages the group to meet at a different home each week, both to see how their co-patients live and to observe their behavior in a natural setting.

Ancillary Treatment Techniques

"The patient is up" and the subsequent go-around are standard procedures in structured interactional group psychotherapy. However, several ancillary techniques have also been utilized from time to time.

The subject session

When appropriate, the group therapist may suggest that a group session be modified, so that another method of patient exploration be used in lieu of the go-around. During the subject session, which constitutes one such modification, the group leader suggests that the group discuss topics which have particular relevance for the patient who is up. Thus, the subject session is still another manifestation of structured interaction, and, as such, it facilitates communication, discussion, and psychic exploration.

At any given session, the therapist may suggest that the group discuss the following subjects, among others: (1) sexuality, infidelity, masturbation, and coitus; (2) manifestations of agression and the warding off of aggressive impulses; and (3) significant temporal events, such as an assassination or a natural disaster.

The following clinical excerpt may help to illustrate the potential therapeutic value of the subject session:

A young woman who had severe guilt feelings about masturbation and was too embarrassed to discuss this either with the therapist in individual session or with the group experienced a strong sense of relief when the therapist introduced this subject at a group session. After she heard several other group members freely admit that they masturbated and describe a variety of masturbatory techniques, the patient was able to discuss masturbation openly for the first time.

Categories

At other times, the therapist may deliberately use provocative words or phrases in an effort to elicit an emotional reaction from the patient who is up. And, once again, this technique is designed to encourage verbal expression and participation in treatment. Although most patients find the category method traumatic and anxiety provoking, they are willing to concede that it forces them to express feelings which would never be verbalized under normal circumstances.

An endless variety of categories can be used for this purpose. The patient who is up is asked to classify other members of the group on the basis of appearance, intelligence, sexuality, etc. In so doing, he is given an opportunity to verbalize his major affective reactions to specific group members. The therapist then encourages the focal member to rate himself in each of these categories. At this point, the patient reveals feelings he has about himself, i.e., his self-image, which he would not touch on normally.

The patient who is up is instructed to discuss his various categories and the criteria he used in making his selections in the after-session. In addition, group members are asked to discuss those listings and categories they found particularly upsetting or pleasant or meaningful and to explore their responses and associations. Those classifications which refer to appearance, intelligence, sexuality, and aggression seem to be the most provocative. The category method should be used sparingly; its frequent use may be too traumatic and may diminish the effectiveness of this technique.

Review sessions

The therapist conducts a review session at his first meeting with the group after he returns from vacation, at his last meeting with the group before he leaves on vacation, and whenever he feels there is a need for such a session during the therapeutic year.

During the review session, all the patients present are discussed. Each patient is requested, in turn, to summarize his present psychological status briefly.

Comments and interpretations may then be made by both the therapist and the other group members. It is important, however, to limit the length of the patient's summary, as well as the subsequent comments and interpretations, so that every patient will have an opportunity to participate. If a session is 1½ hours long, for example, and there are 10 members present, each patient should be discussed for approximately 10 minutes during the formal session in the therapist's office. Patients are instructed to conduct the after-session along similar lines. If the after-session is to last for 4 hours, each patient will be the focus of discussion for approximately 25 minutes.

Carefully structuring the review session in this manner helps to prevent chaos and makes it possible to cover many patients within a limited period of time. When the therapist has returned to the group after a lengthy absence, these conditions must prevail if he is to become acquainted with the current status of each patient and resume his role as the leader of the group.

Psychodrama

Psychodrama may also be used as an ancillary technique in structured interactional group psychotherapy. When he feels that this method may lead to a breakthrough, the therapist asks the patient who is up to step outside the consultation room while he and the other group members devise an appropriate psychodramatic situation for the patient, based on their knowledge of his psychological conflicts. Roles and content are predesignated; one patient may play the role of a mother (or father), another may portray a child, and a third may be a friend or a lover. Once it has been conceptualized, the patient returns to the session, and the psychodrama is enacted. When it has been concluded, the group members and the patient who is up discuss their reactions to the episode.

This technique is most valuable when it is used for patients whose feelings are so deeply repressed they cannot be elicited through traditional treatment techniques:

A 50-year-old depressed patient had not been able to discharge her affective response to her mother's death 10 years previously. Accordingly, the therapist suggested psychodrama as a possible means of facilitating the discharge of repressed material. It was decided that one group member would play the deceased mother returned to visit her daughter, and the patient was instructed to speak to her in any way she chose. Within a few minutes, the patient-daughter had expressed the despair, grief, and anger which were associated with her mother's death via this role-playing technique.

No true and permanent solution can be achieved through abreaction. Nevertheless, it is of value in that it demonstrates to the patient the existence and intensity of his emotions and serves as an introduction to the ensuing working through of what has come to light in the patient's acting out.

Other Methods

Personal movies and photographs

While verbalizing one's past and present life experiences is valuable in itself, seeing movies and photographs of the person involved and the situations described adds a very meaningful dimension to these accounts. This holds true for the patient concerned, for his fellow group members, and for the therapist. Frequently, the members of the group have an intense personal reaction to the photograph of a person they had only heard about, because they have identified with that person or because he or she may have become the target of their strong feelings of hostility and aggression.

Audiotape recordings

A patient's verbal contribution to a group session may be tape recorded, and the recording played back at a later date with remarkable effects. Patients should never be tape recorded without their knowledge and permission; to do so would threaten the privacy and trust which are so important to the doctor-patient relationship. This rarely presents a problem, however. Patients do not object to being taped as a rule, as long as they are aware of it beforehand and are assured of the confidentiality of their communications.

Videotape Recordings

Videotape equipment may also be used to enable patients to see themselves first-hand on a television monitor while they talk, and this device can have equally dramatic effects. In addition, videotape, like audiotape recordings, can be stored and played back at a later date when it seems appropriate to do so.

Dynamic Factors

Transference

It is commonly conceded that the foundation of all psychotherapy is the transference. In individual treatment, the transference is concentrated on the therapist, and identification of the transferential components inherent in the doctor-patient relationship is a prerequisite for the success of treatment. Constructive analysis of the transference is equally crucial to the efficacy of group therapy. In group therapy, however, the cathexis which is directed only toward the therapist in individual treatment is displaced upon other persons in the group (which further dilutes the transference). Concomitantly, transference phenomena become more complicated.

The patient's basic transference—to the therapist—is positive, but temporary periods of hostility or fear of the therapist are inevitable. In group therapy, these negative feelings toward the therapist may be held in check because of the patient's fear of retaliation of other group members, whose feelings are positive. The patient's hostility may then be displaced and redirected toward his fellow group members. On the other hand, the support group members receive from one another may facilitate the expression of hostility toward the therapist.

In any event, it behooves the group leader to keep these complex transferential situations clear and unchaotic. Because transferential reactions, whether positive or negative, are subject to contagion, by which they become greater than the sum of the group's parts, there is a risk attached to their expression in group. This is particularly true when strong negative feelings are directed toward the therapist. It is essential, of course, that the patient eventually express his hostile feelings toward the therapist, since he is the parent surrogate. However, the expression of major transferential reactions—especially negative ones—is best reserved for individual treatment sessions, where they can be analyzed more extensively. The unbridled expression of transference responses in group can produce chaos and the wolf-pack phenomenon, whereby the group gangs up on the therapist or another patient. Whereas such behavior can be extremely destructive in the group setting, it can be dealt with in individual sessions in a most constructive manner.

Interpretation

Interpretation is an index of the skill of the therapist, particularly when it involves elucidation of the transference and other unconscious processes. In group therapy, however, interpretation is not the sole prerogative of the therapist; it may also be made by the other patients in the group. Concomitantly, a patient's behavior may be interpreted in the group session per se, in the after-session, or in sessions which are held while the therapist is on vacation.

When giving interpretations, the therapist needs to beware of unmasking a patient before the group beyond a point the patient can accept. From this point of view, it is preferable that interpretation come from other members, and this occurs constantly as patients respond to the unconscious needs of one another through identification and empathy. Nevertheless, the therapist must evaluate the accuracy of such interpretations. When the interpretations of group members are cogent, the therapist must point out their cogency. When interpretations are insensitive or inaccurate, the therapist must correct them as promptly as possible. If such an interpretation is made during the formal group session, it can, of course, be corrected immediately. If the interpretation is made during an after-session, it may have to be corrected when the therapist sees the misunderstood patient in individual session.

In general, the group members look to the therapist for validation of the interpretations made by their peers, but when a patient speaks with authority (which is especially true of patients who have had some professional training), it may be necessary for the therapist to confront the authoritarian patient with the fact that he is subject to the same misperceptions as other members in the group. Above all, the therapist must never abdicate his role as leader of the group, and his evaluation of the validity of interpretations made by group members must reflect his capacity for leadership.

Dynamics of Group Interaction and Group Interrelationships

Nuclear group member: the therapist surrogate

Every therapeutic group includes several self-appointed group leaders. These patients, who are usually healthier than their peers, tend to function with particular effectiveness as catalysts in group interaction. When the therapist is not present, e.g., in the after-session or during summer meetings, these nuclear or focal members play a meaningful and active role in the group as surrogate therapists. It is the collaboration of these patients that makes structured interactional techniques meaningful in group therapy.

Accordingly, it is important to utilize the skills and participation of the nuclear patient in group therapy, to the extent that it is possible to do so. During those periods when the nuclear patient's relationship with the therapist is a positive one, he can be a potent ally. On the other hand, when he develops a negative transference toward the therapist, he may play a particularly destructive role in therapy. In short, the therapist must be constantly aware of the nuclear patient's psychological status if his skills are to be utilized effectively.

Other factors must be taken into consideration as well. As a rule, patients who assume this nuclear role gain certain unique benefits from group therapy; they achieve a marked increase in self-esteem, and their ego is strengthened considerably. At times, however, the nuclear group member may use his preoccupation with co-patients as a means of evading his own problems and of exposing himself to the group.

The patient, a 28-year-old psychiatric resident, identified closely with the therapist. Because of her innate sensitivity and her psychiatric training, she readily assumed the role of therapist surrogate. And her interpretations of the behavior of other patients were usually accurate. It soon became apparent, however, that these activities, which, on the one hand, helped her to grow and develop both personally and professionally, on the other hand often served to justify her resistance to examining her own problems and resolving her conflicts. Furthermore, her negative sexual transference, which was directed toward the therapist, was acted out with other group members without any attempt to gain insight into her behavior.

At one session, when the patient made an interpretation that was questioned by the therapist, she reacted with violent rage, instead of trying to validate the accuracy of her interpretation. Using her leadership position in the group, she then attempted to mobilize group support for her resistance. And she was stunned when the group refused to cooperate. Finally, her competitiveness with the therapist, as well as her striving for power, were interpreted in a go-around. After this confrontation, the patient's behavior, both in and out of group, began to change rather dramatically. Yet it is safe to assume that, if this conflict had not been exposed and resolved, this patient would have left therapy, feeling justified in her resistance.

Dominant behavior by one group member

Occasionally, a group will include a member whose neurotic need for power causes him to be extremely controlling and dominating. Typically, his co-patients will react to this type of behavior with anxiety and hostility. Only a strong and reasonably secure group member can be expected to challenge such a dominating patient, and at times the group will simply be unable to restrict this destructive behavior. The group will then look to the therapist to control the patient, and the therapist must provide such controls to preserve the group. Not infrequently, the therapist will then become the object, which, in turn, may elicit a strong countertransference. Nevertheless, the therapist must persist in his efforts to encourage the patient to examine the origins of his aggression. For unless he gains some insight into his behavior, such a patient will continue to represent a threat to the survival of the group.

Cooperation among group members

Because of the empathy that exists among group members, they welcome an opportunity to provide practical assistance to one another. From time to time, such opportunities do arise, and, if it seems necessary, the group leader must place restrictions and limitations upon such assistance. For example, when a patient finds himself in economic straits, another group member will usually offer to lend him money. It is the responsibility of the group leader to see that any transactions of this type are kept within the bounds of good judgment, that the amounts involved are not too great, and that the loans are repaid. Whether or not such feelings are verbalized, in the eyes of the group, the therapist bears a good deal of the responsibility for such transactions.

Sexual acting out

Depending on the make-up of the group and the rules set forth by the group leader, there may be a great deal of sexual activity in a group or almost none at all. Most patients are very serious about their group commitment and do not view therapy as a Roman holiday, as an opportunity to engage in unrestricted sexual activity. Since he cannot prevent it, it is usually better for the therapist to be permissive in his approach to sexual acting out in group, but it should certainly not be encouraged. His best position would seem to be, "I do not recommend sexual activity among group members and would like to discourage it on all levels." If such behavior becomes a serious problem for certain patients, the therapist may forbid sexual acting out in group; if it persists, he may then ask those involved to leave the group. When he does take a firm stand in this respect, the restrictions he imposes generally serve to curb destructive behavior.

A married patient who was angry at her husband informed the therapist in individual session that she had decided to seduce a passive male member of her group who was obviously attracted to her. The patient planned to tell her husband about the affair after it had been consummated. The therapist pointed out that such acting out would pose a real threat to her marriage; moreover, it was forbidden on therapeutic grounds. As a result, the patient was forced to deal with her anger toward her husband in a more constructive way.

Pairing is another possible consequence of group therapy. While such behavior is based on a mutual sexual attraction, it would not necessarily be classified as sexual acting out. Nevertheless, it is directly opposed to the philosophy inherent to group therapy. In his volume on group psychology, Freud commented on the effects of pairing on the stability of the group:

Two people coming together for the purpose of sexual satisfaction . . . insofar as they seek solitude, are making a demonstration against the group feeling. The more they are in love, the more completely they suffice for each other. Even in a person who has in other respects become absorbed in a group, when sexual impulsions become too strong, they disintegrate every group formation.

On these grounds, and in light of the fact that such pairing may, in fact, reflect a transitory transference on the part of one partner or another, such behavior should be discouraged.

Evaluation

For obvious reasons, reliable statistics on the efficacy of any one type of psychotherapy are unavailable. Most therapists report empirically on the usefulness of a particular technique, and so it must be with the authors of this chapter. Most patients of the authors share the feeling that structured interactional group psychotherapy constitutes an unusually satisfactory technique. And, since many of these patients are repeaters and have been in treatment with other therapists who subscribe to a variety of techniques, presumably their judgment would have considerable validity. The goals of psychotherapy, whether individual or group and whatever the specific treatment technique employed, are the same: anxiety reduction, personality change, and emotional growth and development. Feedback from patients who have been discharged from structured interactional group psychotherapy indicates that they feel these goals have been attained.

In addition, clinical data are available which clearly attest to the efficacy of structured interactional group psychotherapy.

The fact that, over a period of 30 years, none of the authors' patients have committed or attempted suicide is evidence of the value of this form of treatment in the management of the depressed patient. The extremely low dropout rate (under 5 per cent) is clearly indicative of the acceptance of this treatment modality by an overwhelming majority of patients, regardless of diagnosis. Finally, while conclusive evidence is lacking that structured interactional group psychotherapy influences the duration of treatment, there is no question that the unique techniques employed seem to facilitate the expression of repressed problems and conflicts, and serve thereby to expedite their resolution.

The technique is applicable to other group settings and is easily taught. It has been used with medical students and residents in psychiatry as part of their group experience during training in group psychotherapy (Sadock and Kaplan, 1970). Spitz (1978) reported on its successful use with married couples, a different couple being the focus of discussion each week. Many more applications of structured interaction, in different settings, remain to be tested.

References

Alexander, F. Analysis of the therapeutic factors in psychoanalytic treatment. Psychoanal. Q., *19:* 482, 1950.

Rosenbaum, N., and Berger, M., editors. *Group Psychotherapy and Group Function.* Basic Books, New York, 1963.

Slavson, S. H. *A Textbook on Analytic Group Psychotherapy.* International Universities Press, New York, 1964.

Sadock, B. J. Group Psychotherapy. In *Comprehensive Textbook of Psychiatry,* ed. 3, A. M. Freedman, H. I. Kaplan, and B. J. Sadock, editors, p. 218. Williams & Wilkins, Baltimore, 1980.

Sadock, B. J., and Kaplan H. I. Long-term intensive group psychotherapy a part of residency training. Am. J. Psychiatry, *126:* 1138, 1970.

Spitz, H. Structured interactional group psychotherapy with couples. Int. J. Group Psychother., *28:* 401, 1978.

Wolf, A., and Schwartz, E. *Psychoanalysis in Groups.* Grune and Stratton, New York, 1962.

B.4 Transactional Analysis in Groups

JOHN M. DUSAY, M.D.

Introduction

Transactional analysis (TA) is a technique of psychotherapy that began in the mid-1950's. Eric Berne developed TA as an adjunct to psychoanalysis for specific use in groups, and a total and original theory of personality gradually evolved. During the 1970's, many techniques of the new psychologies which were popular in Northern California (where TA was born) were incorporated into TA's solid theory. TA is now utilized in individual, dyadic, marital and family therapy; in nonclinical consultation settings; and in groups.

Berne's first insight into his theory was provided by one of his patients, who told him the following story: While vacationing at a ranch, an 8-year-old boy in his cowboy suit helped the hired man unsaddle his horse. "Thanks, cow-poke," said the hired man. "I'm not really a cowpoke, I'm just a little boy," answered the assistant. The patient then remarked, "That's just the way I feel. I'm not really a lawyer. I'm just a little boy."

This patient was a successful professional but often acted in treatment and in his everyday life like a little boy. He had a financially successful practice, but, when he gambled, he would take $100 to a casino and, if he lost only $80, he would reason, "I made $20"—a logic system more child-like than grownup. In treatment, when addressed, he sometimes would ask, "Are you talking to the lawyer or to the little boy?"

Through this observation Berne considered the value of dividing the behavior of a person into distinct and separate ego states, which he defined as "coherent systems of thoughts, feelings, and behavior patterns." The initial division of the ego into Child and Adult was soon followed by an additional ego state—the Parent. These three ego states became the basic concepts of structural analysis. When capitalized, Child, Adult, and Parent refer to ego states; lower case implies the ordinary meanings of child, adult, and parent. Shortly thereafter, Berne developed transactional analysis by observing how an individual's three ego states would interact with the three ego states of another person. He found that people may transact on two levels at the same time, leading to his description of psychological games; an orderly series of transactions, with one level hidden from the other, leading to a payoff (Berne, 1964).

Early in 1958, Berne began to meet with a group of professionals who had shown interest in his theory. This group called itself the San Francisco Social Psychiatry Seminars and later changed its name to the San Francisco Transactional Analysis Seminar. The group met without interruption, except for occasional holidays, at Berne's home every Tuesday night until he died suddenly on July 15, 1970, of a myocardial infarct. Renamed the Eric Berne Seminar, the meetings have continued and presently are the longest ongoing seminar in group therapy in existence.

Like many innovators of his era, Berne's training was that of a psychiatrist and a psychoanalyst. His psychoanalytic studies spanned 13 years at the New York and San Francisco Psychoanalytic Institutes. The precursors in Berne's thinking of transactional analysis can be found in a series of articles on the subject of intuition published in the *Psychiatric Quarterly,* from 1949 through 1962. In these articles, Berne focused his interest on the capacities of the ego which seemed to be not strictly rational or conscious. The theme of ego states also has precursors in Berne's association and work with Federn and Penfield. While modern transactional analysts come from various backgrounds, anyone doing TA uses ego states, and, conversely, anyone not dealing with ego states is not doing TA.

One can observe the ego states in action by paying attention to the vocabulary, voice tones, and body languages. The principal ego states, Parent, Adult and Child, are further subdivided and defined as follows: The Parent may function both as Critical and Nurturing. The Critical Parent finds fault, is opinionated, and is moralistic. The Nurturing Parent is caring, giving, and sincerely interested in other people. Since the Adult acts as an impassionate rational computer, it is not further subdivided. The Child has its Free Child aspect, which is natural, joyful, creative, playful, and free; the Adapted Child is sometimes conforming and at other times rebellious. The Adapted Child is continually reacting to other people, and in the process does not do what he or she really wants to do. The elements of modern transactional analysis treatment are illustrated by the following case.

Helen is a 35-year-old single woman whose chief complaint is that she is lonely and gets slightly depressed from time to time. She has a few female friends, none of whom she considers close. She has a secure job as a midmanagement executive in a technological company, has progressed steadily but not spectacularly, and does not feel challenged. She has gradually less contact with her family and has bitter memories of her childhood. The oldest of three children, she considers herself to be the serious one, her youngest sister as the cute, favored child, and a middle brother as the successful scientist, of whom she is jealous. She desires male companionship and has had two brief relationships that were sexual, but both ended unsatisfactorily for her. She has devoted much of her time and energy to psychotherapy, having had a formal psychoanalysis and tried a woman's group and eclectic therapies of a brief duration. She reports feeling disappointed and somewhat bitter about her previous therapies.

During the initial interview she recounted the above history, was tearful and slightly depressed, and expressed marked resentment toward her family, friends, and previous therapists. The transactional analyst quickly noticed that she used the pronouns "I" and "me" quite frequently in her conversation. She talked about "my problems," "my analysis," "my" this, and "me" that. She furrowed her brow and clenched her fists angrily when talking about others and was quite logical and somewhat scientific in discussing theories of her analysis. She said nothing of a complimentary nature about the therapist, and the therapist felt that she did not seem to notice him as a human being. There were no jokes or humor in the interview. The therapist constructed a mental egogram of her at that point. An egogram is a psychological tool which depicts the energy emanating from the five functional ego states. It is arranged as a bar graph to instantly depict one's personality strengths and weaknesses (see Figure B.4-1).

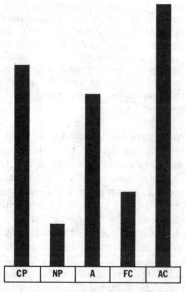

| CP | NP | A | FC | AC |

Figure B.4-1   Egogram.

Helen's egogram represents the relative intensity of energy emanating from her different ego states. Her CP (Critical Parent) is quite high, as she displays a tendency to criticize others. Her propensity to nurture is quite low, as seen on the NP (Nurturing Parent) scale. Her A (Adult), which represents her tendency to think logically, is about average. Her FC (Free Child), which is her spontaneous, fun-loving, and sexual self, is quite low, while her AC (Adapted Child), which conforms to parental messages about her, is very high and is seen in her self-centered, self-conscious approach to life. Helen formed a preliminary treatment contract with the therapist, making new friends and having a sexually fulfilling relationship. The therapist made an intervention and instructed her to finish the interview without saying "I" or "me." Helen looked surprised by this confrontation and found that this simple direction was quite difficult for her.

"How can I ... Oops, there I go again ... Oops—I did it again!"

The therapist persisted by saying, "Tell me what you think or feel about me [the therapist] as a person."

"I didn't come here to talk about you; I came here to have more friends," Helen protested. "Perhaps one could join one of your groups?" she queried. The therapist said, of course, under the promise that she refrain from talking about herself or her problems for the first six sessions (except for a brief introduction). She then asked, "When does my therapy begin?" and the therapist replied, "It has already begun." Helen intuitively sensed this and agreed to come to the group. The therapist then congratulated her by saying, "This has been a tough session for you, but congratulations for deciding to stick it out. The group setting may be quite productive for you, and you are very bright and can contribute greatly to the other members, when you are willing." The therapist knew that she would have to develop her NP if she were going to have friends and also develop her FC if she wanted to experience satisfying sex and spontaneity.

The first two group sessions were uneventful, but during the third session, the therapist noticed that Helen was glancing at her wristwatch, while another group member, Joy, a sexually provocative younger woman who plays a game called Rapo (offering sexual bait and then being incensed when a male notices her), was flirting with a group member.

The therapist turned to Helen and said, "Say out loud what's on your mind." She snapped back, "I'll never get my turn to talk." Rather than reassure Helen, the therapist deliberately had Helen intensify her feeling state, by focusing on the observable behavioral signal she was displaying. Noticing her clenched fists, he said, "Make your fists tighter." She did, and then replied, "I'm angry; you don't pay any attention to me! You like Joy better than me!" The therapist, noticing that Helen was breathing heavily in her accelerating emotional state, had her enhance her rapid breathing, and she said, "You think I'm a piece of shit!"

The therapist arose and went to Helen, saying, "Close your eyes." She did with a pained look on her face. The therapist gently pinched the furrow on her brow (a characteristic body expression of her inner turmoil), intensifying her feeling state, and then said firmly, "Allow this [here and now] feeling to go back through the years of your life [pause] ...."

"You are reviewing similar experiences from your past." When she acknowledged this by external clues, such as nodding affirmatively or looking more pained, she was directed to go back further ... and further ... until she was sobbing profusely and trembling. After a few minutes of expressing this painful feeling the therapist said, "Say out loud what's happening."

"I feel awful; my mind is dark ... It's dark in here," said

Helen in a frightened and sad little-girl voice. "Go on," urged the therapist. She cried for several minutes and then said bitterly, "My father hates me! I'm never coming out of this closet! I'm never coming out!"

Because of the emotional intensity and the absolute pronouncement "never," it was obvious to the therapist that Helen was reexperiencing an important, perhaps the most important moment of an early childhood decision. Later in a rehash, she recalled that this was the day that her baby sister, the cute little one, came home from the hospital; however, this was not the appropriate time for cognitive discussion.

The therapist then offered her another chair, which was placed by another group member directly in front of Helen, who was in her Adapted Child ego state. "Sit in this chair, and in this new position, allow yourself to be a wonderful nurturing mommy or daddy." Helen went to the other chair, and at this time, but not before, the therapist placed his hands on her shoulder in a nurturing and reassuring manner (the early touching was done to enhance the bad feelings).

After a few moments, Helen relaxed and said to the empty chair (symbolic of her Adapted Child ego state), "You're not so bad. You know, you're really quite bright," and she offered a few more nurturing comments. The therapist then instructed her to return to her original chair and respond from the Adapted Child part of her that was in the closet. She smiled briefly, but then that faded as she said, "My daddy doesn't want me." She returned to the nurturing chair and said, "Quit crying, dammit! Shut up!"

Obviously, she was no longer in her nurturing state—she had slipped into her Critical Parent ego state. The therapist, aware of the shift, knew that this was an important moment in the process of her treatment; he brought in a third chair and placed it perpendicular to the other two chairs and said, "Sit here." She did, and he then said, "OK, now *describe* what has just happened." She was encouraged to be in her Adult ego state, the part that rationally observes and discusses what is happening. She began to break the impasse between her Adapted Child and Parent ego states. She said, "I see where my decision comes from, but it's difficult for me to help myself."

At this point the therapist congratulated her for her willingness to work and the depth of her experience. He then opened up the group for mutual sharing of experiences. Other group members congratulated her and supported her by recalling how difficult it was for them to change themselves but offered much inspiration and positive strokes. The therapist then offered cognitive feedback by diagramming her script on the blackboard (see Figure B.4-2).

The script matrix depicts how parental messages were transacted with Helen when she was young. Father from his Parent ego state gave values, such as "Be good," as did mother, but the destructive message called an injunction came from both father and mother's Child ego states. Helen was told in hidden messages (symbolized by the *dotted lines*), "Get lost." After thousands of negative messages from her parents, Helen decided, at a young age, that she was unwanted and unlovable.

While the process of redeciding her script went well, the therapist knew that Helen was not adept or exercised at nurturing (see her egogram) either herself or others.

Patients rarely redecide about their lives and their scripts in a brief period of time because the Adapted Child exercises so much power, and this keeps them stuck.

The group environment provided support and nurturing, whereby Helen received and gave many hugs at the end of her work. Because Helen needed to give and get more

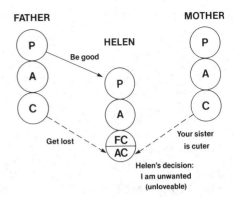

Figure B.4-2   Script.

nurturing, exercises outside of the group were proposed and accepted by Helen. She decided to join Big Sisters and take an orphan to the zoo, although she said, "This does not feel like me." She was reassured that this was not her old style and that she came into treatment for change. Later, Helen called the therapist from the zoo pleading, "She doesn't want to talk to me ... What can I do?" The therapist said, "You are doing fine! Remember, this little girl is as hard to nurture as the little girl inside you. Keep trying."

At the next group meeting, Helen said there were tears in the little girl's eyes when she hugged her and said goodbye. The therapist and the group members knew that Helen was on the way to fulfilling her treatment contract.

Helen continued to see her new friend and found it easier to nurture both herself and the little girl. Gradually, she became more tolerant and loving toward the people in the group—even Joy. She created more outside friendships and ultimately entered into a personal relationship with a man. She is still active in the Big Sisters and seldom gets depressed and lonely anymore.

Ego States and Egograms

The structure of personality is symbolized by the three ego state circles seen on Helen's script matrix. This represents an anatomical approach.

There is also a physiological representation of one's personality which depicts how much energy is available in each ego state, and this is called an egogram. Each person has a distinct, unique balance of the five psychological forces (Dusay, 1972).

A transactional analysis group member asked the others, "How do you see me?" and each group member was asked to privately construct individual bar graphs showing what they thought were her strongest, weakest, and midrange ego states. After comparing results, they were amazed to find that they had consensual agreement as to what were the lowest and highest forces, and near agreement on the midranges. This experiment was repeated frequently by transactional analysts in the early 1970's, and they found that there was 80 per cent agreement on the high and low points, and 70 per cent agreement on the other ego states. Each subject's egogram was reliably consistent over a period of time unless a profound attitude or personality change occurred.

Contract

Simply stated, a treatment contract is an acceptable answer to the question, "How will you know and how will I know when you get what you are coming to the group for?" The answer to this question is worked over in the presence of all group members which allows each member of the group to sort out the vast number of transactions that take place during a group session, and to focus on the stimuli and responses that they consider relevant. All material is not important or relevant, and patients appreciate the opportunity to avoid wasting time on interesting sidelights. They know what each member is aiming for; they then decide their course of action.

Transactional analysis is a contractual type of treatment; Steiner and Cassidy (1969) compared the elements of a patient-therapist contract with a legal contract. Because the four requirements of a legal contract have evolved over hundreds of years of litigation, it is thought that they are necessary and desirable for social intercourse. Retrospective analysis of workable contracts in transactional analysis groups has found these four requirements to be valid for treatment contracts.

Mutual consent

Mutual consent implies that both the patient and the therapist know and agree on what they are working. In transactional analysis, the contract is arrived at by complementary Adult-to-Adult transactions and ends with an agreement. The therapist does not accept just any goal the patient presents, and he does not quietly sit back and allow the patient to think that they are working toward the same goal if they are not.

Consideration

Consideration means that each of the two parties gives the other something for his efforts. The therapist gives his time, skill, and professional knowledge to the best of his ability to the patient. The patient pays the therapist, usually with money or occasionally with other efforts, such as art work. Without the payment of an appropriate fee, readjusted and different for individual patients with varying economic backgrounds, there is a covert Child-Parent situation.

Competency

The therapist must be competent by way of training and experience to perform what he claims he will be doing. If he offers or accepts with mutual consent a schizophrenic's request to work toward not having a relapse and not being rehospitalized, he must have had the training to work with people who have these types of disorders. It is also the therapist's responsibility to judge whether or not there is a probability of attaining the desired goal.

The patient must be competent to enter into a valid contract. If for psychological, chemical, or medical reasons he is unable to cathect Adult at that moment in time, he is not competent and cannot authentically decide on psychotherapy. It is important to discuss the aims and goals of treatment with the parents of minor children or, in the case of people who have had their civil rights taken away from them, the judge, probation officer, or guardian at that time.

Legal object

The therapist is unable to form a valid treatment contract if he agrees to work with a patient toward something that is not legal. If the therapist, by error or by being seduced into some game, does agree to work toward some illegal goal, he will probably lose the respect of his patient. The patient will usually congratulate himself on having found another patsy to watch his maneuvering and game playing.

Script reversal

Berne's major focus was on the understanding of scripts; he placed his emphasis upon understanding and insight. Many contemporary TA therapists are more involved in emotive and action techniques, followed by a cognitive wrap-up. Berne was in contrast to the passive approaches of his era when he would potently deliver counterinjunctions to his patients. This means that Berne would say just the opposite of the negative script injunction. A potent therapist will transact with the patient at a key moment, using as much force as the biological parent used in presenting the negative injunction in the formation of the script. Berne's approach to a "get lost" injunction is seen in the case of Ruth:

Ruth was a young woman who had seriously attempted suicide several times in the past, had frequent psychiatric hospitalizations, and had seen many psychotherapists. She had been unwanted by her father, who had said to her, "Get lost," several times in her childhood as he shooed her out of the room in which he was trying to relax. At one time, when her father was intoxicated, she definitely remembers that he said to her, "I wish you were dead." Since her early childhood, she had been living a constant struggle between getting lost, which she did often, and killing herself, which she had tried seriously several times.

The therapist was somewhat surprised when she unequivocally stated that none of her prior psychotherapists had taken a direct antithetical position to her father (his Child ego state) and had never said to her in dramatic and straightforward terms, "Do not kill yourself." She did recall, however, hearing several statements of concern, as one therapist said, "You must be terribly unhappy to do what you did. Tell me about it." Another therapist took the position that it was her right to kill herself, and he spent time philosophizing about her right to be or not to be. This approach was seen as an Adult-to-Adult philosophical discussion, which was stimulating to the patient, but it did not relieve her of the burden of a life pattern of struggling against suicide.

Following the formation of a treatment contract with a TA therapist affirming her preference to live, he gave her permission to live by saying, "Do not kill yourself—live." The patient responded by saying, "Thank you." This permission was the direct opposite of the negative injunction with which the patient had been struggling all her life. If she ever finds herself standing on a bridge, deciding whether or not to jump, she has at least a strong and well-stated permission to live in her head.

Because the person having psychiatric difficulties is following parental orders that are the cause of his difficulty, the basic task of the therapist is to give the person permission to behave otherwise—that is, in a manner that is autonomous rather than adapted to parental demands. Disobeying parental orders is frightening because no alternative ways of life are known to the person, and because parental retaliation is feared. Therefore, temporary protection has to be provided by the therapist until the person is able to validate his new way of life. Both permission and protection, to be effective, require potency. Potency is a combination of Adult competence, Parent advocacy, and Child zest and optimism. These become the therapist's powerful contributions to the therapeutic process.

When a patient says, "I could have a heart attack over that" or "That makes me sick," the therapist responds with, "Be healthy," and continually assumes an antithetical response to the negative parental injunctions.

Innovative techniques for patients to reverse their scripts continue to evolve and the patient is able to assume personal power for his or her own cure (Goulding and Goulding, 1978).

Script decision and redecision

Redecision is a popular and promising technique utilized by transactional analysts. The pioneers of this approach, Robert and Mary Goulding, began their work with this method in the late 1960's and expanded the theory throughout the 1970's. Redecision is a blend of TA script theory, Gestalt techniques, the work of Perls, and behavior modification. Dusay has incorporated neurolinguistic communication techniques of Bandler-Grinder, hypnosis, and energy theory into the redecision model. At Berne's death in 1970, the human potential movement was fully underway, and many serious students of the more esoteric psychologies were attracted to the solid theory of transactional analysis. Thus, many innovations and applications are seen, especially in the facilitation of script redecision.

Goulding noticed that in Gestalt work a patient would frequently re-experience childhood decision moments. By talking to the Child of the patient in this regressed state, the patient would recognize the power he had as a child when he was making a decision that allowed them to survive with his actual parents. When mother said, "Get lost," the biological child (later becoming the Child ego state) decided that he should get lost, that he is unwanted and, therefore, worthless. Instead of focusing on mother's message, Goulding focused on the response of the patient, the decision. By switching to another chair, Gestalt fashion, the other parts of the Child could aid in bringing about a redecision. It is easier for a person to change after recognizing the power he has in shaping his life, rather than in accepting a position of weakness. This notion of personal power and responsibility for decision is somewhat controversial. Patients do become inspired by the possibility of fulfilling Berne's observation that "anything learned can be relearned."

Steiner (1974) has focused on the debilitating effects of oppressive social institutions, such as racism and sexism, which contribute to human psychological problems. Schiff has emphasized that, in schizoprenics, reparenting is neces-

sary. Yet, in most problems experienced by reasonably functioning outpatients, the notion of personal power and responsibility for change is possible and appreciated. Redecision is based upon this personal power.

Ego state opposition

Ego state opposition (Dusay and Dusay, 1979) is a functional model by which patients can strengthen their weaknesses and undergo the process of redeciding their life course. This is similar to Goulding's mixed structural and function model of redecision impasses but differs in that it is purely functional.

A basic technique for facilitating a function redecision proceeds as follows.

1. In a treatment session a patient is feeling distressed in his characteristic manner (a racket of mad, sad, or scared that has been observed many times by the therapist). A person may have engaged in a psychological game, and, at the concluding payoff, his emotions are intense. Instead of soothing or interpreting what has happened, the therapist working for a redecision actually enhances the painful emotional state of the patient. Noticing tense muscles, clenched fists, rapid breathing, or other somatic components, the therapist either instructs or aids the patient in becoming more deeply emotional. This happens in the here and now of the group session, and, when the patient becomes very emotional, he is ready to move back in time to earlier decisive moments of childhood.

2. The patient is then told to close his eyes and, via a regressive hypnotic technique, is told that his feelings will go back through the years to the earliest experience of this emotional state. Sometimes rapidly, sometimes with more attention to actual suggestions, the patient will re-experience an earlier precursor of the here-and-now feeling. Whether or not the re-experience is actual seems less relevant than the patient's experiential belief that what he is experiencing is the actual precursor. This moment is emotionally charged and seems indistinguishable from what Freud and Breuer termed hyperesthetic memories.

3. In this regressed state, usually between the ages of 2 and 12, the patient is frequently in the presence of their mother or father, or both, and is making major life decisions about self (I am or am not an OK person) and others, usually directed toward the parents (You are or are not OK). The decisions are expressed in the patient's own words, words that are appropriate to the age and situation being experienced. The actual words are less important than the feeling state, and, indeed, the work is just as important even if the therapist does not understand the exact statements, as has occasionally occurred with patients who spoke a different language in childhood (they usually re-experience in their childhood language). The therapist encourages the patient to oppose this negative childhood decision (which is functionally in the Adapted Child state) with the force from another of the patient's ego states. He is instructed to do so by switching to another chair and having a self-dialogue. This process expresses the real problem (in a noncliché sense) and is the essence of self-curing. While the therapist may be working diligently to set up the situation, the patient does the important work. The switching into another chair is where TA script redecision departs from classical hypnosis, whereby the hypnotist would supply the positive suggestion, rather than the patient.

4. Resistances commonly arise when a patient who switches into another chair to confront his childhood deci-

sion actually slips from the curative ego state into a destructive one and reinforces the decision, instead of opposing it. The most important responsibility of the therapist is to be on the alert for slippage, and to skillfully confront the patient or have the patient switch to a new chair and describe what was happening. Other group members are often useful in this regard.

When redecision work is not successful, the usual reason is that the patient is opposing the Adapted Child with the Nurturing Parent in some subtle way. "I'm awful," opposed by "Well, it's not your fault," which is pseudonurturing and needs to be confronted by the adroit therapist. Many times the force opposing the Adapted Child is simply too weak, for now, to bring about a redecision.

When this occurs, a person needs to exercise the low ego state both in and out of the group. When a person leaves a therapy group, he may gradually undo productive work by playing the games that keep him locked into his script. Therefore, ongoing group therapy is important so the patient can build up his strengths.

Research and Evaluation

During TA's developmental years, much reporting was anecdotal individual case histories. These early reports were enthusiastic; however, they lacked the research and other controls necessary for a solid theoretical model. A permanent research committee was established within the International Transactional Analysis Association.

Outcome

TA holds a distinctive advantage in that the process contains a well-stated treatment contract; either the patients gets what they came for, or they do not. In 1968, Berne, Dusay, and Poindexter reviewed their case loads and reported to the San Francisco TA Seminar the finding that 80 per cent of their patients stated that they got what they came for, and their therapists agreed by referring back to their contracts.

Independent investigation then began to review the outcome of TA treatment in a more systematic manner. One important study compared a measurable end point between TA treatment and behavior modification, using a control group. A population of 904 young men with serious emotional or behavioral problems in the California Youth Authority was treated by TA and behavior modification; they were compared with a control group and measured for improvement in mathematical and reading skills and 1-year recidivism rates. Both TA and behavior modification groups improved markedly. The TA treatment group achieved the results in less time than behavior modification, and the parole revocation rate dropped from 43 per cent to 33 per cent over nontreated controls (McCormick, 1973). Interestingly, the TA subjects claimed that TA was more fun and enjoyable.

McNeel (1981) has studied the favorable outcome of script redecision in psychotherapy, and the evidence of change has been reported by Badenoch (1981).

Basic concepts

Because TA theorists claim that the ego states are observable phenomena, they have become a fertile area of research.

Thomson (1972), in his pioneering work, demonstrated that transactional analysis professionals have a high interrater agreement as to which ego state is in operation in a given person, and that naive observers can be trained to correctly identify ego states in agreement with experts.

Dusay (1977) demonstrated that not only can ego states be identified, but they can be measured utilizing the egogram. Trained observers have a high interrater agreement as to the relative amounts of Critical Parent, Nurturing Parent, Adult, Free Child, and Adapted Child emanated when focusing on a given person. Those egogram profiles correspond with clinical problems.

Kendra constructed egograms of suicidal patients from Rorschach Tests and was able to delineate specific features of egograms that were common to that group of psychiatric suicidal patients. His findings confirmed the presence of high Critical Parent and high Adapted Child. The Nurturing Parent and Free Child were extremely low, with the Adult being either high or low.

Heyer (1979) developed an objective questionnaire technique to measure the intensity of ego states and arrive at egogram profiles. His original research was based on a highly researched cross-section sample of the adult population of California (known as the California Poll) conducted in September 1976. A sample of 1,044 persons rated themselves on items measuring ego states and also rated several major political figures (Presidential and U.S. Senatorial candidates). The study found that ego state energy is related to social and demographic characteristics, and that perceived ego state images of candidates have an influence on voting intentions. The egogram questionnaire developed by Heyer is also being used for research on ego states in a variety of settings—including prisons, alcoholism outpatient clinics, growth workshops, and training programs. Couples and families use this questionnaire to discover their psychological compatibilities. The San Quentin prison study revealed that hard-core criminals are low in Nurturing Parent and Adult ego state functions, but above average in Critical Parent, Free Child, and Adapted Child.

Current Status

Eric Berne, the founder of transactional analysis, was a prolific writer who published 64 articles and eight books, and started a bulletin that grew into the quarterly *Transactional Analysis Journal.* The San Francisco Transactional Analysis Seminars boasted eight original members, who met weekly in Berne's home. From this spawned the International Transactional Analysis Association, which has grown to include more than 8,000 formal members in the United States and foreign countries; it is experiencing particularly rapid growth in Europe, South America, Japan, and India.

Berne quipped that professionalism is not as important as curing patients. Berne's original seminar members were mental health professionals and recognized students who developed transactional analysis as an adjunct to their basic training. Berne himself, like many psychiatric innovators, invited a few select persons who were not traditionally trained to his seminars. Indeed, some of the best transactional analysis has been done by paraprofessionals and supervised lay persons. An extreme example of this is incarcerated prisoners who have been trained as group leaders and are running TA groups in prisons.

Berne was a staunch believer in both the stimulating effects of continuing education and the challenges of developing new theories. He encouraged his followers to organize and attend regular local seminars to sharpen their skills. After Berne's death in 1970, the International Transactional Analysis Association created the Eric Berne Memorial Scientific Awards, which are voted upon by the advanced membership each year to recognize the important advances made in the field of transactional analysis.

Berne's zest for expanding the theory encouraged a process of creativity among his followers and was consistent with his own career, which was continually in a process of evolution. TA writings and methods have a wide appeal because they excite the reader's Child, and the simple vocabulary challenges intuitive minds. Berne joked that anything written in the scientific literature or said to a patient in treatment should be understandable by at least two people: the professor of symbolic logic at the Massachusetts Institute of Technology, whom Berne exemplified as the most brilliant person in the world, and a farmer in Minnesota with a third-grade education.

References

Badenoch, A. Redecision therapy: Evidence of change. Trans. Anal. J., 2: 4, 1981.

Berne, E. Concerning the nature of communication. Psychiatr. Q., 27: 185, 1953.

Berne, E. Group attendance: Clinical and theoretical considerations. Int. J. Group Psychother., 5: 392, 1955.

Berne, E. Intuition. IV. Primal images and primal judgment. Psychiatr. Q., 29: 034, 1955.

Berne, E. Intuition. VI. The psychodynamics of intuition. Psychiatr. Q., 36: 294, 1962.

Berne, E. Games People Play. Grove Press, New York, 1964.

Berne, E. Principles of Group Treatment. Oxford University Press, New York, 1966.

Dusay, J. Egograms and the constancy hypothesis. Trans. Anal. J., 2: 3, 1972.

Dusay, J. Egograms. Harper & Row, New York, 1977.

Dusay, J. Eric Berne: Contributions and limitations. Trans. Anal. Bull., 11: 1, 1981.

Dusay, J., and Dusay, K. Transactional analysis. In Current Psychotherapies, R. Corsini, editor. Peacock, Itasca, IL, 1979.

English, F. The substitution factor: Rackets and real feelings. Part I. Trans. Anal. Bull., 1: 4, 1971.

English, F. The substitution factor: Rackets and real feelings: Part II. Trans. Anal. Bull., 2: 2, 1972.

Gilmour, J. Psychophysiological evidence for the existence of ego states. Trans. Anal. J., 11: 3, 1981.

Goulding, R., and Goulding, M., The Power Is in the Patient. TA Press, San Francisco, 1978.

Goulding, R., and Goulding, M., Changing Lives through Redecision Therapy. Brunner/Mazel, New York 1979.

Heyer, R. Development of questionnaire to measure egostates with some applications to social and comparative psychiatry. Trans. Anal. J., 9: 1, 1979.

Kahler, T. The miniscript. In Transactional Analysis after Eric Berne, G. Barnes, editor, p. 222. Harper's College Press, New York, 1977.

McCormick, P. TA and behavior modification: A comparison study. Trans. Anal. J., 3: 10, 1973.

McNeel, J., Redecisions in psychotherapy: A study of the effects of an intensive weekend group workshop. Trans. Anal. J., 2: 4, 1981.

Schiff, J., and Schiff, A. Passivity. Trans. Anal. J., 1: 1, 1971.

Steiner, C. Games Alcoholics Play: The Analysis of Life Scripts. Grove Press, New York, 1971.

Steiner, C. Scripts People Live. Grove Press, New York, 1974.

Steiner, C., and Cassidy, W. Therapeutic contracts in group treatment. Trans. Anal. Bull., 8: 29, 1969.

Thomson, G. The identification of ego states. Trans. Anal. J., 2: 196, 1972.

B.5 Behavior Therapy in Groups

SHELDON D. ROSE, Ph.D.

Introduction

Growing evidence supports the notion that social skill deficits are linked to major psychiatric and interpersonal problems. Research has shown that the level of social competence—based on global measures of educational, vocational, and marital attainment—is related to the degree of psychiatric impairments. A number of authors have shown a relationship between interpersonal deficits and such clinical phenomena as depression and other clinical syndromes. For this reason, social skill training—which includes modeling, rehearsal, coaching, and feedback—provides a key set of procedures in this approach as one means of reducing social skill deficits, a reduction which may prevent and in some cases contribute to the amelioration of psychiatric problems.

Of course, some persons who may not be deficient in specific social skills might still be unable to function without high levels of anxiety or other strong emotional distress. For these, it appears that certain interpersonal and intrapersonal events are accompanied by or evoke irrational or self-defeating emotions. Under intense anxiety, the performance of adaptive or coping behavior is restricted. For these persons, cognitive procedures such as stress inoculation or cognitive restructuring can be combined with social skill training procedures to enhance social functioning and reduce anxiety.

In group behavior therapy, the group is not only the place where training takes place but provides a number of procedures, as well as other advantages for carrying out therapy. Thus, behavior group therapy, as it is described here, combines the advantages of (1) behavior therapy, especially social skills trainings; (2) cognitive therapy, especially cognitive restructuring, stress inoculation, and problem solving; and (3) group therapy, especially the development of cohesion and broad participation, as three major sources of intervention to enhance client social functioning.

The most fundamental notion is that both normal and abnormal behavior is acquired according to the same principles. Treatment consists of a number of strategies or interventions derived from theory for learning new, more adaptive behaviors and cognitions and eliminating or unlearning dysfunctional ones.

Behavior group therapy draws upon the best available empirical research to determine what kind of intervention is best suited to what kind of problem. Of course, the therapist cannot know which research to draw upon until the specific nature of the problem has been ascertained. To determine the problem, data are collected on both the individual and the group before selection of specific interventive procedures. Treatment strategies are tailored to individuals based on individual assessment and assessment in the group.

Assessment, the process by which data are collected, is carried out by means of individual and group interviews, various forms of testing, observations, and other systemic forms of accruing information. Assessment functions to determine the resources available to the client for coping with problems, as well as the nature and extent of problems. The therapist must also assess group problems and group resources. The reason for data collection and problem and resource determination for the individual and group is to select the most appropriate and best demonstrated strategies for dealing with individual and group problems.

Behavior group therapy is a humanistic approach in which individuals and groups contract for mutually determined goals. The client is maximally involved in all decisions concerning not only goal setting but treatment strategy selection. The therapist serves as an active consultant in this process.

Organization

THE GROUP

Since the condition under which therapy takes place is the group, a number of assumptions about the advantages and limitations of the group guide and delineate the therapist's role. Because many problems are social-interactional in nature, the presence of other clients provides an opportunity for practicing new social-interactional skills with peers in a protected setting.

The group gives clients an opportunity to learn and practice many behaviors and cognitions as they respond to the constantly changing group demands. The clients must learn to offer other clients feedback and advice—as a result, developing important skills for leadership. By helping others, clients usually learn to help themselves more effectively than when they are the sole recipient of a given therapy.

In group interaction, powerful norms (informal agreements among members as to preferred modes of action and interaction in the group) arise that serve to control the behavior of individual clients who deviate from protherapeutic norms. If these norms are introduced and effectively maintained by the therapist, they serve as efficient therapeutic tools (Lawrence and Sundel, 1972). The group pressures deviant members to conform to such norms as attending regularly, reinforcing peers who do well, and analyzing problems. Of course, antitherapeutic norms may also be generated in groups as indicated by such behaviors as erratic attendance, non-completion of agreed-upon assignments, and constant criticism of therapists; these norms work against the attainment of therapeutic goals.

To prevent or to deal with such problems, the therapist can call upon a modest body of experimentally derived knowledge about normals and other group phenomena in which individual behavior both influences and is influenced by the various attributes of the group (Cartwright and Zander, 1968). In addition to modifying the antitherapeutic norms of the group, the therapist may also have to help the group to deal with other attributes, such as the status pattern or a broad communication structure in the group. Much of the power of group therapy is lost if negative group attributes are not dealt with.

Another unique characteristic of therapy in groups is the opportunity for peer reinforcement. Each person is given the chance to learn or to improve his or her ability to mediate rewards for others in social interactive situations (with spouse, family, friendship groups, work group). The therapist can structure a therapeutic situation in which each person has frequent opportunity, instructions, and even rewards for reinforcing others in the group. Reinforcement is a highly valued skill in our society; there is some research to suggest that, as a person learns to reinforce others, he or she is reciprocally reinforced by others, and mutual liking also increases.

More accurate assessment can be another major contribution of group therapy. Many aspects of a problem which elude even the most sensitive therapist often become clearly spelled out during an intensive group discussion. The group provides clients with a major source of feedback about what in their behavior is annoying to others and what makes them attractive to others. This is especially helpful when clients cannot pinpoint their own problems.

In addition to facilitating assessment, the group makes available a variety of models, coaches, role players for behavioral rehearsal, manpower for monitoring, and partners for use in a buddy system or pairing off of one client with another for work between sessions.

Since the group provides many of its own therapeutic resources and gives simultaneous treatment to a number of people, this type of therapy appears to be less costly than individual treatment in terms of staff and money. Of course, dual leadership and extensive preparation may increase the cost somewhat.

Finally, the group serves as a control on the therapist's value imposition. Clients in groups appear to be less accepting of the arbitrary values imposed by therapist action than clients in dyads. A group of people can more easily disagree with the therapist than can the individual. The group therapist is constantly forced by group members to make his or her values explicit.

The group is not without major limits. Although a session agenda may provide the therapist with criteria by which excessive wandering to irrelevant topics can be limited, it also may serve to deter the exploration of idiosyncratic needs of any one individual. Each person needs to be alotted some time at every meeting to discuss unique problems. Therefore, no one or two persons can be permitted to dominate it. Some clients may even feel severely restricted by such a concern for involvement of all the other members. Such a problem, however, warrants exploration in the group.

Another disadvantage of the group is the absence of a guarantee of confidentiality. Although all clients contract to hold any discussion of all individual problems in the group in strict confidence, they are not necessarily committed to the professional ethics of the therapist. The absence of this guarantee may sometimes restrict the degree to which some clients are inclined to self-disclosure, or even restrict the degree to which the therapist can urge them to self-disclosure.

THE THERAPIST

At least nine major categories of therapist functions generally found in behaviorally oriented group therapy can be identified. Although there is some degree of overlapping, each category is sufficiently unique to describe separately. These categories include organizing the group; orienting the members to the group; establishing group attraction; monitoring the behaviors determined as problematic; evaluating the progress of treatment; planning for and implementing specific change procedures; modifying group attributes; and establishing transfer and maintenance programs for behavioral and cognitive changes occurring in the group. Each category consists of a series of still more specific activities, some of which will be described below.

Beginning the group

In the initial phase of group therapy, the therapist focuses on three major activities: organizing the

group, orienting the clients, and building group attraction. Organizational activities involve discussion and decision making about type of group, duration of group, length of meetings, number of therapists, location of meetings, nature of fees and deposits, and similar structural concerns. During the pregroup interview and in the first session, the group members may be involved in some of these decisions, such as when and where the group is to meet and the length of meetings. They also may help decide whether new members should be added. In the pregroup interview, clients decide whether the therapist's description of the group's focus adequately meets what they perceive to be their needs. Most intensive therapy groups are 14 to 18 weekly sessions in length, with several booster sessions at 1- to 6-month intervals. Short-term training groups are four to eight sessions. Some therapists have also used open-ended groups for intensive therapy. As clients achieve treatment goals or no longer feel the need for group support, new members are added. The more experienced members remaining in the group orient the new additions. This orientation provides an opportunity for leadership.

Orientation

Orientation refers to those activities in which the therapist informs the client of the group's purposes and content, and the responsibilities of the clients to themselves and to the others. It also involves the process of negotiating the content of the general treatment contract. The contract is a written statement of mutual expectations of clients and therapists (Rose, 1977). In the process of orientation, the therapist—except in open-ended groups—is the major contributor, providing information and case studies as examples.

Building group cohesion

Building group cohesion focuses on increasing the attraction of the group members to each other, to the therapist, and to the content of the program. Increased group cohesion has been found to be positively associated with group effectiveness. Flowers and Borraem have identified eight additional correlates of cohesion: (1) increased attention to the speaker; (2) increased problem disclosure; (3) increased proportion of negative feedback; (4) decreased frequency of group members in negative input or output roles; (5) increased role flexibility during group sessions; (6) increased percentage of client-client interactions; (7) increased number of group members trusted; and (8) increased self-reported session or group satisfaction.

Fortunately, cohesion is amenable to therapist influences. Therapists were trained by Liberman to use social reinforcement and were effective in shaping, modifying, and facilitating verbal behavior reflecting cohesiveness.

Other strategies employed to increase group cohesion include providing food at meetings, varying the content of meetings, providing audiovisual aids, providing incentives for attendance, judicious use of humor, use of group exercises, and goal-oriented interactive games.

Assessment, monitoring, and evaluation are also a part of

beginning the group, but because these activites continue throughout treatment and are so central to the approach to this type of therapy, these are discussed under a separate section.

Assessment, monitoring, and evaluation

Assessment. As defined earlier, assessment is the group activity concerned with determining the behavior and cognitions to be modified, situations experienced as stressful, the resources of the individual and his or her environment that will facilitate remediation of the problem, and barriers to effective treatment.

The assessment process in group therapy cannot be over-emphasized. Group therapists must go beyond preliminary information and initial complaints in determining treatment strategies by careful exploration of detailed information required to decide whether the group is appropriate, the kind of group that is appropriate, the type of goals for which the client can aim while in the group, and the evaluation of whether session and treatment goals are attained. Effective assessment requires pregroup interviews which explore the stressful situations the clients are experiencing and their behavioral, cognitive, and affective responses to those situations. From these interviews and subsequent contacts, information is required about resources and barriers which impinge on the effectiveness of treatment. Interviews should be supplemented by role-play tests, behavioral inventories, checklists, and observations in and out of the group, as a means of zeroing in on specific target areas. Group data such as participation, satisfaction, attendance, and assignment completion, provide a basis of evaluating whether group problems exist and whether group goals are being attained. Group members enhance each other's assessment by being maximally involved as testers and interviewers of each other, as collectors of observational data, as judges of each other's role plays, and as providers of feedback as the basis of goal selection. Such involvement not only increases the interpersonal attraction but mobilizes the full power of the group as the context and means for assessment (Rose, 1981).

Although assessment begins at the pregroup interview, it is constantly refined throughout treatment. In the pregroup interview and early in treatment, members are encouraged to present the reasons they have come to the group. Clients are taught to define their problems in terms of directly observed behavior and descriptions of their inner states (affect and cognitions) as responses to the situations which they perceive as stressful or otherwise problematic. The group members are taught how to help each other to specify the environmental conditions impinging on them in each problem.

One of the most crucial steps in ongoing assessment is the analysis of situations viewed as problematic or stressful by the client. In this analysis, an attempt is made to define a time-limited event in terms of what was happening, who was involved, and where it occurred. Additionally, the clients are asked which moment in time was the most difficult for them. This is called the critical moment.

At the critical moment, the clients are asked to describe behavior, affect, and cognitions. Among specific affectual responses are their satisfaction with their behavioral response and their anxiety or anger. If the client is not at least somewhat dissatisfied with the response, the problem may not warrant working on.

If the problem is that the client does not know how to respond in the specific situation, this suggests problem-solving and social skill training. If the problem is one of self-depreciation or excessive self-demand, then cognitive restructuring is called for. If the situation is unchangeable, e.g., a client has a rigid and highly critical boss, yet he is in a high-paying job for which there are few better possibilities, coping skill training may be useful (e.g., learning to relax when the boss criticizes, learning to avoid certain kinds of stressful experiences). In the case of complex problems, all three approaches may be necessary in order to achieve the client's goal.

Monitoring. Behaviors and the situations in which they occur, once defined, are systematically observed and measured in some way, usually by the client and occasionally by others, prior to the application of any explicit change procedure. For example, some clients will rate their anxiety level four times a day. Others might count the number of minutes of social contacts. Still others might tally the number of urges to withdraw from stressful situations. The process of data collection is carried on throughout treatment and is concluded only at the follow-up interview.

The therapist uses the data as they are collected to evaluate the effectiveness of specific treatment procedures, the group meetings, and the course of therapy. Effectiveness is determined on the basis of whether the goals of a given technique, a given meeting, or a given therapy have, indeed, been achieved. If it is discovered that the format of a given meeting has been partially or totally unsuccessful (because of the high frequency of critical comments on the sessions's evaluation, low participation in the meeting, and failure of most members to complete their weekly assignments), the format can be changed. Changes thus are brought about by a review of data as well as intuitive hunches. Because of the availability of data and the regularity of feedback, change procedures can be designed and implemented as soon as a specific problem and its parameters have been identified.

Evaluation. The therapist and client also periodically evaluate the degree to—and conditions under—which individual treatment goals are achieved. Evaluation of data related to weekly goal achievement (for example, assignment completion, satisfaction, attendance, participation) provides the therapist with a basis for looking with the group at alternative group strategies or programs for more effective strategies. Evaluation of progress in terms of data-related long-term goals provides clients and therapist with a measuring stick against which to consider change in individual treatment goals or strategies, additional treatment, early termination, and similar issues. Furthermore, by keeping a record of ongoing progress, the therapist and others with whom data are shared can ascertain what kind of clients can best use the procedures commonly found in various models of group therapy. Each therapist can expand the knowledge base further if research controls are established. In behavior therapy, if all treatment steps and problems are explicated, the total treatment of each group and each client can be viewed as an experiment in which the client and group are observed before, during, and after treatment. Variations of this time-series model without a control group have been suggested by a number of authors as a means to strengthen the conclusion of a casual connection between treatment and outcome. Such designs as the multiple baseline, the ABAB model, and other time-series designs are especially suited to small samples.

Therapeutic planning

Therapeutic planning in groups has two components; individualized and group planning. Group planning is preceded by an analysis of the data about individuals and the group to determine common skill deficits. On this basis, training programs are then selected—for example, problem solving, giving and receiving feedback, relaxation, role playing, cognitive self-analysis, and other skills which are, in varying degree, commonly deficient among the members but which are required to mediate the individualized therapy.

These basic therapeutic skills are taught through group exercises and other interactive procedures, usually in a 6-hour marathon session at the beginning of therapy. In some cases, these exercises may be incorporated in each of the first six to eight sessions for 15 to 30 minutes.

Individualized treatment planning involves developing a highly individualized plan for each client, in consultation with the therapist and the group, in which individual situations are worked on. It is determined whether social skill training, problem solving, cognitive restructuring, or other techniques used in the group might be the most appropriate set of strategies for resolving that problem.

Social skill training

Combs and Slaby define social skills as "the ability to interact with others in a given social context in specific ways that are societally acceptable to values and at the same time personally beneficial, mutually beneficial, or beneficial primarily to others."

Social skills involve several critical assumptions. The first is that interpersonal behavior is based on a distinct set of skills which are primarily learned behaviors. Thus, how one behaves in an interpersonal situation depends on the individual's repertoire of social behaviors. The second assumption is that socially skilled behavior is situationally specific. It is important to recognize that cultural and situational factors determine social norms or what an indivdiual believes may be expected of him or her. Third, effective functioning (making a friend) under a set of social circumstances is a powerful source of reinforcement for continued functioning under these circumstances. Finally, the absence of such skills results in social punishment and in avoidance of future situations.

Bellack and Hersen describe three sets of concrete activities that make up the components of social skills—conversational skills, social perception skills, and skills unique to special problem situations. With regard to conversational skills, Bellack and Hersen point out that every social interaction is dependent on one's ability to initiate, maintain, and terminate a conversation. With regard to accurate perception of the social situation, the following skills have been identified as relevant: listening, getting clarification, maintaining relevancy, timing, and identifying emotions. Lastly, it is important to attend to special problem situations which are particularly difficult because they are stressful, even though they may be infrequent. Such situations place unique demands on the individual, such as dealing with impositions of others, job interviews, or an oppressive employer.

Research on social skills training has revealed no specific intervention strategies which are universally effective across different subject populations and different problems. Whereas McFall and Twentyman found that coaching (instructing a client how to perform in a specific situation) and rehearsal (role-played practice) were important components of assertive training, and that symbolic modeling (observing others) contributed little, Eisler, Hersen, and Miller found modeling and instructions to be the most critical elements in social skills training with psychiatric clients. It appears that different training components are effective in producing different aspects of social skills, and that results have different effects depending on the subject population. In general, it appears that a complete treatment package is important when teaching complex response patterns.

Prior to the initiation of social skills training, the therapist discusses with members the rationale of the procedures and provides examples. Where possible, the therapist draws upon those members who have used the procedures to share their evaluation of these experiences with the group.

In teaching social skills, the therapist initially enlists the group members in helping each client, one at a time, to determine in a specific situation at a specific moment what is to be achieved. The group members are asked to provide suggestions as to how that set of goals can be achieved. The members help each client evaluate these suggestions by asking questions about relative risk, appropriateness, compatibility with personal style, and probable effectiveness. It is the client with the problem who determines the final over-all strategy.

Usually, the therapist or a group member demonstrates (or models) the desired verbal and nonverbal behavior in a brief role play. The client, in consultation with the group, evaluates how realistic the modeled situation was and articulates what is useful in the demonstration.

The client then practices or rehearses the situation, utilizing, as nearly as possible, the agreed-upon behaviors. In a series of rehearsals, the difficulty and complexity of the situation are gradually increased. Where difficulty in carrying out the strategy is observed, the client may be coached or assisted by the therapist or another member. If coaching is used, it is usually eliminated in subsequent rehearsals. Following each rehearsal, the client receives an evaluation from the other group members as to what was done effectively and what could have been done differently. After several increasingly difficult rehearsals, the client gives himself a homework assignment to try out some of the new strategies rehearsed in the group, to practice a given role of the new strategies rehearsed in the group, to practice a given role play, to observe the client's own self in a new situation, or to keep a diary. Homework is an integral part of this approach, and is used as a means of increasing time spent on therapeutic endeavors and for generalizing in-therapy achievements to the real world.

Cognitive restructuring

In describing their cognitive responses during stress situations, clients often reveal self-defeating thoughts or severely distorted beliefs about themselves in relation to the world about them. In some cases, these cognitions seem to generate so much anxiety for an individual that the client would be unable to make use of social skills training in developing and trying out specific alternatives for coping with stress as it occurs in the real world. Under these conditions, some form of restructuring of cognitions may be necessary. Cognitive restructuring refers to the process of identifying and evaluating one's own cognitions, recognizing the deleterious effect of maladaptive cognitions, and replacing these cognitions with more appropriate cognitions.

Just as in social skills training, the provision of a rationale for cognitive restructuring is an imperative first step. As a part of this step, clients are provided with examples, evidence of effectiveness, and an overview of the major steps. Members are encouraged to provide to others their own examples of the relationship between cognitions, anxiety, and behavior. An example of a rationale commonly used in groups is the following.

No one is free from stress. The way we view ourselves, what we say to ourselves, what we expect from ourselves—all this may strongly influence how stressful a given situation becomes and how anxious we may feel. One person might view as a terrible tragedy the sight of his car being towed away for a parking violation and might brood about it for a week with an intense headache; another person in the same situation might reflect casually that it was an expensive parking fee, pay the fine, and vow to be more careful in the future. The situation is the same, but the stress experienced is dramatically different. Changing the first person's view of the situation to a more realistic appraisal may result in reduced anxiety, better problem solving, and, in general, more comfortable living.

The following step is to identify each client's particular self-defeating or irrational cognitions through analysis of logical inconsistencies and long-range consequences of pervasive cognitions. This is done through the analysis of cognitive responses to stress situations brought in by the clients, who are interviewed by the other members of the group. The group provides each participant feedback on the accuracy of their cognitions.

Group exercises may be first used to teach clients to differentiate between self-defeating and coping statements. Additional exercises are sometimes used to encourage clients to learn how to identify and analyze their own cognitions. Group participants provide each other not only with feedback but with repeated and varied models of a cognitive analysis for each other.

Often, convinced recognition of the self-defeating cognitions is sufficient to warrant change, but more

often in clinical experience, further steps must be employed. Thus, the subsequent step is to solicit ideas from the client and from other group members as to potential self-enhancing or coping cognitions which facilitate problem solving or effective actions.

After the client decides on a set of accurate and comfortable cognitive statements, cognitive modeling is used in which the client imagines the stressful situation, experiences the initial self-defeating statements, stops himself or herself, and replaces the self-defeating remark with a coping statement.

In cognitive rehearsal, the client goes through the same steps as the model but adapts his own style. Afterward, the client gets feedback from the group. The client may need to be coached during the first few trials. Finally, when feeling comfortable, the client practices the entire process silently (covert rehearsal).

Usually, after several trials in the group, an assignment to practice a number of times at home is developed with the client. Ultimately, it must be tried out in the real world.

Thus, in the final step, homework is developed at the end of one session and is monitored at a subsequent session. Assignments are usually developed in pairs and discussed in the larger groups. Homework is developed at successive levels of difficulty each week. For example, it might initially focus on learning to discriminate in general between self-defeating and self-enhancing or coping cognitions. Later, the focus might be on identifying and evaluating the clients' cognitive responses to their own situations, or shifting from the practice of self-defeating responses to coping skills.

Stress inoculation

This procedure is quite similar to cognitive restructuring but goes beyond it to teach physical as well as cognitive and social coping skills. Designed by Meichenbaum and Cameron, stress inoculation is aimed at providing a client with a set of skills to deal with future stressful situations. Stress inoculation has three important facets: orienting the client to the nature of stressful reactions, cognitive and overt modeling and rehearsing of various physical and cognitive skills, and helping the client to apply these skills during exposure to highly stressful situations. This approach has been used to aid abusive clients and law enforcement personnel in anger control (Novaco, 1977) and to teach others how to manage anxiety, stress, tension, headaches, and pain.

Coping skill training

In addition to overt interactive responses which are usually taught through social skill training procedures, a number of other more general behavioral strategies have been found effective in coping with both specific and general stress situations. These include: relaxation, deep breathing, inquiry, and (in some cases) avoidance of the stress situation (Barrios and Shigetomi, 1979).

Relaxation and deep breathing are taught to the group as group exercises. The skills are demonstrated, members practice the skills in pairs and give each other feedback, and, finally, with the help of instructional tapes, they practice the skills at home. Once learned, the group discusses when and where such procedures should be used.

Teaching clients when to use inquiry (collection of information) in stress situations is taught as each person brings in a stress situation. The question is always asked: What information do you need to reduce the ambiguity of this situation? Avoidance, too, is often looked at as one alternative response in every stress situation. However, the question must be asked as to whether the costs or risks of avoidance are greater than a more confrontative approach or a cognitive coping or physical coping strategy.

One additional cognitive coping strategy, systematic problem solving, is taught universally in group therapy.

Problem solving

Several studies have shown that emotionally distressed individuals are not very efficient problem solvers. Emotionally distressed individuals tend to use more impulsive and aggressive solutions to problematic situations, and are less capable of means-ends thinking than their normal peers (Shure and Spivack, 1972). The term "problem solving" has been used by helping professionals to explain a particular systematic process between therapist and worker which leads to the resolution of problematic situations experienced by the client.

In problem-solving training, the client learns systematically to work through a set of steps for analyzing a problem, discovering new approaches, evaluating these approaches, and developing strategies for implementing these approaches in the real world. In groups, problem solving is taught through problem-solving exercises in which each person brings a problem to the group and the group goes explicitly through the various steps mentioned above. It is also demonstrated when group problems arise and must be dealt with. Both social skills training and cognitive restructuring involve the client in the major steps of the problem-solving process.

Group procedures

These can be distinguished from individual intervention in that instructions are for interactive or cooperative activities which usually modify the group structure. Member-to-member discussion would be used as a group interventive technique involved in most other more specific procedures, which include recapitulation, subgrouping, fishbowl, leadership training, group exercises, and the buddy system (Rose, 1977). Most of the procedures discussed earlier—such as modeling, rehearsals, coaching, problem solving, and brainstorming—are also interactive in nature and, as used in group therapy, make use of the many members' ideas, experience, information, and leadership.

Group and individual procedures are often used together to modify group attributes. These include the level of group cohesion, the distribution of group participation, the agreement to certain group norms, the status of various members in the group, and the domination of a given member over others in the group. It is this concern for influencing group phenomena to mediate the modification of individual behavior that distinguishes group from individual therapy.

Modification of group structure, such as the communication pattern among members, was illustrated in a group of six members in which data revealed that two members spoke almost 60% of the time and one less than 5% of the time. After seeing the data, they agreed participation was a problem and developed a plan to implement at that meeting. The more active members agreed to reformulate the previous speakers' position before making a point of their own recapitulation, and the less active members agreed to write down any thought they had relevant to the subject if they were disinclined to speak up. The leader agreed to call upon them to review their notes. The group practiced the complex plan for the following 5 minutes, and decided to use it only twice a meeting for 20 minutes, since it was somewhat disruptive. They also agreed to end it once the distribution of participation was somewhat more even. Thus, the plan utilized problem solving, recapitulation, cueing by the leader, and rehearsal.

Transfer and maintenance of behavioral change

Transfer of change or generalization involves the application of those strategies designed to facilitate the transfer of learning occurring in the treatment situation to the real world of the client. There are two major types of procedures for transfer. The first are intragroup procedures, such as behavioral rehearsal, which simulates the real world and represents a preparatory step toward performance outside the group, and the second are extragroup procedures, such as the behavioral assignment in which the client tries out the rehearsed behavior in the community. Other extragroup techniques include meeting in the homes of the clients and using the buddy system outside of the group.

Maintenance of change refers to strategies oriented toward maintaining the goal level or quality of behavior achieved during the course of treatment long after treatment is terminated. Several techniques are used. Among them are the gradual fading of the treatment procedures and thinning of the reinforcement schedules, i.e., reducing frequency and regularity of rewards and overlearning the new behavior through frequent trials. Overlearning of simple tasks is probably not sufficient. It is also necessary to review summary rules or cognitive strategies in order that the more complex patterns of functioning be maintained. In groups, this review is often carried out at the end of each meeting.

In preparing for termination, the attraction of other groups is increased relative to the therapy group. Clients are encouraged to join non-therapeutic groups in order to practice their newly learned skills under less controlled conditions. Greater reliance is placed on the decisions of the clients, as they increasingly perform the major leadership tasks in the group. The role of the therapist shifts from direct therapist to consultant. These activities serve to make termination easier on the clients, and they permit them to function independently of a therapist. This independence is necessary not only for the maintenance of changes beyond the end of the group, but in making the client more comfortable in dealing with new problems, should and when they happen. Clients are prepared for potential setbacks, unsympathetic relatives and friends, and unpredicted pressure through role play of situations simulating the above conditions. It should be noted that preparation for the transfer and maintenance of change is found throughout treatment. As early as the third or fourth meeting, partners are working with each other outside of the group, rehearsals are occurring within the group, and behavioral assignments are given to practice the desired behavior outside of the group.

Conclusion

Some empirical support does exist for most of the components of behavior group therapy. Preliminary data suggest that these components in combination do add to the effectiveness of the program. The behavior and cognitive model of group therapy— which combines social skills training, cognitive restructuring, coping skills training, problem solving, and group process modification—offers a promising set of alternatives to the treatment of clients in groups with complex and varied problems.

References

Barrios, B. A., and Shigetomi, C. C. Coping skills training for the management of anxiety: A critical review. Behav. Ther., *10:* 491, 1979.

Cartwright, D., and Zander, A., editors. *Group Dynamics: Research and Theory.* Harper & Row, New York, 1968.

Eisler, R. M., Frederisken, L. W., and Peterson, G. L. The relation-ship of cognitive variables to the expression of assertiveness. Behav. Ther., *9:* 419, 1978.

Fremouw, W. J., and Zitter, R. E. A comparison of skills training and cognitive restructuring: Relaxation for the treatment of speech anxiety. Behav. Ther., *9:* 248, 1978.

Glalss, C. R., Gottman, J. M., and Shmurak, S. H. Response-acquisition and cognitive self-statement modification approaches to dating-skills training. J. Couns. Psychol., *23:* 520, 1976.

Goldfried, M. R., Linehan, M. M., and Smith, J. L. Reduction of test anxiety through cognitive restructuring. J. Consult. Clin. Psychol., *46:* 32, 1978.

Lawrence, H., and Sundel, M. Behavior modification in adult groups. Soc. Work, *17:* 34, 1972.

MacDonald, M. L., Linquist, C. U., Kramer, J. A., McGrath, R. A., and Rhyne, L. L. Social skills training: The effects of behavior rehearsal in groups on dating skills. J. Couns. Psychol., *22:* 224, 1975.

Meichenbaum, D. *Cognitive Behavior Modification.* Plenum Press, New York, 1977.

Novaco, R. W. Stress inoculation: A cognitive therapy for anger and its application to a case of depression. J. Consult. Clin. Psychol., *45:* 600, 1977.

Rose, S. D. *Group Therapy: A Behavioral Approach.* Prentice-Hall, Englewood Cliffs, NJ, 1977.

Rose, S. D. Assessment in groups. Soc. Work Res. Abstr., *17:* 29, 1981.

Safran, J. D., Alden, L. E., and Davidson, P. O. Client anxiety level as a moderate variable in assertion training. Cog. Ther. Res., *4:* 189, 1980.

Schinke, S. P., and Rose, S. D. Interpersonal skill training in groups. J. Couns. Psychol., *23:* 442, 1977.

Schwartz, R. M., and Gottman, J. M. Toward a task analysis of assertive behavior. J. Consult. Clin. Psychol., *44:* 910, 1976.

Shure, M. B., and Spivack, G. Mean-ends thinking, adjustment and social class among elementary school-aged children. J. Consult. Clin. Psychol., *38:* 348, 1972.

Taylor, F. G., and Marshall, W. L. Experimental analysis of a cognitive-behavioral therapy for depression. Cog. Ther. Res., *1:* 59, 1977.

Thorpe, G. L. Desensitization, behavior rehearsal, self-instructional training and placebo effects on assertive-refusal behavior. Eur. J. Behav. Anal. Mod., *1;* 30, 1975.

Wolfe, J. L., and Fodor, I. G. Modifying assertive behavior in women: A comparison of three approaches. Behav. Ther., *8:* 567, 1977.

B.6 Existential Group Psychotherapy

WILLIAM V. OFMAN, Ph.D.

Introduction

The legacy of Descartes, Cartesianism, is our being suffused with the implicit, hardly questioned ideas of dualism, reductionism, determinism, and mechanism, ideas which lie in our very language (Corey and Maas, 1976). These ideas form the grammar of our appreciation of persons, psychodynamics, personality structure, and psychotherapy; our view of interpersonal relationships; and—centrally—our calling persons neurotic or sick. In short, Cartesianism provides the foundation upon which group therapy rests.

Koch wrote that the Newtonian-Cartesian legacy is obsolete (Koch, 1981). Eschewed by the physical scientists and philosophers of science almost as soon as it was imported to the behavioral sciences, it persists there with unquestioned acceptance. Psychology is in the unenviable position of holding to philosophical foundations which were "vacated by philosophy almost as soon as the former had borrowed them ... [and] are now seen as shallow and defective by all save the borrowers" (Koch, 1981). Allen Wheelis wrote of the scheme of things which, having begun as the possibility of the way things are, finally became our world, became self-evidently true. The positivist, Newtonian-Cartesian view seems accepted so naturally and automatically that one is actually not aware of an act of acceptance having taken place.

It is in the bastions of normal science as translated by the human sciences that the anachronistic scheme of things is held with the tenacity of an infant grasping its pacifier. And, via the media—and the psychological media in particular—the person is infected by this view. The patient comes to group therapy as the embodiment of the influence and power of this view as it is assimilated into that person's life.

One of the major points of emphasis of existential psychotherapy is the struggle against the implicit paradigmatic assumptions which persons hold, belief systems of which persons' behavior in group therapy is emblematic. It is on the basis of these held assumptions that persons suffer loneliness, encapsulation, and the psychopathology that is a sequent to the system which is its genesis—the Cartesian scheme of things.

There can be no escape from the responsibility of a philosophical position. The therapist who frames the person in terms of, say, a conversion or projection is making a metaphysical statement and thus teaches and reinforces that position from which the patient suffers in the first place. The patient suffers his or her view of the world, of the body, of others. The work of group therapy is the illumination of the person's view of the way things are and the way the person's suffering is a function of this view.

Humanistic existentialism, the basis upon which this chapter is written, includes the work of Sartre, de Beauvoir, Camus, and Barnes.

Concepts

In existential approaches, the centripetal concepts are the idea of human consciousness and intentionality; the derivative constructs are freedom, responsibility, lucidity, and authenticity; and the applied concepts are radical self-declaration, symmetry, affirmation, and engagement (as opposed to retroflexion).

Person as consciousness

The world is divided into two elemental forms, Being-in-itself (all of nonhuman things and animals) and Being-for-itself (human, self-reflexive, transcendent consciousness). This way of thinking about persons is not merely a philosophical dilettantism, a nicety; rather, the existential revolt to which the above schism refers sees the definition of human consciousness as foundational to its aim—a change in our view of ourselves and of our world; and, as a function of such a changed view, the person's position, vis-à-vis the person and others, is clarified.

The root concept of the schism in nature into Being-in-itself and Being-for-itself is designed to permit of a different consciousness of the self—of what a person is.

Beings-in-themselves are determined, can be described fully and completely, and belong to the essentialistic order of things. Being-for-itself—human consciousness—is different in kind. Human consciousness is a negation: it injects a film of nothingness between itself and its objects of purview.

This nothingness is freedom, its syntax is intentionality, and its grammar is responsibility.

In the human sense, existence precedes essence; this is the first principle of existentialism (Sartre, 1967). Importantly, the phenomenological tradition upon which existentialism is built—beginning with Brentano, through Husserl, Heidegger, and Sartre—had as its main task a radical break with essentialism via the pivotal idea that consciousness has no interiority, no content (Tillich, 1961).

The architecture of consciousness is thus an emptiness. Cleansed of essentialistic engrammata residing in the mind—which drafted the person as a determined being—consciousness must always be a consciousness *of* something. This concept breaks with the insular notion of former conceptions (resident still in the Freudian paradigm which emphasizes intrapsychic events) which emphasized the discontinuity between the world and human consciousness, a world of appearances and realities. Consciousness, having no interiority, being conscious of something, is thus always in relation to its objects; to the external world. Consciousness thus cannot be separated from being, from the world, and from the world of others. A consequence of this view is that, because of the intentionality of consciousness, the person is in direct contact with the world. The pivotal point is as follows: That which the person sees is the thing that presents itself. It is real, and is not merely an appearance or a distortion.

This is the uniquely human event from which all else flows. It is a radically new definition of the person, a definition which rests on triple pillars: freedom, intentionality, and a connected-with-the-world-and-with-others dyadic circuit.

Being-in-the-world

Since the basis for existential group psychotherapy is the concept of intentionality and its sequent, the personal myth, the concept of intentionality must be understood. Underlying this concept is the principle of Being-in-the-world: The person is inextricably wedded to the world which is around the person. The world frames, outlines, and permits of the person's existence. There is no person and the world, there is a person-in-the world.

Thus a table is not in consciousness, a table is in space, beside the window. Consciousness is, therefore, a positional consciousness of the world.

When a person attempts to examine consciousness itself, there appears a lack of knowing what to do. As in sensory deprivation experiments, the person hallucinates a world, else he would stand alone, isolated, wrapped before a cement wall where the self meets only the self. The whole being of the person is in the world, inextricably connected to it and to others.

This notion has decided consequences as to the manner persons shall be thought about in group interactions. The fact that person A in a group is identified, stably, as A (A is a kind man, for example) does not imply that he is that person under different circumstances, or to person B. This point is analogous to the issue of the bifurcation of nature to which Whitehead addressed himself—to the paradox of the world of objective, scientific explanation versus the issue of the person in the human, immediate, lived experience. The principle is as follows: No object, person, or event exists without a context. The person thus sees different aspects of reality under different circumstances and in different contexts. The person is aware of absolutely real things in others and in the world, but is related to them in a special way both contextually and intentionally.

How does this idea work in a group setting? When a member of a group expresses a subjective complaint about the self—not about the body, about another member of the group, or about the therapist—the person retroflexively withdraws from an authentic Being-in-the-world position and creates the self into a pure subject. This maneuver is the magical retroflexive transform—foundationally inauthentic— which is the hallmark of personal difficulty. It should be noted that a child or a naive subject rarely performs such a maneuver; such a person complains about the others in the world. The child never says "I have feelings of anger" (only therapists speak that way); the child says, "I don't like you!" The former is a retroflexive statement; the latter is a connected statement referring to a person who-is-in-the-world and, in this case, in the world of others.

Further, when the child or patient says, "You are mean," this person tells what his world is like. Indeed, the basic proposition posited in humanistic existentialism psychotherapy is that violation is the seminal injury, the basic ensickening act. Violation is the breaking of a person's subjectivity via the covert denial of the validity of the person's vision. Van Den Berg points out that the therapist joins the patient's relatives and friends in their violation by the therapist's lexicon of symptoms and labels (nosology) which are mainly "a dictionary of rejection." This leads to a crucial therapeutic issue: How should the group therapist understand the person who reports that the world or that "Mary, sitting opposite me," is different today than she was yesterday, or that she is "angry" or anything else? Is the therapist (or other group members) going to further engage in the very process which brought the person to therapy in the first place by further violation? Or can the therapist, together with the climate built in the group, affirm the person's reality?

Much depends upon how the therapist interprets the fact that the person sees that which the person, in fact, sees, and that the person speaks the truth. If the therapist holds to one side of Whitehead's bifurcation of nature—the quotidian Cartesian world of scientific or objective explanation properly belonging to the nonhuman world—then the therapist will attempt to dissuade the patient's perception. In this mode, the therapist will not apprehend or appreciate the patient's subjective world but will, instead, objectify that patient and state that the patient is distorting, is paranoid, projecting, etc. Even worse, the therapist will marshall the group's support around this position. In doing so, the therapist disconfirms (violates) the person's perception, rejects the patient, and further promulgates an already weakened self-confidence and reality sense. By this tack, the therapist echoes the original provocative violating act which led the person to become a patient.

The group therapist in the humanistic existentialism mode is interested in the person as the person is; the primary interest is in the phenomena as they are.

Thus, there will be an acceptance and respect for that which the person reports about that person's world and about the person's perceptions of the therapist or about other group members. There will be acceptance and affirmation of the person's vision not because it is therapeutic or beneficial (that would be a frank manipulation and, therefore, inauthentic), but because the person's vision is truth. One may, if one accepts the common Cartesian mode, assume a self-conscious, reflective, uninvolved, intellectualized approach to the person's vision, but it must be noted that such an approach disturbs the objects and events of the person who is speaking.

The analytic mode reduces things to a position wherein events and persons are apprehended without feelings and without emotion, a mode reserved for the laboratory, not the group room. The humanistic existentialism therapist remains, above all, true to the facts as they are happening—to the facts of immediate, unself-conscious experience. One rarely, in the lived world, sees objects or persons as pure objects. We see things within their context and in connection to ourselves, in a unitary manner which may not be broken down. If one does not see the significance of an event, nothing is seen. In a deeper sense, we see our intentions; that is what it means to be human.

Intentionality

The concept of Being-in-the-world attempts a preliminary correction to the Cartesian dualism. The basic correction, however, is in the concept of intentionality—a centripetal concept which leads the therapist to understand the self as it is presented in the therapy group.

The person is a Being-in-the-world who intentionally organizes the world into that person's world. Importantly, this organizing process is prereflective; it is immediate—unself-conscious—and it is the very structure of direct, lived, experience. It is also the first look, as it were, at the world. Although this concept of prereflective versus reflective modes is a difficult one, it is central. The making of the world into "my world" occurs immediately, without a free interval. The moment we are aware of anyone or anything, of it, the world is already ordered, organized according to our particular and fundamental intention.

An analogy may be drawn here: Just as existence precedes essence, the organization via intentionality precedes any aware cognition. To be in the world is to have already apprehended it; the very instant that Being-for-itself exists, it is already related to the world because consciousness has no interiority—since it is a nothingness—and is conscious of the world and of things in it. Awareness is impossible without its object. The person exists irrevocably in context, in situation, engaged in the world, and in the world of others.

The concept of intentionality provides a special view of motives, of feelings, and of emotions. Motives are not events which direct behavior. The person's motivation depends upon that person's aims, upon the person's intentionality in the world. The person does not first select a motive and, on that basis, a goal; rather, it is the other way around. And the person's aims are part of that person's way of organizing reality, the person's unique way of being in the world.

Both motives and emotions are related to an immediate assessment (intentionally determined) of the person's total situation. This situation is seen in the context of an organizing fundamental intentionality, in the personal myth.

The concept of intentionality thus provides the group therapist with a most useful centripetal perspective. The therapist needs to ask—and help the members of the group ask themselves and each other—questions designed to elicit explicitly aware answers to fundamental issues which are illuminated by the person's transactions in group. Objective reality seems singularly ambiguous. The person's assessment of it—and the seeing of it is that very assessment—is that which gives reality meaning (Keen, 1970).

It is the therapist's nonjudgmental interest in the way behavior illuminates the group member's intentionality, and the person's becoming explicitly aware of his or her intentionality, that are the work of the group and the coin of the therapist. Moreover, illumination and explicit awareness are entirely sufficient. That which the person does with that awareness ought not, perhaps, be the therapist's business. If it were, therapy would be reduced to teaching and manipulation, and to the admonition (of which the patient already suffers in full measure): "Change! You indeed are not good the way you are!"

Intentionality and intersubjectivity

Thus far, the individual nature of experience and of awareness has been stressed. There is an amendment needed to the idea that the conscious act is always intentional, that one is not merely aware, but that one is aware of this or that. This amendment takes shape as the following: Not only is one conscious of something, but one is conscious of something as something, and this awareness, in addition to being intentional, is also symbolic. The symbolic amendment has profound consequences for one's thinking about interpersonal processes. It means that a person is not merely aware of something for the self, but that the person is aware of something as being for us. Consciousness, thus, in addition to being intentional is, at its root, an intersubjectivity. It is a knowing for us.

It is intuitively evident that the very act of naming something implies a mutuality. A person who names anything names it for another, or else there would be no need for that activity. Naming a pen a pen is merely another way of stating that the pen is a pen for you and for me. Thus, naming is an intersubjective, mutual occurrence, since every symbolic formulation implies a real or a posited other for whom that name or symbol is intended to have meaning. One does not simply cry, one cries to, for, or about someone.

We are, it seems, incurably bound to the world and to each other in a dyadic circuit. We are thus never angry; we are angry at someone. We are never afraid; we are afraid of something or someone; none of us is afraid of the unknown; we are afraid of that with which we people the unknown. We are not simply depressed; we are depressed when, by, and about. One might even say that depression is the residue of feeling when the authentic responses are shorn from those to whom they belong. There are no villages of feeling which are insular from the rest of the world.

Awareness, consciousness, and mutuality or intersubjectivity are inextricably intertwined. They are, in fact, aspects of the same uniquely human orientation toward the world, the orientation which involves others.

Derivative Concepts

Freedom

The issue here is on what basis will the therapist see and respond to patients and thus—for metacommunication is always a factor—teach them about themselves and reality.

Much of the therapist's response depends on how the person is conceived: Whether the therapist holds that for some actions, the person could have chosen otherwise; or whether the therapist holds that the perception of freedom is illusory, that all the causes of a person's behavior—although unknown at the present—can ultimately be known, and, when they are thus known, it will become quite clear that human choices and human freedom are not and never have been real. Psychoanalytic systems fall into the latter category and are joined with even greater fervor by the behaviorists (Barrett, 1979).

The definition of determinism—based on "if all factors were known"—leaves the issue itself empty of all verifiability and meaning. The concept is neither an empirical nor an analytic one. It is in principle unfalsifiable because the determinist can always hide behind the cloak that the totality of all the antecedent circumstances for any act is unspecified. It is the remnant of the borrowed philosophy of science, clung to by the workers in the human sphere but quickly abandoned by the lenders themselves (Barrett, 1979).

The human issue, however, hinges upon how the group therapist considers any human action: whether it is an act that is involved or a reflex, an involuntary movement. Both activities are available to recent corpses, as well as sentient humans. As these behaviors are not intended to accomplish anything, they are not acts. Acts, human acts, have goals and purposes. Acts have reasons for their being. While acts are caused—upon this there is no disagreement—the humanistic existentialism therapy holds that the cause is integral to the person and to the person's freedom itself. The cause is not something external to the person. Thus a cause or a motive is seen as forged by the person. Out of the cornucopia of events and tasks available to the person, the person freely chooses and assesses certain ones as the cause and motive for any action. An act is caused, but it is undetermined, because it is the person who has determined the motive underlying it on the basis of that person's fundamental intention.

Freedom, however, is human freedom in the sense that it is a freedom of choice among alternative possibilities which may be mutually exclusive and certainly reciprocally limiting. The obstacles to action (others, things) are the resistance the world offers—the formless mass—out of which human freedom congeals its intentional projects.

Being free, undetermined by outside forces, the person is inexcusably responsible. A basic and difficult principle is that a person's being is individual freedom; the person is fully responsible for all acts—for the past, present, and the future—and is determined by nothing.

The acceptance of this principle and its declaration to others—for it is via declaring oneself honestly to another that one comes to an authentic explicit awareness of oneself—is authenticity, a major goal of existential group therapy. This concept implies a proximate lucidity of the person to the person, a renouncing of physiology or history (we make and remake our history to suit our present tasks), of others, or of unconscious motivation as an explanatory or justifying principle for action.

Reality as the existential correction

The existential correction to the Cartesian dualism—with its disastrous translation into psychotherapy as a position based on reductionism, determinism, mechanomorphic thinking, and a doubting of one's perceptions—is the phenomenologically based, humanistic existentialist position's response to the basic question of "What is real?"

The humanistic existentialist position is that the real is located in the raw, immediate, nonreflective experiential world of the person who is speaking. This person's world is something of which the group therapist has to be exquisitely mindful. It is not to be violated via a priori judgments as to what is cause, what is effect, what is complex (thus needing reduction), what is more basic or fundamental. The person's experience and responses to the therapist or to other members of the group are to be taken as absolutely real. They are merely emblematic of the way that person has organized reality, and in this respect, even though this person leads a different existence from others, he or she is no different from anyone else.

The humanistic existentialist position is that one can see reality anytime one chooses to look. It is right there in the group, among us, in the phenomenally given world. This is the lived world; it is the matrix of our existence. It is the only source of meaning and intelligibility available to the person in the real world and in the forge of the therapy group. To skip over this world to a world behind the scenes—a world of science or unconscious motivations (which are in principle and unknowable to the person)—results in the criticism of most of psychotherapy available to-day: that in the plethora of facts there is irrelevancy and confusion (Koch, 1981).

A central therapeutic element here is as follows: That via the therapist and other members in the group, self-knowledge is illuminated by an insistence upon an explicitly aware and careful description of the person's perceptions of—and reactions to—the others in the group here and now. The humanistic existentialist approach to group therapy emphasizes the point that explicit awareness is the antidote to self-deception and insists upon this: That specificity is the essence of reality.

The focus is upon free, immediate, and full description—as opposed to interpretation—of the person's perception, of the person's deep subjectivity (Poole, 1972). Interpretation and hypotheses are then needed only when there is a failure of adequate description.

The ubiquitous emphasis upon feelings and emotions and their expression in group is in terms of their illuminating the person's world, not as foundational events in themselves. The person's way of seeing the group therapist, others, the way things are felt, the way emotion is activated, illuminates, at any instant, the intentionality of the person in the world.

Feelings are understood as accompaniments to intentionality, while emotions are its instrumentality. The inchoate body is seen as being manifested—as embodying—the person's fundamental way of being.

Conclusion

The idea of a basic project or overarching intentionality, or a fundamental personal myth, is the matrix—the centripetal concept—which is foundational to the work of the existential therapy group. Without such a centripetal concept, the patient and the therapist may find themselves in a kind of Brownian motion, as responding to personal transactions in a deterministic, atomic fashion.

The group is the medium whereby the shape of the personal myth is sublimated out of the plethora of seemingly unrelated and disconnected behaviors and feelings, where it is seen, accepted, and finally embraced by the person. This is the way a person comes together.

In sum, the world can only advise—and vaguely at that—and then only if the person asks it pertinent questions. These questions are asked only in terms of the centripetal personal myth. The therapy group provides the prepotent field where evidence of this myth is available.

These ideas are founded on the phenomenologically based humanistic existentialist conception of the unity and imminent translucency of the person himself, and to others via authentic self-declaration. Persons can know—if demystification occurs—what they are about. But it seems it cannot be done in isolation. What is good for the patient has to be what the therapist openly struggles to attain. There cannot be dissonance here or dissembling, for, if there were, the patient would perceive it and learn that.

We are a conversation. We need each other. The actualization of this need and the creation of an authentic environment for its satisfaction are what the existential group is all about.

References

Barrett, W. *The Illusion of Technique.* Anchor Books, New York, 1979.

Boss, M. *Existential Foundations of Medicine and Psychology.* Jason Aronson, New York, 1979.

Bugental, J. *Psychotherapy and Process.* Addison-Wesley, Reading, Mass., 1978.

Corey, D., and Maas, J. *The Existential Bible.* Na Pali Publishing Company, Honolulu, 1976.

Keen, E. *Three Faces of Being.* Appleton-Century-Crofts, New York, 1970.

Koch, S. The nature and limits of psychological knowledge. Am. Pschol, *36:* 257, 1981.

Košik, K. *Dialectics of the Concrete.* Reidel, Boston, 1976.

Lemiell, J. Toward an idiopathic psychology of personality. Am. Psychol., *36:* 276, 1981.

Lyon, J. *Experience.* Harper & Row, New York, 1973.

Ofman, W. Existential psychotherapy. In *Comprehensive Textbook of Psychiatry,* A. M. Feedman, H. J. Naplan and B. J. Sadoch, editors, ed. 3, p. 838. Williams & Wilkins, Baltimore, 1980.

Percy, W. *The Message in the Bottle.* Farrar, Straus, & Giroux, New York, 1975.

Poole, R. *Towards Deep Subjectivity.* Harper, New York, 1972.

Sartre, J. P. *Essays in Existentialism.* Citadel Press, New York, 1967.

Solomon, R. *The Passions.* Anchor Press/Doubleday, Garden City, NY, 1976.

Tillich, P. Existentialism and psychotherapy. Rev. Exist. Psychol. Psychiatry, *1:* 1961.

B.7 Psychoanalysis in Groups

ALEXANDER WOLF, M.D.

Introduction

All group therapies share three fundamental ingredients: (1) a group therapist and at least two patients; (2) multiple interaction among the group members; and (3) limits on what takes place. Psychoanalysis in groups, one form of group therapy that was pioneered in 1938, shares these three parameters. There is, however, an additional ingredient basic to psychoanalysis in groups: the exploration and working through of intrapsychic unconscious processes.

The therapeutic group

In order to practice group psychotherapy, the therapist must have a group. One therapist and one patient do not make a group. A therapeutic group demands at least three persons, two of them patients and the third a therapist. There is no psychotherapy without a therapist. And, there is no therapeutic group if two of the members are therapists and the third is a patient; this is a group setting, but the treatment is individual. Two patients and one therapist or a number of patients and one or two therapists provide structurally for the simultaneous presence of hierarchical and peer vectors. The therapist fills the need for a responsible authority figure. Two or more patients afford an opportunity for peer relatedness.

The presence of authority in the person of the therapist and of peers in the persons of patient group members provides for an interplay of vertical and horizontal interactions that elicits parental and sibling transferences. The distortions projected onto the peers are generally diluted versions of more intense projections onto the therapist. The claim is sometimes made that these dilutions interfere with the emergence of intense transferences to the therapist and, therefore, promote resistance. It seems, however, that, where transferences to peers as parental figures are worked through, the patient sooner or later is confronted with his projections onto the therapist. Having worked through, if only in part, the less threatening aspects of parental transference onto his peers, the patient is able to more easily face the authority of the parent invested in the therapist. There are occasions when a peer, because of his particular character structure, will elicit a more threatening transference than the therapist, but this kind of distortion is diluted by reality. The peer is, in fact, only a peer and, therefore, more devoid of parental authority than he seemed at first.

In the therapeutic group, the focus of attention moves from one patient to another. This is the principle of shifting attention. No one patient has the exclusive attention of the therapist. The more patients there are, the greater is the diffusion of attention from the therapist as well as from patients. For many, this shifting of attention gives them time to assimilate and work through whatever insights they have obtained. For others, it represents some freedom from continuous scrutiny, which in individual treatment can be experienced as immobilizing. For still others, it becomes a form of resistance, a way of avoiding examination of their intrapsychic distortions.

Shifting attention can be a means of working through the demand that one be the only child in the family, a problem that is sometimes not adequately challenged in the dyadic therapeutic relationship. Group therapy, with its insistence that there are others besides the self, provides a medium for working through the irrational transferential demand that no one else be heard.

Another consequence of group structure is the phenomenon of alternating roles. Each patient is required by the presence of others to listen, to try to understand them. New kinds of activity, feelings, or responsiveness are induced. A patient would not necessarily experience these reactions if he were the therapist's only patient. In the group, each person listens, gives counsel, tries to understand, reacts, feels empathic, becomes annoyed, and elicits reasonable and irrational responses. He seeks help and offers help. He experiences interaction on a peer level, an experience that is not available to him alone with a therapist. In individual treatment, the difference in status and activity between patient and therapist is so marked, and the roles of helper and helped are so clearly defined, that a patient has less chance to alter both his role and his activity. As soon as other patients enter the treatment structure, the role limits and dimensions are enlarged by new kinds of activities.

Multiple interaction

Here again, the structural situation encourages group members to respond to one another. Patients become involved with each other as well as with the therapist. In nonanalytic group therapy, the interaction is largely phenomenological and deals with manifest content. There is much acting and some acting out of a verbal nature. Here-and-now responses take precedence over an examination of historical determinants. There is preoccupation with group dynamics: Cohesion, what the group is feeling or doing, group themes, and climate. Special topics may be discussed, and patients protest if a member tries to divert the group from a prevailing subject. Group roles, group rituals, group traditions, and a group history emerge in the course of interaction. To some extent, these phenomena determine the ways in which patients and therapists behave over a period of time.

In the multiple interaction that prevails in group therapy, a homogeneity tends to develop in which group members join or submit to whatever theme, climate, or tone is set by a dominant member. On the other hand, attention may suddenly shift from one theme or member to another without an in depth examination of how or why this phenomenon occurred. Patients counsel or advise one another and suggest alternative solutions to each other's current dilemmas. There is more emphasis on what the group is or is not doing than on the individual. When the therapist encourages the group to function in this way, it remains homogeneous and nonanalytic. Group members under such influence identify with one another, rather than differentiate themselves. The result is that the group becomes more cohesive as treatment emphasizes the likenesses among patients. Group conventions take precedence over individual differences, and patients conform to group rules. Personal exception is rejected and unrewarded.

Homogeneity versus heterogeneity

All therapeutic groups have relative degrees of homogeneity and heterogeneity. Nonanalytic group therapies tend to sponsor homogeneity. A group therapist may select patients with similarities: A shared psychovisceral symptom, a common diagnostic category, a similar chief complaint. The psychoanalyst in groups tries to provide more diversity in organizing his groups. Although he acknowledges certain similarities among patients, he is alert to each patient's uniqueness and is sensitive to each member's right to be different. For there is psychopathology in the formation and cohesion of a homogeneous group that too often rejects the stranger as deviant. The psychoanalyst in groups sees a positive value in the complementarity of differences, in man and woman relating constructively to one another just because they are different, of parents and children breaking the generation gap. He sees homogeneity as insular, isolated, snobbish, and antisocial.

If there are several homosexuals in the group, for example, the analyst is not only aware of their manifest similarities but alert to the differences in historical development that led to the underlying psychopathology. Given a group of alcoholics or obese patients, the analyst is cautious about making an interpretation that assumes his observation is equally insightful for all members. Rather, he sees the end product of homosexuality, alcoholism, or obesity as having divergent origins and different bases for its persistence, despite similarities in operational forms.

When group members and the analyst, even in the most homogeneous group, examine each other deeply, they find that each person is different from his neighbor in his history, his development, and his psychodynamics. A working out and working through takes place that makes each patient more interesting to the next. A regard for one another in difference becomes more appealing than the superficial pseudocollusion of similarity and identification. Divergence in healthy resources for gratifying and realistic involvement—not just differences in pathology—can be the basis for mutual interest and acceptance. The novelty that stirs the membership to try to understand and accept their differences represents a reciprocity based on contrast. While the members study one another in depth, they nevertheless discover and grant each other areas of commonality.

Further, in psychoanalysis in groups, the exploration of intrapsychic processes enables the patient to understand in greater detail the nature of his submission to members of the nuclear family and members of his current group. He is encouraged to find his way out, to recover his repressed ego. The psychoanalytic group sponsors his individuation, his nonconformity, and the recovery of his lost self.

Limits

One of the characteristics of emotional disorder is

the pursuit of limitlessness. The patient often tries to overcome his anxiety in an inappropriate way. The search for absolutes or for immortality is one such irrational aim, and it is related to the irrational hope for omnipotence. Treatment needs to be limited in duration, in number of sessions in a week, in the length of each session, in activity, and in participation. The therapist's and the patient's agreement to limit themselves is a commitment to reality. The ingredient of limits is essential to all forms of psychotherapy.

Number of patients. It is not easy to define limits. One therapist may be unable to treat more than six or seven patients in a group. Another may find it congenial to work with numbers up to 10, 12, or 15. It seems doubtful that one can practice psychoanalysis in a group made up of more than 12 or 15. As already pointed out, a definite lower limit for the size of a group does exist: three, one therapist and two patients. The author's view that the upper limit ought to be eight or 10 is not a rigid one; he has worked with groups of 12 to 15. But he is not aware of analytic groups larger than 15, and questions whether it would be possible for an analyst to follow adequately what was going on in such a large group.

Time. Group meetings are most effective if they last between 1½ and 2½ hours. Just as the regular session should be limited in time, so should the alternate meeting. Although a group may have an alternate session that lasts longer than usual, the members inevitably resist unduly prolonged sessions.

Moreover, it makes sense to limit the length of time a patient remains in any given group. If he does not appear to make some progress in 6 to 12 months, continuing in that same group seems of doubtful value. A time limit should be placed also on his remaining in his particular group for more than 4 years. Beyond this time some patients seem to deteriorate in their capacity for cooperative endeavor with the same group of participants. Such members might well be referred elsewhere for treatment.

Activity. Sometimes the analyst in groups is too permissive of patient activity. He needs to take a stand against sexual relations and physical aggression among group members. A monopolist may, for example, dominate a group, with insistent demands that he always be heard at the expense of the others. Or a masochist, by assuming the position of scapegoat, may repeatedly invite group members' aggression.

Families. Psychoanalysis in groups should be limited to patients initially unknown to each other. Such a view excludes family members, as well as married couples, from analytic groups. It is not appropriate to make parents and children or husbands and wives aware of one another's unconscious processes. There are too many potentials for mutual destructiveness in such exposures. It is, however, possible to do group therapy with families and married couples when the therapist plays some interpretive, supportive, guiding, and mediating role.

Most married couples get along without full awareness of the details of their history or of one another's unconscious processes. The exposure of these details might threaten the stability of a marriage. For most couples, the less they know about the significance of one another's dreams, the better the marriage. It is a rare couple, but there are a few, who, the more they know about one another in terms of unconscious processes, the better they get along. These unusual married couples may do well in psychoanalysis together.

Kinds of patients. Limits need to be imposed on the introduction of certain kinds of patients to psychoanalytic groups. Not everyone is suitable for such therapy. Severe alcoholics who cannot come to meetings sober need to be excluded, as do drug addicts who come to sessions under the influence of drugs, seriously handicapped stutterers, the mentally retarded, epileptics, hallucinating psychotics, the actively deluded, suicidal and homocidal patients, the psychopathic, cardiac patients who develop pain under emotional stress, patients more than 50 or 60 years old, adolescents less than 18, the very seriously depressed, and the manic. Such patients can be better treated in nonanalytic group therapy. If they improve, they may become suitable for psychoanalysis in groups.

The therapist. The analyst must also impose limits on himself. He should be available to patients for the whole of their appointed time. He should neither keep them waiting to start a session nor see them beyond the time of the regular meeting. He needs to deny himself sexual and aggressive acting out with patients. At the sessions the analyst may not himself be disturbed, unable to concentrate, intoxicated, drugged, hallucinating, delusional, very depressed, or suicidal. He must have undergone psychoanalytic training and have been an analysand in individual and in group analysis.

Whether he admits it or not, every therapist has a point of view, a philosophy—a therapeutic personality. Regardless of any assumed manner determined by theory or technique, his underlying commitment and his behavior are revealed to the patient. His position with regard to the human condition shows itself in the appearance of his consulting room, the clutter or neatness of his desktop, the kind of wardrobe he has, the paintings on his walls, the color and light in his office, the quality and volume of his speech, and how and whether he responds to phone calls during sessions. The patient experiences him in what he selects to analyze and in what he seems to neglect, in whether he engages vital or trivial issues, in whether he engages vital or trivial issues, in whether his attitude is welcoming or rejecting at first meeting, and in whether his greeting is warm or distant. The therapist indicates his approach to life by his hopefulness or cynicism, and by whether he attends the patient's association or pursues his own fantasies. His preferences are demonstrated in whether he asks the patient to use the couch or the chair, whether he prefers to see the patient alone or in a group, and whether he asks to see members of the patient's family or not. Every therapist betrays to his patient his sense of what he believes is relevant and irrelevant. He exposes himself and his values to the patient not only by the content of what he says but also by how he says it, and by the way be behaves.

Exploration of latent material

Group therapy that introduces psychoanalytic means is concerned not only with the manifest, but with understanding the latent in patient interaction and function. The analyst takes the lead in the search for unconscious processes by promoting free association, the analysis of dreams, resistance, and transference. The search for unconscious motivation and processes leads patients away from the here-and-now and into the there-and-then, into historical determinants. Group therapy is converted into psychoanalysis in groups only when this element—the investigation of intrapsychic material—is introduced.

Under such circumstances, the other parameters take on new depth and meaning. Hierarchical and horizontal vectors cease to be merely current experiences with authority and peers, but instead acquire parental and sibling transferential qualities that are reexperienced; and conscious plans are then introduced to work through these distortions.

The intercommunication characteristic of multiple reactivities is no longer promoted simply for cohesive socialization, which admittedly has its psychotherapeutic benefits. Interaction is also used to proceed from the interpersonal to the intrapsychic, from the manifest to the latent. The pursuit of the intrapsychic in the interpersonal stresses self-knowledge that can lead to personal integration. This personal integration can lead to more wholesome social integration. Nonanalytic group therapy frequently imposes a more superficial social interaction that can disregard the personal psychodynamics of the individual.

In nonanalytic group therapy, the patient may be either well served or victimized by the principle of shifting attention. The patient overly concentrated on may welcome a respite from group examination. Still another member may find himself too frequently bypassed. Little if any time is spent in a study of each member's psychodynamics in provoking the response he gets and the latent nature of these reactions. The contrast when psychoanalytic means are introduced is striking. The patient who is focused on may be masochistically provoking whatever latent sadism exists in other members. Manifestly he is a monopolist, but on a deeper level he may be trying to exclude his younger siblings from getting parental attention. He may be demanding attention in an oral-incorporative way, or he could be receiving much attention because of his narcissism, his exhibitionism, or his phallic overbearance. There are multiple possibilities. The bypassed member may be latently the good child quietly waiting his turn—hurt, disappointed, and enraged at being neglected. He may be frightening to the other patients, who vaguely sense in his silence an enormous hostility they are afraid of tapping. Here, too, the bypassed patient, like the monopolistic one, may have any one of a series of unconscious determinants that require exploration in depth.

In group psychotherapy, with the principle of alternating roles, members are sometimes asking for help, sometimes giving it. In psychoanalysis in groups, some members use the role of helper as a way of resisting treatment. The same is true of those who are always helplessly demanding. The analytic group searches for the historical determinants that have imposed this particular repetition-compulsion in order to work it through.

The analyst in groups introduces an activity not generally available in other group therapies: He interprets the nature of unconscious processes in the interaction among the patients and between the patients and the therapist. The patients in time learn how to understand the latent meaning of their contributions and make significant interpretations as well; their impressions are sometimes appropriate, sometimes not. Unconscious material is worked out and worked through. The patient develops insight, which helps him to understand his disability. He is thereby able, with the support of the analyst and the other patients, to struggle to resolve his difficulties.

The nonanalytic group psychotherapist may use many of the means of the analyst. But unless he emphasizes an exploration of latent content, he is not practicing psychoanalysis in groups. The analyst in groups does not limit himself exclusively to the search for unconscious manifestations. If he entirely neglects manifest behavior, he is practicing individual analysis in a group setting. Analysis in a group requires attention to horizontal and peer vectors, to multiple reactivities, and to unconscious processes, with special emphasis on the last. But individual similarities, manifest behavior, and group dynamics are neither neglected nor denied.

Psychoanalysis in Groups versus Individual Analysis

Multiple reactivities

Multiple reactivity, a characteristic of group therapy, is given fuller play in a heterogeneous group than in a homogeneous group. It is not present in the dyad except to the extent that the therapist is able to evoke diversified reactions. It is available indirectly in the dyad when the patient talks of his responses to persons outside the treatment milieu. But then the therapist is required to see through the analysand's subjective distortions in his accounts of events outside the consulting room. In the group the analyst is a direct observer of how the patient reacts to others in a multiplicity of situations. Through the variety of their provocations, the group members evoke a larger picture of the patient's disorder. At the same time, they call for a more inclusive reconstruction in the face of a greater variety of appropriate and inappropriate expectations.

The patient in a group has an opportunity to take part in an invaluable exercise not available in the dyad. He becomes aware that all people do not necessarily react as he does to the same provocation. He finds that, when he feels one way, others feel differently; when he wants to share a feeling, another person wants to retire in self-examination; when he is feeling warm, the object of his empathy is about to castigate him for his offensiveness during a previous encounter. But he does not learn that there is never any complementarity of interaction. He learns, in fact, that there are as many mutually responsive interactions as there are antagonistic ones.

Multiple transferences

The analytic group speedily and successively furnishes the patient with a number of evocative stand-ins who excite multiple transferences more readily than the analyst alone. Each group member invests every other member with a variety of transferences in the course of every group session. In dyadic treatment, such a variety of misperceptions of the analyst does not occur in a given therapeutic hour. The fluctuating distortions in the group follow from the multiple interaction in which the relationships among members change from time to time. Transference is more inflexible in dyadic analysis. Similar shifting of transferences to the analyst may be seen in one-to-one treatment only if the patient is very unstable.

Some patients homogenize the whole group into a single transferential figure. This coalescence is a phenomenon that, of course, does not occur in individual treatment, at least not in the treatment setting. When it occurs in the group, the members are misperceived as one parent and the analyst as the other. Very likely, similar distortions are made in social situations, but the individual analysand is generally not aware of them. The distortions can be dealt with in the group, since the difficulty becomes manifest. The patients must be urged to react to the other members as individuals, to distinguish one patient from the other, to look for differences in them, and to see them in reality.

Sibling transferences. In dyadic analysis, parental transference is usually the prevailing distortion. Transferences to siblings tend to be disregarded or casually discussed as being less noxious because they do not as a rule manifest themselves in the same deeply felt way. In the analytic group, the presence of peers provides the stimulation for the evocation of sibling transferences, and they can be readily seen, examined, and resolved. The availability of peers provides the opportunity to work out and work through problems with members of the family beyond the parents. Group members are not always perceived as familial surrogates, but, because this distortion is a generally recurrent finding, it needs to be looked for.

Parental transferences to peers. Transferences to peers may have a parental as well as a sibling quality. The investment of co-patients with mother and father distortions is usually experienced as less formidable than when the therapist is perceived as a symbolic parent. Because the peers are also perceived in reality as less authority laden than the analyst, the parental transferences to them are less intense and more easily resolved. Some patients who assume aggressive or dominating roles may elicit strong parental transferences, but even here the awareness of their relative equality in reality as peers reduces the distortive predisposition. The preliminary experiencing and working through of mother and father distortions invested in peers makes it easier to resolve the same distortion when patients begin to undertake, as a later experience, the resolution of the more difficult parental transference to the analyst seen in the hierarchical vector.

Transferences to the therapist. In the group setting, the transferences to the therapist are more fixed than those made to co-patients. Transferences are more stable with relation to the analyst because his role is more consistent than that of the patient, who plays multiple roles and elicits, therefore, a multiplicity of transferences. In dyadic analysis, transferences to persons other than the therapist are only approximately or inaccurately understood because the analyst is dependent on the patient's filtered reports of interpersonal exchanges. In the group, these same transferences are present within the treatment setup. Transference to the therapist is less attended at first because patients find it easier to work out whatever distortions they make with peers seen in the hierarchical vector than with the reinforced authority of the analyst. In dyadic treatment as well, if the analyst first works out and resolves transferences toward persons in the patient's life outside the consulting room, it then becomes less difficult to work through transference to the therapist. If the strategy is transposed—if the analyst tries to work out and work through transference to him as an introductory procedure—he usually encounters greater resistance.

Countertransference. No analyst is totally free of transference or countertransference involvement. To the degree it is present, the therapist experiences trials and crises in his struggle to understand the patient and to see him objectively. In the group, the analyst's inappropriate behavior is more quickly seen by patients, who demand more germane responses from him. As a result, there is protection against the misperceptions of the analyst. A patient alone with such a therapist has no co-patient allies to support him in confirming his belief that the analyst is distorting reality.

Occasionally, the therapist's countertransferential difficulty takes the form of compulsively trying to induce a transference neurosis in the patient. By so binding the patient to him in a symbiotic tie, he may in some instances remove the patient from productive and invigorating relations with his peers. The analytic group tends to counteract such exploitation.

Analysis of transference. Transference is dealt with somewhat differently in individual analysis and in group analysis. In dyadic treatment, the analysis of transference tends to be one of the major functions of the therapist. The patient often plays a lesser part in this activity. In the group, however, patients call attention to each other's misperceptions and make proposals for more realistic alternative ways of functioning.

This willingness among group members to consider and admit to their multilateral distortions refines and enriches the insight into the multilateral nature of transference. The provocative nature of each member in eliciting the transference of each patient is observed more clearly in the group than in dyadic analysis, where the therapist is more reluctant to admit to his inciting role. This denial cannot be so readily maintained in the group in the face of a number of patients concertedly pointing out how his behavior provoked particular patient response.

In the group, transferences are generally interpreted as bilateral or trilateral. In individual analysis, they are generally analyzed as emanating only from the patient. The therapist is supposed not to transfer or countertransfer, which is an illusion.

In dyadic analysis, the rigidity of transference generally exceeds its duration in the group. Its persistence in individual treatment is promoted by the one-to-one situation and the separation from peers, thereby inducing a sometimes persistent and prolonged transference neurosis or psychosis. In the group, patients are invested with mother surrogate and father surrogate distortions, but, because they are also seen in reality in the horizontal vector and because they can move so freely in reacting subjectively from one patient to another, their transferential misperceptions are less virulent, more moderate, more yielding, and more readily relinquished for reasonable alternatives. Quantitatively and qualitatively, patient-to-patient transference is different from that of patient-to-analyst.

Displacement

Group members frequently displace affect onto one another as a means of evading their responses to the analyst. This displacement is both expedient and resistive. An individual analysand may describe his attitude toward a person outside the treatment room, when, in fact, he is reporting how he feels about the analyst. In the group, a member may in the same way be responding to a fellow patient or to all his co-patients as stand-ins for the therapist. There is greater likelihood of secreting displacement in dyadic analysis becuse the inciting cause that leads to such proxy formation is often not discernible.

Support

A patient experiences a greater sense of security in a group because there is a probability there of finding co-patients who encourage his healthy or disturbed aspirations. The analysand in a dyad is usually less sure of getting support for his strivings when he is dependent on only one other person.

Relief and assistance are necessary requirements in all treatment. They are means by which the faltering resources of a patient may be promoted. By having his positive potentials encouraged, the analysand is stirred to show his disorder, his pathology, his gradually recalled history, and his suppressed feeling. The analyst's support is circumscribed because it is derived from the hierarchical position and because it is offered in kind, in degree, in quality and quantity that he believes to be relevant and required. He may deny offering this relief in the concern that it may deepen the patients' symbiosis.

In the group, sustenance is derived from other patients as well as from the analyst. The helpful function of co-patients is particularly apparent at the alternate meeting. Members often reveal problems there for the first time. Then only through the support of fellow patients is the exposed material presented at the regular session with the analyst. Some members need to be encouraged by the analyst in the dyad before they are able to reveal a difficult history or problems in the group. There are more chances of finding greater and various kinds of support in the dyad or the group in multiple therapeutic settings. The patients and the analyst offer different kinds of help. Co-patients' support is more spontaneous, more impulsive, and more compulsive. The analyst's is more purposeful, more useful, and more discriminatingly applied.

Indeed, the most moving experience in the group is not the comfort offered to the ailing but the attainment of fulfillment in reality, the triumph over the neurotic adaptation, the conscious alternative choice over the obsessive one. It is a moment that comes when the previously estranged group members accept and enjoy one another, when they treat each other like human beings, instead of brutes.

Interpretation

The analyst guides the group members from multiple interaction to the search for unconscious motivation, from the manifest to the latent. By this means, the historical bases for the activity are brought into consciousness. Patients who object to the movement from manifest behavior to the investigation of unconscious motivation and persist merely in catharsis or verbal acting out of affective interaction are in resistance. When they accept the idea of the relevance of the latent material, they begin to offer interpretations of their own. Some of these interpretations are most valuable. In the main, however, they are not systematically timed. An analyst may carefully consider when to introduce an interpretation, but a patient reacting spontaneously is liable to be wild, and a poorly timed interpretation is only partially heard or not heard at all.

Accountability

The patient in individual analysis is generally not held accountable for his wildest fantasies of love or hate, of sexuality or homicide. The analyst fosters this illusion to enable the patient to speak freely and regress with the assurance of support and without fear of retaliation. No such security in illusion is available in the group. Expressed fantasies, dreams, thoughts, and feelings are met with all sorts of emotional reactions: fear, anger, rivalry, hostility, rage, anxiety, sensuality, etc. This responsiveness makes each member aware that, although he is always free to say what comes to mind and heart, he is accountable for what he says and does.

There is, therefore, more at stake in speaking up in the group. It becomes more hazardous, for there are always consequences. The wonder is that patients nevertheless do speak up. They always have allies, frequently the very members to whom they are being reactive. This setup is much more reality oriented than is the individual setting, where the benignity of the analyst sponsors the illusion of nonaccountability.

In a way, it is dangerously irresponsible for the therapist to permit this kind of illusion to go on for too long without limiting it, without showing the patient the consequences of his thoughts and feelings, especially if he tends to express them or act them out beyond the consulting room. The analyst's leniency, permissiveness, and forbearance cannot be limitless. Group members quite appropriately hold each other responsible. This is salutary, for it seems to be more realistic to do so. At the same time, group members are enormously tolerant in the recognition of the value of regression as long as it is in the service of the ego. The nonisolatedness of the interaction in a group, when compared with the dyadic setting, supports the need to be aware of the other, the necessity to maintain communication. If treatment deprives a patient of awareness of the consequences of his expressions, it denies him orientation, a place among his fellows, an ego. Whatever he says becomes a whisper lost in the wind, and he becomes equally uncertain of his place.

Group analysis also cultivates a sense of social responsibility among patients. This is one of its values. The conditions that the dyadic therapist demands of the analysand relate mostly to paying a fee, not physically hurting the analyst, and not damaging his furniture and books. The largely tolerant stance of the analyst occasionally institutes or maintains in the analysand a frustrating inclination to take favor as his due and to complain if it is not always as immediately available as a pacifier. If the analyst does not frustrate and analyze this inappropriate anticipation, the exploitative patient's abrasive and inordinate claims for support are intensified. In the group, no member can maintain such exemption from obligation without protest from the others. This protest is wholesome. The demanding, dependent patient is required to react with increasing resourcefulness, autonomy, and responsibility if he hopes to develop better relations with others. This pressure to relinquish the dependent tie to a parent surrogate is a valuable influence in resolving a persistent transference neurosis.

Control

Psychoanalysis in a group would become untenable and dissolve if every member were emboldened to act impulsively on every flash of feeling or thought. The group limits acting out that endangers the mutual effort to resist the gratification of archaic longings. And it is necessary to limit certain activities to meet the needs for some social order in the group.

Impulsivity and compulsivity require a study of just how, when, and where this insufficiency or excess of inhibition developed. If few controls were imposed on a patient by his nuclear family, he may choose an individual analyst in the hope that the surrogate parent may likewise exercise little discipline. If the inducement to acting out took place with nonfamilial figures outside the home, he may choose group therapy. Or, the opposite may turn out to be the case. The patient may choose an individual analyst in the wish of finding a parental substitute who will limit his impulsivity, his pathological repetition. If the peers in the nuclear family insufficiently controlled him, he may seek in group therapy peers who will help to limit him.

Repetitive patterns and flexibility

Repetitive patterns may become apparent in dyadic analysis before they do in a group. This is true in part because the analyst tends to be more experienced as a single parental surrogate. Therefore, the repetitive transferential distortion manifests itself more obviously in dyadic analysis. But transferences also emerge in the group. They appear, however, in more variety because more transference figures are available from the outset. Because of their multiplicity, it may seem, at first, more difficult to designate the various transferences in the group. As a result, the impression may be that the patient has less rigidity than was at first thought. But the fact is that in the group he is exposing a larger variety of transference reactions. As treatment goes on, the inflexibility of these transferences becomes clearer.

In dyadic analysis, the patient is not required to make many flexible adaptations to the changing expectations of persons. The individual analyst does not usually make the multiple demands for health that members of the group do. Of course, they also have irrational expectations of mutual adjustment to one another's pathology.

Dyadic analysis tends to expedite the development of transference. One-to-one treatment promotes the evocation of repetitive patterns with the idea that an unvarying relationship between patient and therapist is essential to ultimate change. Diversified responses tend to be regarded as resistive to the repetition of transference and its final resolution. The individual therapist sees the constancy, regularity, and routine of characteristic distortion as the essential basis for therapeutic intervention.

The dyadic analyst, therefore, is doubtful about the value of psychoanalysis in a group, since uniformity of response seems not to occur, and group patients appear not to persevere in their reactions. The analyst may believe there is too little assurance in foreseeing how patients will respond to one provocation or another. But if he affords himself any clinical experience in a group, he encounters a real and characteristic continuity of reaction in each patient, even among the most heterogeneously stimulating membership.

The heterogeneity of a group makes room for the patients' more flexible choices. For the impulsive member, there are patients whose rigidity helps him to exercise greater control. For the superego-ridden member, there are patients in the group who support his right to allow himself more privilege. The mutual support of peers provides a less severe and more permissive influence than the illusory and actual authority of the analyst, whose interventions are experienced as more unequivocal.

The coexistent and synchronous presence of horizontal and vertical vectors is also a factor that promotes flexibility in response. If only one of these dimensions is available, as in dyadic analysis or in a leaderless group, there is less flexibility and greater rigidity.

Hierarchical and peer vectors

The phenomenon of transference in psychoanalysis in groups can be made more intelligible if one understands that the group provides for the simultaneous presence of peer and hierarchical relationships. By supplying a lateral vector as well as the vertical vector found in dyadic analysis, psychoanalysis in groups provides the patient with the freedom to relate to peers. These horizontal relationships may be facile or awkward, depending on each member's history. One common dilemma with sibling surrogates involves rivalry.

In dyadic treatment, the vertical dimension prevails, with the analyst seen as a parent surrogate. In the power-invested one-to-one climate, it may not be easy for the analysand to convey what he would like to say. In a group, the access of peers in some measure shrinks the ominous influence of the leader, and interaction among the members is usually freer. However, the opposite may occur. The analyst may be easier to talk to than the co-patients. A patient may coalesce the members into a single parental surrogate figure so that even fellow patients are misperceived as being in the vertical vector.

If the analyst is dogmatic, the peers support each other judiciously and injudiciously in defying his predominance. For some of the patients, this support is salutary; for others, it is obsessive. In any event, it challenges the analyst, who is thereby less able to dominate the membership of the group.

Effective treatment leads to a sense of equality between patient and analyst. But actual parity cannot be achieved in dyadic analysis. It can, on the other hand, be accomplished with one's peer in a group setting. The achievement of a sense of equality in the group enlarges the hope and the feasibility of parity between analysand and analyst. In dyadic treatment, where the patient is always being assisted by the analyst, a healthy sense of equality in difference is more difficult to achieve. Fortunately, only a few dyadic therapists regard the patient as infantile and helpless and see themselves as models—dead certain and infallible. In the act of practicing psychoanalysis in groups, the therapist rejects such assumptions about his patients and himself. He sees wholesome potentials and sources of help among group members. He does not see himself as the only source of assistance, insight, innovation, and inducement to healthful change.

The dyadic therapist's all-knowing position tends to sponsor illusion. Because he is the only other person available to the patient, the latter is dependent on the analyst's views. The analysand has only the therapist's associations for testing reality. Group members, however, provide multiple others to define the nature of reality and of unreality.

Equality, freedom, and hostility

Whenever there is superiority and inferiority among persons, with limited independence for the inferior, enmity and hatred can be anticipated. Disaffection occurs when impartial opportunity is not available. The vertical character of dyadic treatment denies the analysand's feeling of parity. If the analyst stresses the analysand's disorder, the patient more than ever feels disparate, inadequate.

Parity, independence, and freedom are more readily experienced in the group. There, patients have more room to ventilate, less acute anger, more em-

pathy, more compassion, and more realistically positive affect than in the dyad, where angry and warm feelings are most commonly dependent, child-like, and distorted—that is, one-sided.

On occasion, however, members of groups are inappropriately harsh and cruel with one another. Good treatment must not entail trial and punishment. The adherents of such a principle, whether patients or therapists, have residual unresolved sadomasochistic difficulties. The aggressor is acting out a negative transference, and his prey a compliant one. When this phenomenon takes place in a group, the therapist must analyze the bilateral distortions early to save the participants from damaging one another. Tolerance and compassion cannot develop during prolonged mutual attack. They grow only in a more wholesome atmosphere. Repetitive anger does not lead to mutual regard unless a member has never been allowed to express negative feelings. But if he is encouraged to ventilate his hostility, he will later be obliged to redeem himself, before other patients will trust his good will. Malice is usually met with resentment, open or concealed. The group analyst needs to be watchful for ways and means to deal with the disorder of hate.

Retaliation and fulfillment

In the psychoanalytic group, there is more response to both transferential and realistic expectations. It is the analyst's function to analyze the mutually hurtful character of bilaterally fulfilling archaic needs and to promote the gratification of more realistic requirements. The illusory exemption from retribution and the frustration of antiquated expectation that theoretically prevail in dyadic analysis may not always be a salutary influence. The analyst's need to overprotect a patient from his peers has something to do with his concern that they will damage each other. Patients, in fact, turn out to be not so hurtful. They demonstrate their healthy resources and their potential for growth in the decent and tolerant ways they treat each other.

There is an inclination in some quarters to regard the interaction between patients as just as significant and valuable as that between analyst and patient. Interaction among group members is generally less intense. In dyadic and group analysis, the authority of the leader is both real and illusory. To regard the leadership of the therapist in the dyad as an illusion and the authority of co-patients as genuine, or the opposite, is to misconstrue the quality of leadership in the dyadic and group settings.

Psychoanalysis in groups is effective because, in part, it does not deny the participant his freedom to examine his many-faceted affect about genuine and illusory hierarchial figures and peers. He has more of a chance in a group to retort and to gratify himself in fact and in fantasy in both the peer and hierarchical vectors. These gratifications, both wholesome and sick, in which he is supporter and supported, heard and hearing among his fellows, have an important place in group analysis.

Genetic and current material

Interaction among patients followed by free association often leads to the recollection of significant genetic material. Either the interaction spontaneously generates free association, or the analyst promotes it. By this means, history is made available in the group, unless the analyst or the resistive patient rejects it for an exclusively here-and-now experience. At times, the therapist may have to initiate the process of cultivating an interest in free association to early derivatives and their history, making clear the relevance of the past to its repetition in the present. If the analyst evades this responsibility, the patients will also do so and become less resistively involved in here-and-now expressions of affect, thought, and behavior.

In dyadic analysis, preoccupation with current events in the patient's life outside of the therapeutic milieu is resistive. In the dyad, the interaction is largely in terms of transference and the emerging transference neurosis. In the group, current events in and outside of therapy play an integral part in analysis. The impromptu thought and feeling, the extemporaneous, and the present occasion are subject to examination and are explored for understanding. In the dyad, even in responses to the analyst, the preoccupation is with history, partly on theoretical grounds, and partly because the therapist believes he cannot or should not interact.

Data

In dyadic analysis, the material for study is provided as a sequel to the actual event—that is, it is furnished out of recollection of the experience. The only original and verifiable data that are experienced are provided in the patient's responses to the analyst. In the group, the stuff of analysis is available not only in terms of historical recollection but also on the basis of interaction with co-patients. The accent in the group is on bilateral interaction, which is then enlisted for understanding the unconscious urges and motives that generated it. The engaged group members join in an exploration and analysis of the shared experience. In dyadic analysis, an interaction outside the treatment room can be comprehended only by hindsight. In the group, the participants can be seen in action, direct observation can be made of how the episode began, and a detailed study can be made of the motives of the provocateur as well as those of the reactor. Group members tend to object to overlong, repeated stories, whether historical or current in nature. In the therapeutic dyad, an obsessive concern with the analyst can also turn into an insulating, symbiotic, and illusory experience.

Resistances and defenses

Resistance yields more readily to psychoanalysis in a group. Patients directly challenge one another's resistive maneuvers. They do not permit a member to escape in sleep. They do not for long permit a non-participant to continue silent. They vigorously demand an end to resistive operations. They push for change and new activity, demand interaction, object to anyone's retirement or dominance and to obsessive intrapsychic preoccupation or grossly fantastic ways of nonrelating. They press for coexistence, verbal intercourse, and plain speaking.

By sustaining and criticizing one another, patients penetrate defenses more readily. Some therapists believe that defenses are weakened under attack in the group, but that the anxiety underlying these defenses needs to be analyzed only in the dyad. The analyst in a group may on occasion be obliged to support a defense at a particular moment. But the idea that defenses may be resolved in the group but the subjacent anxiety may not seems to be a fallacious view of the nature of the group experience. In the dyad, the technical skill and timing required for dealing with defenses are the analyst's. In the group, the breaching of defenses of certain patients often promotes corresponding breaches among the more defended, who experience vicariously the understanding, progress, and working through of the need to maintain certain inappropriate defenses.

Silence

Therapists are familiar with the resistive significance of silence and are usually impatient with it. However, it has other dimensions in the group. Silence is not necessarily resistive; on occasion, it represents periods of renewal, integration, meditation, or deep feeling without the need to express, act, or respond immediately to the other. While one member is quietly examining a problem by himself, another may be unavailable in resistance. Still another may be too apprehensive of exploration for the moment, and two others may be involved in an intense interaction and invite analytic inquiry. The group analyst can turn productively from one patient to another while some are provisionally silent.

If an analysand is making himself known and requires a listening silence, it is necessary for the analyst to be quiet. His inactive attention is required by the patient as an act complementary to his own. The analyst's being quiet looks like passivity on a manifest level; it is, in fact, his chosen activity appropriate to the patient's needs.

Anxiety

Anxiety emerges when defenses or resistances are attacked or dissolved. Some patients feel little apprehension in the bipersonal situation but are obviously threatened at the idea of entering a group. Often they are symbiotically tied to a mother surrogate and fearful of the environment and persons apart from her. Other patients who were historically in disease in the nuclear family or with an original parental figure, and more secure in circumstances outside the family, frequently find the group more reassuring than the analyst alone. They appreciate the alternate meeting more than the session when the analyst is there. The therapist may feel the same way. Depending on his original history, he may be more or less nervous in the dyadic or in the group situation. The analysand needs to be encouraged to examine the source of his anxiety and to resolve it in the setting in which he experiences it. If he does not do this, he is liable to avoid the circumstances in which he develops anxiety, evade confrontation, and escape resolution.

Every patient experiences anxiety. The therapist needs to know whether his apprehension is determined by realistic perception or by transference. Psychoanalysis in groups provides three means for the elucidation of transference, the anxiety associated with it, and the defensive operations used to suppress the anxiety: the consultation with the analyst alone, the regular meeting, and the alternate session. In these three settings the therapist can examine the differences in anxiety in various transferential relations.

In dyadic analysis, there is anxiety in the transferential impression of threat from the analyst as parent, generally the mother. A sense of being threatened by forces outside the analytic situation, whether in fact or in illusion, is derived from the patient's associations. In the dyad, it is hoped that the analysand will become conscious of his anxiety in the society external to the analysis, and that he will be disinhibited enough with his therapist to tell him of his feelings. In the dyad, there is a greater need to become aware of anxiety stirred beyond the couch; in the group, anxiety can be revealed more easily and quickly in the course of interaction.

Some patients are more anxious in the dyad and more relaxed in the group. Alone with the analyst, they are more apprehensive about closeness to the parental surrogate, about his intensive scrutiny of their strong and ambivalent feelings about him, and about the possibility of isolation with him and its attendant regressive possibilities. In the group, there is more hope of flight from exploration and, as a result, less anxiety. For other patients, the co-patient peers are more anxiety provoking. It may be that for most patients, given a choice of milieu, they would choose the dyad over the group as less anxiety inducing. The belief that in the group there will be less skillful intervention, less benevolence, and more eruption impels most patients to seek individual treatment. In some measure, a patient's choice of milieu is dependent on his history with parents and siblings, as well as on currently popular styles of therapeutic intervention.

Shifting attention

The experience of attention shifting from one member to another in psychoanalysis in groups diminishes anxiety by providing respites from exclusive and sometimes oppressive examination. In dyadic analysis, the patient is continuously under scrutiny. This scrutiny may produce defensiveness and resistance—a reaction to analytic pressure that can at times be incapacitating. The group, on the other hand, permits the patient periods of time for repose—to reflect on

what he has just previously experienced, to consider what interpretations have been made to him, to speculate on alternatives in the process of working through—and, after being helped, he can turn to others and offer help. The shifting of attention is itself an alternative way of conducting oneself. It confronts the patient with the reality that he need not compulsively engage in a limited kind of activity.

Alternating scrutiny gives the patient an opportunity to show himself at a speed that is not too overwhelmingly anxiety provoking for him. In the therapeutic dyad, he is under continuous scrutiny, and is required to expose himself. In the group, shifting attention away from him without the ongoing expectation that he make himself known may provide opportunities for resistance.

Timing

One criticism of group analysis is that a member may awkwardly or discordantly offer some insight that the recipient is by no means prepared to accept at the time. The judgment is made that a precipitate or untimely offer of understanding may be too hurtful to a patient who may not be able to cope with the anxiety provoked by the confrontation. The author's experience is that group members are, in general, able to deal with insights offered by co-patients either by resisting them or by gradually accepting them. When the therapist errs in the timing of a confrontation, the analysand becomes more disturbed because the understanding comes from a figure in authority.

The analyst in groups soon learns that it is not he alone who has the delicate touch, the exquisite empathy to know just when and how to offer insight. Surely some members are at first indifferent and unconcerned with others, but a larger number have from the start a sensitivity to their feelings. At times the analyst may be overprotective with a patient in the group, doubtful about his capacity to tolerate some newly offered interpretation. He may under such circumstances inappropriately postpone the acquisition of insight.

A co-patient does not have the expertness in timing interpretations that the skilled analyst has. But it is a common experience to find untrained members making very valuable observations about one another with an intuition and an acuity that are surprising. It is not that psychoanalytic theory and practice just come naturally to them. It is their good sense, directness, spontaneity, naturalness, enthusiasm, and artlessness, free of analytic jargon, and their obvious wish to help, that give them the capacity to be reparative. The affective pitch of reaction is also a factor in their reaching one another.

In dyadic analysis, it is the therapist's exclusive jurisdiction and responsibility to determine when to offer a piece of insight. His mistakes in timing are burdened with his authority. Excitation, insight, and confrontation by group members are both more readily resisted and at times more welcomed because they come from peers. If dyadic analysts alarm patients less with their confrontations, it may simply be that they make fewer interpretations and are more guarded than necessary. If individual analysts are careful about poorly timed offers of insight, they may be just as reserved in tendering properly timed comments, thereby delaying the progress of an analysis. In the group, the therapist can more securely turn over the experience of interaction to his patients, who provoke less anxiety than he does. He need not then be fearful that their attentions will be hurtful. He is also free to step in more discreetly and discriminatively at those times when his interposition can be most beneficial. A member may at times become distributed by a poorly timed response of a co-patient, but interaction among peers usually animates, sustains, and augments the progress of group members.

Activity and passivity of the analyst

There is dissimilarity in the functioning of the analyst in the two settings. In the group, patients turn more to each other for affective interaction, for understanding, for confrontation and insight. In the dyad, the analysand has only the analyst to look to for such responses, but the analyst reacts in these ways only when in his clinical judgment they are indicated. As a result, the therapist in a group can generally be more of an uninvolved and reasonable onlooker as interaction goes on about him. In the dyad, where every response is turned on him, he is expected by the patient to become more engaged than he may think appropriate. Here it is more arduous for the analyst to sustain a detached, reasonable, and regardful stance. The reverse may be true for those therapists who become more insulated and detached in dyadic sessions, and more affectively and inappropriately engaged at group meetings.

In dyadic treatment, the therapist may be obliged to be more animated, to cultivate the interaction that is inherent in a group. The group analyst may reduce his exertions because the group members foster the interaction.

Therapists, like their patients, choose to function in one setting or the other because they are able in one more than in the other to be more passive or active. An analyst may be more stirred, more quickened, more incited in one milieu and more immobilized, almost paralyzed, in the other. But one needs to explore the reality, the unreality, and the relationship to treatment goals of particular activity and passivity. In dyadic analysis, the analysand is generally more active and the therapist more passive. But if the patient is passive, it may be necessary for the analyst to become active. The very passive neutrality of orthodox analysis may require revision in the face of clinical experience with group analysis, in which forced interaction has shown itself to be productive. The dyadic analyst may find that, if he penetrates resistance more actively by provocation and by encouraging interaction, he will expedite treatment.

Where analysis takes place

Analysis takes place largely through the interventions of the analyst. For certain patients, generally in the early phases of therapy, the most striking progress may not come in the dyadic interviews or in the group meetings the analyst attends but at the alternate sessions. This advance occurs without analytic intervention. Such improvement becomes analytic when the character of the unconscious material is explored and made conscious, when the significance of the repressed material is grasped in terms of the total experience, and when the latent posture and design that produce the anxiety are analyzed.

A most significant function of the analyst is to promote the activity of the analysand in interpersonal relationships beyond the therapeutic dyad. Some analysts too nondiscriminatively prefer to limit the analysand to his one-to-one involvement with the therapist. They make the analytic relationship too exclusive of connections with others. This treatment has questionable validity because it may insulate the analysand in symbiosis. It limits the patient's choices, freedom, and growth; it circumscribes his activity within the therapeutic frame; and it negates the value of transactions beyond the dyad. The same thing may take place in group analysis if the leader interferes with the patient interaction beyond the group, rejects the alternate session, and supports responses primarily to himself.

Selection of material

In any setting, access to underlying psychodynamics and psychopathology is always incompete, and the emphasis is chosen by the therapist. In dyadic analysis, the choices are directed by the character of the actual or subjective anxiety the patient experiences with the analyst, the analysand's capacity to trust his therapist, and his relative certainty of nonreprisal. In group analysis, the selection of material is defined by the patient's security that he will not be seriously hurt by the other members or the therapist, and to the extent that he can look for assistance and relief from them. What the patient consciously and unconsciously exposes may differ from dyadic to regular to alternate meetings. His choice depends on the nature of the material, the kind of patient he is, the make-up of the group, and the attitudes of his co-patients and of the leader.

In any form of psychotherapy, the totality of a patient's responses is not available. It is not selective of the therapist to be occupied with catching each and every response the patient makes. It is grandiose to have to be all knowing and aware of the slightest detail. Treatment is discriminating, selective, choosing to attend this process and phenomenon, and rejecting or analyzing another as resistive. In dyadic analysis, for example, the analyst may choose the patient's transference to him for study. Or, he may scrutinize among the patient's free associations those elements that illuminate his realistic circumstances outside the treatment room. But the therapist is in a position to explore only those reactions and recollections the analysand presents. In the group situation, a wider range of material is presented. The analyst may choose to scrutinize whatever transferential response or defensive operation he believes is appropriate to work with at a certain time. He exercises his judgment in opting to examine this or that maneuver at the heart of things, one of the interconnecting elements that may explain the historically derived current behavior. He pays less regard to a multitude of other patient reactions; if he did not, he would fail to function effectively as an analyst. If he attends everything, he is swamped and misses the core in a mass of less relevant detail. He has to be selective. He has to choose for examination the gist of things that fits each analysand, depending on his phase of evolution and growth.

Focus on interaction

In dyadic treatment, the analyst may promote the patient's responses to him, concentrating on the analysand's disturbed reactions to him with a view to resolving them. In the group, many of these responses are directed toward co-patients, and there is intense affective interaction, both realistic and transferential. Such profoundly emotional interaction rarely occurs in dyadic treatment, where the analyst circumscribes such an eventuality by his remoteness. He rather permits the patient's affect simply to unfold without himself becoming emotionally involved. He cannot become involved without jeopardizing the treatment relationship. He certainly cannot become inappropriately enmeshed. In the group, however, patients may be supported in response to one another and encouraged to interact without acting out. This interpersonal engagement has value. The therapist can preserve his reasonable, examining role. In the therapeutic dyad, such a posture tends to block the affective interpersonal exchange that occurs in a group setting.

Dependence on therapy

The morbid clinging to the therapist that can develop in the course of treatment is more ominous in the dyad than in the group. It is more of a hazard, at least in its intensity and depth, in the one-to-one setting, not infrequently becoming a transference psychosis and removing the patient from reality. In a group, a member may become neurotically needful of the group, the leader, or one or another patient, but the analyst and co-patients push for interaction with others in and out of the group, which operates to resolve pathological dependency. This is valuable in exploring and working through the most serious transference neurosis.

There is a danger that some therapists may tend to develop in their groups an unhealthy association, in which patients may be encouraged merely to act out, rather than work through. Here regression is extended and appreciated, and the leader supports the patient's illness and entrenches his transference neurosis. The dyadic or group setting may be used by the analysand or the analyst to sponsor dependent ties or to resolve them. Treatment can become habituation, whether in the dyad or the group.

Working through

The necessity for working through is often neglected in treatment, particularly by group therapists, probably because so many of them repudiate psychoanalysis or are inadequately analyzed themselves. As a result, they are confused about the analytic process and are unable to formulate a unified theory of analysis for members of a group. Their perplexity is evinced in the multiplicity of group therapies reported in the literature. The enormous volume of material made available by interpersonal reaction in group therapy may be disequilibrating to some group leaders and may make them feel that working through is not achievable.

Clinical experience seems to indicate that working through can be effected in a group. The profusion of material can make it easier to discover the repetitive core of psychopathology, even the transference neurosis, and can facilitate working through. Recurrence is characteristic not only of psychopathology but also of treatment. After ventilation and insight into the psychodynamics and the psychopathology, the therapist again and again suggests more reasonable alternative choices. Only in the group is it possible to work through the bilateral and multilateral—entwined neurotic manipulations involving two or more patients. The resolution of various facets of the disorder of members at different phases in their treatment is useful in making clear the analyst's recurrent preference for reality over illusion. It is this reiteration that promotes the working through of compulsive and archaic yearnings toward the final choice of more reasonable alternatives.

A good many patients come to psychoanalysis in groups after a failure to respond to individual treatment. Frequently they have developed an increasing dependency on the therapist, with a deeply entrenched transference neurosis or psychosis. Such patients often demand concurrent individual sessions immediately after their transfer to an analyst in groups. They do so out of anxiety about breaking the symbiotic tie to the mother surrogate. The group analyst must resist these maneuvers. Instead, he must help such patients develop some independence, stronger egos, and responsibility for themselves. If group members insist that such patients function with them and the therapist resists the wish for exclusive individual support, these patients become more securely involved with their peers, more removed from the mother tie, increasingly independent of the therapist, and more self-reliant. They become less needful of the therapist in an infantile way, and more relaxed with group members and in social situations apart from the therapeutic group. A significant derivative of the group analytic experience is that each patient becomes more ego oriented.

Termination

It is probable that successful conclusion of treatment is more easily attained in the group because it fills the therapeutic need for interaction and engagement apart from the analyst. It is the judgment of the therapist that generally determines when a patient is ready to end treatment. But, on occasion, the leader may not be fully aware of the extent to which a member has improved. Then other patients may call his attention to the fact that a progressing member has made substantial gains. A patient may feel freer to show his good resources at alternate sessions than at regular meetings, and so the leader may not be as aware as the members of the patient's considerable improvement. What requires resolution in such a case is the patient's hesitation to show his effectiveness in the presence of the group leader.

Resistance to ending treatment may be a problem not only for the patient but for the therapist as well. The observing group members help to reduce the patient's or the analyst's resistance to termination. This validation by the group does not depreciate the competence of the analyst. It simply offers him another impression on which to base his estimate and assessment. In dyadic treatment, the material is always derived from the analysand, except in the relationship to the analyst. The patient is a partial and one-sided source of enlightenment. Group members offer more evidence and reasoning for reaching a conclusion as to the propriety of ending at any given time. The patient considering termination usually seeks the opinion of the analyst. If his wish to leave is resistive, he commonly looks to his peers for allies who will support his inappropriate flight from treatment.

The recovery of one patient heartens another member with the hope that one day he, too, will be well. The release of one member is a stimulus and a promise to the others. Such an experience is not available to the patient in individual treatment. Only the member of a therapeutic group can observe another patient's getting well. The improvement of one induces the rest to try harder to attain similar well-being. The departure of a recovered patient may remotivate another at a time when he is feeling despondent. The more disconsolate are stimulated by being witness to another's restoration. They become more inquiring and searching about how this particular co-patient managed to get well in order to achieve the same for themselves. They may become more rivalrous with the departing or remaining members in the competition for return to health. This competition may have its resistive aspects. If one member is discharged as well, another may insist that he, too, has been cured when he is still quite ill. It takes little examination by the group and the analyst to expose this resistive maneuver.

Controversial issues

Individual versus group stimuli

The members of a group provide the patient with more stimuli than does the analyst alone in the dyadic relationship. The analyst is also the focus of more stimulation in the group than in one-to-one treatment. This situation poses a problem. Do these multiple stimuli produce more diversion, more shifting of attention, and less careful examination of each patient than he might receive in individual treatment? It is quite possible. The answer depends in part on the competence, skill, and leadership of the therapist.

In a group, each patient receives not only the analyst's attention but also the critical responses of a number of other members whose observations are insightful. In this respect the patient has the advantage of being stimulated and observed by multiple resources not available to him in the dyad. Thus the diversity made available by group members may be used to enrich whatever the patient presents, whether fantasy, dream, conflict, or external problem. In the group there may be less focusing than in analytic dyads but more stimulation to a wider canvas of psychopathological and healthy reactivity.

Homogeneity versus heterogeneity

The presence of both men and women is a more therapeutic milieu than a unisexual and more homogeneous group. In a group containing both sexes, more unconscious psychodynamics, psychopathology, and healthy resources of each patient become manifest. The variety in the membership promotes mutual interest, diverse stimulation, complementarity, and multiple transferences. The differences among the patients demand a healthy struggle to cope rationally with divergent points of view, to resolve disagreement in appropriate, reality-bound compromise.

If it is true that heterogeneity facilitates treatment, it is relevant to examine which setting, individual or group, provides more homogeneity. There is more sameness and more consistency of response in dyadic analysis than in group analysis, even if the analyst organizes the group on some homogeneous basis. The group cannot react as a single individual, even though it may at times seem to be doing so. In reality, some members seem more committed to their archaic needs, whereas others struggle more for the healthy alternative. There are myriads of still other differences among all patients. In contrast, the analyst follows a fairly uniform course. His commitment, his value system, his stance, his reactions, and his offers of understanding all have a particular aim and direction, and produce more homogeneity in the dyad than in the group.

It is a formidable task for an analyst to homogenize a group, to impose his authority on an assemblage of patients. The patient in a dyad is much more liable to succumb to his dominations. A therapist may try to impose on a patient a limited responsiveness, such as here-and-now reactivity, or demand that he express only his feelings and not his thoughts or associations. He may circumscribe productions only to historical data, focus on motivation, stress ego functions, or press for strictly conscious and reality-bound material. In doing any of these, he demands of the patient a homogeneous way of operating. Such a fixed way of functioning is not analytic, for it does not facilitate choice. Instead, it promotes repetition-compulsion. The therapist who inflexibly defines what may be explored over time homogenizes and circumscribes treatment.

Isolation versus socialization

Isolation and socialization are consequences as well as sources of intrapersonal and interpersonal dynamics. A good many individually but inadequately analyzed patients are poorly adjusted in their relations with groups of people. After extensive individual treatment they sometimes find themselves to be more lonely and unsocialized than before. They may then seek out a group therapist to help them resolve their withdrawal and to promote their socialization. Previously committed to intrapersonal preoccupation, they may be propelled into ever more disengagement.

The analyst in groups is aware that patients may socialize in mutually destructive ways that are resistive and acting out. He guards against such abuse of socialization by analyzing these operations and supporting the wholesome qualities of social intercourse.

The feeling of abandonment is more vividly experienced by the patient when he is placed in an analytic group. In individual treatment, he has the therapist all to himself, at least in fantasy, and in reality the illusion is fostered by isolating one patient from the next. A group member repeatedly talks of his sadness, anger, or sense of isolation when the therapist or a meaningful co-patient seems to prefer another member. Because the therapist is less available, because he is not exclusively possessed, the feeling of being isolated recurs more frequently in the group. Therefore, the analyst can more easily pursue the interpersonal dynamics that led to the real and unreal sense of isolation. He can also explore the genetic determinants that led to the intrapsychic dynamics that now keep the patient in isolation. And the patient has group members with whom he can work toward a more gratifying socialization.

It is always enlightening to the analyst to find how often the problem of isolation presents itself when a patient moves from individual analysis to treatment in a group. The therapist may have been unaware of the extent to which this was a problem. The previous dyadic setting, in which the patient had the analyst to himself, prevented the emergence of this difficulty. The experience in a group vividly promotes the appearance of a sense of isolation for all to see. The patient sets himself apart by reproducing in repetition-compulsion his refusal to participate, or by reproducing his competition with a parent or sibling who is favored by another familial figure whose appreciation or affection he wants.

Traditionally, socialization is regarded as a resistive maneuver, and it may so become. This need not be so as long as socialization is examined and analyzed for its resistive components. Socialization is a phenomenon that occurs to some extent in all group therapy. In psychoanalysis in groups, however, the issue of whether socialization is obstructing the analytic process or making it more manageable needs to be explored. It seems that socialization has a humanizing and a restorative value. But social intercourse may enable patients to resist the search for latent mainsprings. Therefore, the analyst needs to be alert to the way in which patients use the alternate session, the post-session, clique formation, and subgroup dating.

The alternate meeting

Many group therapists reject the alternate meeting. They see it largely as encouraging patients to act out. There may be greater opportunity for acting out when alternate meetings are made available, but alternate sessions are not proposed for the purpose of acting out, nor are patients encouraged to act out. They are, in fact, urged not to do so. Attempts are made to analyze imminent acting out. When it takes place, it is analyzed in order to interrupt it. All else failing, it is forbidden.

The alternate meeting has important advantages. One of these is spontaneous mutual support among members of the group, an advantage that appeared quite naturally in the earliest post-sessions. At these meetings, thoughts, feelings, and activities emerged that were different from those at regular sessions. By comparing and contrasting behavior at regular and alternate meetings, therapists found quantitative and qualitative differences in the two settings and were able to examine these differences productively.

Only the therapist is sufficiently trained to conduct the systematic intervention of treatment. Patients are not expected to be therapists with one another. If they try to assume such inappropriate roles, they are in resistance. They are generally incapable of making the skilled observations required of the therapist. Therefore, treatment in this sense does not go on at the alternate meeting. Patients may attempt to conduct themselves as therapists for one another, but such behavior is usually rejected and resisted. They tend to interact spontaneously. They do not know one another's diagnoses, and they are unaware of what stage of treatment each member is in. The therapist has a plan in mind for the treatment of each member. The patients do not.

The therapist at regular meetings demands that the patients do analytic work. Patients also offer each other insight at alternate sessions, but there the pursuit of mutual understanding and insight is not so intense or concentrated. Patients in the alternate meeting experience one another as trying to be helpful. This diffused helpfulness is experienced in the regular meeting as well. But under the therapist's influence there is an effort to work more analytically in his presence. He is the primary source of insight and of pressure to give up archaic means. He induces them to apply themselves more vigorously to the task of getting well.

If the analyst tries to use a patient as a co-therapist, he is misusing the patient in countertransference. Whenever the analyst so misuses a group member, the patient may be induced to play this role at alternate meetings as well. But being a co-therapist should be neither his role nor his responsibility. He is in treatment to get well, not to become a therapist. The analyst has no objection to the members being helpful to one another. They do, in fact, repeatedly offer one another useful support and understanding. But whenever a patient compulsively tries to exercise the role of co-therapist, he is in resistance to his more realistic position as patient. Nevertheless, patients often turn to one another for emotional sustenance in anxiety and depression. When the analyst is unavailable—on vacation, for instance—patients are obliged, as at the alternate meeting, to turn to one another for understanding, maintenance, and relief. Such assistance is useful and often insightful. Even at regular meetings, patients offer one another interpretations. The analyst welcomes such expositions as long as they are not pursued compulsively as a way of resisting analysis.

Group dynamics

There are some positives in homogeneous group responses. Co-patients are often helpful to one another, sustaining in critical situations, compassionate, insightful, and empathic. In spite of variations in their history and character, they frequently identify with and feel for each other. To the degree that this takes place, members are constructively homogeneous, and the group leader can endorse such wholesome mutual support and positive interaction. But it does not seem technically possible to incorporate into treatment the idea that, when patients love one another, there is a good reparative result. The therapist cannot in treatment create an atmosphere of love. To try to do so would deny the possibility of technical intervention determined by insight into psychodynamics. It is valuable when patients relate to each other positively and support one another's weakened egos, but such mutual sustenance should not be confused with psychoanalytic treatment.

Anger at therapist. Occasionally, co-patients support one another in expressing negative feeling toward the therapist. This type of support is extremely productive for those members who are not likely to assert themselves when alone with the analyst. An alliance enables them to do so until they have sufficient ego strength to stand up to the therapist alone. This group dynamic may be encouraged in general, but it seems inappropriate for each patient to experience anger at the group leader at the same time. Nor does it seem at all likely that each member is in that phase of a transference relationship when the expression of negative feeling is indicated.

Demand for participation. Another example of useful group dynamic pressure occurs when the whole group demands the participation of a silent or withdrawn member. Although such authority directed at a detached patient may, in fact, lead to his engagement, it seems to be an especially non-analytic means to penetrate resistance. Are there not analytic devices more appropriate than aggressive group demand? Might not an occasional patient take flight in the face of such mass pressure?

A group demand seems dedicated to pressing members to do something. If it appears so, very likely several aggressive patients are leading the pack while the others are submissively following.

Even if the group dynamic demand that a member give up his resistance works under the influence of the united power of the group, the precedent seems dangerous. The idea has too many overtones of brainwashing, or forcing an individual to yield to group demand. The effect may well be de-egotizing and may lead to a split ego.

Therapeutic value. The leader's or the group's preoccupation with group dynamics is not psychoanalytically therapeutic. The group psychodynamicist tends to neglect psychoanalytic confrontations and individual insights for observations about what the group as a group is doing. He may neglect the individual's unconscious psychodynamics and psychopathology.

The leader who is repetitively engaged in pursuing group dynamics tends to homogenize the group, to treat it as a whole. In doing this, the therapist may be motivated by anxiety in coping with a triad or a multivariable condition. He may be more secure in creating the illusion that he is in a dyad. In the dyad, he may be immersed in the illusory security of a relationship with his mother, a transference neurosis. Or, he may be in a homosexual relationship with the group homogenized as symbolic father. He may be excluding one parent or the other or disregarding a sibling with whom he is in rivalry.

The group psychodynamicist tends to use group dynamic terms and concepts and to use phrases like "group ego," "group id," "group superego," "group mind," "collective unconscious," "collective consciousness," "group resistance," and "group transference." All these terms are distortions on the part of the leader.

A group may be reparative or destructive, but this is a matter of chance and must be distinguished from psychoanalytic therapy, which is a series of technical interventions, such as making the unconscious conscious, working through resistance, and transference.

An emphasis on group dynamics is antianalytic, a distraction from analytic work, because it focuses primarily on the group rather than on the patient. The interpretation of group dynamic phenomena in therapy does not treat the patient. No means has yet been devised to psychoanalyze a group. The individual is not analytically reconstructed by mystical interventions dedicated to treating the group as a whole, despite the ingenuity of Ezriel, for example.

The group psychodynamic view is a mystique because it claims to heal by group cohesion and group atmosphere rather than through the individualized and expert attention and intervention of an analyst. The group is invested with a magically healing power it does not possess. It has no inherent benevolent influence that enables it to apply its magnetic authority. Such a belief in the group is sorcery, incantation. The group dynamicists overvalue cohesion and climate, and they undervalue analysis.

The group dynamicist's dedication to the group leads to a denial of each member's individuality and differences. It tends to promote a pathological homogeneity, rather than interactive and complementary heterogeneity. It would influence the patient by group dynamics, rather than by understanding. It is repressive-inspirational, rather than psychoanalytic. In the group dynamic view, the manifest is seen as the individual patient's and the latent is regarded as the group's activity as a whole. This is, of course, a reversal of the analytic view, in which the group's activity would be conceived of as the manifest and the patient's unconscious contribution to the group's activity as the latent.

Ego strength. Whenever a patient has ego weakness,

he is inclined to deny his own perceptions, judgment, choices, wishes, and aspirations and to yield to those of the other. Sometimes this other assumes gigantic proportions, especially when it is the homogeneous group dynamic pressure of co-patients. To the extent that a patient has good ego strength, he has the capacity to respect his own ego resources and pursue his own inclinations in the face of group dynamic domination. To the degree that the group leader supports the group dynamic position, he imposes on the individual ego a di-egophrenic problem—a split-ego problem. In doing this, he limits personal development, weakens ego resources, and cultivates borderline pathology.

Health does not come from submission to group fiat. And healthy cohesion does not depend on a denial of individuality and a wholesale acceptance of group standards. It should not be necessary to split one's ego in order to be accepted by a group. Any treatment based on submission to an authoritarian group is dictatorial. Reconstructive change is not achieved by capitulation to a dominating group but by careful analytic work. The patient cannot appropriately avoid conflict by obediently conforming to the common point of view.

The psychoanalyst is, therefore, opposed to routine group dynamic interpretations, which do injury to already damaged egos. If the therapist does not recognize individual variations and does not promote each patient's autonomy, if he chooses to make group dynamic observations, he guides the members toward a homogeneity in pathology instead of toward the more wholesome possibility of interactive diversity. He prevents group members from attaining the independence and freedom that are the goals of good treatment. An analyst who endorses group dynamic consensus creates di-egophrenia by not promoting the privilege of each patient to differ with the majority. In so doing, he allows an authoritarian group to dominate the individual. The group psychodynamicist is satisfied with the emergence of group themes. The psychoanalyst is not content with this. He goes beyond the manifest conformity to get to the latent individual uniqueness of each patient.

Free association

Analytically trained therapists are often doubtful about whether patients can associate as freely in a group as in a dyad. True, there are more interruptions of free association in the group. But to look upon unrestrained, unbounded, and indefinite free association as fitting is to misunderstand the function of free association and the nature of analytic treatment. It is better to employ free association selectively, with recognition of when it is expedient. It is neither possible nor advisable to associate freely at all times. Discontinuity and bounds are essential in treatment, as they are in life.

The dyadic analyst may be doubtful of the effectiveness of group analysis because he does not believe the patient can associate freely when he is interrupted

by co-patients. In reality, free association may be hindered by co-patients at certain times and helped at others. Where a patient is delving into as-yet unexplored latent material, he usually stimulates and wins the attention of the other members and is, therefore, emboldened to go on. When he continues to reproduce the same psychopathology in free association, co-patients become disinterested with the recurrence and appropriately try to stay his repetition and ask for a more mutually invigorating alternative. When his free association is moving him to the disclosure of appropriate, noncompulsive possibilities, his fellows are hopefully but quietly attentive, in the expectation that he will have the freedom to make a nonobsessive choice. When his stream of consciousness appears to be running down into estranging autism, co-patients resist his self-destructive and isolating free association.

In dyadic analysis, the therapist interprets the free association of the analysand, whose associations are less free to the extent that he is aware of them. In group analysis, the patient not only freely associates but is required to operate with an awareness of the others. Although this obligation may appear to limit the freedom of his stream of consciousness, the demand for mutual awareness promotes his good health. Unrestrained free association without the checking of feedbacks in reality leads to disequilibration and derangement.

In analysis, whether individual or group, the patient is expected to reveal the truth about himself. In the dyad, the analyst is not required to expose himself. In the group, all the members are encouraged to show themselves and interact in an open way. The result is that every patient becomes aware of the effect he has on others in a way that is not available to him in dyadic treatment. Each member finds out what his own provocative role or behavior patterns are.

The group analyst's preoccupation with interruptions of free association may represent his wish to conduct individual analysis in the group setting. But such a commitment prevents the leader from using the resources of his assembled patients and interferes with proper treatment of them. The interruptive contributions of fellow patients not only clarify the presentation of a given patient but may be used as free associations in themselves. In discussion of a dream, for example, the free associations of various members stir the further exposure of the dreamer's unconscious material. They also give the analyst more hints for understanding the dream, and clues to the psychodynamics and psychopathology of the others, which can be multilaterally interpreted.

The analyst's conception of fellow patients' communications as interruptive denies to the group the value of multilateral analysis. Instead, it imposes individual treatment in a group setting and encourages a rivalry to interrupt one another, becoming a competition to be heard by the analyst.

Encouraging patients to enter in with their own free associations, which are also acknowledged and examined, promotes the feeling that all are in analysis, rather than just a single member at a time in rotation. It is, therefore, necessary for the analyst to deal with any presented material as interactional, so that the number of patient interrelationships is enhanced. In so doing, he augments, rather than circumscribes, all the streams of consciousness in the group. The analyst's aim to give space to each patient in which to associate freely is commendable. But by limiting the free play of the others, he really hinders the achievement of his goal. In group analysis, all the analysands should be encouraged to be collaborative and active participants.

Dreams

Dreaming and dream analysis are most valuable in treatment, whether in the dyadic or group setting. But dreams are dealt with in different ways in the two climates. In one-to-one therapy, the analysand associates freely to his dream, and the analyst seldom reveals his own associations. They are withheld—or are only partly revealed in a refined product—in his interpretations and other responses. In the group, the dreamer at first associates freely to his dream. The co-patients then associate to the dream, both as it belongs to the dreamer and as if the dream were their own. Then everyone tries to interpret the dream and the significance of each patient's subjective associations as applicable to himself. In this way, the therapist avoids individual analysis of each member's dream in turn and encourages multilateral group analysis. He may enter the interpretive process from time to time to integrate what has been said, to underscore an essence, to make a point more intelligible, or to suggest an exploration of neglected elements in the dream when they seem to be meaningful.

Analysands who evade unconscious processes in the dyad may not present dream material. They justify their opposition by contending that they do not see any value in dream analysis. This resistance can be resolved more readily in the group than in the dyad, for in the group the patients witness another member's presentation of a dream, its analysis, and the member's greater understanding and forward movement in treatment.

Some group therapists do not press for dreams in the group. In fact, they seem to reject the analysis of dreams. But in most groups a number of members quite spontaneously tell their dreams, so it is more difficult for the therapist to discourage them in that setting. He is more obliged to pay them some attention. Even in a group, however, if the analyst frustrates the emergence of dreams, they are likely to be recounted less and less often until they are entirely abandoned.

Transference

Transference neurosis. A deep transference neurosis is less likely to develop in a group than in a dyad. In individual analysis, the patient is readier to submit, to regress, and to accept frustration. In the group, this readiness is less apparent. Besides, the presence of a father figure and sibling surrogates in group members attenuates the formation of deeply symbiotic ties to the analyst as a mother figure. The provision of an alternate meeting further attenuates the possibility of a strong attachment to the therapist. If no alternate sessions are provided, or if one or more individual meetings a week with the analyst are routinely used, there is a greater tendency for a transference neurosis to develop. The development of a deep maternal transference is also attenuated by the presence of other members who act as auxiliary egos to enable the patient to free himself from a regressive dependence on the analyst as a mother surrogate.

A large number of patients in groups are borderline psychotic, and are already in a transference psychosis to the mother figure that is projected almost everywhere. For these patients, there is no need to promote further regression. To do so would produce a further break with reality. For neurotic patients in whom the therapist believes a regression in the service of the ego is indicated, one or more individual sessions a week can be provided to serve such a purpose. But this is not necessary for most patients.

Lateral transference and lateral countertransference. In the therapeutic group, patients may gratify one another's archaic needs in a way that would be inappropriate in individual sessions, where such behavior on the part of the therapist would be regarded as countertransferential. Patients sometimes bring in food or drink. And on rare occasions some members feel obligated to prepare a dinner for co-patients at an alternate session.

There is a greater likelihood that members will gratify one another's transference expectations in any group therapy than in individual analysis, where the therapist is aware, in general, of the inappropriateness of fulfilling the patient's archaic longings. To distinguish the analyst's countertransference from a member's similar response, the therapist may find it practical to designate such reactions coming from co-patients as lateral, peer, or horizontal countertransference.

Since group members are under no injunction to treat one another therapeutically, their spontaneous and compulsive responses to one another always contain lateral transferential and countertransferential components. If members fulfill in some degree one another's inappropriate expectations, how can they help one another? To the degree that in peer transference and countertransference there is frustration of each other's archaic longings, there is propulsion to other and more mature alternative choices. To the extent that there is regression-inducing fulfillment of horizontal transference expectations, bilateral analysis of the interacting patients is indicated. For the patient who is seeking historically predetermined satisfaction, it becomes necessary to provide insight into the current inappropriateness of his compulsive pursuit of outmoded predilection. For the patient who is obsessively and unconsciously in lateral countertransference, it is necessary to discover the underlying peer transference on which his horizontal countertransference is based. Then it becomes equally possible to work through his present, persistent transferential distortion.

Even what manifestly seems to be a reasonable suggestion from one patient to another, such as a proposal for a more appropriate choice alternative to his pathology, may mask lateral transference and countertransference. It needs, therefore, to be explored for such unconscious content.

A patient is especially likely to step in prematurely between two vigorously disagreeing group members who are misperceived as contesting members of the nuclear family. His efforts to interrupt the disharmony with pacifying gestures or precipitate analysis are less appropriate to the needs of the antagonists than to his own anxiety over a projected insoluble quarrel in his original family. At the opposite pole is the patient who transferentially detaches himself from any contention among others for fear that he may be accused of taking sides, or that he may be caught in the cross fire.

The same kind of anticipatory intervention or disengagement may take place in the face of a positive exchange between co-patients. The interrupting member may be trying to separate the positively engaging members, who are projected as parents or as parent and sibling. He may be hoping to be included. He may wish to exclude one of the partners and to possess the other. Disengaging or retiring members may feel they have no right to be included in loving parental exchange or tender parent-sibling shows of affection.

A patient's lateral transferences and countertransferences make his responses one-dimensional in character. But as long as the group is heterogeneous, as it should be, the multiplicity of the members' peer transferences and countertransferences militates against the fulfillment of archaic longings. The variety of responses in sickness and health leads to a minimal gratification of outdated necessities and to an openness to new ideas. These multiple reactions are influences against any one patient's one-dimensional prevalence in horizontal countertransferential pathology. As a result, it is difficult in the therapeutic group to fulfill a patient's transference needs because the group's heterogeneity makes such varied demands of the individual member.

Transference dilution. The criticism has been made that depth analysis is not possible in a group because the intensity of transference to the analyst is diluted by the presence of co-patients. It has been the author's experience that, where regression, as in the transference neurosis, is in the service of the ego, such transference reactions are both achieved and worked through. The intensity of a member's transference neurosis may be diluted by its direction to a co-patient rather than to the analyst, but the experience and resolution of transference aimed at a peer facilitates both its subsequent emergence and ultimate resolution when invested in the group leader. It is as though the prior activation and working through of parental transference directed toward a peer becomes a practice ground for its later emergence and resolution

with the therapist. In this sense, transference dilution need not be regarded as a limitation of psychoanalysis in groups, but as an asset.

Also, a good many patients enter a group after failures in prolonged individual analysis and are in obvious unresolved transference psychosis after long regressive experiences. For them it becomes necessary, even essential, that the misperception of the therapist in the parental position be diluted by intensified but less noxious peer interaction. Here again, transference dilution is in the service of the ego, and the co-member peers enable the patient to free himself from the intensity of his transference psychosis.

Activity

Acting and acting out. Because of his training, the analyst is not likely to act out. There are occasions, however, when he is predisposed by his own or a patient's disequilibrium to act out. If this happens, he loses his reasonable, examining, discerning, and objective role. In the group, he is required, even forced, to retain a regardful and watchful role because the patients sustain one another with refuges in reality. They maintain one another in resisting the inappropriateness of the therapist's acting out.

The members of every therapeutic group sooner or later set bounds on their acting out. Prime movers for this restraint are the wholesome, realistic aspirations in each patient and the prophylactic factors in various ego functions. Another mainspring inheres in the projection of influential power, of living by the rules of law and order, of what is right and wrong, of superego values, which act to curb irrational behavior. The analyst, his attendance at regular meetings, and his vaguely felt presence at alternate sessions or afterward all exert a limiting influence as well. The members are aware that their activity will sooner or later be revealed. Apprehension over such an outcome is also a factor in controlling acting out.

Certainly, there is less activity in the dyad than in the group. The essential point is not whether there is more or less activity in one setting than in the other. As long as there are patients in therapy, there will be acting out. The issue rather seems to be that the therapist is alarmed at the prospect of acting out taking place among his patients. In the dyad, acting out is prevented by the analyst, but the patient may act out outside the analytic chamber without the therapist's knowledge for some time. Acting out in the group is more easily exposed and discovered, and it can be more readily worked through.

In psychoanalysis in groups, there is more activity of all kinds than in individual analysis. There is more expression of warmth, affection, helpfulness, anger, aggression, hostility. The analyst is obliged to interrupt an interaction from time to time by offering interpretation, insight, and analysis. On occasion, when analysis fails in its object to limit acting out, he may have to forbid it. At the outset, patients may object to the analyst's denying them in this way and to the imposition of control, but in time the interdiction offers them so much relief from anxiety that they show their appreciation for the limits that are set. A good deal of the activity, however, is not acting out at all but a healthy consequence of wholesome group interaction. Acting out in the group is, in part, a result of intensely affective mutual stimulation. If the therapist persists in his interpretive analysis of what is going on, acting out can be controlled.

Self-imposed limits to acting out. If the therapist does not intervene to interrupt acting out, even the most dramatic kinds, group members sooner or later set their own limits. In the most seriously disturbed acting-out groups, the members inevitably turn to the analyst and ask him to help them set limits. Ultimately, there is always such frustration between members who act out that the parties to it inevitably turn to the other patients and to the analyst for control and insight. Patients who act out at alternate sessions sooner or later turn to the analyst, asking him to set limits and to seek greater understanding of the nature of their behavior.

Action groups. In the last 40 years, group therapy has led to movement from lying on the couch to being seated in a circle. And in more recent years there has been a leap into vigorous action. There is an increasingly anarchic rejection of reasonableness and reality. Whereas psychoanalysis has always sought a controlled, systematic regression in the service of the ego, the disciples of action promote irrational feeling, acting out, and assault on order—all in the name of love. Such destructive activity is a call for infantilism, for regression without thought, in the name of freedom from the bourgeois values of the Establishment. This kind of activity is a repudiation of all that years of careful analysis have taught—the necessity for dispassionate study of the patient. It makes a virtue of his illness. It puts pseudo-love and its destructiveness above therapeutic reconstruction. It tells people to embrace one another without understanding. It says people can understand nothing. Therefore, they must give up as hopeless their historical aim of knowing one another. All they can do is act—act blindly but feelingly. This unthinking activity is destructive not only of the other but of the self.

What followers of group-therapy-as-feelingful-action seem not to grasp is that, if feelingful action is the magic road to recovery, there is no further necessity for scrupulous training. Already, the group therapy movement is heavily weighted with dianeticists, scientologists, activists, zenists, and affectivists, who mindlessly lead loving and fighting groups into psychotic acting out. These leaders do not wish to be burdened by what they regard as the formalized disabilities of learning. It is easier to act swiftly and ruthlessly without the handicap of second thoughts or even first ones. What a patient needs, however, is thoughtful consideration. He turns to the analyst for insight, not rebellious exercises. There is serious danger that the group therapy movement will be taken over by the revolutionary know-nothingism of the affect-action promoters, for whom "id is beautiful."

Conclusion

The assumption by some dyadic analysts that psychoanalysis in groups cannot be effective because patients are too unaware of each other's realistic necessities and lack the capacity to grasp and deal with their archaic needs is not confirmed by clinical experience. On the contrary, analysands attain in groups an unusual facility for multilateral examination, for insight, and for mutually enhancing conduct.

In a group, no single member becomes the focus of analytic attention to the exclusion of others. Consideration by the members and the leader moves from one patient to the next so that cyclic oscillation of activity and rest, disinhibition and restitution, take place. No member is obliged to engage in only one kind of activity or to play an assigned, homogeneous role. In the analytic dyad, it is difficult to change his repertoire, for he is always in the position of being helped by a helper. In psychoanalysis in groups, he is expected and even required to play a multiplicity of emancipating parts.

Much of this chapter is based on a chapter which appeared in the first edition of this book and which was coauthored by Alexander Wolf and Emanuel Schwartz (the latter is now deceased).

References

Kadis, A. L., Krasner, J. D., Winick, C., and Foulkes, S. H. *A Practicum of Group Psychotherapy.* Harper & Row, New York, 1963.

Locke, N. *Group Psychoanalysis.* New York University Press, New York, 1961.

Markowitz, M., Schwartz, E., and Liff, Z. Nondidactic methods of group psychotherapy training. Int. J. Group Psychother., *15:* 220, 1965.

Mullan, H., and Rosenbaum, M. *Group Psychotherapy.* Free Press of Glencoe, New York, 1962.

Rosenbaum, M., and Berger, M. *Group Psychotherapy and Group Function.* Basic Books, New York, 1963.

Schwartz, E. K. Leadership and the psychotherapist. In *Topical Problems of Psychotherapy,* B. Stokvis, editor, p. 72. S. Karger, Basel, 1965.

Schwartz, E. K. Group psychotherapy: The individual and the group. Acta Psychother., *13:* 142, 1965.

Schwartz, E. K., and Rabin, H. M. A training group with one nonverbal co-leader. J. Psychoanal. Group, 2: 35, 1968.

Schwartz, E. K., and Wolf, A. Psychoanalysis in groups: Resistances to its use. Am. J. Psychother., *17:* 457, 1963.

Schwartz, E. K., and Wolf, A. On countertransference in group psychotherapy. J. Psychol., *57:* 131, 1963.

Schwartz, E. K., and Wolf, A. The interpreter in group therapy: Conflict resolution through negotiation. Arch. Gen. Psychiatry, *18:* 186, 1968.

Wolf, A. Short-term group psychotherapy. In *Short-term Psychotherapy,* L. R. Wolberg, editor, p. 219. Grune & Stratton, New York, 1965.

Wolf, A. Group psychotherapy. In *Comprehensive Textbook of Psychiatry,* A. M. Freedman and H. I. Kaplan, editors, ed. 1, p. 1234. Williams & Wilkins, Baltimore, 1967.

Wolf, A., and Schwartz, E. K. *Psychoanalysis in Groups.* Grune & Stratton, New York, 1962.

Wolf, A., and Schwartz, E. K. Psychoanalysis in groups: As creative process. Am. J. Psychoanal., *24:* 46, 1964.

Wolf, A., Schwartz, E. K., McCarty, G. J., and Goldberg, I. A. *Beyond the Couch.* Science House, New York, 1970.

B.8 Recent Advances in Psychoanalysis in Groups

IRWIN L. KUTASH, Ph.D.
ALEXANDER WOLF, M.D.

Introduction

The thrust of psychoanalysis in groups is that the creative growth of the individual ego is primary. Group psychotherapy is a misnomer for a technique that, while conducted in a group, is designed to aid an individual; it is a treatment of ailing individuals in a group setting, not a treatment of ailing groups, since only individuals have intrapsychic dynamics.

Basic Design

GROUP SIZE

Eight to 10 members are today considered the ideal number for psychoanalysis in groups. Believing that most families consist of between three and eight members, with the majority today four or five, a group of eight to 10 provides transferential room for the nuclear family, as well as some extrafamilial significant others. With fewer than eight members, there is often not enough interpersonal provocation and activity, leading to dead spots in spontaneous interaction. With more than 10, it is difficult for patient and group therapist alike to keep up with what is happening. However, some individuals feel lost even in a group as small as eight, because they were neglected in a family that may have numbered as few as three; an experience in a group setting where the leader can assure them a prominent role can provide a new constructive experience.

Several people who had previously found themselves overwhelmed in large groups were placed in a group with three or four individuals, a minigroup. The smaller size of the group was never mentioned as the reason for the invitation to these groups. These patients found themselves participating more and feeling a unique freedom. They were at last in a setting without overpowering mother, father, or sibling figures; simultaneously, they did not feel lost in the crowd. At a later date, additional members were added, including less passive potential transferential mothers or fathers. At this point, their egos were more secure from their previous experience with the leader as a "good parent." They felt his respect for their participation and the regard of siblings who were not perceived as overpowering or parental favorites. The larger group then became the arena for their further growth.

HETEROGENEITY AND COHESION

Since treatment, in large part, constitutes analysis of transference, it is advantageous to place the patient in a group setting in which he can project father, mother, and siblings as well. This can best be accomplished in the heterogeneous group. Furthermore, heterogeneous groups reflect a microcosm of society, and they tend to reproduce the family. Since the family probably ushered in the patient's neurosis, it is the logical agency for checking it. Despite the fact that, at first, many patients do not cope successfully with dissimilar character structures, the battle can best be won where it was apparently lost. In psychoanalysis in groups, the early precipitation and recognition of multiple transferences are facilitated by the presence of numbers of provocative familial figures in the persons of the various members.

Once having assembled a heterogeneous group, however, the battle is not yet won. Homogeneous structure or heterogeneous structure can be a consequence of the position taken by the therapist. The imposition of a make-believe unity is a projection of the therapist. When the therapist turns the group as a whole into an earlier familial figure of his own, it may be termed the leader's group-as-a-whole transference.

What often passes for concurrence in the group is itself the expression not so much of constructive cohesion as it is of diegophrenic pathology (Wolf, 1981). The split ego is so characteristic of our time that many patients passively follow the more assertive leaders, lending to the group the appearance of cohesion. This manifest accordance, so liable to be sponsored by the therapist as a salutary group climate, needs to be analyzed as it shows itself in each dominant-submissive relationship. Each group may have one or two members whose personalities strongly sway the others. They are frequently the most verbal and active, but are not necessarily reparative in their insensitivity to others. In order to support weakened egos, it is a function of the therapist not to be misled by an apparent appearance of uniformity and to analyze any compulsive passivity or leadership. Individuality can lead to greater group cohesiveness than efforts toward homogeneity, since a person needs to appreciate himself before he can truly appreciate others.

CLOSED VERSUS OPEN-ENDED GROUPS

Psychoanalysis in groups is a totally open-ended approach, unlike a laboratory or time-limited group. People join and leave as they are ready, not as part of a whole-group readiness phenomenon. If the individual in any way goes through stages in group by the nature of his individuality, these stages will occur for each person at different times, based on when he or she joined, how strong his or her ego was to begin with, and his or her personal rate of progress. Furthermore, as in psychoanalysis per se, these phases of therapy are based on individual dynamics, ego strength, and individual rate of growth. It is like an illustration often given a patient at the beginning of treatment when he or she asks how long it will take: "If someone asked me how long it would take them to get to any location in the city, I would tell him, it depends on where you want to go and how fast a walker you are." For an entire group to go through therapy at the same pace, some would have to walk too fast and some too slow; where they would all end up would be a compromise.

In psychoanalysis in groups, the group is self-perpetuating. Although there is a transplanting of patients, the groups do not entirely disband as a rule. Patients may join and leave.

Dreams and Fantasies in Groups

As in psychoanalysis per se, in psychoanalysis in groups, dreams and fantasies are of the utmost importance. In groups, dreams can have even more utility in one sense. They can elicit unconscious free associations, not only from the dreamer but from other group members as well. In psychoanalysis in groups, patients are requested to recount recent dreams, recurrent dreams, and old nightmares. They are asked to free associate around the dream content and finally to speculate about and interpret the dream. In lieu of dreams, the therapist encourages the group to present fantasies, reveries, and daydreams. He asks group members to avoid censorship of fanciful speculation about one another's productions. In this way, the dynamics of the dreamer are analyzed, as well as those who associate to another's dream.

The essential difference between analysis of dreams in individual therapy and in psychoanalysis in groups is that, in groups, individuals can associate to others' unconscious productions, as well as their own. Here it is the analyst's job to translate their associations in regard to the associators' dynamics and only secondarily to those to whose dream he associates, i.e., he is taking another road to each individual member's unconscious, through associations to the unconscious production of others.

For the dreamer himself, dreams are discussed because they reveal essential unconscious data reliably and with such a demonstrative and liberating effect. The analyst must ask for them in detail.

Dreams are also valuable therapeutic adjuncts in the clarification of transference. A member may, for example, project an associated woman patient in a dream in a dual role, both as a menacing figure and a lovable one. He may do this before free association or biographic acknowledgment has given us any indication of his mother's ambivalent attitude toward him. Interpretation of the dream enables him and the group to discover a destructive mother image with which he compulsively invests the woman. As he recognizes the transference features of his vision of her and sees her, in fact, as a friendly associate, he is able to divest her of her threatening aspect; she becomes more lovable. As he progressively analyzes the compulsive character of his attachment to her, he dispels even this maternal hold, and she becomes simply an engaging friend, stripped of maternal qualities but with an attractiveness of her own. In these instances, reality proves much richer and more rewarding to the patient than his illusion.

Analysis of Resistance

Resistance in groups manifests itself in the forms encountered in individual analysis, but the group setting provides a special environment that lends itself to the elaboration of resistive forms peculiar to it.

For the patient "in love with" the analyst, being in the group is enlightening. She may become as emotionally attached to another group member as she was to the analyst. Her "unfaithfulness," the rapidity and completeness with which she moves from one man to another, confronts her with the irrational and compulsive character of her behavior, and the nature of her activity becomes obvious to her as transference.

Another manifestation of resistance is the compulsive missionary spirit. Here the provider persists in looking after group members in a supportive, parental way, using this device subtly to dominate and attack the other members and to repress more basic pathology. The group resents this false charity and demands and evokes more spontaneous participation by rewarding the messianic for unguarded slips of feeling, and by rejecting dogmatic helpfulness. This does not imply that warm and spontaneous offers of assistance are rejected; rather, as long as supportiveness is not compulsive but thoughtfully sympathetic, it is welcomed as a sign of good health.

Voyeurism is resistance that is more general in psychoanalysis in groups. Some patients try to escape personal examination and engagement by retreating; they seem willing and even eager to allow others full interaction, while they assign to themselves a tremulous watchfulness. The group, however, has little tolerance for nonparticipants. It engages the voyeur by its welcoming self-exposure. It moves him by inviting and provoking him to become involved in the warm emotional life of the new family. His resistance begins to melt when the sideshow to which he was drawn by dubious motives becomes a wholesome drama in which he is impelled to take a legitimate part.

Hiding oneself behind the analysis of others is also a common form of resistance in psychoanalysis in groups. This resistance is characterized by a concentration on the neurotic behavior of other patients and is accompanied by an evasion of analysis directed toward oneself. Such a patient cleverly shifts attention from himself to the associator in order to defend himself against disturbing examination. He manages to redirect the group's attention to any individual who dares to analyze him. He handles what is said of him, for example, by remarking that his critic had an interesting overtone in speech that he ought to examine. By endless devices, he deflects what could add up to deeper insight, tackling his examiner. The other patients, however, gradually dissolve his resistance by expressing their appreciation for his incisiveness and by simultaneously demonstrating to him that, behind his emphatic lecturing, he makes himself inaccessible to the helping hands of the group for fear of humiliation. It is pointed out that fear of his vulnerability to parental substitutes in the group is forcing him into this compulsive role. To the extent that the members understand the frantic insecurity that underlies his bravado, they extend a reassuring friendliness that enables him to relinquish his insistent critical study of others for self-examination.

Transference

One of the most important aspects of psychoanalysis in groups is the identification and resolution of transferences. Under the therapist's leadership, patients discover the extent to which they invest one another with early familial qualities. In the group setting, when a member may not only project a significant historical figure onto the analyst but may also single out members of the group for the same purpose, the field for transference is appreciably extended. Some individuals, in fact, immediately re-create their own original family in any small cluster of strangers.

The discovery and analysis of transference is the most important work of psychoanalysis in groups, since it repeatedly interferes with the patient's true estimate of reality. Transference prevents each member from being able to accept another by conferring traits on him which originally stood in the way of a full relationship to a member of his original family. Accordingly, patients need to be made aware as to its derivation, qualities, and purpose.

While in individual psychoanalysis a patient may project onto the therapist at different times father, mother, or sibling images, the analyst is less likely to spontaneously arouse these multiple investments than is a group of people with variously stimulating personality peculiarities. The central or thematic transference reaction, most generally elicited, appears as a reproduction of a relationship to a more significant parent with whom the patient was more ambivalently and affectively bound. Lesser peripheral or penumbral transferences, appearing with more subtlety and often altogether neglected in individual analysis, reproduce more conflicting but less painfully traumatic relationships to the less significant parent and siblings. The multiplicity of ways in which a patient dresses up the other members accurately reanimates the old family, disclosing in the action both his history and the richly divergent facets of his personality.

An element in the group setting that facilitates the analysis of transference is the confrontation of each member with his disparate projection on the same person. It is often baffling in individual treatment to try to convince a patient that his estimate of the analyst is far from realistic but is, rather, a reproduction of an unresolved, conflictual attitude toward a parent. The neurotic person stubbornly insists that his feelings for and impressions of the therapist are accurate. While the analyst may grant their tenability, he has great difficulty in persuading the patient that they are also an attempt to maintain archaic familial constellations. The patient's obstinacy melts more easily in a milieu where he is faced with divergent impressions of the same person, projected by many present; he is forced to re-examine his perceptive faculties. He cannot maintain so readily his critical obstinacy that the analyst is brilliant, strong, and all-providing when another patient insists just as mulishly that the doctor is stupid, weak, and unreliable. He is obliged to reconsider his original investment of the therapist for possible misrepresentation. And, in his reactions to other patients, he is also forced to reinvestigate his projective devices.

There is another element in the group setting which is conducive to the fuller evocation of transference possibilities. This is the variously provocative characteristics of the multiple personalities in the group. The disparate personalities in the group furnish a larger number of exciting agents, whose particular differences elicit wider and more subtle facets of transference than are attainable by the analyst alone. With little effort on his part save mere attention, the therapist can discern how naturally one patient animates another into revealing peripheral sides of neurotic investment that would otherwise be missed. Each patient's provocative role should also be explored in terms of the healthy and neurotic responses he elicits. Members are asked to assist in discovering one another's inflammatory tactics so that the therapist can distinguish between what is truly provocative, originating in the provocateur, and what is neurotically derived from the reactor.

ANALYST'S TRANSFERENCE

Countertransference is thought by many to be the analyst's transference. The distortion is perceiving the patient or patients in a group as if he, she, or they were members of the analyst's original family. Distinction needs to be made between the therapist's transference and his countertransference. Who the analyst represents to the patient is the patient's transference; who the patient represents to the analyst is the analyst's transference. It is not sufficient knowing who the analyst is to the patient or the patient to the analyst; the connection between the two must be known as well. If the analyst is to the patient a mother, and the patient is to the analyst a child whose archaic needs he gratifies, we have fulfillment of the transference demand of the patient, and we have countertransference in the analyst. If, on the other hand, the analyst is to the patient a mother, and the patient is to the analyst a mother whose archaic needs he frustrates, we have cross-transference, not countertransference.

The following terminology has been coined to cover some important types of analyst's transferences: direct transference, projected identification transference, and introjected transference (Kutash). In direct transference, the analyst or group therapist invests the patient or group members with qualities linked with early familial figures from his or her original family. In projected identification transference, the analyst or group therapist identifies with the patient or patients and projects his own early feelings from his own original family onto the patient, thereby getting vicarious transference satisfaction through seeing that person gratified. In introjected transference, the therapist takes on the role of his own parents in the manner in which he ministers to the patient or group who he has come to see as early familial figures. He or she acts as his own parents might, as leader of a re-created original family. The analyst who experiences feelings of betrayal might find he is the victim of an introjected transference reaction.

COUNTERTRANSFERENCE

Countertransference is what is says—namely, activity of the analyst in response to the transference of the patient which the analyst fulfills. Countertransference is descriptive of behavior induced in the therapist which is responsive to transference and provides the patient transference satisfaction. In every transference of the patient, there is an implicit demand on the analyst that he fulfill or satisfy some aspect of it. This is transference expectation. While transference reactions of the patient may facilitate therapy, countertransference reactions interfere because they fulfill illusion and deny reality. Countertransference is the therapist's unconscious, involuntary, inappropriate, and temporarily gratifying response to the patient's transference demands. It is irrational and ultimately disagreeable to both analyst and patient. Countertransference results in oscillation between gratifying and frustrating the patient; while probably present to a degree in all therapy, some patients elicit more and some less.

Alternate Session

The alternate session is a scheduled meeting of the members of a psychoanalytic group without the therapist. Such sessions are scheduled to alternate with regular meetings when the therapist is present. The therapist asks the group to meet without him once or twice a week, usually in the homes of the various patients. In this way, an atmosphere is provided in which free interaction and participation are stimulated. They are not restricted to carry on the analytic process in the alternate sessions; nevertheless, the alternate session frequently becomes an extension of the regular session and tends to preserve its atmosphere and interaction, with patients speculating about each other and the absent therapist.

One purpose of the alternate session is to facilitate interaction in the absence of the therapist. Members learn that they can disagree and still be friends without the continuous guidance of authority. Many patients seem freer to interact at alternate meetings, when transferences to the therapist are less threatening. And projections developing at the alternate sessions are attenuated by peer realities.

The alternate sessions provide an opportunity for the patient to be helped by his peers and to exercise, as well, a constructive role as a helper. In this respect and in others, the alternate meeting comes closer to an experience in life, where the patient plays a great variety of roles, as husband or wife, parent and child, employer and employee, ally and antagonist, giver and taker, and helper and helped.

Together, the two climates represent a field which cannot be experienced in one or the other group atmosphere alone. By comparing differences in conduct and analyzing the transferences involved, the patient is able to work through more completely in both settings.

Disequilibrium, Equilibrium, and Malequilibrium in Groups

The interpersonal environment of the contemporary group can fall into a generally destructive balance or pattern of interaction, a generally constructive balance or pattern of interaction, and, perhaps most insidious, a generally comfortable but stultifying balance or pattern of interaction. These three group situations have been termed group disequilibrium, group equilibrium, and group malequilibrium (Kutash, 1980). Group disequilibrium takes the form of a transferential, pathogenic, uncomfortable, re-created family; group equilibrium takes the form of a comfortable, transferential family with a new look; and group malequilibrium takes the form of a pathogenic but comfortable family.

GROUP DISEQUILIBRIUM

Just as an individual may re-create his pathogenic family, there is the ever-present danger that the group, functioning as a re-created family, may become pathogenic as a family. Without adroit management, some groups end up this way. The therapist must watch for the elaboration of self-sufficient, inbred, and incestuous trends that bind members together as neurotically as in the original family.

A recovering patient, for example, may be attacked as unready for discharge by a compulsively overprotective member who is parentally antagonistic. If a man and woman gravitate toward one another with erotic interest, they may be invested with father and mother roles, and other patients may react to them with detached respect, voyeuristic and aggressive interest, or moralistic disapproval that corresponds to earlier ambivalent curiosity and condemnation with regard to intimacy between the parents.

Occasionally, a member or two will exhibit some reluctance to permit a patient who has recovered to leave the group. They demonstrate the same kind of envy or jealousy earlier directed toward a sibling or parent, and feel the family group or parental therapist is favoring the cured member, which his own performance does not deserve.

Another unfavorable situation which may arise in a group is the development of intense neurotic resistance, accompanied by hostile bilateral transferences, and the formation of allies in groups of two or three, leaving some individuals isolated except for a relatively warm relationship to the analyst. Sometimes even this association becomes strained, because the patient blames the therapist for his having been exposed to such a trying antagonistic environment. Such forms of resistance need to be analyzed; otherwise, the group may fall apart. Attendance may become low and demoralize those present. The therapist, while taking an analytic view of absenteeism, confronts those who stay away repeatedly with attempts to understand their flight. He explores transferences that force aggressors into belligerent roles, and points out their illusory character. He is equally vigilant with regard to projective devices that impel the compulsively withdrawn to retreat further or to submit to the domination of other members. He seeks to uncover the causes for resistance to participation on deeper levels, pointing out explicitly the destructive character of particular defenses and encouraging free emotional ventilation.

All else failing, the analyst may be obliged to remove a patient here and there, one at a time, at varying intervals, introducing each retired member into a more constructive group. Such a crisis can usually be avoided by not organizing a group with a majority of strongly sadomasochistic patients, or with consciously or unconsciously closed and rejective patients. Too many such members in the same milieu provide an unfavorable climate for the evocation of the positive resources that need to be expressed if the group is to proceed efficiently.

GROUP EQUILIBRIUM

Group equilibrium is achieved when the group constructively re-creates the family but with a new look. By cultivating a permissive atmosphere in which mutual tolerance and regard can fluorish, the earlier prohibitive character of the original family is projected with less intensity and is more easily dispersed. Furthermore, the general acceptance and sense of belonging that follow make it possible to achieve a similarly easy transition to correspondingly untroubled social relations beyond the confines of the group. The other patients, out of their numbers, provide more familial surrogates for transference evocation. Each member comes to the realization of the extent to which he re-creates his own childhood family in every social setting, and of the extent to which he invests others with inappropriate familial substitute qualities. The number of participants also clarifies the variety and multiplicity of central and penumbral transferences. Whereas in individual analysis the therapist tries to see clearly what perceptual distortions the patient makes of outer reality and what internal factors contribute to this social disfigurement, the analyst is often misled, because he does not see the patient in action. In psychoanalysis in groups, the therapist is also interested in what is happening at the

moment, so that the patient's unconscious warping of fact can be observed in motion. He can then be confronted with his projective trends and the inciting role he plays in precipitating the environmental disturbance he resents so much.

An illustration of how a group helped an individual to see his misperceptions of the present as if it were the past is offered to show the usefulness of psychoanalysis in groups for this purpose, and to show how group equilibrium can emerge from group disequilibrium.

A group member was transferentially viewed by one younger male member of the group as an immovable controlling figure (his father). A second younger male group member also viewed him as very controlling and irritating but also experienced a positive feeling that he would like to help him to feel free to be less controlling (feelings he felt for his father). A younger female group member saw the person as manipulative and subtly controlling (this was like both her parents). A fourth group member saw him as talking down to her and treating her as if she were unintelligent (again like her parents); and yet a fifth group member saw him as a warm good father (the father she never had). When the first four members described, all began to express their feelings to this member, who was the recipient of so much transference, and they told him how he should behave; as a group, they thus became transferentially his mother, who always did control him and tell him how to act. He vehemently resisted their efforts. Only after each father transference was explored one by one and the group came to see the defensive nature of this man's controlling behavior—warding off his own mother, while his transference to the group was clarified—did progress for many group members occur. Many individuals came to see how they related to present-day figures as people from their past.

The group setting thus facilitates the emergence and acceptance of insight by confronting each member with his disparate investments of other patients and the therapist. When a patient joins a group, he finds that each patient, unconsciously warps his perception of the therapist and of the other patients as well. He begins to question the reality of his view of people in the group; and, as he discovers and studies his transferences, he also becomes aware of his provocative role.

Resistances seem to melt easily in this potentiating, catalytic atmosphere of mutual revelation in the group. The necessity of exposing oneself to another person without a corresponding disclosure by the therapist makes some patients self-conscious; however, each member is stimulated by the partial but always increasing self-revelation of another to expose more and more of himself. The discovery that the next person not only comes to no harm in showing himself but wins social approval besides encourages one to uncover as well. The general feeling of shared divestment in a benevolent atmosphere enables a patient to show himself more freely. This experience is confirmed by the psychic climate of an ongoing group, and, after 3 or 4 months, each new member becomes part of the operation.

Another constructive advantage offered by a group that is in equilibrium is that it removes the patient from the danger of prolonged dependence on the therapist. In the isolation of private treatment, the analyst can encourage the patient to pursue his deepest personal longings. It may turn out that these aspirations are egocentric and that indulging them leads to detached, antisocial self-assertion. The gratification of his particular yearnings can amount to being allowed to exploit familial substitutes for neurotically satisfying ends. Humoring these impulses is bound to bring the patient into provocative, neurotic conflict with his associates, who will not tolerate such infantile actions. The group process encourages reliance of one person on the next and more quickly demands and gets an abandonment of prolonged, possessive, and parasitic attachment that excludes the possibility of mature kinship.

Finally, one of the most valuable aspects of psychoanalysis in groups that are in equilibrium is that it facilitates giving up the ideal of having a relationship with the single-parent analyst. Instead of offering the questionable shelter of a private relationship to one omniscient ego ideal, it presents the patient with a group of persons in whose common effort he can join. Whereas the basis of a private relationship may well be evasive of social reality and tend to create an aura of isolation, the group serves in just the opposite way. Instead of enhancing the average patient's tendencies to neurotic isolation and his anarchic wish to act out his pathology, psychoanalysis in groups may help him realize his full potential as a social being. This is an added bridge to the establishment of healthy social relationships outside of analysis. Rather than strengthening the egocentric idea—typified in the neurotic's mind by the notion of the omnipotent therapist—psychoanalysis in groups helps to resolve the false antithesis of the individual versus the group by giving the patient a conscious experience that his fulfillment can be realized in a social or interpersonal setting without his losing his individuality.

GROUP MALEQUILIBRIUM

Group malequilibrium occurs when group members are all comfortable with each other but do not in any way challenge each other's defenses. The group itself is in an unhealthy or stultifying balance. Conflict-laden topics are avoided, and everyone, in an unconscious deal, avoids stressful but potentially growth-inducing material. An example of a patient in such a group is the following:

The patient whose love for the emotional climate of the group borders on the ecstatic. He revels in the luxury of what he considers an absolutely honest relationship. He is in a family whose projections, having become at last analyzable and understandable, no longer alarm or hurt him. The danger in his case is that he runs from real life to the fabricated safety of an unreal laboratory. He finds the group warmer and saner than most associations on the outside. He

needs to be instructed on how to carry the affective closeness he has consummated in the group to larger segments of society, beyond the confines of his fellow members.

This last is a common objection to working in concert with other patients: How can one transpose the good fellowship of the group to areas outside it? Group analytic technique offers the patient a means of making conscious those trends that stand in the way of his vigorous affective contact with others, whether loving or hating—hating, because there are some psychopathic influences in the world which can appropriately be hated.

The following case is also illustrative of malequilibrium in a group.

A woman patient was placed in a group and arrived at her first meeting with a long cigarette holder and a very theatrical air and dress. After attending the session, she told the therapist, "This is not my kind of people; haven't you a group of people who have more in common with me?" The therapist, who was seeing a number of artists and theatre people, was about to start a new group. He invited this woman and several other patients who seemed compatible into the group. Everyone immediately hit it off, laughed, joked, and had a marvelous time. No one talked about themselves, their feelings, associations, or their dreams.

The group described above was eventually disbanded and its members placed in more heterogeneous groups, groups where the cultivation of the group came through the promotion of differentiated, complementary and uncomplementary, agnostic and anti-agnostic, conflictual and nonconflictual personalities. People, through their growing individuality, learned—through differences in realistic perception and unrealistic misperception—to appreciate one another's mutually proffered gifts of vision and the treasures of each other's perceptions.

Conclusion

Therapists who emphasize group process and group dynamics, as well as those who emphasize the psychoanalytic treatment of the individual in interaction and his intrapsychic life, wish to create a climate which supports the progressive evolution of each patient in a therapeutic group. The current emphasis on group process and group dynamics not only fosters resistance, but also creates a diegophrenogenic impact on every member and provides a pseudocohesion to which each participant submits. A genuine cohesion follows only after the liberation of the suppressed ego in each patient and the working through of his individual resistances and transferences. An appropriate regard for each other can follow only after a member has realistic regard for himself. With the emphasis on the primacy of the individual in psychoanalysis in groups, it is, therefore, not the aim to lead the group into the chaos of every man for himself. Psychoanalysis in groups is an approach which emphasizes harmony growing out of disharmony, reciprocity growing out of antagonism, ego growth through persistent emphasis on supporting the suppressed ego, self-respect and respect for others in the course of the struggle, appreciation of differences, and a sense of mutual regard as treatment goes on. Indeed, psychoanalysis in groups, with its emphasis on protecting and promoting the wholesome uniqueness of the individual, is perhaps more relevant in contemporary society than it has ever been.

References

Kutash, I. L. Prevention and equilibrium-disequilibrium theory. In *Handbook on Stress and Anxiety*, I. L. Kutash and L. B. Schlesinger, editors, p. 463. Jossey-Bass, San Francisco, 1980.
Kutash, I. L., and Schlesinger, L. B. *Handbook on Stress and Anxiety*. Jossey-Bass, San Francisco, 1980.
Schwartz, E. K., and Wolf, A. On countertransference in group psychotherapy. J. Psychol., 57: 131, 1964.
Wolf, A. Psychoanalysis in groups. Am. J. Psychother., *3:* 525, 1949.
Wolf, A. Diegophrenia and genius. Am. J. Psychoanal., 40: 213, 1981.
Wolf, A., and Schwartz, E. K. *Psychoanalysis in Groups.* Grune & Stratton, New York, 1962.

B.9 Short-term Group Psychotherapy

SIMON H. BUDMAN, Ph.D.
MICHAEL J. BENNETT, M.D.

Introduction

Group psychotherapy has been viewed as a treatment modality of extended duration. This is true in spite of the fact that the average length of outpatient mental health treatment in this country is about 3.4 per year visits at community settings and 8.4 visits per year at private practice settings. These figures, combined with the fact that the dropout rate from group psychotherapy in some studies has been as high as 50% (Baekeland and Lundwall, 1975), may indicate that many patients referred for what is described to them as long-term group treatment choose to vote with their feet. That is, they may neither need nor want 2 or more years of group psychotherapy to deal with the problems for which they sought help. Furthermore, in this era of accountability, wild inflation, and staggering medical costs, it will become increasingly difficult for the practitioners of long-term psychotherapy approaches to convince third-party payers to support years of treatment when briefer therapies have been often found to be as efficacious (Johnson and Gelso, 1980; Smith et al., 1980).

History

The forerunner of most short-term group treatment approaches—and probably of long-term group therapy as well—was the work in the early 1900's by Dr. Joseph Pratt, a Boston internist who organized groups for tubercular patients. Following Pratt's lead, a voluminous literature has developed regarding short-term groups with one type of medical patient or another (Mone, 1970; Ohlmeier et al., 1973; Keegan, 1974).

A variety of brief therapy or counseling groups have been developed over the years for homogeneous groups of patients with particular types of problems, such as stressful life circumstances, disturbed adolescent males, and prospective counselors.

It is only in the last several years that a literature has begun to appear which examines brief group approaches for less specialized outpatient populations (Bernard and Klein, 1977; Imber et al., 1979; Budman et al., 1980). At least in part, this change is presumably due to the fact that the encounter group movement—which reached its peak in the early 1970's—left a legacy of enthusiasm and hopefulness about the possible impact of brief group intervention approaches (Bernard and Klein, 1977; Sabin, 1981).

Additionally, there has recently been a burgeoning of interest in time-limited individual psychotherapies (Sifneos, 1972; Mann, 1973; Davanloo, 1980). This rising tide of interest and increased theoretical understanding of brief treatment has obviously begun to spill over into the group therapy area.

Unifying Elements in Short-term Group Therapies

There are at least 6 elements common to all modes of short-term group therapy.

Focality of treatment

According to many sources (Ursano and Dressler, 1974; Small, 1979) the single most important factor which differentiates long- and short-term therapies is the more limited focus found in the briefer therapies. Whereas long-term treatments often have as their implicit or explicit goal a major and general restructuring of personality or character, briefer therapies have more limited and some would say more realistic goals. Short-term inpatient groups might have a goal such as helping patients deal more effectively with life on the ward. The crisis group has as its central purpose helping members handle a particular crisis in their lives; the short-term young adult and midlife groups focus upon common adult developmental themes; and short-term couples groups focus on the marital relationships of members.

Rapid group cohesion

Unless there is a quickly developing sense of cohesiveness and trust in a short-term group, it is unlikely that the group will be viewed by members as providing a valuable therapeutic experience. In part, the clear and limited focus of the group helps to initiate a sense of cohesion. Also, the therapist may contribute to the cohesiveness of the group by aiding members in seeing ways in which they are similar and ways in which they are working together on the common group task.

For young adult and couples groups in the Harvard Community Health Plan short-term group program, a pregroup workshop serves to prepare potential members for the group itself (Budman, 1981). Such a preparatory experience enhances cohesiveness by helping members to meet and become familiar with one another under less anxiety-provoking circumstances than would ordinarily be the case in the early stages of a therapy group. Furthermore, pregroup preparation and screening have reduced the group dropout rate from 17% to below 1%. This further enhances early group cohesion in that dropouts tend to be demoralizing to a group and often lead to further dropouts.

Members of short-term groups wish for these groups to become cohesive rapidly and, therefore, seek out similarities and parallels. It is nearly invariable that group members will search for and find striking (and at times obscure) background similarities. For example, in one couples group nearly every member had had at least one alcoholic parent; in one young adult group most members had at some point in their lives had a weight problem or eating disorder.

As Robert Frost so eloquently put it, "Something there is which doesn't love a wall." If the task and the time limit are clear and the therapist is supportive of the group pulling together, members will attempt to tear down the interpersonal walls and become a cohesive unit as quickly as possible.

Relatively circumscribed and brief time limits

Butcher and Koss (1978) have described brief therapy as being about 25 sessions or less in duration. This time frame is probably a reasonable one for short-term group treatment as well. Although the literature includes time-limited therapy groups which are 18 months in length, this period is well out of the realm of short-term treatment.

It is imperative that potential short-term group members be made aware of the time limits immediately upon being offered and again upon entering the group. Furthermore, the more important the time limit is as a theme in the group, the more the therapist is advised to stick to that limit. In general, in a closed group (where all members begin and end together) the time limit assumes greater importance than in an open group, where there is much coming and going.

Active therapist

In some long-term group therapy approaches, the therapist is advised to be minimally active, except for occasional deep interpretations (Malan et al., 1976). This type of an approach paradoxically fosters a leader-centered focus as members struggle to get more from the therapist. Such a preoccupation with the leader would work against the goals and foci of most short-term therapy groups. Rather, the leader in such a group should be relatively active, clear, and direct in assisting members to stick to the group task and in working on their individual goals in the group. Transferential issues and characteristic modes of dealing with authority figures may certainly arise within the context of the group; however, to allow these to become the central themes is not productive.

A here-and-now or there-and-now orientation

The dominant motif in most short-term group therapy is the patient's current life situation or current life patterns. Although the therapist may flexibly weave in the examination of some historical material if this seems appropriate, for the most part, the orientation should be present centered. This may include looking at the patient's pattern of relating to others within the group, as well as what is occurring in the patient's life outside of the group.

Patient selection

Evidence is growing that the major determinants of outcome in brief therapy and perhaps psychotherapy in general are the pretherapy characteristics of patients entering this treatment (Gomes-Schwartz, 1978).

For some practitioners of brief individual therapy (Sifneos, 1972), criteria for treatment are quite stringent. However, it seems that most outpatient neurotics can profit from a short-term group approach as long as several criteria are met. The patient should be willing to try group therapy; the patient should have some history of relatively good ability to relate within a group setting; the patient should not be psychotic or borderline; and the patient should not be violent.

In a research study of pregroup patient characteristics and their relationship to outcome, Budman et al. (1980) reported:

> Overall, our findings seem to point to our dropouts and low changers . . . as more disturbed, schizoid and isolated people, who might be described diagnostically as borderline or character disorders. High changers appear to be more in the neurotic range. Although they come into the group hurting and symptomatic, they begin treatment with a liking for people, friendships and a base from which to operate when interacting in the group.

In dealing very briefly with a group of 5 to 10 people wanting help, the last thing the therapist needs is a patient who is highly destructive or represents a serious management problem. If such a patient is not screened out in the interview or pregroup workshop, the therapist should not be hesitant in removing him or her in the early stages of the group. The duration of a short-term group is simply insufficient to deal with such a patient, and his or her continued membership will be a loss to all.

The Harvard Community Health Plan Short-term Group Therapy Program

The short-term group treatment program which will be described is one component of a spectrum of services which has evolved over the past 11 years at the Kenmore Center of the Harvard Community Health Plan (HCHP), a prepaid group practice type health maintenance organization (HMO) in Boston. Given the challenge of caring for a defined population, with all members entitled to outpatient and inpatient mental health services, the development of high-quality, effective methods of treatment has been attempted, while containing costs. Certain assumptions underlie the description which follows:

1. Large numbers of people in a general population require some mental health services. This is clearly demonstrated by epidemiological studies and borne out by experience; approximately 12 to 15% of plan members use specialized mental health services in a given year; an undetermined additional number benefit from mental health care offered by primary care physicians and nurses, a function backed up and supported by Harvard's (integrated) Mental Health Department.
2. With early access, facilitated by low barriers to referral and use of services, and favorable attitudes on the part of members and referring providers, most patients can be helped by timely, focal interventions.
3. In a closed system, where continuity of health care is a given, members will use mental health services at times of need, repeatedly if necessary, and continuous treatment will be required for only a small percentage of those needing help (Bennett and Wisneski, 1979).
4. Group methods have an important place in the spectrum of mental health services. Currently 25 to 30% of treatment is done in groups. Of these, the vast majority are short term (15 sessions or fewer).

Operating as part of a comprehensive service program, brief groups have been used to serve the needs of patients who are dealing with problems of living, crisis situations, or problems in adult development. The three types of group used most commonly are:

1. Couples groups: 15-session groups for couples in conflict, where the goal is to identify areas of dissonance and to promote improved communication.
2. The crisis group: an eight-session biweekly group run jointly with the nurses of the triage (walk-in) unit, designed for those with previously healthy psychological functioning who are responding to overwhelming, usually acute, situational stress.
3. Adult developmental groups: for patients who are dealing primarily with the tasks and transitions of adult life; homogeneous for age, these are mixed groups serving 8 to

10 adults with varying character structure, presenting problems, and diagnoses; there are 3 main categories within the adult developmental groups: young adult (twenties to midthirties), midlife (35 to 50), and late midlife (50 and older).

SHORT-TERM GROUP TREATMENT OF COUPLES

Since 1976, the Kenmore Center of the HCHP has run short-term, time-limited (15-session) groups for couples in conflict. These groups generally include 4 or 5 couples between the ages of 30 and 50.

Prior to beginning a short-term couples group, 6 to 10 couples who have generally been seen several times for evaluation or treatment by individual therapists in the mental health department are assembled for a pregroup workshop. The purpose of this workshop is both as pregroup preparation and as screening for the group itself.The workshop is highly structured and lasts approximately 1½ hours. Couples have the opportunity to get some idea of what the group experience will be like (even though the group is far less structured), and the therapists have the opportunity to screen out any couples who do not appear to be appropriate for or well suited to the group. Using this mode of pregroup preparation and screening, the HCHP dropout rate among couples who choose to begin the group is far less than 1%.

The major focus of the couples group is on communications within a given couple and the interactions between group members which can shed light upon the marital difficulties being experienced. The male-female co-leaders of the group are fairly active; however, there is an attempt made to encourage and support group input and group interaction. This is far preferable to simply doing conjoint couples therapy within a group context. That is, input from group members to other members or couples is viewed as having great value, and the leaders do not do all the work with a given couple as the others sit back and observe.

The leaders help the group maintain an awareness of when the group will end and a sense of pressure to accomplish as much as possible in the sessions remaining. The following clinical example from the sixth session will give the reader some sense of the interaction within these couples groups.

Sandy, a women in her late forties, said that she had been having terrible difficulties over the previous 2 weeks with Jack, her husband. Although for the first several weeks of group meetings they had felt that they were talking more with one another, things now were at a new low. This couple, the J.'s, were approximately 10 years older than most of the other couples in their group and had in general been very warm, supportive, and almost parental to other group members as they expressed their marital difficulties. Fred and Linda, another couple, attempted to get clarification from Sandy and Jack about what specifically was going wrong, as did several other group members. Jack (who was a very humorous and witty man) launched into an extremely funny and overdramatized story explaining how he and Sandy always fought about different aspects of the business which they run jointly. At this point, nearly every member of the group made suggestions to them about the business and possibilities for lessening the conflict which this generated. "Let Jack run the business and have Sandy work for someone else" offered Phil. "No, it would be better if Sandy ran the business" said Linda. After about 10 minutes of suggestions, each of which were promptly rejected by the couple as impossible, one of the leaders laughingly asked if the members would like to fill out ballots about what Sandy and Jack should do. All the members (who had been through a very similar pattern of help-rejecting-complaining in another couple several weeks previously) realized that there was no real solution to be offered. Phil asked what was actually going on. Jack replied, "I guess the truth of it is that I am simply an unmitigated bastard and make Sandy's life miserable because I'm so awful." Sandy smiled and said that this was so and that she wished Jack would finally shape up after 17 years of marriage. The female leader of the group asked Sandy what she herself needed from the relationship, to which she again replied that she just wanted Jack to shape up. Again, the leader asked her about her (Sandy's) own needs. She would only talk about what Jack did to her. She also said, "My mother and sister were mentally ill and gave me lots of trouble, and Jack always gives me lots of trouble." She looked sad and uncomfortable. Almost immediately, Jack launched into an explanation of how difficult he made life for Sandy. The leaders and several of the members pointed out to the J.'s that, whenever someone in the group became upset, they would set up a distraction. It became much clearer over the course of the meeting (much of which was devoted to this couple) that Jack's *mea culpa* ("I'm so awful") routine was his way of protecting his wife. She, in turn, was terrified of her neediness and acted the role of the poor, beleaguered women for whom life would be wonderful if only her husband would stop being so difficult. He could not give directly nor could she take directly.

Although much of this particular session focused on a given couple, all of the members were highly involved. There was a great deal of feedback and comparisons made by other couples. The two therapists clearly led the session; however, much of the active input came from the membership.

THE CRISIS GROUP

The crisis group is a biweekly, eight-session, open group for adults in crisis, which has been in operation in the Kenmore Center continuously since 1971. The group is run jointly by the Mental Health Department and medical nurses attached to the triage (walk-in) area. It is a readily available, cost-effective treatment resource. In addition, it serves as a major training opportunity for medical staff in the evaluation and management of crisis states.

Crisis group candidates are referred directly to the group from medical providers or from a mental health provider who has seen the patient on referral. The emphasis is on ready and early access. A group candidate is a man or woman, 17 or older, who has experienced the acute onset of significant symptomatology or functional impairment in response to an identifiable situational problem or event, most commonly a loss or series of losses. The patient is not actively suicidal, homicidal, psychotic, or currently abusing alcohol or drugs. He or she is willing to be treated briefly, in a group, and can agree on a focal objective. An intake interview is performed by either the mental health therapist or nurse co-therapist, focusing on the problem which provoked the crisis and establishing a working alliance and a treatment goal. The therapist defines and accounts for the crisis, relating the current event to relevant biographical data. The evaluation and dynamic formulation are shared with the patient in everyday language. The group is described, questions are answered, the prospective member is told what to expect and what will be expected of him or her. Ordinarily, the first session follows in 1 to 3 days.

Meetings are held in the health center twice weekly for 1½ hours. The average group size is six to 10 members, who attend for eight sessions and then terminate. Therapists rotate, with termination of therapists overlapped, so that one of the two finishes after every fourth session. Content is centered on the there and now, especially on the problem which provoked the symptomatic response. There is only secondary emphasis on group process. Leaders are active, often directive. Over-all the tone is warm and supportive. There is little reliance on medication.

The patient is helped to see his or her problem in perspective, linking symptoms to causes: "You are irritable with your children because you cannot express your anger at your husband to him directly." A psychodynamic explanatory formulation, made during the evaluation, often reduces the mystery of the crisis and helps the patient to begin the process of mastery through understanding. Such formulations may or may not be pursued and elaborated upon in the course of the group, where the focus tends to be on active resolution, rather than insight. Frequently, advice and suggestions are offered, regression and passivity are discouraged, and the patient is encouraged to take steps which will resolve the crisis situation. The willingness of therapists and other group members to share the patient's feelings of distress is tempered by an insistence that he or she move forward, utilizing the group, family, or friends as needed. The time limit is kept in mind, and is a powerful motivating force.

In fostering the group culture, leaders discourage a therapist-centered orientation, transference is not permitted to build, and members are encouraged to relate to each other. Extragroup contacts are neither encouraged nor discouraged, and occasionally group members will assist each other in practical ways outside the group, such as offering phone numbers for times of need. Occasionally, groups meet informally after treatment ends.

The milieu constitutes a holding environment in which a member may take what he or she needs and give to others as well. The group is health, rather than illness, centered. Excessive dependency is discouraged, and regression is opposed. Members are encouraged to do the work and then move on. As with all treatment modes at the Harvard Community Health Plan, termination is viewed as less than absolute, since plan members know the department is there for future use as needed.

The following case exemplifies the process. It also demonstrates a common pattern. States of crisis, in which there is a sense of being overwhelmed and normal adaptive mechanisms fail, are often the result of repeated or cumulative stress, rather than single stressful events. They are also, as Mann (1973) suggests, related to core issues of self-esteem which emerge repeatedly through life and take a variety of forms. Depending on the severity, duration, and specific nature of the stresses involved, there may be a concomitant sense of fragmentation, a feeling of loss of integrity, self-worth, or cohesion. The most common complaint is an inability to cope or function.

Ann was a 38-year-old computer programmer referred by her primary care provider because of feelings of rage and periods of uncontrollable tearfulness and agitation interfering with her ability to work. Her stresses were multiple:

1. An immigrant whose family still lived in Scotland, she had learned almost exactly a year earlier that a beloved younger sister whom she had helped to raise had inoperable cancer. She had visited the sister months earlier to say goodbye but had been prevented from speaking openly because the sister's husband and her doctors had decided to withhold the truth from her.

2. Two months prior to her presentation, she had learned that her ex-husband, who had left her for another woman 6 years earlier, was about to have a child by his new wife. The patient's only child, a son, was having marked problems accepting this.

3. Escalating work conflicts with a female supervisor had culminated in her being suspended. The patient, who had been active in promoting union interests, felt that she was being scapegoated. The supervisor was seen as cold and unsympathetic to the patient's reaction to her sister's illness, a fact known at her place of work.

In the group, Ann was soft spoken and self-effacing, giving practical suggestions to others at times, often choosing to remain silent. Through her positive relationship with the (male) co-therapist, she was encouraged to share her feelings, especially in regard to two other patients, both of whom complained bitterly about being hurt by their husbands and, in both cases, having old resentments stirred up toward hurting and neglectful fathers. Gradually, Ann began to connect current feelings of hurt and betrayal with childhood memories. Her beloved father had abruptly died when she was 3, leaving three children to be cared for by her aloof and rejecting mother. Feelings of sadness, hurt, and anger at her father were mobilized, and Ann could connect her own memories of loss with her concern over the imminent loss which her sister's three children would have to bear. Her supervisor's behavior, previously seen as personally rejecting, could be viewed in more objective fashion and became a problem to be solved, rather than a source of personal hurt. As her self-esteem improved, she became more vocal, demonstrating wit, wisdom, and genuine warmth; she began to speak of her accomplishments overcoming early trauma, poverty, relocation, and divorce. She spoke with pride of her current efforts to educate herself (as a part-time student). In her final session, she began to speak of herself as attractive, bright, and competent. Less self-preoccupied, she began to help others in the group.

SHORT-TERM GROUPS BASED UPON AN ADULT DEVELOPMENT MODEL FOR PSYCHIATRIC OUTPATIENTS

If psychiatric services are readily available and affordable, many who elect such services will be seeking relief not from major psychiatric illness but from the assorted problems of living, including those which occur more or less predictably (and normatively) at the nodal points in adult development. Short-term groups, homogeneous for age, can help to identify and mitigate obstacles to continuing growth in such individuals. Also, by capitalizing upon the healthy thrust to maturity in the motivated patient who is not seriously disturbed, the group can help to relieve symptoms and facilitate behavioral and intrapsychic change.

The three brief modes most commonly used in the short-term group setting are: young adult (twenties to midthirties), midlife (35 to 50) and late midlife (50 and older) mixed groups. These groups have certain features in common: (1) Treatment is planned to be brief; (2) Members are encouraged to apply what is learned to their outside lives and make changes in behavior during as well as after treatment; (3) Both the structure and content of the group are oriented toward the specific tasks and life stage issues concerned; (4) The groups are health, rather than illness, oriented; and (5) Character change, per se, is never the objective.

Midlife group

Midlife is characteristically a time of reassessment. Accomplishments and failures are examined under the pressure of the passage of time, and normal people seek to come to grips with their own mortality and imperfections, as well as the limits and imperfections in the world. In the face of real and anticipated loss, depression is common, and its resolution requires facing destructive elements in oneself, tolerating ambivalence, ultimately seeking to balance hatred and jealousy with caring and concern for others. There is an accompanying shift in narcissism, in which one's hopes and aims are invested in the coming generation, termed by Erikson as achieving a state of generativity. Failing this, the individual becomes self-preoccupied and stagnant. The key to navigating this period of life is to be able to activate strengths and inner resources from the past; in this process, a reworking of old hurts and conflicts may be necessary.

Midlife group candidates present with a variety of symptomatic problems, character types, and diagnoses. The common denominator is active reassessment and a sense of being stuck, as well as an acceptance of the need to examine and change something within. In order to highlight the reality and relevance of time and the need to settle for limited goals, the group is time limited. Focus alternates between the there-and-now and the here-and-now. Commonalities such as aging parents, growth of children, the limits of career and other achievements, and the feelings and thoughts provoked by group interactions are all grist for the mill. Personal mythologies and cognitive perceptions are elaborated, clarified, affirmed, or questioned by the group; feelings of shame and doubt, associated with split-off or rejected parts of the self, are shared and often traced to old hurts. The normative nature of the tasks and the need for meaningful connections with others are reinforced by the group mode. The possibility of new beginnings emerges as the group ends, even as the ending underscores the need to mourn what has been lost or what will never be.

Late midlife group

As life begins to draw to a close, individuals struggle less with the world within and more with external realities: deterioration of the body, declining powers, economic problems, intergenerational conflict, and loss of sustaining others. For such patients, the group mode is especially relevant for two reasons. First, a wealth of experience and wisdom can be pooled in dealing with universal problems; second, impoverishment of sustaining figures often creates a state of true isolation, and the group presents available objects to be used to meet a variety of needs.

Referrals are made in the context of some specific problem of late life mastery, manifested by symptoms of anxiety or depression or the aggravation of a physical disorder. In contrast to young adult and most midlife groups, the format is open, and members can come as often or as seldom as they choose, with the 20 sessions per year mental health benefit operating as a resource to be apportioned. The leader is viewed as a physician who provides a stable, reliable setting where patients can help themselves and others.

The focus in the group is here-and-now, with a minimal focus on group dynamics and a de-emphasis on termination. Anxieties regarding death are rarely dealt with directly, although they frequently are part of derivative discussion. Members rarely exceed the 20 sessions per year limit, but since they may return again and again, they do not terminate in the usual sense.

Young adult groups

Regardless of presenting complaints, the overriding developmental issue for this population is that characterized by Erikson as achieving intimacy. The consequence of failure is termed distantiation. Having separated from family, the young adult seeks to (re)establish meaningful, fulfilling, and appropriate relationships, especially with one or more love objects. Such relationships require that one be reasonably open, self-disclosing, and assertive. A firm sense of identity, the ability to tolerate closeness and to risk loss, to trust oneself and others, is essential. Patients often present after a loss, when the event underscores concern over how they are managing this part of their lives, or they may come in because of growing loneliness and a sense of isolation and failure at loving. In the group, patients can reframe their distress in interactional rather than idiosyncratic terms. They can work toward overcoming patterns of excessive self-protection, hyperindependence or defensiveness, which are based upon discomfort with real needs for

and from others, shame over perceived faults or lacks, and transferential binds stemming from unresolved family issues. The leader's role is to help the milieu to develop, to keep the group focused on the time limit, and on the need to pursue limited goals. The therapist also attempts to help group participants perceive the relationship between group events and the problems which brought them to treatment.

The following account is drawn from the tenth session (out of 15) of an eight-member young adult group.

Alice announced that she had been fired from her job and would be moving to Los Angeles in 2 weeks, leaving her only 1 more meeting. The group responded with sadness, and several members commented on her importance to the group, expressing the wish that she stay. Alice was pleased and excited about the move, although concerned that she might be repeating a pattern of flight. She described in detail the circumstances of her job loss, and most members responded with sympathy and support. Her contributions to the group were again praised, especially her softening an earlier pattern of abrasive and provocative behavior which tended to drive others away (a problem which had led her to seek therapy). Throughout this, Alice did not comment on her own feelings about leaving the group. When asked directly about this by Joan, the nurse co-therapist, she initially focused on her feeling that the loss was a familiar one, that it seemed like "someone is always leaving me, or I leave them." Ed and Winston became angry at Alice's perceived undervaluing of the group. Then Alice softened, expressing her sadness and sense of loss, and began to review her gains. This prompted Alice to say that she had also been reviewing her experience in the group, and she had found herself feeling excited and pleased about it in a recent discussion with a friend. She could not explain her improvement but knew that she was feeling symptomatically improved and more at peace with herself. After a brief silence, Winston turned to Roger, who had remained characteristically aloof, and asked him to open up, since the group was coming to an end. This was seconded by Ed, who observed that Roger looked flustered and uncomfortable, not his "usual buoyant self." Roger acknowledged his concern that time was running out and he had to open up, saying he had been having sleepless nights all week in considering doing so. He then proceeded to share more than he had previously. He told the group that he had been raised in a small town in Vermont and that his sensitivity and bookishness had made him an outcast. He acknowledged for the first time that he was homosexual and spoke of his self-consciousness, the lack of understanding in his family, and his resultant inhibition and unassertiveness. The group thanked him for trusting them. Roger than expressed his great relief and began to smile. Bob, the only black member of the group, compared Roger's experience to his own, as the only black in an all-white school. Roger became embarrassed at the attention he was receiving and stated that he could tolerate criticism by withdrawing, but he did not know what to do with approval. He managed to sit with his discomfort and tolerate the closeness. Many of the group members were leaning forward; the tone was warm and caring. In response to Roger's comments about his self-consciousness, Judy began to speak about her discomfort with her appearance, especially a gap between her front teeth. As the meeting came to a close, several members commented on the closeness and sharing.

References

Baekeland, F., and Lundwall, C. Dropping out of treatment: A critical review. Psychol. Bull., *82:* 738, 1975.

Bennett, M. J., and Wisneski, M. J. Continuous psychotherapy within an HMO. Am. J. Psychiatry, *136:* 10, 1979.

Bernard, H. S., and Klein, R. H. Some perspectives on time-limited group psychotherapy. Compr. Psychiatry, *18:* 579, 1977.

Budman, S. H. Avoiding dropouts in couples group therapy. In *Questions and Answers in the Practice of Family Therapy,* A. S. German, editor, p. 57. Brunner/Mazel, New York, 1981.

Budman, S. H., Bennett, M. J., and Wisneski, M. J. Short-term group psychotherapy: An adult developmental model. Int. J. Group Psychother., *30:* 63, 1980.

Budman, S. H., Demby, A., and Randall, M. Short-term group psychotherapy: Who succeeds, who fails? Group, *4:* 3, 1980.

Butcher, J. N., and Koss, M. P. Research on brief and crisis-oriented therapies. In *Handbook of Psychotherapy and Behavior Change,* S. L. Garfield and A. E. Bergin, editors, John Wiley & Sons, New York, 1978.

Davanloo, H., editor *Short-term Dynamic Psychotherapy.* Jason Aronson, New York, 1980.

Donovan, J. M., Bennett, M. J., and McElroy, C. M. The crisis group: An outcome study. Am J. Psychiatry, *136:* 906, 1979.

Gomes-Schwartz, B. Effective ingredients in psychotherapy: Prediction of outcome from process variables. J. Consult. Clin. Psychol., *46:* 1023, 1978.

Imber, S. D., Lewis, P. M., and Loiselle, R. H. Uses and abuses of the brief intervention group. Int. J. Group Psychother., *29:* 39, 1979.

Johnson, D. H., and Gelso, C. J. The effectiveness of time limits in counseling and psychotherapy: A critical review. Counsel. Psychol., *9:* 70, 1980.

Keegan, D. L. Adaptation to visual handicaps: Short-term group approach. Psychosomatics, *15:* 76, 1974.

Kibel, H. D. A conceptual model for short-term inpatient group psychotherapy. Am. J. Psychiatry, *138:* 74, 1981.

Malan, D. H., Balfour, F., Hood, V., and Shooter, A. Group psychotherapy: A long-term follow-up study. Arch. Gen. Psychiatry, *33:* 1303, 1976.

Mann, J. *Time-limited Psychotherapy.* Harvard University Press, Cambridge, MA, 1973.

Mone, L. C. Short-term group psychotherapy with post-cardiac patients. Int. J. Group Psychother., *20:* 99, 1970.

Ohlmeier, D., Karstens, R., and Kohle, K. Psychoanalytic short-term group psychotherapy with post-myocardial infarction patients. Psychiatr. Clin., *6:* 240, 1973.

Sabin, J. E. Short-term group psychotherapy: Historical antecedents. In *Forms of Brief Therapy,* S. H. Budman, editor, p. 271. Guilford Press, New York, 1981.

Schwartz, M. D. Situation/transition groups. Am. J. Orthopsychiatry, *45:* 744, 1975.

Sifneos, P. E. *Short-term Psychotherapy and Emotional Crisis.* Harvard University Press, Cambridge, MA, 1972.

Small, L. *The Briefer Psychotherapies* Brunner/Mazel, New York, 1979.

Smith, M. L., Glass, G. V., and Miller, T. I. *The Benefits of Psychotherapy.* Johns Hopkins University Press, Baltimore, 1980.

Ursano, R. J., and Dressler, D. M. Brief vs. longterm psychotherapy: A treatment decision. J. Nerv. Ment. Dis., *159:* 164, 1974.

B.10 Self-help Groups

STEPHEN A. COLE, M.D.

Introduction

The past decade has seen a burgeoning of self-help organizations in general, but particularly in the health care field. This phenomenon has arisen primarily through the action of grassroots mutual aid activities, with the support of private insurance companies and the federal government, to promote more effective health care, health maintenance, and an awareness of preventive medicine.

Definition

Self-help groups (SHG's) are organizations of people with similar mental, physical, or psychological conditions, afflictions, or perceived abnormalities. Self-help groups serve a need felt but not met by other religious, educational, community, or health-related institutions. Prior to participation, these "defective" people often consider themselves inferior and may likewise be stigmatized by the wider society (Goffman, 1963). Clubs are usually begun by assertive persons with the particular condition, who then recruit like-minded volunteers willing to meet regularly to discuss the meaning of their shared condition, as well as to define steps each can take to come to terms with their common problem. As a rule, self-help groups meet within the community in public settings, such as churches, schools, or spaces provided by public agencies. While they may meet in members' homes, the formality of a neutral setting may add to the sense of ongoing purpose. Members discuss their experiences with the illness or defect, exchange advice, and often offer encouragement to one another. Professional health care workers are frequently invited to be guest speakers. Newsletters may be published to foster greater unity of outlook, keep members informed of coming events, and educate the public. Self-help groups are usually non-profit, although some have nominal dues to cover operating expenses. Many are connected with national organizations bearing the same name, but usually retain considerable local autonomy.

Individuals who join self-help groups may want primarily to solve problems but frequently also join for the group experience itself or to make new friends. One study of women's consciousness-raising groups found that their reported level of problems-in-living was comparable to people who joined growth centers, and that a substantial proportion were in concurrent psychotherapy. In general, those who join self-help groups appear to be better educated and more satisfied with professional help than people who do not join.

It is now generally believed that SHG's provide their members with an important source of social support, which appears to be protective against the untoward effects of highly stressful situations (Cobb, 1976). Health professionals are wondering now whether the problem of non-compliance will be at least partially resolved through patient participation in self-help groups (Green et al., 1977). Guttmacher, Navarro, and others have warned that an overemphasis upon individual self-care and mutual aid will result in blaming the victim, and thereby relieve health care institutions from accountability for providing primary care which meets real patient need. On the other hand, the self-help movement offers patients the opportunity to become both further informed and more highly motivated in matters of health care, and to participate in the formation of health care planning and policy.

Dynamics

CATEGORIZATION

Self-help groups can be categorized according to six major concerns (Katz and Bender, 1976; Killilea, 1976; Gartner and Riessman, 1977; Cole et al., 1979):

1. Groups concerned with the behavior change of people with addictions include the Anonymous groups, Take Off Pounds Sensibly (TOPS), Weight Watchers, SmokeEnders, and Synanon.

2. Groups concerned with providing members with social support and new coping strategies include Alanon, Parents Without Partners, Recovery, Inc., and Friends and Advocates of the Mentally Ill.

3. Groups involved in enhancing the process of primary care include Emphysema Anonymous, The Arthritis Foundation, The American Diabetes Association, and The Lupus Foundation.

4. Groups concerned with rehabilitation include Mended Hearts, Stroke Club, United Ostomy Association, and the International Association of Laryngectomies.

5. Groups concerned with social survival include the National Organization for Women, Welfare Rights Organizations, the Gay Activists' Alliance, and the National Alliance for the Mentally Ill.

6. Groups concerned with personal growth and self-actualization include consciousness-raising groups, Integrity Groups, and the La Leche League.

THE PROCESS OF CHANGE

The recognition and use of peer group experience

to produce change in attitude and behavior was suggested by Adler, Sullivan, and Lewin. Adler believed that people improved in therapy by integrating their private interests with community feeling. Sullivan recognized the important effect upon an individual's self-esteem of the reflected appraisals of others. Lewin held that people were more likely to make important adjustments in their lives when they belonged to a group of others in the process of making similar changes.

Groups under stress and in situations where there is a scarcity of resources pull together and adopt problem-solving orientations as long as their efforts are at least moderately successful. An important step is to involve individuals in the issue being discussed. The more central an issue is to an individual's deeply held values and the more frequently others try to convince them of the issue's importance, the more likely they are to adopt it as their own. Some people will take greater risks when the action in question is confidently advocated by a trusted group member. Self-help groups are led by volunteers who encourage members to help one another, urge maximal participation of each in the groups' activities, and recognize the importance of self-education and self-determination. The very act of helping others may lead to important behavioral changes or "self-persuasion through advocacy" (Riessman, 1965).

A crucial variable affecting individual participation, group productivity, and morale is the opportunity for members to participate in decision making—to take the pledge together. This principle is exemplified by Alcoholics Anonymous (AA) as members take the pledge of sobriety and together agree to follow the Twelve Steps. The degree of individual behavior change may be enhanced even further by group discussion and public commitment, supplemented by group consensus regarding a particular course of action, in this case the promise to remain sober.

Thus, during World War II, Lewin found that a group decision process was 10 times more likely to influence housewives to change their patterns of eating and baby feeding than a course of formal instruction. Group discussion methods were also found more effective than formal instruction in persuading shop foremen to change their rating practices of workers. In a study described by Green and co-workers, asthmatic emergency room patients were organized into small groups and given five health education sessions, after which the group as a whole was directed to agree on the most effective means of managing the acute effects of their illness. Four months later, those patients who had received the service had visited the emergency room half as frequently as the patients in the control group (Green et al., 1977). Similarly, Caplan and co-workers compared the impact of a short-term, six-session support group experience upon the adherence of hypertensive patients to their regimens with patients receiving standard health instruction and those receiving treatment as usual (patients attended the support groups as dyads, the other person usually being the spouse). A statistically significant improvement in adherence was found for patients in the support groups and health instruction classes taken together, as compared with the control.

Small organizations can only continue to pursue their goals by actively recruiting new members, and by teaching them the group's norms, goals, and problem-solving strategies. The goals, however, must be such that they remain forever unattained, since final resolution would threaten the group's further existence. Since there will always be people with addictive conditions and chronic illnesses, and those who feel a sense of social stigma due to their condition, this will guarantee a potential supply of new members. Likewise, the beliefs that one bears the cross of alcoholism for life and that the road to recovery lies through public surrender of control over the bottle to a "power greater than ourselves" and the pledge to follow religiously the Twelve Steps and Twelve Traditions, serve to tie the person to AA and thereby assure the organization's continued existence. The longevity of AA is in no small measure due to its having developed this tradition, which is effectively passed on to every new member who joins and takes the pledge of sobriety.

These traditions are passed on to new members through written materials describing the organization's purpose, through formal initiation rites, and informally through preceptorship or sponsorship with one of the group's elders. Thus, as members grow with the organization, they may be given greater responsibilities and accorded commensurate respect, having risen from the inferior position of novitiate or child to that of priest, elder, or parent to succeeding generations of alcoholics.

SOURCES OF CHANGE

The sources of individual change in self-help groups may be viewed from emotional, cognitive, and behavioral perspectives (Barish, 1971; Borkman, 1976).

Emotional

The group experience provides warmth, empathy, understanding, and encouragement. As a nurturing peer, friend, or sibling-level subsystem, it offers its members co-equal, unconditional care and concern. As self-help groups serve to help members make the transition from the margins of society toward more normative social roles or toward a more normal definition of a deviant social status, they may provide the powerful primordial social bond, *communitas*, thus affording the opportunity for people to become peculiarly spontaneous, free, and open with one another.

Cognitive

The experience helps to validate members' sense of self-worth by providing the opportunity to perceive oneself among others with similar conditions, rather than in comparison to normals without the condition. By thus providing members with a new reference group among whom the open declaration of deviance becomes a declaration of commonality and community, there occurs a considerable reduction of felt alienation and anomie.

Behavioral

Strengthened by these emotional and cognitive changes, members are free to provide one another with mutual help. They exchange coping strategies (experiential knowledge), give advice, share equipment, teach one another skills, and make friends. In this way, self-help groups become an arena for social experimentation and relations.

COMPARISONS WITH OTHER CHANGE-ORIENTED GROUPS

Self-help groups, in contrast to encounter groups and therapy groups, appear to effect change through a critical alteration in self-perception made possible by the shared condition and group support. Encounter groups emphasize the expression of intense interpersonal feelings and critical comments, and often exert pressure on members to solve problems. Only in the behaviorally oriented self-help groups are members held accountable for making substantive behavioral changes. In the large majority of self-help groups, members are encouraged to set personal goals but are rarely brought severely to task for not accomplishing them. Therapy groups emphasize shared self-disclosure, interpretation, guided fantasy, and even psychodrama. Since self-help groups frequently are leaderless, group processes requiring central control (e.g., interpretation, behavior prescription, feedback, punishment, confrontation) are seldom practiced.

What has been described of the self-help process is a non-directive, non-threatening process of reorientation occurring within a safe, comfortable, and reassuring human group, emphasizing the importance of mutual aid. As such, it is the very antithesis of professional help, for persons seeking aid from professionals place themelves in subservient positions, where they feel compelled to accept the professional's definition of the problem and the way toward its solution. While pointing the way toward recovery or normality, the professional also provides the patient access to expert advice and the latest technology. Early outcome research indicates that participants in self-help groups report enhanced self-esteem and self-respect, a greater sense of self-reliance and mastery, and a greater level of empathy for others (Lieberman and Borman, 1979). Self-help groups thus provide no specific advice but, rather, a sense of realistic hope, and often provide cause for optimism which may lend demoralized and despairing individuals the will to participate more actively in their own care.

Professionals and Self-help Groups

There would be little point in writing a chapter on self-help groups in a book directed primarily toward working clinicians if the crucial issue of professional involvement in what is essentially a nonprofessional arena were not addressed. While many self-help groups specifically exclude professional participation except for providing consultation (particularly the consciousness-raising groups and the Anonymous groups), others were started by professionals, and many more actively seek professional advice and board membership. There remains an important and substantial segment of potential self-help consumers whose condition renders them either incapable of initiating or maintaining group activities (e.g., stroke victims and persons with schizophrenia, dementia, or retardation) or unmotivated to begin them (e.g., the often demoralized relatives of these persons). In these instances, there appears to be a definite need for ongoing professional support and assistance.

Possible professional roles include the following (Gartner and Riessman, 1977; Silverman, 1980):

REFERRAL

Realizing that many self-help group members have positive attitudes toward professionals, physicians and other health care workers are beginning to refer persons with addictions and chronic, debilitating conditions to self-help groups.

CONSULTATION

Many self-help groups welcome speakers on topics of concern to their members. These groups may actively seek out professionals with relevant expertise, or the professionals themselves can initiate the contact.

BOARD MEMBERSHIP

Many health professionals serve as members of professional advisory boards. In this capacity, they are occasionally called upon to provide the membership with advice and guidance.

LEADERSHIP AND GUIDANCE IN THE START-UP PHASE

Here, professionals may provide facilitator training, teach self-help skills, accelerate the feeling of mutuality, serve as role models, and further engender an over-all vision. Professionals can also provide important information, correct misinformation, and help identify priorities and goals (Cole et al., 1979; Silverman, 1980). A particular difficulty which professional facilitators encounter is not being able to relinquish the leadership role. One's primary purpose here is to encourage member initiative and to train members as group facilitators and leaders, as authority is eventually transferred from professional to member control and leadership. Experienced group therapists may find this process to be particularly difficult, while experienced agency consultants, accustomed to brief encounters, may find the process more congenial.

The following guidelines for facilitator intervention have been written to further clarify the kinds of intervention appropriate for self-help groups.

1. Display an attitude of warmth toward group members, and an interest in group members' problems which is communicated by feedback statements such as, "My understanding of what you are concerned about is . . . ."

2. Keep group members actively involved with one another by encouraging them to talk with one another about their problems.

3. Encourage group members to help one another by sharing similar experiences of living with the particular condition or illness.

4. Foster the notion that group members are experts in the art of coping with some aspect of their shared condition.

5. Reframe member narratives with an emphasis on how group members share the responsibility for both contributing to problematic situations and potentially changing them for the better.

6. Stress the positive rather than the negative aspect of member motivations and intentions.

7. Encourage group members to seek more effective means of coping with their condition.

8. Refrain from dominating the group process, and prevent any one individual from dominating the group.

9. Correct possible errors in group members' scientific knowledge about the etiology, diagnosis, prognosis, and treatment of the particular condition or illness, and suggest consultation with the appropriate health professional.

10. Suggest that members invite guest speakers and contact other self-help organizations with similar goals.

As with other task groups, the primary goals of the first meeting are to establish an atmosphere of trust and to set group goals. In the case of the latter, this would mean learning more about the shared condition and how the members might learn to cope more effectively with their problems. The professionals may introduce themselves in a more personal fashion than in therapy groups (perhaps recounting some of their own experiences) so the group members might feel more disposed to disclose their own concerns. Written materials may be handed out, including names of relevant professional and lay resources and organizations which might serve as sources of consultation or speakers, and a list of topics pertinent to members' mutual concerns (e.g., medical aspects of their condition, community supports, how family and friends can help, the health consumer movement, and how to become an activated patient).

The first few meetings invariably focus upon members' experience with the illness. These discussions are often quite lively and intense, as some members begin sharing their doubts, uncertainty, hopelessness, guilt, and shame for the first time. Facilitators should assume the attitude that no situation is hopeless and that most things can in some way be improved, whether by reframing the problem and its meaning, eliciting previously unsought assistance, or trying out a new problem-solving strategy. Facilitators should focus on the positive, giving members credit for accomplishing what they have tried, attributing poor outcomes to situations or actions rather than traits of the person, and assuming good intentions and a common interest in discovering new ways to deal with old problems.

In the first several meetings, facilitators should suggest that the mutual aid sessions be punctuated by more formal instruction (conducted by the group facilitators or selected outside speakers) about the biomedical and behavioral aspects of the particular condition and the resulting problems which it poses for both patients and their significant others.

A strong sense of morale and commitment most often develops in these groups, arising from the sharing of common problems. This bond will be heightened further as members give and receive emotional support, information, and advice. This expression of group consciousness and loyalty often occurs sooner than in more traditional therapy groups, where the sense of shared condition and purpose may be neither recognized nor encouraged.

The facilitator's goal is to stimulate an active process of mutual give and take so that the group can assume a caring and supporting function. The group process should more closely resemble that of a community meeting than a therapy group, as members' suggestions are not interpreted but acted upon. For instance, members who ask for refreshments to be served or for a newsletter to be published should be encouraged to head up ad hoc committees for these purposes. To ensure that early initiatives of this kind are successful, it is important for the professionals to make sure that those appointed to such positions have some leadership experience. It may require the utmost in clinical sensitivity and tact to make this determination and then to either gently discourage volunteers who are not ready to shoulder the responsibility or to appoint members with greater competence.

When working to withdraw as primary group leaders, professionals should constantly promote member initiatives to encourage indigenous leadership. Should professional domination continue for too long, the group will remain passive, because the professional leaders have not relinquished their superior positions in favor of peer relationships. Eventually, a point will be reached when the professionals will begin to assume consultant roles and suggest that the group meet for alternate sessions, either in the community or within the health care setting. Formalization of the self-help group may be enhanced by securing positions for elder group members in the volunteer service of the clinic or hospital staff.

Clinical Examples

COMMUNITY INVOLVEMENT GROUP AND STROKE CLUB

In 1974, a Community Involvement Group to accelerate the rehabilitation of recovering stroke victims was established at the New York Veterans Administration (VA) Medical Center. Recognizing these patients' loneliness, isolation, and discouragement—a direct result of their suddenly disabling condition, which abruptly removed them from their working and social world—the group's leaders set out to help them find active alternatives within the community. This group emphasized role playing, structured discussions, and exercises, such as preparing meals. It was led by professionals, yet permitted the sharing of experiential knowledge during regular meetings of stroke victims. As the group neared the end of its third year and members became more competent and

independent, it was decided to start a stroke club for the graduates.

Composed of persons whose disabilities impaired their walking and talking, initiation and maintenance of the stroke club required professional and institutional support. The VA offered free transportation to the monthly meetings at the hospital, and also provided secretarial help and volunteer staff to serve refreshments (which were purchased through funds donated by members and the VA service organizations). With a mailing list of approximately 200, there are now nearly 50 active members. Members live in all five boroughs of New York City, and have participating family members. Non-veterans living in the surrounding community have also been accepted as members.

There is a specific program for each meeting, which generally features a speaker from the hospital professional staff or from one of the agencies working with the handicapped, in addition to parties, dinners, and outings. It took approximately a year for natural leaders to emerge and assume responsibility for planning and running the meetings. Members look forward to these monthly get-togethers and report a new sense of importance, independence, and individuality.

PATIENT-FAMILY SUPPORT PROJECT FOR VICTIMS OF SCHIZOPHRENIA

Rationale

Ongoing outcome research studies suggest that the course of schizophrenic illness can be improved through the combination of neuroleptic medication and social skills training for the patient, combined with health education classes and self-help groups for their relatives and family crisis intervention for the whole family (Anderson et al., 1980).

Workers from the Social Psychiatry Research Institute in London have demonstrated in three separate studies that relapse rates of patients with schizophrenia are higher when family members demonstrate a higher level of expressed emotion (EE), as measured by counting audiotape remarks which indicate criticism of or overprotectiveness toward the patient. Such relatives may regard the patient as indolent (and hence are overcritical) or incurable (hence overprotective). They may then become intrusive, intolerant, oversolicitous, resentful, and guilt provoking. This is all thought to come about because the relatives fail to appreciate and fully understand that the patient is suffering from a disease which produces varying degrees of disability, which are modifiable through medical and social intervention.

Hogarty has shown convincingly that the single most important factor preventing relapse is maintenance of an adequate level of neuroleptic medication. In addition, patients who have been stabilized on neuroleptics are less likely to undergo relapse if they have not had a relapse for 8 months, and if they have been involved in concurrent social therapy (pragmatically oriented individual and family case work).

Medication is thought to exert a protective effect by lowering the patient's level of brain dopamine, thereby lowering the state of arousal and rendering the patient less vulnerable to stressful life events and high EE family responses. The medication may also enable schizophrenic patients to learn new behavioral repertoires through social skills training. Social skills training is designed to improve patients' level of posthospital functioning, and to lower their chances for relapse by giving their family members less opportunity to be critical.

The key to the success of such a program is arranging an intervention which helps the patient's relatives (1) to come to a more accurate understanding of schizophrenia and its treatment and (2) to adopt more tolerant and realistic attitudes toward the patient's at-home behavior. Health education has been employed in many programs which assist patients and their families to understand and cope with the vicissitudes posed by chronic illness and disability. Health education is also seen as a way to increase patient satisfaction and ensure better patient compliance with prescribed medical regimens. Were health education to be provided within the supportive setting of a self-help group composed of relatives with the shared problem of a schizophrenic family member, group members might be more likely to take the first step toward assuming more realistic attitudes toward the patient and his illness.

Multiple family groups have been utilized in the treatment of schizophrenia for nearly 25 years. Their clinically demonstrated effectiveness is thought to spring from a combination of skillful professional leadership and social support. Here, families may receive the benefits of both family therapy and a self-help group. However, if the professionals conceive of their roles as instructors and facilitators (rather than as therapists), they may wish to remove the patients from the group in order to maintain a group focus on mutual learning, rather than immediate control of disorganized behavior (Atwood and Williams, 1978). In a multiple relatives' group, family members with high EE may learn more successful management techniques from low EE group members. This is the rationale for the Patient-Family Support Project, begun at the New York Veterans Administration Medical Center in 1980.

Project description

Eligible patients are recruited from the inpatient service, providing they are under age 50, meet the standards for DSM-III schizophrenia, and have no history of alcoholism, drug abuse, organic brain dysfunction, or mental retardation. Patients are invited for social skills training once in remission from acute psychosis and to medication clinics upon discharge. Relatives are invited to join the education and self-help group (the Relatives Support Project) at the same time the patient joins social skills training. A few group members have been referred directly by relative group members, even though their sons or daughters are not inpatients.

All meetings take place on the same alternate Wednesday evening. As a reminder, postcards are sent to each patient and set of relatives several days before the meeting is held. Patients meet first with the project psychiatrists for medication and then report to the occupational therapist for social skills training. Simultaneously, the relatives meet with the psychiatrist and social worker in a 1½-hour combined class on schizophrenia and its management and self-help group.

The membership is open to any relative of a veteran who suffers from schizophrenia, and the Relatives' Support Group has grown steadily from its inception at a rate of approximately two new families per month. The professional facilitators encourage particularly articulate and skillful group members to lead the session, usually with a description of their own story, focusing primarily on how their views of the disorder and their coping strategies have changed since joining the group. Other relatives are urged to ask questions and describe how the discussions related to their situation.

Primarily for the benefit of new members, the professionals lead the group once every few months and provide relatives with the latest theories and research bearing on the etiology, diagnosis, course, medical treatment, social management, and rehabilitaion of schizophrenia. Members are then provided with handouts emphasizing the main points of the lecture material. These sessions become increasingly lively as the elder members become accustomed to actively participating, which is encouraged and positively acknowledged by the professionals. Other faculty who have spoken on specific topics (e.g., the dopamine theory of schizophrenia) have been impressed with the group members' intensity and seriousness of purpose. In addition, contact has been made with the New York Chapter of Families against Mental Illness and with the National Alliance for the Mentally Ill. As a result, project professionals have spoken at the organizations' meetings, and representatives of the aforementioned oganizations have attended meetings of the relatives' group.

Current plans center around involving certain of the group elders in more formally recognized leadership positions, as the group itself evolves from one dominated by professionals to a true self-help group. Even now, these members are particularly helpful conducting the group process and keeping high EE members from dominating the group discussion with countless illustrations of unsuccessful attempts to help their relatives. A planning committee will be established to decide on the meeting format, contact speakers, collect dues, and provide refreshments, thereby gradually assuming acknowledged leadership of the organization. Institution professionals who initiated the project will continue to serve as consultants and as teachers of group skills to the indigenous leaders.

Conclusion

Self-help groups are a most valuable adjunct to modern medical practice. Although never intended to replace professional health care, patient response to them has been so overwhelming that they must be reckoned with. It is to be hoped that, in this consumer era, more professionals will become aware of the value inherent in self-help group membership. Self-help groups offer people with chronic conditions a support system which may protect them from emotional stress and provide them with the motivation to make the first steps toward change. The time has surely come for group therapists to become acquainted with the special techniques for consulting to and facilitating the initiation of these unique autonomous organizations.

References

Anderson, C. M., Hogarty, G. E., and Reiss, D. J. Family treatment of adult schizophrenic patients: A psychoeducational approach. Schizophrenia Bull., 6: 490, 1980.

Atwood, N., and Williams, M. E. Group support for the families of the mentally ill. Schizophrenia Bull., 4: 415, 1978.

Barish, H. Self-help groups. Encycl. Soc. Work 2: 1163, 1971.

Borkman, T. Experiential knowledge: A new concept for the analysis of self-help groups. Soc. Sci. Rev., 50: 445, 1976.

Cobb, S. Social support as a moderator of life stress. Psychosom. Med., 37: 300, 1976.

Cole, S. A., O'Connor, S., and Bennett, L. Self-help groups for clinic patients with chronic illness. Prim. Care, 6: 325, 1979.

Gartner, A., and Riessmann, F. Self-help in the Human Services. Jossey-Bass, San Francisco, 1977.

Goffman, E. Stigma: Notes on the Management of Spoiled Identity. Prentice-Hall, Englewood Cliffs, N.J., 1963.

Goldstein, M. J. New Developments in Interventions with Families of Schizophrenics. Jossey-Bass, San Francisco, 1981.

Green, L. W., Werlin, S. H., Schauffler, H. H, and Avery, C. H. Research and demonstration issues in self-care: Measuring the decline of mediocentrism. In Consumer Self-care in Health. United States Government Printing Office, Washington, D.C., 1977.

Katz, A., and Bender, E. I. What makes self-help groups tick. In The Strength in Us, A. katz and E. I. Bender, editors, p. 79. Franklin Watts, New York, 1976.

Killilea, M. Mutual help organizations. In Support Systems and Mutual Help, G. Caplan and M. Killilea, editors, p. 37. Grune & Stratton, New York, 1976.

Lieberman, M. A., and Borman, L. D. Self-Help Groups for Coping with Crisis. Jossey-Bass, San Francisco, 1979.

Riessman, F. The "helper" therapy principle. Soc. Work, 10: 27, 1965.

Sagarin, E. Odd Man In: Societies of Deviants in America. Quadrangle Books, Chicago, 1969.

Silverman, P. R. Mutual Help Groups: Organization and Development. Sage, Beverly Hills, CA, 1980.

B.11 Sensitivity Groups, Encounter Groups, Training Groups, Marathon Groups, and the Laboratory Movement

LOUIS A. GOTTSCHALK, M.D., Ph.D.
EDWARD M. HOUSER, M.S.W.

Definitions

TRAINING LABORATORY

A training laboratory is an educational procedure that aims to create a situation in which the participants, through their own initiative and control but with access to new knowledge and skilled professional leadership, can appraise their old behavior patterns and attitudes, and look at new ones. A laboratory recommends a temporary removal of the participants from their usual living and working environment, where attempts to re-evaluate attitudes or to experiment with new behavior patterns might involve risks and possible punishment. It provides a temporary artificial supportive culture (hence the designation "laboratory") in which the participants may safely confront the possible inadequacy of their old attitudes and behavior patterns and experiment with and practice new ones until they are confident in their ability to use them.

The assumption of the laboratory method is that skills in human interactions are best learned through events in which the learners themselves are involved. The training activities, therefore, are social experiences in which the trainees take part and then reflect on their patterns of participation. Essentially, the laboratory scene provides an occasion for experimental learning.

SENSITIVITY TRAINING

Sensitivity training is any of a set of experiences, including but not restricted to the training group, attempting to help each participant recognize and face, in himself and in others, many levels of functioning (including emotions, attitudes, values, and intellect); to evaluate his behavior in light of the responses it elicits from himself and others at these various levels; and to integrate these levels into a more effective and perceptive self. The term sensitivity group is used interchangeably with the term encounter group.

TRAINING GROUP

The T-group is a relatively unstructured group in which individuals participate as learners. The basic data for learning come from the participants themselves and from their immediate experiences within the group as they interact with each other in the effort to create from their own resources a productive and meaningful group. The experience is designed to provide a maximal opportunity for the participants to expose and analyze personal behavior and group performance, to learn how others respond to their behavior, and to learn effective personal and group functioning.

MARATHON GROUP

This term is used to describe a sensitivity training group that meets continuously for periods of time ranging from approximately 10 to 45 hours. The purpose of this technique is to heighten the impact of sensitivity training by not interrupting the interactions being generated within the group. Members leave the room only for absolutely necessary reasons. Marathons have been used in weekend laboratories, where the total amount of time available is short, and in longer term laboratories, as a device to move the group to a greater depth of involvement and group interaction. Proponents of such groups report heightened emotionality, a greater expression of negative feelings, and a decrease in defensive role playing because of fatigue and nearly constant pressure to be more open.

A variation on the marathon is the weekend encounter group, whose sessions are 3 or 4 hours in length but occur several times during each day and evening of the weekend, with time out for eating, exercise, and sleep. In such a group there are usually many opportunities for formal and informal pairings, triads, and quartets. These small groups, plus the varied activities, allow for normal social relationships. Many trainers believe that, rather than detracting from the pressure-cooker formula of the marathon, these more informal groups allow less threatening relationships to develop. These relationships are then deepened during the formal sessions. The theory is that the participants develop more trust during their informal encounters and, therefore, relax their guard because of lessened fear, rather than heightened external pressure.

Group leaders have experimented with different time formats to ascertain the optimal approach to sensitivity training.

TRAINER

The trainer is the experienced educator within a sensitivity training group who serves as a resource to the group. Since the primary social learning data for the participants come from their own involvement with each other and with the group, the role of the sensitivity training group trainer is different from that of the usual role of an educator. He cannot assume the role of the expert, controlling and directing the group, without making the group dependent on him, thereby undercutting the experience of group responsibility and participation that is supposed to be the primary source of learning data. The trainer, therefore, is supposed to serve as a facilitator, helping the group to make its own decisions and to use its own resources. He does this by calling the attention of the group from time to time to the behavior being exhibited and the relationships emerging in the group and by helping the group to clarify its own goals and procedures. The trainer focuses primarily on here-and-now events and relationships that have been experienced within the life of the group.

Laboratory Training

Classically, three different group activities have been subsumed under laboratory training: (1) the sensitivity, personal encounter, or training group; (2) the task-oriented group involving structured group exercises aimed at teaching group function skills; and (3) intervention laboratories that are established for functional work groups in the community or industry. All three types of group activities may overlap or may be conducted separately.

T-GROUPS VERSUS TRADITIONAL GROUP THERAPY

The overlap between T-groups and group therapy is considerable, and at times they are indistinguishable. The problem is compounded by the fact that T-group leaders vary so much among themselves that one cannot really describe a model or typical T-group. One can only describe typical differences between T-groups and group therapy. In the early days, the distinctions between the two kinds of groups seemed fairly clear. But both the T-group and group psychotherapy have been changing over the past 30 years. Now examples can be cited of therapy groups that follow the T-group pattern and vice versa.

Participants

Traditionally, the T-group is designed for normal people with good ego defenses and good ego-coping skills who can readily learn from experience. The group therapy participant, on the other hand, is selected because he has deficient ego skills and an inability to learn from immediate experience.

Although T-groups may be made up of non-related persons, they may also be concerned with groups of people who work together or have some other ongoing association. Group therapy, in contrast, has traditionally been conducted with persons who had no extra-group relations.

Although T-groups and their variants are used as therapy groups for normals, therapy groups are also used for non-patients, such as wives of alcoholics and parents of neurotic children. The distinction between education, training, and therapy becomes blurred, as does the distinction between patients and non-patients.

Goals

The T-group seeks to heighten interpersonal coping skills, sharpen interpersonal perception, and increase self-awareness and the authenticity of life experiences. In group therapy, these goals may be seen as prerequisite learning that will enable the patient to work out his emotional problems.

However, many T-group trainers have disdained group process or group growth, and see their goal as solely personal change. On the other hand, many group therapists see individual change as accomplished only through effective group process. Hence, their therapeutic effort is directed at maximizing group process. In this instance, the T-group and the therapy group have reversed the traditional stances of both fields.

Leadership

In the T-group, the trainer or leader is seen as a catalyst who may become fairly assimilated into the group—at least in theory. In group therapy, the leader is traditionally a therapist who not only catalyzes group process but also has a responsibility for making the group experience a therapeutic experience for each patient. The therapist can never fully shed his role, even if he attempts to do so.

Yet some T-group trainers see the leadership function as indispensable for effective T-group function; these trainers act in very authoritarian or autocratic roles that give little control to the T-group participants. Other trainers work toward total assimilation and actually give up leadership role and function. Likewise, in group therapy, therapists maintain various degrees of leadership, ranging from those who do individual therapy with a patient while the group watches to those therapists who deal only with group process and never with individual patients. Yet other therapists of existential persuasion move toward assimilation into their therapy groups, with virtually total abnegation of the therapeutic role. In addition, there have been experiments with alternative sessions of therapy groups where the therapist is not present and even experiments with leaderless therapeutic groups.

Duration of the group activity

Typically, T-groups meet for relatively short periods of time from 1 day to a month or two. The therapy group may meet for 1 or 2 hours in weekly sessions over a long period of time, even 4 or 5 years in extreme instances.

There has been emphasis in the laboratory movement on follow-up work. The first T-group experience may be only a part of the task, to be followed by many months of subsequent meetings with the group membership. On the other hand, some therapy groups are conducted on a short-term basis, such as crisis intervention groups, diagnostic intake groups, and marathon therapy groups.

Content of discussion

The T-group has been seen primarily as an arena for the elaboration, analysis, and discussion of conscious thought and feeling, interpersonal interaction, and here-and-now issues. The therapy group has been concerned with the genetic there and then, the intra-personal, the preconscious, fantasy, and dreams. The T-group focuses on "how we function in this group"; the therapy group focuses on "using that group to see how I function."

T-group emphasis on the conscious here and now has remained a major focus, but many trainers have expanded the repertoire of the T-group to the exploration of dreams, fantasy, and primary intrapersonal experiences as relevant to the major focus of the T-group. On the other hand, much of family therapy and group therapy has moved to a here-and-now focus and to an exploration of the interpersonal, with a de-emphasis of the genetic there and then and purely intrapersonal experience.

GOALS AND PURPOSES

Sensitivity training may range in goals between two extremes: (1) the mainly agency-oriented or task-oriented training, so structured as to enlighten the participants concerning more effective communication, problem-solving methods, and leadership patterns, primarily for the purpose of better influencing the environment, particularly other people; and (2) the communion-oriented training, so structured as to give participants a variety of experiences, often nonverbal, which put each participant in touch with inhibited sensory and emotional facets of his personality, not for purposes of influencing people but for purposes of improving his capacity to be closer to others.

Common to both types of groups, regardless of the amount of cognitive and sensory input, is the laboratory or experiential method—learning by doing, practicing, trying different ways of relating to other human beings, getting immediate feedback. Personal growth labs, ordinary marathons, encounter groups, and nude marathons theoretically fall more toward the communion end of the continuum.

TECHNIQUES

Regardless of its type, an experiential group devoted primarily to the actualization of the participants uses certain fundamental attitudes and processes to help its members grow.

The facilitator

The facilitator or trainer is probably the single most influential factor in the group. He interacts as an actual member of the group, although he has the additional responsibilities of seeing that the other members are supported or confronted when necessary, and that the group process continues to offer the members opportunities for growth. He sets the example for emotional expressiveness by his spontaneous affective and intellectual behavior toward the other participants, but he does not behave primarily as a teacher who gives didactic inputs. It is his own openness, his daring to reveal his own feelings and to confront others about theirs, his staying in the here and now that sets the tone for the group and encourages the participants to drop their stereotyped social roles.

Intervention

Interventions unfreeze the attitudes and definitions of people toward themselves and others that block and inhibit their natural growth. In general, as Tate noted, there are two main types of intervention in the group: contrasting and substitution. Contrasting interventions are usually verbal; substituting interventions are usually nonverbal. Contrasting interventions are cognitive; substituting interventions are experiential. Contrasting interventions involve a verbal comparison by a group member or the facilitator between what is actually happening in the group and what another member perceives is happening. Substituting interventions involve introducing experiences for group members from which they may grow. Contrasting interventions help a group member to understand so that he can improve his behavior. Substituting interventions may improve his behavior but not his understanding; what are substituted are experiences he has missed, usually in his early life, or has had infrequently in his development. Substituting interventions provide the participant with new information about himself. Contrasting interventions, on the other hand, usually provide no new information, but help the participant become better at discriminating the veracity of information he possesses.

Stimulation

The facilitator can use some exercises or devices to stimulate experience in the areas of cognition, perception, emotion, and sensation. But the greatest influence for change is the democratic and accepting attitude of the facilitator and the group, rather than any gimmick or device. The exercises are intended only as boosters to launch the group or individual into the orbit of an experience. There are literally hundreds of experiential stimulators. Only a representative few are discussed below.

Cognition stimulation. One of the simplest of the diagrams that explain the purpose of sensitivity training is the Johari Window, so-called because it is the brain-child of Joseph Luft (Jo) and Harrington Ingham (Hari) (see Figure B.11-1).

Sometimes simple explanations of interpersonal exchanges can become meaningful when put in terms of the Parent, Adult, and Child of Berne's transactional analysis, as explained by Harris. By encouraging a group member to question the values and assumptions of the critical or ignoring Parent and the overly rebellious, indulged, or adjusted Child, the facilitator can often make astoundingly good sense for that group member out of an apparently complicated interpersonal or intrapersonal situation.

Perception stimulation. One of the best devices to enlarge one's perception is role playing, which can be done in a number of ways.

One can, for example, follow Shapiro's theory of a number of subselves in the individual—reminiscent of Federn's 1943 concept of multiple ego states in every person—and encourage a member who is having an intrapersonal conflict to role play it by himself (the facilitator acting as coach), using several chairs to represent the selves in conflict and moving from one chair to another as he speaks extemporaneoulsy for each subself. Gestalt therapy methods also fit this category of perceptual expansion. Role training is a psychodramatic technique in which, with the help of other group members, one can play out a conflicted relationship, ask others to play the same scene—handling it as they perceive it—and then try out some of the suggested solutions.

Affect stimulation. The general verbal techniques used by the facilitator to stimulate affect are to keep asking participants for feelings, rather than thoughts, and to serve as a model by showing his own feelings. An attitude of unconditional acceptance and the practice of active listening for feelings as well as for content encourage the expression of affect.

If a member starts to cry, a sympathetic participant may shut off the crying member's feelings too quickly

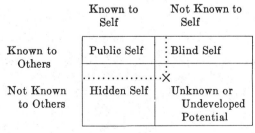

	Known to Self	Not Known to Self
Known to Others	Public Self	Blind Self
Not Known to Others	Hidden Self	Unknown or Undeveloped Potential

Figure B.11-1   The Johari Window is used to explain the purpose of sensitivity training in cognitive terms.

by moving in right away with the Kleenex or a physically comforting gesture. It is often better to let the weeping person experience his sadness in depth before making the comforting gesture.

One method of breaking through the ideational shield into affective states is to have the facilitator sit in front of a group member, take his hands, and ask him how he feels. As the member begins to talk, the facilitator makes him repeat emotional phrases by telling him, "Say it again," sometimes feeding him what he intuitively senses would be appropriate phrases, which the group member may feel free to repeat or reject. By having the group member talk constantly on a feeling level, the facilitator frequently breaches the barrier to affect, and much emotion pours out.

Sensation stimulation. Gestalt therapy has particularly emphasized getting in touch with the senses in order to function fully as a person. Perls had a famous dictum: "You must lose your mind to come to your senses."

The child in each person can be revived joyously if he allows himself to re-experience child-like modes of relating. Perls, Hefferline, and Goodman developed special exercises to revive the senses of taste, touch, smell, sight, and sound. Encounter groups have taken these and similar experiential exercises into their repertoire of anti-repression devices. In one exercise to help revive the sensation of taste, the group members eat a silent meal together, concentrating on the food, its taste, and its texture. Smelling various substances while blind-folded or paying attention to the smells of the earth, grass, flowers, and trees may make group members feel more alive again by re-establishing their union with nature, a union often repressed from childhood.

An artist may make a great contribution to the experience of a group by pointing out different designs, shadings, colors, and textures in the environment, or by sitting in a group and drawing his impressions of members, their poses, and their interactions and then discussing his perceptions with the group. Group members often benefit from being encouraged to look at each other, to consider carefully which side of another person's face seems more dominant, and to examine the texture of someone's skin.

Nonverbal techniques for special situations

Some nonverbal exercises are helpful for group members who need to experience and fulfill directly, more than to talk about, some deeply personal need.

The outsider. He seems to stay aloof from the group, he does not join in, he does not respond to encouragement by the group to participate. Particularly—but not necessarily—if he himself admits to feeling left out, the following exercise can be explained to him, and the group can then carry it out without words.

The group forms a very tight circle, with arms locked around each other. The outsider is placed physically outside of the circle and is told that he must break through to the center in any way he chooses, except that he may not physically hurt anyone. The group cohesiveness ensures his having to work hard to get in.

The non-truster. Several simple experiences may become turning points in the non-truster's group life. In one, the subject, eyes closed, stands 18 inches or more in front of someone strong enough to support him. Facing away from this partner, at a signal or when he and his partner are ready, he falls backward into the arms of his catcher, who must, of course, not let him down. After several instances of giving himself in this vulnerable way to another person, the non-truster is much more likely to allow himself to be vulnerable in other ways with the group.

Another exercise that develops trust is the blind walk, in which one person, eyes closed, is led by his partner through a house, outside into the garden, up and down steps, and so forth. The non-truster completely relies on his partner not to let him trip or hurt himself. This exercise is particularly helpful for people who are anxious about being dependent or submissive.

The timid person. A humorous and noisy exercise to use when someone in the group speaks timidly or seems unable to show aggression or self-assertion is the karate-chop experience. In this exercise, the facilitator or an assertive group member stands facing the timid person, and the two pretend to be karate antagonists, making fake karate chops and kicks at each other, without touching but yelling the karate "Hai!" as loudly as possible with each chop. The group vocally encourages the timid one to yell more loudly, to be "vicious," and to let go. The usual result of such an exercise is increased acceptance by the timid person of his aggressiveness.

General group inhibition or warm-up. A series of 2- to 4-minute nonverbal exercises helps in warming up a cold group. The following are a few suggestions:

1. The group members choose partners. One rolls up in a ball on the floor, and his partner unravels him while he resists strongly. Then the partners reverse roles.

2. One partner plays dead and takes on the waxy flexibility of the catatonic. The other partner places him in different positions, finally putting him in an appropriate rest-in-peace position.

3. Partners, lying on their stomachs and facing each other, arm wrestle while making great grunts and groans of anguish.

4. Partners sit on the floor back to back, arms engaged, and try to "talk" with their backs.

5. Partners sit facing each other, eyes closed, and explore each other's hands, arms, faces, necks. Or they "talk" with their hands.

6. Partners lie with heads on each other's shoulders, bodies at 180 degrees to each other, eyes closed, listening to music while each has a fantasy about the other. When the music stops, they share their fantasies, first with each other and then with the group.

After each of these exercises, the partners talk to each other about their experiences. During the exercise itself, however, no words are said, although appropriate sounds are permissible.

Sociometric feedback

The following problem is posed to the group:

All of you have been together on a ship that has just sunk. You [point to one member] have just found a small life raft capable of holding three other people. Ahead is an island on which you can live fairly comfortably; but, because it is out of the shipping lanes, you will have to be there at least 6 months. What three other people in this group will you ask to join you on the raft, row to the island, and live there together? What do you expect of them during that 6-month period? [Build in your own questions.]

Each person in the group announces his choices and talks about his decision with the group. Often someone is left out by everyone else. This can be turned into a growth experience for the person left out as he discusses his feelings and gets honest feedback from the group about why he was avoided. The difficulties and style of choosing companions with whom to live become sources of confrontation and feedback.

Group cohesiveness and humor

This exercise is a delightful version of the island fantasy, particularly after the group has become fairly cohesive and needs a release from tension. The group members lie on the floor in a close circle, with their heads as the axis in the center, bodies extending out, eyes closed. They are asked to have a fantasy about their life together on a lush tropical island, where food, water, and weather are no problems. Once someone starts the fantasy, each person spontaneously adds whatever occurs to him. The project usually becomes a warm, affectionate, sometimes moving, often hilarious experience of joy, humor, and closeness. The facilitator may bring the exercise to a close by some appropriate fantasy, such as the group's being picked up by a passing ship. Very often no one wants to leave the island.

TECHNICAL AND POLICY ISSUES

Sociopathic leadership

What about ensuring against sociopathic leadership? There is no clearly identifiable professional or institutional base for the recruitment, training, and practice of laboratory practitioners. Trainers are recruited from a variety of disciplines, backgrounds, and experiences. Their training is varied. Their practice is extremely variable. Within the laboratory movement, this variability is perceived both as a strength and as a weakness—but it does present problems. Without an identifiable discipline, there are no norms for performance, no explicit forms for evaluation. Instead, shifting social sanctions support or undermine the context of training laboratory practice. The lack of disciplinary identity also presents problems in terms of clinical issues. The laboratory movement has yet to acquire a professional status. The issues confronting professionalization are complex, for the movement does not have a relatively uniform ideological base, nor are its goals confined to a narrow range of clinical or organizational concerns. Consequently, the laboratory movement has continued to develop apart from more structured and institutionalized concerns of university departments, well-delineated research fields, and the clinical professions. Schools of education and schools of business administration represent the major sources of institutional and professional support.

Strong leadership

If one is a participant in a group with a strong, professionally trained leader, how does one distinguish the group process from group therapy? As noted earlier, the boundaries between the training group and the traditional therapy group are blurred. This blurring of distinctions can have some serious consequences for some group participants. In contrast to most psychotherapies in which a patient asks to be changed in some respect—to be relieved of distressing symptoms or what he regards as personality or behavioral deficiencies—the training group participant does not regularly frame his goals in such terms. Rather, he may want to learn about groups, his behavior in groups, and how to improve his functioning in groups. When the training group is under way, a participant may find that he is being induced to change in ways he did not anticipate. He may find that the trainer and various group members are calling on him to stop certain ways of behaving, talking, thinking, and feeling, and that different ways of behaving are being prescribed. The pressure of the group and trainer may not necessarily be in the same direction. Or, the trainer's silence may mistakenly be taken as a sanction, endorsement, or recommendation for behavioral change made by one participant with regard to another. Some of the T-group participants may become seriously upset under such pressure to alter their identity, especially when they do not recognize this identity as a problem or difficulty and when they have not even thought of trying to modify some aspects of their identity.

Authenticity

Regardless of the type or caliber of leadership and intensive group experience, what is authenticity with respect to personality? A key goal of all laboratory training has been called authenticity in interpersonal relations. This term signifies a relationship that enables each person to feel free to be himself and communicate openly with himself and others. Authentic, in this sense, refers to conscious or readily accessible emotions and thoughts, and not to those that are unconscious and, hence, not easily available to awareness. Thus, a person could be encouraged to be more open and express some usually withheld hostility. This change could be labeled as becoming more authentic from the viewpoint of laboratory training, but underlying this hostility might be discovered, possibly through psychoanalytic therapy, a more valid emotional love and yearning for others but an anxiety over revealing it. The hostile emotion would then be a defensive emotion—the psychological mechanism of turning into the opposite. Although authentic, in the sense of being part of the individual's personality facade or character armor, the hostility would not typify the deeper, basic emotional need of the person.

Authenticity relates in part to what one is really like behind one's facade. One's facade, however, is also very much a part of oneself, and many people fail to realize that this facade was socially acquired and need not, in every respect, be ready for the rubbish heap. Characteristic ways of relating to one another may be socially useful and reflect conventional ways that human beings, in Western culture, relate to and communicate with one another. Many of these traits can be so inflexible and ritualized that the more spontaneous, emotion-laden, or healthy impulsive aspects of a person are never permitted to appear. On the other hand, indiscriminate, sensual, aggressive, disorganized, and chaotic thinking or other kinds of expressive behavior are not necessarily more authentic.

FACTORS AFFECTING OUTCOMES

Several recent research studies have focused on the effects that various factors can have on the outcome of laboratory training groups. Group leadership, pretesting, subject attitude toward the type of group approach utilized, locus of control, and the cognitive style of the trainee are some of the areas which have been examined.

The impact of group leaders on laboratory training groups is one of the variables looked at in the major Stanford study of encounter groups. Six different leadership types are identified and their short-term and long-term effectiveness described. Leader types are labeled Energizers, Providers, Social Engineers, Impersonals, Laissez-faires, and Managers. Providers, individually focused leaders who gave love, as well as information and ideas about how to change, were most effective in producing positive changes and minimizing negative outcomes.

Those leaders described as Managers, who exercised an unusual degree of control over how, about what, and for how long members interacted with one another, were shown to be the least positively effective. The study sought to identify specific effects of group leaders in terms of value and attitude change, behavior change, effect of leader behavior on self-esteem, changes in perceptions of others, and effect on external relationships. Four basic dimensions underlie various leader behaviors: stimulation, executive function, caring, and meaning attribution. Beneficial effects are associated with caring and meaning attribution while excessive stimulation and inordinate attention to executive function are associated with negative outcomes. Over-all attempts to relate particular areas of change with style of leadership were disappointing. Systematic relationships between leader style and outcome effects were few except in the area of values and attitudes. It is perhaps more useful to think of effect of leadership in terms of over-all impact on learning rather than in terms of specific ways in which people may change.

The TIE (Talent in Interpersonal Exploration Groups) project at Berkeley, California, also investigated the effect of leadership in laboratory training groups. One of the members of the project staff, Charles Alexander (1980), has discussed the effect of leader's confrontation and member change. Alexander concluded from his study that the most effective group leaders practice positive confrontations. They are perceived as highly energetic, supportive, and flexible in their style. They provide stimulation for the group, opportunity for emotional expression, and closeness.

Other studies of the effect of leadership on outcomes have included investigation of the sex variable, the effect of

leadership experience in maintaining a therapeutic orientation in encounter groups, the effect of natural social skills on success in volunteer student leaders, and the usefulness of tape recordings as a replacement for group leaders.

Summary

To summarize the assets and liabilities of the T-group methods, one may state that the T-group presents a powerful means of involving people in human behavioral analysis. The method provides possibilities for a highly significant contribution to the humane quality of existence in Western culture and its various work and community components. The training laboratory has potential as a powerful instrument. Its liabilities lie in the area of utilization, as with any powerful instrument. Without adequate training, supervision, and guidelines, a powerful instrument may be destructive, just as a valuable drug may have undesirable effects if used unwisely or in incorrect doses. The liabilities are not intrinsic deficits; rather, they are deficits of training, experience, clarity, and precision of goals. They can be avoided. Leaders within the laboratory movement are addressing themselves to the task.

Of more concern are the peripheral and derivative products of the laboratory movement—groups that have picked up bits and pieces of the laboratory movement but without the democratic concerns of the originators, without the clinical experience of the early leaders, without the informal communicative guidelines that tend to keep professionals within a self-corrective framework, and without the continuous inquiring, self-critical, self-evaluative, and research perspective.

SENSITIVITY TRAINING AS BRAINWASHING

Sensitivity training has sometimes been attacked by ultra-conservative groups as a form of Communist brainwashing. But brainwashing is the use of educational procedures, including some principles of psychology and psychiatry, to interfere with normal, healthy interpersonal relationships, particularly at the individual level, for the purpose of physically and ideologically manipulating the recipients. Sensitivity training, on the other hand, is the use of educational procedures, including some principles of psychology and psychiatry, to develop open, accepting, and spontaneous interpersonal relationships, particularly at the individual level, for the purpose of helping people to understand both individual and group behavior, thereby freeing them from being manipulated or manipulating without their knowledge, and to experience warm personal relationships with other people.

The purpose of brainwashing is indoctrination, leading to the acceptance of a closed system of values. The purpose of sensitivity training is the development of awareness and acceptance of the feelings of oneself and others and the acceptance of responsibility for one's own acts, leading to clearer, independent thinking and realistic behavior. With sensitivity training, a person develops a better understanding of group dynamics and individual motivation.

Both brainwashing and sensitivity training are usually carried out in small groups of 10 to 16 people.

The main difference between brainwashing and sensitivity training lies in their purposes. Brainwashing is an agency-oriented method to bring people into a completely dependent and selfish relationship with the ideological leaders while breaking down kinship among peers so that the individuals composing the group can be manipulated at the leader's will. Sensitivity training is a communion-oriented method that encourages responsibility for one's own actions, a spirit of inquiry among group members, a sense of empathy and identity among peers, a spirit of collaboration with each other and with the leader, a strong sense of belonging and participation. The result of brainwashing is distrust, defensiveness, isolation, and lack of empathy. The result of sensitivity training can be increased trust, openness, a sense of belonging, and empathy.

POPULARIZATION OF AWARENESS TRAINING

Large-scale awareness training programs have evolved from the original T-groups. Organizations such as Silva Mind Control, Actualizations, Lifespring, and Erhard Seminars Training (est) are examples of this phenomenon. Some have become multimillion dollar businesses (Puishes, 1980).

The est organization has attracted much attention, perhaps because it was one of the earliest and most successful. Several books and a number of articles have been written about est, thus making it considerably easier to discuss than are the others. One need not apologize for success. However, serious concerns have been raised about some aspects of the est program.

Tens of thousands of people have taken the est training since its inception in 1971. Many of the trainees have been satisfied with the difference in their lives through "enlightenment" or "transformation" which is accomplished in 60 to 70 hours over two consecutive weekends with optional follow-up seminars.

The est approach draws from a combination of Eastern philosophy, transactional analysis, Gestalt therapy, Jungian psychology, psychoanalytic theory, Scientology, Mind Dynamics, meditation, and positive thinking. The seminar trainers, as described by those who have participated in the program, seem to fit somewhere between the types of leadership described as Energizers and Managers. Such leaders are characterized as charismatic; as intense emotional stimulators; attached to an articulated belief system;

emotionally tied to the founder of their school of thought; as religiosity, proselytizing; as ready, willing, and able to lead participants and to turn them on the road to salvation; and as exercising unusual degrees of control on how, about what, and for how long members interact with one another. A relatively large percentage of participants in groups conducted by these types of leaders were identified as casualties.

References

Alexander, C. Leader confrontation and member change in encounter groups. J. Humanistic Psychol., 20: 41, 1980.

Anderson, J. D. Growth groups and alienation: A comparative study of Rogerian, self-directed encounter, and gestalt. Group Organizat. Studies, 3: 85, 1978.

Argyris, C. Reflecting on laboratory education from a theory of action perspective. J. Appl. Behav. Sci., 15: 296, 1979.

Back, K. W. The small group: Tightrope between sociology and personality. J. Appl. Behav. Sci., 15: 283, 1979.

Bednar, R. L., and Kaul, T. J. Experiential group research: What never happened! J. Appl. Behav. Sci., 15: 311, 1979.

Blair, M. C., and Fretz, B. R. Interpersonal skills training for premedical students. J. Counsel. Psychol., 27: 380, 1980.

Bradford, L. P. Biography of an institution. J. Appl. Behav. Sci., 3: 127, 1967.

Carkhuff, R. R. Rejoinder: What's it all about anyway? Some reflections on helping and human resource development models. Counsel. Psychol., 3: 79, 1972b.

Cooper, C. L. Risk factors in experiential learning groups. Small Group Behav., 11: 251, 1980.

Curran, J. P., Gilbert, F. S., and Little, L. M. A comparison between behavioral replication training and sensitivity training approaches to heterosexual dating anxiety. J. Counsel. Psychol., 23: 190, 1976.

DeJulio, S. S., Lambert, M. J., and Bentley, J. Personal satisfaction as a criterion for evaluating group success. Psychol. Rep., 40: 409, 1977.

Galinsky, M. J., and Schopler, J. H. Warning: Groups may be dangerous. Soc. Work, 22: 89, 1977.

Glass, L. L., Kirsch, M. A., and Parris, F. N. Psychiatric disturbances associated with Erhard seminars training. I. A. report of cases. Am. J. Psychiatry, 134: 245, 1977.

Goodstein, L. D., and Dovico, M. The decline and fall of the small group. J. Appl. Behav. Sci., 15: 320, 1979.

Hartley, D., Roback, H. B., and Abramowitz, S. I. Deterioration effects in encounter groups. Am. Psychol., 31: 247, 1976.

Kilmann, P. R., and Sotile, W. M. The marathon encounter group: A review of the outcome literature. Psychol. Bull., 83: 827, 1976.

Kinder, B. N., and Kilmann, P. R. The impact of differential shifts in leader structure on the outcome of internal and external group participants. J. Clin. Psychol., 32: 857, 1976.

Kirsch, M. A., and Glass, L. L. Psychiatric disturbances associated with Erhard seminars training. II. Additional cases and theoretical considerations. Am. J. Psychiatry, 134: 1254, 1977.

Monti, P. M., Curran, J. P., Corriveau, D. P., and DeLancey, A. L. Effects of social skills training groups with psychiatric patients. J. Counsel. Clin. Psychol., 48: 241, 1980.

Puishes, D. S. Erhard seminars training (est): A theoretical and empirical inquiry. Diss. Absts. Int., 40: 3417, 1980.

Scheidlinger, S. Therapeutic group approaches in community mental health. Soc. Work, 13: 87, 1968.

Simon, J. Observations on 67 patients who took Erhard seminars training. Am. J. Psychiatry, 135: 686, 1978.

Smith, P. B. Are there adverse effects of sensitivity training? J. Human. Psychol., 15: 29, 1975a.

Smith, P. B. Controlled studies of the outcomes of sensitivity training. Psychol. Bull., 82: 597, 1975b.

Zander, A. The study of group behavior during four decades. J. Appl. Behav. Sci., 15: 272, 1979.

B.12 Psychodrama

ZERKA T. MORENO

Introduction

Psychodrama represents a major turning point away from the treatment of the individual in isolation and toward the treatment of the individual in groups, from treatment by verbal methods toward treatment by action methods.

Psychodrama and Universals

The objective of psychodrama was, from its inception, to construct a therapeutic setting that uses life as a model, to integrate into the setting all the modalities of living—the universals of time, space, reality, and the cosmos—including all the details and nuances of life.

TIME

To what extent does time enter into and function in psychotherapeutic settings? Man lives in time—past, present, and future. He may suffer from a pathology related to each dimension of time. The problem is how to integrate all three dimensions into significant therapeutic operations. It is not sufficient that they figure as abstract references; they must be made alive within treatment modalities. The psychological aspects of time must reappear in toto.

The past

In orthodox Freudian psychoanalysis, time is emphasized in terms of the past. Freud found going back and trying to find the causes of things of particular interest. Psychoanalysts went back further and further—into the womb and, if possible, even beyond that—until they tired of this futile search.

The present

However important the past is as a dimension of time, it is one sided, neglecting and distorting the total influence of time upon the psyche. Time has other important phases, one of which is the present, the here and now. In 1914, Jacob L. Moreno began to emphasize the dynamics of the present and all its immediate personal, social, and cultural implications from the viewpoint of the therapeutic process as it takes place in connection with patients in patient groups—the encounter.

The encounter is a telic phenomenon. The fundamental process of tele is reciprocity—reciprocity of attraction, rejection, excitation, inhibition, indifference, and distortion.

The future

Until recently, the future has also been neglected as a dimension of therapeutic time. Yet it is an important aspect of living; we certainly live a good part of our lives with an eye on the future.

It is one thing to consider the expectancies of future happenings and another to simulate them, to construct techniques that enable one to live in the future, to act as if the future is on hand. With therapeutic future techniques, one can act out a situation expected to happen tomorrow, a meeting with a new friend or an appointment with a prospective employer, to simulate the morrow as concretely as possible so as to predict it or to be better prepared for it.

Many patients suffer from an employment or an unemployment neurosis. They are anxious about getting a job, or about an interview with a boss to ask for higher wages. In psychodrama, the therapist rehearses such a patient in advance for what may happen; it is a rehearsal for life. This rehearsal-for-life technique is also effective with patients concerned over affairs of the heart—whether it be a prospective marriage, a divorce, or a new baby. The problem is how to integrate these expectancies and concerns of the patient into the therapeutic operation as actualities so as to be of value for both client and therapist.

SPACE

Space, too, has been almost entirely neglected as a part of the therapeutic process. If you go into a psychoanalyst's office, you find an abstract bed, a couch, but the rest of the office space is not related to the therapeutic process. The patient is language centered, and the therapist is centered to listen. If you go into an office in which one of the current varieties of psychotherapy is practiced, you may find only a chair. The space in which the patient experiences his trauma has no place in that setting.

The idea of a psychotherapy of space has been pioneered by psychodrama, which is action centered and which comprehensively tries to integrate all the dimensions of living into itself. When a patient steps into the therapeutic space, the therapist insists on a description of the space in which the ensuing scene is to be portrayed—its horizontal and vertical dimensions, the objects in it, and the distance and relationship of the objects to one another. The configuration of space warms up the protagonist to be and to act as himself in an environment modeled after that in which he lives.

REALITY

Reality has undergone quite a change in the last 40 years. As psychiatry takes place more and more in the community, rather than in hospitals, reality begins to attain new meanings. The trend is very much along the lines of confrontation and concretization.

Infra reality

The reality of a psychoanalyst's office, from the point of view of therapy, is reduced, an infra reality. The contact between doctor and patient is not a genuine dialogue but is more of an interview, a research situation, or a projection test. Whatever is happening to the patient—for example, a suicidal idea or a plan to run away—is not a phase of direct actualization and confrontation but remains on the level of imagining, thinking, feeling. To an extent, this is also true of the reality in the office of the patient-centered, existential, or interview therapist.

Actual reality

The next step is the reality of life itself, of the everyday lives of all people: how they live in their own homes, in their businesses, and in their relationships to all those who affect their lives—their husbands, wives, children, employers, teachers, clergymen—and to the world at large.

The manner in which they live in reality, their relationships with the significant people in their lives, may be defective or inadequate, and they may wish to change, to attempt new ways of living. But change can be both threatening and extremely difficult, to such an extent that they stay in their familiar ruts, rather than risk a calamity they cannot handle. Thus, a therapeutic situation is needed in which reality can be simulated so that people can learn to develop new techniques of living without risking serious consequences or disaster, as they might if they first tried the techniques in life itself.

Surplus reality

Surplus reality represents the intangible dimensions of intrapsychic and extrapsychic life, the invisible dimensions in the reality of living that are not fully experienced or expressed. The therapist uses certain operations and instruments to bring out these dimensions in therapeutic settings.

Role reversal. One of the most popular surplus-reality techniques in psychodrama is that of role reversal. If a husband and wife fight in the reality of daily life, each remains in his own role, in his own life situation. The perceptions, expectations, fears, and disappointments of each remain unchanged. And even if both parties come to some point of agreement, they still maintain the same relative status: The husband remains the husband, the wife remains the wife. But in role reversal the wife takes the part of the husband, and the husband takes the part of the wife. Not only must they do this nominally, but each one must try to feel his way into the thinking, feeling, and behavior patterns of the other. This technique is particularly useful in situations that are provoked by stress.

It is not always easy to establish identity with one's own self at a certain time in one's life, to recapture one's own feelings and behavior in a crucial episode—as a child or adolescent, for instance—but it is at least plausible. How then can one establish identity with another person, as one is requested to do in role reversal? It is possible, especially with two people who have lived a long time in intimate ensembles, such as husbands and wives, mothers and children, fathers and sons, sisters and brothers, or very close friends.

Auxiliary ego. One of the basic instruments in constructing a patient's psychodramatic world is that of the auxiliary ego, the representation of absentee people or of delusions, hallucinations, symbols, ideals, animals, and objects. They make the protagonist's world real, concrete, and tangible.

Bodily contact. In the course of making the protagonist's world real and dynamic, numerous problems emerge, as in the use of bodily contact, for instance. Bodily contact has been, to some extent, a taboo in all psychotherapies. Yet, when a nurse sees a patient suffering, she cannot help but touch him and say, "Now, Jack, don't worry; it will be all right." Her touch may mean more to the boy than the words she speaks—not in a sexual way but as a maternal, protective approach to him.

A psychoanalyst who would become in any way physically personal with his patient would be ostracized. But in the psychodramatic approach to human relations, the therapist is interested in following the model of life itself and, within limits, in making therapeutic use of the bodily-contact technique. This technique is obviously contraindicated if it is used to gratify the need of the therapist, but it is indicated if it gives the patient, not only in words but in action, the warmth and immediacy of pulsating life in an area in which he is in need.

Role playing. This is another important surplus-reality technique. Here a person may be trained to function more effectively in his reality role, whether he be employer, employee, student, instructor, parent, child, mate, lover, or friend. In the therapeutic setting of psychodrama, the protagonist is free to try and even to fail in this role, for he knows he will be given the opportunity to try again, to try another interpretation and another, until he finally learns new approaches to the situations he fears, approaches that he can then apply in life itself.

Other techniques. There are still many other effective surplus-reality techniques, such as the empty chair (empty crib, empty pew, empty bed, etc.), the high chair, the magic shop, dream enactment, God technique, existential validation, and the therapeutic community.

WARMING UP

It would be difficult to find an adult who has not witnessed at some time or other an act of warming up. An automobile engine warms up when it is started; track athletes warm up prior to a race; some people make circular motions before signing an important document; singers vocalize before singing a solo. Every act of man begins with warming up.

There is a circular quality in the relationship of warming up and spontaneity. Warming up initiates spontaneity. Spontaneity, in turn, shortens the period of warming up. At times, warming up and spontaneity are so entwined that they seem to be both cause and effect. In a sense, the shorter and more controlled the process of warming up becomes, the greater the degree of spontaneity. Also, the shorter the period of warming up, the more efficient the personality becomes in meeting life situations. The more quickly one can make adjustments prior to beginning a task, the less trial and error is involved in shifting gears, especially in proceeding from one task to another.

One of the goals in creating a good personality is to be aware of and to appreciate the effect of warming up. Efficient warming up may also reduce emotional anxiety. Take, for example, the ubiquitous intrusion of the telephone call. Answering a telephone permits very little opportunity for warming up to the voice on the other end of the line. The usual reinforcement clues, such as the speaker's appearance and the location of the conversation (one expects to talk of bowling in a bowling alley), are absent. The abrupt ring of the telephone, the voice not always clear, the face unseen, and the disruption of one's activity are not designed to aid the answering party in warming up to the conversation. Emotional anxiety may result, therefore, if the individual does not possess adequate spontaneity and an efficient warming-up technique suited to telephone conversation.

Warming up does not mean the same thing as conditioning. Conditioning implies a set relationship between a stimulus and a response. A person may become conditioned to respond to the telephone's ring by arising and answering the call with little or no apparent thought. However automatic that response becomes, he is still confronted with a warming-up task the moment he picks up the telephone. In his conversation he makes preliminary adjustments, and the manner in which he makes them produces reciprocal adjustments in the person calling him. Both prior to the call and during the call, the warming-up process is operating. A conditioned response produces only a singular behavior pattern. Warming up both prepares the subject for the act and is highly involved in structuring the act as it proceeds from singular act to singular act. As the individual warms up to the telephone conversation, he becomes more spontaneous. As he becomes more spontaneous, he continues to warm up to the situation.

CREATIVITY-SPONTANEITY-CULTURAL CONSERVE TRIAD

Creativity

Creativity manifests itself in any series of creative states or creative acts. One example is the creation of new organisms capable of surviving on land at the time that animal life was confined to the sea. A new animal organism arose when it underwent, through the evolutionary process, certain physical changes. This process may be called biological creativity. A second example is the Sermon on the Mount as it emerged, however unformed, for the first time from the mind of Jesus. This is a form of religious creativity. A third illustration is musical creativity, such as the music of

Beethoven's Ninth Symphony at the moment it was being created by him in contrast to the same music as a finished product, separated from the composer himself.

Spontaneity

Creativity is a sleeping beauty that, to become effective, needs a catalyzer. The arch catalyzer of creativity is spontaneity, a form of energy that is unconservable. It emerges and is spent in a moment; it must emerge to be spent and must be spent to make place for new emergence, like some animals that are born and die in the love act. It is a truism to say that the universe cannot exist without physical and mental energy that can be conserved. But it is important to realize that without the other kind of energy, the unconservable one, the creativity of the universe could not start and could not run. Creativity would come to a standstill.

Spontaneity operates in the present. It propels a person toward an adequate response to a new situation or a new response to an old situation. Thus, while creativity is related to the act itself, spontaneity is related to the warming up, to the readiness for the act.

Here follow three types of spontaneity: The first type is a novel response to a situation that is not adequate for that situation. Psychotics, for example, may state that two times two equals five, certainly a novel response but hardly adequate. Children, too, burst with spontaneity and have a wide range of novel experiences, but the creative value of their responses is often doubtful, at least from the point of view of the adult world, just as the creative value of the novel responses of psychotics is doubtful from the point of view of normal people.

The second type of spontaneity is a stereotype variety. It consists of a response that is adequate to the situation but that lacks sufficient novelty or significant creativity to be fruitful for the situation. The comedian's repetitive reaction to a situation soon loses its novelty, and, although it may continue to provoke some laughter, it loses spontaneity with each repetition.

The third type of spontaneity is the high-grade creativity variety of genius. In this type an adequate response is accompanied by characteristics that are both novel and creative. The resulting phenomenon may be in the form of an act or a substantive article, such as a poem, story, art object, or piece of machinery. To be truly spontaneous, the results must be in some way new and useful for some purpose.

Cultural conserve

The finished product of the creative process is the cultural conserve, the latter word coming from *conservare*, to guard. The cultural conserve is anything that preserves the values of a particular culture. It may take the form of a material object—such as a book, film, building, or musical composition—or it may appear as a highly set pattern of behavior—such as a religious ceremony, theatrical performance of a written play, fraternity initiation, or inaugural ceremony for the President of the United States. As a repository of the past, cultural conserves preserve and continue man's creative ego. Without them, man would be reduced to creating spontaneously the same forms to meet the same situations day after day. For example, a cultural conserve such as the dictionary makes it unnecessary for men to redefine words every time they wish to communicate. In addition to providing continuity for the heritage of human existence, the cultural conserve plays an even more significant role as the springboard for enticing new spontaneity toward creativity.

There is a danger in the overreliance of mankind on the cultural conserve. This danger is inherent both in the conserve's state of finality and in its abuse by mankind. Once conserved, spontaneous creativity—however supreme it may be in itself—is, by definition, no longer spontaneous.

ENCOUNTER

In the center of the group process is the concept of the encounter. The term "encounter" covers numerous areas of living. It means to be together, to meet one another, the contact of two bodies, seeing, observing, touching, feeling the other person, withdrawing and uniting, understanding one another, intuitive insight through silence or movement, language or gestures, kiss or embrace, becoming one.

Encounter is a unique experience that occurs only once and is irreplaceable. A touch and contact between two bodies, as in a psychodrama session, is a personal outburst of interaction that is unrehearsed. It is a challenge not only to the acting protagonist but also to all the participants. They witness an experience in the making. Encountering is, therefore, at the core of psychodramatic experience. The encounter comes first. Perception or interpretive analysis comes second. It cannot be exchanged through other forms of expression, other individuals, a book, or a letter.

Encounter means that two persons not only meet but also experience and comprehend one another, each with his whole being. It is not a circumscribed contact like a professional meeting of a therapist with a patient, nor is it an intellectual contact (teacher and pupil) or a scientific contact (a transaction between an observer and an object). The participants in an encounter are not pushed into the situation by an external force. They are there because they want to be there. The encounter is unprepared; it is not conducted or rehearsed in advance. There is in every encounter an element of surprise.

Encounter is essentially different from what the psychoanalysts call transference, and it is also different from what the psychologists call empathy. It does not negate transference, and it does not negate empathy. Rather, it includes transference and empathy and gives them their natural function in the entire process. It moves from I to Thou and from Thou to I. It is two-feeling. It is tele.

TELE

Tele, a term introduced by Moreno (1940), describes such affects as group stability, group cohesion, and group integration. Previously, it has been used not as an isolated term but always in various combinations: telencephalon, telepathy, telephone, television, and the like. Taking over such concepts as transference from the individual situation would not have satisfied the requirements of the group situation. By definition, transference tends to produce dissociation of interpersonal relations. In contrast, tele strengthens association and promotes continuity, security, stability, reciprocity, and cohesiveness of groups. In the construction of a conceptual framework, it is advantageous to introduce concepts that are indigenous to the field, rather than to force alien concepts on a new situation.

Tele is the constant frame of reference for all forms and methods of psychotherapy, including not only professional methods of psychotherapy like psychoanalysis, psychodrama, and group psychotherapy, but also nonprofessional methods like faith healing, and methods that have apparently no relation to psychotherapy, such as Chinese thought reform.

Neither transference nor empathy could explain in a satisfactory way the emergent cohesion of a social configuration. Social configurations consist of two or multiple ways of interaction. They are social wholes, not the point of view of one particular person. Empathy and transference are parts of a more elementary and more inclusive process, tele. It is an objective social process functioning with transference as a psychopathological outgrowth and empathy as an aesthetic outgrowth. The process of reciprocation does not enter into the meaning of empathy, and transference is considered the factor responsible for dissociation and disintegration in social groups. Tele is the factor responsible for the increased mutuality of choices surpassing chance possibility, and responsible for the increased rate of interaction among members of a group.

Tele is the interpersonal experience growing out of person-to-person and person-to-object contacts from the birth level on and gradually developing the sense for interpersonal relations; some real process in one person's life situation is sensitive and corresponds to some real process in another person's life situation, and there are numerous degrees, positive and negative, of these interpersonal relations.

ROLE

Role can be defined as the actual and tangible form that the individual self takes. The role is the functioning form a person assumes in the specific moment he reacts to a specific situation in which other persons or objects are involved. The symbolic representation of this functioning form is perceived by the person and by others. The form is created by past experiences and the cultural patterns of the society in which the person lives, and may be satisfied by the specific type of his productivity. Every role is a fusion of private and collective elements. Every role has two sides, a private and a collective side.

Role versus ego and self

It has been hypothesized that understanding of human behavior is more easily facilitated by means of the role concept than by any other concept. It is a more operational concept that the concept of ego, and more descriptive than the concept of self.

The tangible points of crystallization of the ego are the roles in which it manifests itself. The roles and the relations between them are the most important phenomena within a given culture. It is simpler to speak of the roles of a person than of his ego. Ego has mysterious, metapsychological side orientations. But the expression of behavior in terms of roles is not new. The universal cultivation of drama has made this a part of our common-sense knowledge. Dramatists have repeatedly described in literary terms what today is defined in technical terms. However, such roles as King Lear, Macbeth, and Romeo are not created before the eyes of the audience. The step from the texts of the playwrights to scientific texts requires a return to the original formation of a role in *statu nascendi*.

The approach to the problem of verifying the role process is most promising in experiments with roles in laboratory settings. In such settings, persons are placed in an experimental climate with the task of improvising and creating roles on the spur of the moment. The people who are used for these experiments are required to use their spontaneity, rather than their memory. A psychodramatic theatre can be easily transformed into a laboratory setting by the adequate selection of subjects, controls, recordings, and trained observers.

Role playing comes before the emergence of the self. Roles do not emerge from self; the self emerges from roles. This is, of course, a hypothesis that appeals only to the sociometrist and the behavioral scientist, but that may be rejected by the Aristotelian, the theologian, and the metapsychologist. The sociometrist will point out that the playing of roles is not an exclusively human trait, that roles are also played by animals. They can be observed taking sexual roles, roles of nest builders, and leader roles, for instance.

Role reversal

Role reversal is important both as a learning technique for children and adults, and as a method of therapy for individuals and social groups. Role reversal is the heart of role-playing theory as demonstrated in psychodrama and sociodrama.

Here are some hypotheses about the nature of reversal:

Role reversal increases the strength and stability of the child's ego. Ego is here defined as identity with himself.

Role reversal tends to diminish the dependency of the child on the parent, but it tends also to increase his ability to dominate the parent because the child has gained a profound knowledge of him through inside information.

Frequent role reversal of the child with persons superior in age and experience increases his sensitivity for an inner life more complex than his own. In order to keep up with them on their internal role level, which is far above the overt level of the role, he has to be resourceful. He becomes prematurely skilled in the management of interpersonal relations.

The excess desire to reverse roles with the mother is due to an early appreciation and perception of her roles. Frequency of role reversal with the father increases as the perception of the father's roles becomes clearer to the child.

The technique of role reversal is more effective the nearer in psychological, social, and ethnic proximity the two individuals are: mother-child, father-son, husband-wife.

Role reversal is an effective technique for socializing one ethnic group to the other. The greater the ethnic distance between two social groups is, the more difficult is the application of role reversal.

The empathy of individuals or representatives of groups for the internal experiences of other individuals or representatives of groups—what they feel, think, perceive, and do—increases with the reciprocal perception of the roles in which they operate. Therefore, the training of auxiliary egos and doubles, as well as of psychotherapists in general, is in the direction of increasing their sensitivity.

The empathy of therapists increases with their training in role perception and role reversal.

Role reversal is a risk, and is at times contraindicated when the ego of one person is minimally structured and the ego of the other is maximally structured. Psychotic patients like to play the part of authorities—nurses, doctors, policemen—or of ideal persons—for instance, they like to play God. But when faced with an actual person who embodies authority, they resent interaction and role reversal.

Role reversal is without risk when the two persons who reverse roles with one another are solidly structured.

Rules and Techniques

Psychodrama may be applied as a method of individual treatment—one patient with one director or with one director and an auxiliary ego, or one patient and the director. It may also be applied as a method of group treatment with other patients in the group serving as auxiliary egos for one another. In this fashion, even individual-centered sessions involve other members of the group. They, in turn, derive therapeutic benefit from this auxiliary ego function, thus intensifying the learning of all those present.

RULES

Action

The patient acts out his conflicts, instead of just talking about them. To this end, a special vehicle or psychodrama stage is ideal, since the special vehicle makes for more intense involvement. But the process sometimes has to take place in an informal room or space when no such specially designed vehicle is available. The process also requires a director or chief therapist and at least one trained auxiliary ego, although the director may be forced to act as an auxiliary ego when no one else is available. Maximal learning is achieved whenever such trained assistant-therapist-actors are used.

Here and now

The patient acts in the here and now, regardless of when the actual incident took place or may take place—past, present, or future—or when the imagined incident—which may never take place—was fantasied or when the crucial situation, out of which this present enactment arose, occurred. The patient speaks and acts in the present and not in the past, because the past is related to memory. Speaking in the past tense removes the subject from the immediacy of experience and turns him into a spectator or a storyteller, rather than an actor.

Subjectivity

The patient must act out his truth as he feels and perceives it in a completely subjective manner, no matter how distorted it appears to the spectator. The warming-up process cannot proceed properly unless the patient is accepted with all his subjectivity. Enactment comes first, retraining comes later. The therapist must give him the satisfaction of act completion first, before considering retraining for behavior changes.

Maximal expression

The patient is encouraged to maximize all expression, action, and verbal communication, rather than to reduce them. To this end, delusions, hallucinations, soliloquies, thoughts, fantasies, projections—all are allowed to be part of the production. Restraint has to come after expression, although restraint should never be overlooked. Without, however, getting expression in toto, restraint can be at best only partial.

Inward movement

The warming-up process proceeds from the periphery to the center. The director, therefore, does not begin with the most traumatic events in the patient's life. The beginning is on a more superficial level, allowing the self-involvement of the patient to carry him more deeply toward the core. The director's skills are expressed in the construction of the scenes and in the choice of persons or objects needed to assist the patient in his warming up.

Patient choice

Whenever possible, the patient picks the time, place, scene, and auxiliary ego he requires in the production of his psychodrama. The director serves as dramaturgist in assisting the patient or protagonist. The director and protagonist are partners; at any one moment the director may be more active, but the protagonist always reserves the right to decline the enactment of a scene or to change it.

When the interaction between patient and director becomes negative, with the patient resisting the director as well as the process, the director may do any one of the following: (1) Ask the patient to designate another director if more than one are present; (2) Ask the patient to sit down and watch a mirror production of himself by an auxiliary ego or egos; (3) Turn the direction over to the patient himself, who may then involve others in the group as auxiliary egos; (4) Ask the patient to choose another scene; (5) Explain to the patient why he chose the scene, even though it may not be carried out now; (6) Return to an enactment of the scene at a later time if the patient needs it; and (7) Insist on its enactment if the benefits to be derived for the patient are greater than his resistance.

Restraint

Psychodrama is just as much a method of restraint as it is a method of expression. The repressiveness of our culture has attached to expression a value that is often beyond its actual reward. A greatly underestimated and disregarded application of psychodrama lies in such methods as role reversal and the enactment of roles that require restraint, retraining, or reconditioning of excitability. One thinks especially of the chronic bad actor in life, the delinquent or psychopath, whose ability for self-restraint has not been strengthened by his warming up to stresses in life.

Acceptance of inexpressiveness

The patient is permitted to be as unspontaneous or inexpressive as he is at the time. This rule may seem to be a contradiction of the maximal expression rule, but only apparently so. Maximizing the patient's expression may also refer to his inability to express, his withdrawal, his submerged anger, etc. The therapist must first accept this inability and help the patient to accept himself. Then, gradually, the therapist tries to release the patient from his bonds by such methods as asides, soliloquies, and doubles.

The fact that a patient lacks spontaneity is not a block to psychodramatic production. It is, indeed, the reason for the existence of auxiliary egos—who are trained to support, assist, and strengthen the patient—and techniques such as the soliloquy, the double, the mirror, and role reversal. The person who is unable to be spontaneous as himself, in his own roles, may become extremely spontaneous in role reversal—in the role of his wife, father, baby, or pet dog. His expressiveness grows as his spontaneity increases.

Expressiveness at any price is not necessarily spontaneous. Producing a steady flow of words and actions may be a cover-up for genuine feelings. A patient may be entirely spontaneous, on the other hand, while sitting quietly in a chair or observing others around him.

Interpretation

Interpretation and insight giving in psychodrama are of a different nature from those processes in the verbal types of psychotherapy. In psychodrama one speaks of action insight, action learning, or action catharsis. It is an integrative process brought about by the synthesis of numerous techniques at the height of the protagonist's warm-up. Psychodrama is actually the most interpretative method there is, but the director acts upon his interpretations in the construction of the scenes. Verbal interpretation may be either essential or entirely omitted at the discretion of the director, because his interpretation is in the act. Verbal interpretation is frequently redundant.

Even when interpretation is given, action is primary. There can be no interpretation without previous action. Interpretation may be questioned, rejected, or totally ineffective, but the action speaks for itself. Furthermore, interpretation is colored by the orientation of the therapist. Thus, a Freudian will interpret from a different framework from an Adlerian, Jungian, or Horneyan. But varied interpretations do not in any way change the value of the production itself. They merely put interpretation on a less important rung. At times, indeed, interpretation may be destructive, rather than constructive; it may be that what the patient requires is not analysis but emotional identification.

Cultural adaptations

Warming up to psychodrama may proceed differently from culture to culture, and appropriate changes in the application of the method have to be made. It may be impossible to start a psychodrama in the Congo by verbal exchange; it may be necessary to start with singing and dancing. What may be a suitable warm-up in Manhattan may fall flat in Tokyo. Cultural adaptations must be made. The important thing is not how to begin but what one begins.

Three-part procedure

Psychodrama sessions consist of three portions: the warm-up, the action, and the post-action sharing by the group. Disturbances in any one of these areas reflect on the total process. However, sharing may at times be of a non-verbal nature. The most suitable way of sharing with a protagonist is often a silence pregnant with emotion, going out to coffee together, or making plans to meet again.

Identification with protagonist

The protagonist should never be left with the impression that he is all alone with his type of problem in the group. The director must draw from the group, in the post-action discussion phase, identifications with the subject. This will increase cohesion, broaden interpersonal perceptions, and establish anchorages in the group for mutually satisfying relations among group members.

When no one in the audience openly identifies with the subject, the protagonist feels denuded, robbed of that most sacred part of himself—his private psyche. Then it is the task of the director to reveal himself as not merely in sympathy with the protagonist, but as being or having been similarly burdened. It is not analysis that is indicated here but love and sharing of the self. The only way to repay a person for giving of himself is in kind. Doing so frequently warms up other persons in the audience to come forward in a similar manner, thus involving the audience in a genuine warming up, which once more includes the protagonist and helps to establish closure.

Role playing

The protagonist must learn to take the role of all those with whom he is meaningfully related, to experience those persons in his social atom, to experience their relationship both to him and to one another. Taking this still a step further, the patient must learn to become in psychodrama that which he sees, feels, hears, smells, dreams, loves, hates, fears, rejects, is rejected by, is attracted to, is wanted by, wants to avoid, wants to become, fears to become, or fears not to become.

The patient has taken unto himself, with greater or

lesser success, those persons, situations, experiences, and perceptions from which he is now suffering. In order to overcome the distortions and manifestations of imbalance, he has to reintegrate them on a new level. In role reversal, an excellent method, he can reintegrate, redigest, and grow beyond those experiences that are of negative impact, free himself, and become more spontaneous along positive lines.

Flexibility

The director must trust the psychodrama method as the final arbiter and guide in the therapeutic process. This imperative is so universal that it finds confirmation among psychodramatic director-therapists. When the warm-up of the director is objective, the patient and the group feel the spontaneity of his presence and his availability for their needs. Stated another way, when there is no anxiety in the director's performance, the psychodramatic method becomes a flexible, all-embracing medium leading systematically to the heart of the patient's suffering, enabling the director, the protagonist, the auxiliary egos, and the group members to become a cohesive force, welded together to maximize emotional learning.

TECHNIQUES

Therapeutic soliloquy

A therapeutic soliloquy is the portrayal by side dialogues and side actions of hidden thoughts and feelings, parallel with overt thoughts and actions.

Self-presentation

The protagonist presents himself, his mother, his father, his brother, his favorite professor, etc. He acts all these roles himself in complete subjectiveness, as he experiences and perceives them.

Self-realization

The protagonist enacts, with the aid of a few auxiliary egos, the plan of his life, no matter how remote this plan may be from his present situation. For instance, a patient is actually an accountant, but for a long time he has been taking singing lessons, hoping to try out for a musical comedy part in summer stock, planning eventually to make the theatre his life's work. In psychotherapy he can explore the effects of success in this venture, possible failure and return to his old livelihood, or preparing for still another career.

Hallucinatory psychodrama

The patient enacts the hallucinations and delusions he is at present experiencing, although they may not be so designated by the director. The patient portrays the voices he hears, the sounds emanating from the chair he sits on, the visions he has when the trees outside his window turn into monsters that pursue him. Auxiliary egos enact the various phenomena expressed by the patient and involve him in interaction with them, so as to put the phenomena to a reality test.

Double

The patient portrays himself, and an auxiliary ego also represents the patient, establishing identity with him by moving, acting, and behaving like him.

Multiple double

The protagonist is on the stage with several doubles of himself, each portraying another part of the patient—one as he is now, another as he was 5 years ago, a third as he was when at 3 years of age he first heard that his mother had died, another how he may be 20 years hence. The multiple representations of the patient are simultaneously present and act in sequence, one continuing where the other left off.

Mirror

When the patient is unable to represent himself, in word or in action, an auxiliary ego is placed on the action portion of the psychodramatic space. The patient remains seated in the group portion. The auxiliary ego re-enacts the patient, copying his behavior, trying to express his feelings in word and movement, showing the patient, as if in a mirror, how other people experience him.

The mirror may be exaggerated, employing techniques of deliberate distortion in order to arouse the patient to come forth and change from a passive spectator into an active participant—an actor—to correct what he feels is not the right enactment and interpretation of himself.

Role reversal

The patient, in an interpersonal situation—for instance, in a scene with his mother—steps into his mother's shoes while the mother steps into those of her son. The mother may be the real mother, as is done in psychodrama *in situ*, or she may be represented by an auxiliary ego. In role reversal, the son is now enacting his mother, the mother enacting the son. Distortions of interpersonal perception can be brought to the surface, explored, and corrected in action. The son must warm up to how his mother may be feeling and perceiving him. The mother goes through the same process.

Future projection

The patient portrays in action how he thinks his future will shape itself. He picks the point in time—or is assisted by the director to do so—the place and the people, if any, with whom he expects to be involved at that time.

Dream presentation

The patient enacts a dream instead of telling it. He takes the position he usually has in bed when sleeping. Before lying down and taking this position, he warms up to the setting separately. The director asks him when and where he had this dream, what the room looks like, the location and size of the bed, the color of his pajamas, whether he wears top and bottom or sleeps in the nude, whether he sleeps alone, with the light on or off, with the window open or closed, and how long it normally takes him to fall asleep. In the lying position the patient is asked to breathe deeply and evenly, as he does in sleep, to move in bed as he does ordinarily while asleep, and to relax and let himself drift off as though into sleep.

Dream presentation is the unique contribution of psychodrama to dream therapy. One can go into enactment over and beyond the actual dream, include actual and latent material, and, even more important, retrain the dreamer, rather than interpret the dream for him. Interpretation is in the act itself.

Therapeutic community

This is a community in which disputes and conflicts between individuals and groups are settled under the rule of therapy, instead of the rule of law. The entire population, patients and staff alike, is responsible for the welfare of every other person, each participates in the therapeutic process, and all have equal status.

Hypnodrama

Hypnosis is sometimes induced on the psychodrama stage. The hypnotized patient is free to act and move about. He is given auxiliary egos to help him portray his drama. Hypnodrama is a merging of hypnotherapy with psychodrama.

Psychodramatic shock

The patient is asked to throw himself back into a hallucinatory experience while it is still vivid. He does not describe it; he must act. He puts his body in the position in which it was then, in the space he was in, at the time of day or night when this incident actually occurred. He may select a staff member to re-create the hallucinatory involvement.

The patient may resist being placed again into the horrifying experience from which he has just emerged. His natural bent is to forget, not to talk about it, to leave it behind. He is full of fears that his new-found freedom may be shattered. The mere recall frightens him, and the idea of enactment frightens him still more. The psychodramatic director explains that the purpose is to learn control, not merely to relive the experience, and that reenactment will help him build resources against recurrence.

Once the patient has warmed himself up again into the psychotic state and has thoroughly enacted it, the director stops him and helps the patient realize that he can construct his own inner controls.

Improvisation

The patient is brought into the psychodrama theatre or the life situation without any prior preparation. The director has structured the situation in advance with the aid of auxiliary egos. The subject is then asked to warm up to the situation as he would if it were actually happening to him.

Numerous sets of standard situations have been devised, and they enable the director and group members to get a profile of the action potential of the individual that paper-and-pencil tests are unable to uncover.

Didactic psychodrama

In this teaching method, auxiliary egos, nurses, social workers, psychologists, and psychiatrists take the role of a patient in a situation of everyday occurrence, such as a patient who refuses to obey rules as they are applied in a hospital or clinic. The psychodrama students also take their own professional roles. The training situations are structured according to typical conflicts with which they are familiar or which they are likely to face in their professional roles. Several versions of how to deal with the obstreperous patient can be represented by various students. Real patients need not be involved.

Psychodrama and narcosynthesis

Under the influence of drugs, the patient relives certain experiences or, after having undergone drug therapy, needs to integrate his experience as it unfolded inside of him while he was unable to communicate those experiences. There are two variables: the drug and the enactment of the inner worlds. The question here is which variable contributes what to the treatment.

Family psychodrama

Husband and wife or mother and child are treated as a combine, often facing each other, rather than separately, because separate from each other they may not have any tangible mental ailment. In the course of this approach the family members may reverse roles, double for each other, and, in general, serve as each other's auxiliary ego.

Videotape and television in psychodrama

Television is a medium in which interpersonal action of the moment is the final desideratum. It is a medium which is continuously changing, and in which the attention of the participants is shifting from one task to another without warning. Under these conditions, split-second judgment and responsive spontaneity will be most rigorously challenged. One of the earliest studies of the use of videotape and television for group psychotherapy and psychodrama was made by Jacob Moreno in 1942.

Psychodrama's main features—the group or audience, the director, a staff of egos, the emergence of one or more protagonists, and the dramatic action between them—can be maintained in television productions. It is of great therapeutic value that the total process of interaction between group members is televised.

Conclusion

Psychodrama is a form of psychotherapy which is modeled after life. It offers great flexibility for growth and emotional learning. Man, in the psychodramatic situation, is free from the fetters of facts and actualities, although not without the highest respect for them. He has a good foundation to believe that things are changing, as science has repeatedly taught us. In psychodrama, he can take his own dreams, hopes, and aspirations and create his own new world. This is not a plea for escape from reality but just the opposite—a plea for creativity in a psychodramatic world which one day may become true.

Much of this chapter is based on the original work of the late J. L. Moreno, M.D., as it appeared in the first edition of this textbook.

References

Allport, G. W. Comments on: J. L. Moreno, transference, countertransference, and tele—their relation to group research and group psychotherapy. Group Psychother., 7: 307, 1954.

Bischof, L. J. *Interpreting Personality Theories.* Harper & Row, New York, 1970.

Dreikurs, R., and Corsini, R. J. Twenty years of group psychotherapy. Am. J. Psychiatry, 110: 567, 1954.

Ezriel, H. A. Psycho-analytic approach to group treatment. Br. J. Med. Psychol., 23: 59, 1950.

Fromm-Reichmann, F., and Moreno, J. L., editors. *Progress in Psychotherapy.* Grune & Stratton, New York, 1956.

Moreno, J. L. Interpersonal therapy and the psychopathology of interpersonality relations. Sociometry, 1: 9, 1937.

Moreno, J. L. Mental catharsis and the psychodrama. Sociometry, 3: 209, 1940.

Moreno, J. L. The philosophy of the moment and the spontaneity theater. Sociometry, 4: 206, 1941.

Moreno, J. L. *Psychodrama.* Beacon House, New York, 1946.

Moreno, J. L. *The Theater of Spontaneity.* Beacon House, New York, 1947.

Moreno, J. L. *The First Book on Group Psychotherapy.* Beacon House, New York, 1957.

Moreno, J. L., editor. *International Handbook of Group Psychotherapy.* Philosophical Library, New York, 1966.

Moreno, J. L., and Dunkin, W. S. The function of the social investigator in experimental psychodrama. Sociometry, 4: 392, 1941.

Moreno, J. L., and Fischel, J. K. Spontaneity procedures in television broadcasting with special emphasis on interpersonal relation systems. Sociometry, 5: 7, 1942.

Moreno, J. L., and Moreno, Z. T. *Psychodrama.* Beacon House, New York, 1959.

Sacks, J. Group psychotherapy and psychoanalysis, historical note. Group Psychother., 13: 199, 1960.

B.13 Co-therapy

MAX ROSENBAUM, Ph.D.

Introduction

A sense of excitement continues to pervade the field of psychotherapy, especially group psychotherapy, which today is accepted as a major treatment modality for people who suffer from emotional disturbance. Indeed, in the treatment volume which follows the DSM-III guide, group psychotherapy is recognized as a major therapy approach. As a less costly alternative to individual psychotherapy, it is appealing to medical economists, especially as the nation moves toward some form of national health insurance. Further, in many reports on group psychotherapy, it is almost assumed that the reader will know that co-therapists were involved in the leadership of the group. Only when one reads the report does the fact of co-therapy become clear. Co-therapy is practiced much more than most therapists are aware. Most therapists face difficulty as they approach work with groups of patients. As a result, they tend to seek techniques that will ease the practice of psychotherapy, and, as therapists try to ease the emotional burden they face and to function more efficiently as therapists, they are more and more drawn to the idea of co-therapy, a technique that, although apparently recent, has actually been practiced in many forms since the outset of dynamic psychotherapy.

Additionally, because of its very structure, group psychotherapy has encouraged the use of co-therapists, though co-therapy is by no means restricted to groups. Since the therapist-patient relationship is no longer one-to-one but is, rather, one-to-a-group, the group members are more responsive to the idea of another therapist coming to the therapy group.

The use of more than one therapist at a time in individual or group psychotherapy has been given many names: co-therapy, dual leadership, role-divided therapy, three-cornered therapy, multiple therapy, three-cornered interviews, cooperative psychotherapy, conjoint therapy, and joint interview. Anywhere from two to 10 therapists may work with a single patient, and groups of therapists may join groups of patients.

For the most part, clinical practice validates the use of a co-therapist as an aid to therapy. The co-therapist appears to enhance group process and increase interaction. Also, the co-therapist often increases the validity and intensity of the interpretation. Patients are more prone to accept two interpretations that are consonant than one solitary interpretation. One of the side benefits is that the group therapist becomes accustomed to co-therapy and may be responsive to the idea of having a co-therapist for an individual session. Additionally, sometimes the presence of another therapist helps break through a therapeutic impasse. This use of another therapist in individual therapy and family therapy is called multiple therapy, and is an aspect of co-therapy.

The use of co-therapists aids group therapy in several ways. First, the patient has another figure to whom he may transfer. This added person causes an imbalance in the traditional transference response of patient-therapist. The presence of other group members has already modified the traditional transference response, and the presence of a co-therapist simply modifies it further. Second, more movement is promoted in the therapy group. Third, the group members appear to move toward greater depths. Fourth, co-therapy offers an effective method to break through blockages. Fifth, one therapist may undercut while another supports the patient's defenses. Sixth, one therapist is able to take more risks in depth interpretation, since another therapist is present as a kind of ballast, especially in work with psychotic patients, where a therapist may fear the loss of his own psychic balance as he enters the world of the acutely disturbed.

One of the important features of co-therapy is that psychotherapists can balance one another and ameliorate discouragement so that there is an atmosphere of hope. There is always the danger of equating diagnosis and prognosis. A patient diagnosed as having process schizophrenia may not receive psychotherapy if the psychotherapist believes that patients who suffer from schizophrenia cannot benefit from psychotherapy. If a climate of hopefulness is established, the expectation of positive results may play a large part in successful psychotherapy.

Reasons for Co-therapy

MacLennan (1965) observed that, in some places, co-therapy is used routinely without any awareness of its dynamic implications and consequences. But therapists must have a theoretical rationale to justify the use of co-therapists, which may be based on the following.

TRAINING THERAPISTS

As group therapy becomes more and more popular in private practice, clinics, and hospitals, administra-

167

tors display a certain urgency to train future group therapists quickly. And, although co-therapy seems to be excellent on-the-job training, administrators must clearly delineate the co-therapists' roles in such a training situation. If they do not, tremendous rivalry comes to the surface. Often the more experienced therapist runs the group while the trainee just sits at the feet of the master. Worse yet, the trainee finally becomes the experienced co-therapist and begins training juniors. He may never, alone, lead a group of his own or withstand the pressures to which he is exposed.

SIMULATING A FAMILY

Many advocates of co-therapy feel that the patient can use the group as a second family, often a more helpful and healthy family than the original one. With the helpful reassurance of the second therapist, the patient can try to cope with unresolved problems toward the dreaded parent or, in some cases, an overwhelming sibling. For example, a patient can confront a feared parent in the person of one therapist only because he feels that he has another therapist to whom he can turn. The second therapist is somewhat like the parent who supports the child while the other parent is angry. Of course, in some situations both parents turn on the child, but there are no reports in the literature of both co-therapists being destructive.

Groups led jointly by a man and a woman therapist seem logical in this concept of the group as a second family, especially in view of the wide agreement that a basic value of group therapy is that the patient can experience and work through multiple transferences. Many therapists believe opposite-sex co-therapists activate sexual transferences, the rationale being that co-therapy permits the patients to identify with a therapist of the same sex and to clarify problems with a therapist of the opposite sex.

Certain patients may profit from the use of therapists of different sexes. For instance, patients ranging from juvenile delinquents, who have not been exposed to a man and a woman living together in marriage, or, to a couple with healthy differences as to how they perceive the world, may be able to work out their oedipal problems and their distorted perceptions of the man-woman relationship if they have a man and a woman as co-therapists. Some therapists find that teenagers profit from observing the substitute parent figures in the persons of the man and the woman co-therapists as they disagree with one another and yet present themselves as adults who are able to communicate with each other. The larger question here is whether group psychotherapy is the appropriate setting for corrective experiences in living. This question is particularly pertinent in community health programs and in work with socially deprived patients from broken or unhappy homes.

Co-therapy is also of benefit in many community psychiatric clinics, where a population of elderly patients is attracted. These patients are seen as chronic complainers who have minimal insight and little possibility of change. When they are seen in individual psychotherapy, the therapist becomes frustrated, and the patients become increasingly depressed.

A very innovative use of a family group occurred in Waverly, Tennessee, after a tank car exploded and treatment was required for the disaster victims. The burn patients' families were seen in a group utilizing an educational model. There were seven burn patients, all men, and they and their families were invited to group sessions. These were weekly sessions, 90 minutes in duration, and the group met for 8 weeks. The families were predominantly rural, southern fundamentalist in religious belief, who tended to distrust psychiatry. The liaison psychiatrist and the hospital chaplain co-led the group and provided continuity and direction in a complementary fashion. The representatives of each medical specialty involved in the care of the burn patients were present for most of the meetings. The results were successful, and most of the pressing emotional problems were worked through in the group (Campbell et al., 1980).

ECONOMY

Many of the economic reasons advanced for co-therapy, some of which sound rather mercantile, are not supported by full consideration of the theoretical implications. For example, some of those who advocate co-therapy feel that co-therapists can treat larger groups. This argument denies the importance of intimacy. Many patients suffer from intimacy problems and would prefer to obscure these problems; large groups meet this preference. Also, advocates of larger groups assume that the therapists possess an enormous capacity to comprehend the dynamics of an expanded group, thus endowing them with extraordinary strengths. Actually, patients may so maneuver co-therapists that they engage in rivalry, thereby masking the patients' own conflicts.

CONVENIENCE

Some therapists advocate co-therapy because it gives them more freedom. One therapist can lead the group while the other is absent because of illness, emergency, or vacation. This argument ignores the patient, who may not express but almost invariably feels a sense of rejection when the therapist is casual about his own presence and does not appear to be very committed. When a patient is absent from scheduled group meetings, many therapists are outraged and wonder about the patient's commitment, although they themselves find all sorts of rationalizations for their own absence and lack of commitment.

MUTUAL SUPPORT

Some therapists welcome the idea of co-therapy as a means of coping with their own anxiety about their adequacy as therapists. A mutual support mechanism is at work here, and patients often spot the mechanism and wonder about the unresolved anxieties of the group leaders. Actually, some therapists are not prepared for the groups they undertake to lead, so they invite another therapist to help them cope with the task. One therapist who works with schizophrenic patients both in groups and in individual sessions routinely invites a co-therapist to work with him when he enters the patients' intense fantasy life. He is fearful that he may become psychotic, and so he wants the control of another therapist.

When a group approach is used with regressed psychotic patients, some group therapists have recommended that the group be no larger than four patients. Once the regressed phase of the acute psychosis has been resolved, the group size may enlarge to nine or 10 members. The mutual support of therapists to one another is matched by patients who also desire support and protection of their very shaky egos. Kibel (1981) has noted that schizophrenic and borderline psychotic patients experience a therapist quite differently when placed in a group.

SELF-THERAPY

The therapist who contemplates co-therapy must be on guard, since some therapists have a neurotic need to pair off with one another. They use co-therapy as therapy for themselves. For psychotherapists to work out their countertransference problems at the patients' expense is exploitation of patients. Some therapists who are fervent supporters of co-therapy completely ignore their own marital distress and loneliness, which are quite obvious to observers, as they recruit male or female therapists to work with them in groups. And lonely therapists often become intrigued with marathon therapy.

Selection of Co-therapists

No firm rules for the selection of co-therapists can be set down. Co-therapy is still very much an art, and many variables are involved. Clinical experience indicates that certain therapists are more at ease in co-therapy relationships than when they lead a group alone. Some workers speak of the value of mutual and spontaneous choice as sometimes more valuable than pairing based on objective criteria, but it seems more likely that spontaneous pairing may not survive the rigors of hostility between co-therapists.

In institutional settings, co-therapists are rarely selected with care. Too much attention is paid to the training needs of the institution, and very little attention is paid to the specific anxieties and problems of the proposed co-therapists. Those who are new to co-therapy have to prepare by reading the literature and working with a supervisor even before co-therapy begins.

Equal clinical experience seems to be important in a co-therapist team. There is then a tacit acknowledgment that therapists of equal skill are working with each other, rather than for each other.

In Malan's study of psychotherapy at Tavistock Clinic, he was not especially encouraging about results in a long-term follow-up study (Malan et al., 1976). But what is most striking was the rather impersonal stance of the therapists. Whether this reflects the culture—Great Britain—or a rather guarded style of group therapy, the co-therapists did not seem to stimulate one another to a more productive outcome (Bloch and Reibstein, 1980).

The use of co-therapists to relieve one another's anxiety or despair has a long history. When working with acutely psychotic or very depressed patients, the co-therapists give one another constant support (Emery et al., 1980).

COMPATIBILITY OF THERAPISTS

Careful attention should be paid to the personality characteristics of therapists who plan to join one another as co-therapists. Most important is compatibility of temperament. Both therapists must be comfortable with intimacy and able to accept their differences. Over the years, experienced therapists establish a style, and co-therapists respect each other's style. Ideally, their styles blend together, so that a smoothly working team of co-therapists has its own style. A degree of trust must be present, because on occasion a therapist may interpret or react in a manner that makes no sense at all to his co-therapist. Sometimes, when they lack regard for each other, co-therapists engage in rivalry for the patients' affections. Or they may engage in games or ploys that, exciting at the outset, later prove to be obstructive. In these situations, therapists end up performing for patients, not treating them.

The issue of compatible pairing of therapists becomes critical if therapists attempt to work with acutely disturbed patients.

In private practice, co-therapists often pair on the basis of personal friendship. Such pairing does not appear to be wise. The ostensible convenience may prove to be an obstacle when fantasy material comes to the surface and intense transferences develop. Because of their friendship, one therapist may avoid significant material. Openness and honesty must be present in the co-therapy relationship. Personality differences can be resolved as they occur, and the therapists can serve as healthy models for patients. Lack of authenticity often results in a floundering group that comes to a rapid end.

However, none of the aforementioned observations precludes co-therapists from developing friendships. Similarity of background, geographic isolation, and a variety of situational circumstances may, in fact, promote close friendships. But a friendship between therapists has an impact on the group, and the therapists should be aware of this fact.

COMPATIBILITY OF PATIENTS AND THERAPISTS

The limited psychotherapeutic research data available suggest that black clients prefer and work better with black counselors than with white counselors. Some research studies suggest that more positive relationships result when the therapist and the patient are of the same race. But in co-therapy, is it advisable to pair therapists of different races, religions, or cultural levels? One major metropolitan psychiatric center makes an effort to use therapists of different races to dissolve ethnic isolation. The ethical problem is one for the reader to evaluate.

Active members of the women's liberation movement have claimed that many male psychotherapists are guilty of male chauvinism. These women search for sympathetic therapists. Their comments have the familiar echo of comments made during the 1930's and 1940's by members of the political left, who claimed that psychotherapists were out to convert them to an acceptance of the capitalist system. Their psychotherapists had to pass political tests of acceptability.

Class differences have as much validity as ethnic and religious differences in the selection of therapists. Yet too much attention to the manifest material obscures the psychological reality that the patient responds to in terms of his own unconscious.

MALE-FEMALE CO-THERAPISTS

A man-woman pairing is often effective. Here one must not be thrown by surface appearances. Sometimes the man is quite feminine, and the woman is quite masculine, with the patients becoming quite confused.

The co-therapists serve as models for the group. If co-therapists of opposite sexes have unresolved problems concerning male and female roles in the culture, chaos will rapidly ensue. One extremely dominating woman therapist consistently espouses co-therapy and invariably chooses a passive male as her co-therapist. In another instance, an experienced but rather grandiose male therapist consistently chooses very attractive and rather seductive women as co-therapists, almost as if he were showing off a mistress. Because of his prominence and the teaching position he enjoys, his patients and the psychiatric residents he trains rarely challenge him as to his behavior. A follow-up study by this writer indicates that many of his patients have deep fantasy problems and confuse marriage with harem-type living.

In some instances, a husband and wife do co-therapy as a matter of convenience. They may, in fact, be creating the ideal family, with themselves as idealized parent models. One couple, both of whom had been previously married, were unconsciously drawn to the practice of co-therapy. They acted out a model for patients who had had unsuccessful marriages, as though they were telling patients that they—the co-therapists—could relate together in a second marriage, and, therefore, so could the patients. There is no objection to this technique if it is conscious. Unfortunately, the therapists were not aware of what they were doing. Their therapy is the creation of an extended family.

Sometimes a nurse is chosen as the female co-therapist. Since she generally ranks low in the hierarchy of a hospital setting, she may be supportive only and may pass on feelings of inadequacy to the women patients in a group. Selection of co-therapists should be intelligent, not a hit-or-miss selection of whatever staff is available.

Some groups of aged patients receive tremendous stimulation from exposure to male and female co-therapists, who apparently renew the aged patient's interest in heterosexuality. In many cases, paraprofessionals can supply a similar corrective emotional experience in group work with this patient population.

Relations between Co-therapists

The idea of a co-therapy relationship promotes anxiety in the majority of psychotherapists who have been practicing individual or group psychotherapy. Co-therapy demands maturity and sensitivity in both therapists. Besides having to define interaction in the group, therapists are confronted with many of their own unresolved problems in a co-therapist relationship. A quality of strain exists at the outset and possibly throughout the co-therapy relationship, as unresolved transference phenomena come to the surface. But in the same way that anxiety serves as a stimulus for change, the acknowledged tension between co-therapists may further therapeutic change.

Most therapists find it difficult to visualize their impact on a group. Videotape may capture some of what is going on. But when another therapist observes a working therapist within the group setting, all kinds of unresolved feelings become apparent. The group therapist who has successfully masked omnipotent behavior, a need to be seductive, a need to avoid anger, or a need to stimulate hostility will almost certainly have his behavior and needs exposed when another therapist joins the group. Of course, the therapist with problems of omniscience may select as a co-therapist someone who will not rock the boat.

For the most part, group therapists resist the exploration of their own countertransference problems as they come to the fore in the group. The co-therapist may quickly perceive the problem, and this perception may threaten one or both of the therapists. A therapist in training may be reluctant to confront his co-therapist mentor. Or the trainee may have the neurotic need to confront the senior therapist. Some therapists experience difficulty leading groups and they turn to the co-therapist as a lifesaver. Although reluctant to acknowledge their need, these inept therapists want another therapist to help with the pressures and anxieties that develop in the group.

Both complementary and symmetrical behavior are at work in co-therapy. In complementary behavior, each person's behavior complements or fits the other's behavior, as when one person teaches and the other serves as the student, or when one leads and the other follows. In symmetrical behavior, two people engage in the same type of behavior. In this situation, their behavior is both competitive and equalitarian, and the interaction is on a level of parity; in short, it is the behavior of two people who are equals. An effective co-therapy team works on a symmetrical pattern. Some teams may work effectively in a complementary fashion, but their goals appear to be more limited, since one therapist dominates the other. Pairing an experienced and an inexperienced group therapist produces a complementary pattern at the outset. As the team matures and grows in its work together, the move is toward a symmetrical pattern. But some teams never outgrow the complementary pattern.

In clinical practice one therapist can supplement and complement the skills of the other therapist. Co-therapists should be able to accept each other emotionally, understand each other's methods of working in a group setting, and share common aims and goals of treatment. Emotional acceptance and mutual respect are prime requisites. Neither therapist should feel a necessity to mold the behavior of the other, to be defensive with the other, or to use the group and its members to resolve competitive strivings.

On occasion, co-therapists maintain a social contact outside of the group, which invariably affects their behavior in the group. The administrative hierarchy of the institution also affects the group and the co-therapists. Some psychiatric residents in training use co-therapy as an opportunity to attack their mentors—verbally and nonverbally—while both are with the group. Some staff members are fearful of reacting genuinely in the group because of some unresolved reaction to a co-therapist who is perceived as a superior—either intellectually or administratively more powerful. And a senior therapist with power problems of his own may have great difficulty in accepting the contributions of a junior member serving as a peer co-therapist. The patients observe all this interaction whether they comment on it or not.

All the differences that co-therapists feel about the administration of the group and the group process should be clarified before the first group meeting. Obviously, not all the issues will be resolved before the first group session, but a quality of authenticity must be present between the two therapists. The optimally functioning co-therapy group reflects the comfort and openness that exists between the leaders.

Relations with Patients

In leadership of a group, the therapist assumes certain responsibilities. He enters into a therapeutic contract with the patients. The contract is modified when co-therapists work with the group. The patients may become quite confused, unless the therapists clearly define their areas of responsibility and what the patients can reasonably expect from each group leader. Ideally, the co-therapists should work out their relationship and responsibilities before they decide to lead a group, but theory is often complicated by fact. Huxley, the biologist, refers to the finest theory defeated by the ugly fact. This is very much the case with co-therapy. All too often, the resistances of patients to the group experience are founded in the resistances of co-therapists to the exploration of their own problems in interaction. Even before they organize a group, both therapists should, ideally, interview and screen potential members of the group. From the outset, then, the patient is prepared for the experience of co-therapy. The patient may also be able to establish transference reactions from the first contact with the therapeutic situation.

Often, therapists overlook the fact that they are being carefully observed by patients in the group setting. These same patients compare reactions while out of earshot of the therapists. Co-therapists should take note of their behavior, particularly if patients meet on their own before or after the regularly scheduled group meeting or if they arrive at or leave the group meeting together.

In private practice, the question of fees should be clarified before a patient enters a group led by co-therapists. There are no definite rules concerning payment. Some therapists are paid directly by the patient; others divide the fee equally.

If a patient wishes to have an individual session with one of the therapists, both therapists should know about it. Otherwise, the patient may trap one therapist into his patterns of resistance.

A therapist's personal preference for a patient is quickly noted by the group. In the same way that a therapist may unconsciously keep patients in individual therapy because of his unresolved problems in sharing them with a group, he may unconsciously resent sharing patients with a co-therapist. Many patients are still working through their unresolved need to separate their parents. And some of these patients may try to separate the co-therapists—by creating emergency situations, for example. In such a situation, both therapists should meet with the patient in an individual session (Spitz et al., 1980).

In the course of a group experience, changes occur in the lives of therapists. A team of therapists described a long-term, continuous therapy group of convicted pedophiles on probation; they were being treated as part of a project to study the effectiveness of analytic group psychotherapy for sex offenders. One therapist, who had been conducting the group for 3 years, accepted a position in another city. At the time, his co-therapist was a third-year resident in psychiatry who had been a group member for 1 year. The transference phenomena became very intense among the group members and the therapists because of the change in leadership of the group.

The death of a leader also has a strong impact on a group. In 1947, Rosenthal described her experience with a group led by Paul Schilder, one of the pioneers in group psychotherapy. She participated for many consecutive months in the group psychotherapy sessions conducted by Schilder before his death. It thus devolved upon her to help adjust these abandoned patients to the death of the father figure, a task beyond the psychological means at her disposal. Since the early work of Rosenthal that described the impact on the group of the death of a leader, there have been many situations where groups have suddenly lost a group therapist through death or illness. The use of a co-therapist would appear to spare patients the extreme pain of the loss of a therapist.

Techniques

Probably the most elaborate description of co-therapy was written by Demarest and Teicher (1954), and their description is still valid. It was based on an experience with a group of five hospitalized schizophrenic patients who were in intensive psychotherapy for a period of 1½ years. Demarest and Teicher stated that their hypotheses should be viewed within the framework of the

widely accepted ideas that the goal of therapy is to enable

people to effect changes in life patterns and that transference is the enabling instrument, the working tool, which allows therapy to accomplish this goal.

Demarest and Teicher observed that, in group therapy, transference occurs on many levels of relationship:

patient-patient, patient-therapist, patient-group, and therapist-group. Where there are co-therapists, it also occurs on the therapist-therapist level.

They defined transference as

the process in which a person projects a pattern of adaptation which was learned, developed, and adopted in a previous significant life situation from that previous situation to a current life situation; he then displaces the affect of the previous situation from that situation to the present situation.

Demarest and Teicher's group of five patients met twice a week for 1¾-hour sessions. Although the therapists attempted to establish a careful balance—matching patients on the basis of verbal ability, type of illness, educational background, and motivation for psychotherapy—the balance did not work. There were too many external variables. Even so, they derived that the presence of male and female therapists made it possible for each patient to structure a family group, which allowed him to act out family conflicts and set up familial constellations in which problems of sibling rivalry and of mother-son and father-son struggles could be perceived and worked through. Furthermore, having therapists of both sexes allowed a patient to act out his problems with each sex in relation to the opposite sex.

When the woman therapist went on vacation, the group members expressed transference reactions toward the mother deserting them and displaced their aggression to the male therapist, who remained as group leader. Thus Demarest and Teicher noted: "The absence of one therapist became a valuable device with which to precipitate feelings and fantasies on the therapist-group transference level that could not be experienced or expressed in the presence of both therapists."

The important feature is that the therapists worked within a consistent theoretical framework. One of the values of co-therapy is that it offers the possibility of more valid and objective observation and evaluation of different levels of the transference phenomenon. In the therapist-patient relationship, there is a process of working through, and generally only one therapist is centrally involved. The co-therapist is able to observe the relationship and the manner in which it expresses itself. Thus, one therapist can continuously check on the other.

Bardon (1966) notes that male and female co-therapists are usually reacted to as father and mother figures, respectively, and feels that patients work through their transference feelings toward the mother and father figures more rapidly in co-therapy than in one-to-one therapy. His groups of six to eight patients were composed of university students, with a generally equal sex distribution in the groups. His orientation was psychodynamic, and the goal was a recon-

struction of the patients' personalities. He found that the patients developed transference reactions to the actual relationship between the co-therapists and expected the co-therapists to show the same problems in their relationship that the patients' parents did. Consequently, the transferences developed not to the therapists as individuals but to their joint presence and interaction with each other.

Proponents of conjoint therapy, in which a patient works individually with one therapist and in group treatment with another, say that this type of therapy helps the patient work through his unresolved intrapsychic conflicts related to his relationship with one or both parents. Here, again, the suggestion is made to use therapists of different sexes. The hope and purpose is to bring oedipal and preoedipal problems to the surface much more quickly than in either individual psychotherapy or group therapy led by one therapist. The belief is that no transference deadlock will develop.

When co-therapists work with married couples, one therapist often serves as a balance wheel for his co-therapist, especially when unresolved problems of the therapist come to the surface. The expectation is that the co-therapists will not join in the neurotic behavior and attack either the group members or one another. In family therapy, the co-therapists can help pick up faulty patterns of communication in the family, but the primary emphasis is on interaction phenomena. Unconscious conflicts or transference phenomena are largely ignored.

There is a difference between an active co-therapist who takes responsibility and an observer who does not take responsibility for the patients in a group. However, the observer is a person to whom patients do react and transfer. In the overemphasis on the interactional, the intrapsychic is often ignored. But the patient is always reacting, even if he does not care to share his reactions with the observer therapist or active co-therapists.

The more structured situational approach to co-therapy does not seem to be as relevant as the intrapsychic approach. To say that a male and a female therapist will serve as father and mother figures ignores clinical experience, especially with acutely disturbed patients, who often perceive the therapist of the same sex as father and mother. In essence, situational arrangements overlook the patients, particularly in clinical work with sex offenders. Also, transferences are not diluted. Therefore, the situational approach cannot be used exclusively.

The use of co-therapists in a time-limited group appears to be a frequent practice. Friedman and Cohen (1980) treated five women in an eight-session miscarriage peer group which met each time for an hour. The group was organized because of a belief by the group leaders that a miscarriage often constitutes a major life crisis, and the group leaders, a psychiatrist and a medical educator, both female and working in a university medical department, organized a homogeneous group in which all of the members shared a common life experience. The focus of the group was educational and therapeutic and was on the specific life crisis—the miscarriage. The emphasis was upon support and rapid symptomatic relief. The co-leaders of this pilot project report that the members of the group derived substantial benefit from the therapeutic process. Since they also observed that there was a good deal of anger and blame— "both husbands and obstetricians are frequent targets of externally directed rage"—it is worth conjecturing as to whether the group might have functioned even better with co-leaders who were male and female.

Conclusion

The therapist who practices co-therapy rapidly comes to grips with his unreal and overidealized expectations. The most experienced therapists have difficulty as they embark on this new collaborative venture. One therapist plus one therapist does not necessarily add up to better treatment. The new team of co-therapists may become quickly disillusioned. Whether they are able to persevere and ask for help from one another is a test of their maturity. Unresolved problems of sibling rivalry and status needs rapidly come to the fore, and can be handled with adequate supervision. However, therapists are not there to treat one another. Doing so is an abuse of the patient's trust. The therapists' primary responsibility is to the patient; and on occasion, co-therapists have to be reminded of this responsibility.

References

Agazarian, Y., and Peters, R. *The Visible and Invisible Group.* Routledge & Kegan Paul, London, 1980.

Bardon, E. J. Transference reactions to the relationship between male and female co-therapists in group psychotherapy. J. Am. Coll. Health Assoc., *14:* 287, 1966.
Bloch, S., and Reibstein, J. Perceptions by patients and therapists of therapeutic factors in group psychotherapy. Br. J. Psychiatry, *137:* 274, 1980.
Campbell, D. R., and Sinha, B. K. Brief group psychotherapy with chronic hemodialysis patients. Am J. Psychiatry, *137:* 1234, 1980.
Campbell, T. W., Brock, G., Van Gee, S. J., and Greefield, G. Use of a multiple family group for crisis intervention. Gen. Hosp. Psychiatry, *2:* 95, 1980.
Demarest, E., and Teicher, A. Transference in group therapy: Its use by co-therapists of opposite sexes. Psychiatry, *17:* 187, 1954.
Emery, P., Levitan, J., and Gadlin, W. Modified group therapy for psychotic and depressed patients. Group, *4:* 21, 1980.
Friedman, C. T. H., Procci, W. R., and Fenn. A. The role of expectation in treatment for psychotic patients. Am. J. Psychother., *34:* 188, 1980.
Friedman, R. R., and Cohen, K. The peer support group: A model for dealing with the emotional aspects of miscarriage. Group, *4:* 42, 1980.
Ireland, M. S., and Brekker, J. The mandala in group psychotherapy: Personal identity and intimacy. Arts Psychother., *7:* 217, 1980.
Kanos, N., Rogers, M., Kreth, E., Patterson, L., and Campbell, R. The effectiveness of group psychotherapy during the first three weeks of hospitalization. J. Nerv. Ment. Dis., *168:* 487, 1980.
Kibel, H. D. A conceptual model for short term inpatient group psychotherapy. Am. J. Psychiatry, *138:* 74, 1981.
Loeffler, F., and Weinstein, H. M. The co-therapist method: Special problems and advantages. Group Psychother., *6:* 189, 1954.
MacLennan, B. Co-therapy. Int. J. Group Psychother., *15:* 154, 1965.
Malan, D. H., Balfour, F. H. G., and Hood, V. G. Group psychotherapy: A long term follow-up study. Arch. Gen. Psychiatry, *33:* 1303, 1976.
Ormont, L. Principles and practices of conjoint psychoanalytic treatment. Am. J. Psychiatry, *138:* 69, 1981.
Spitz, H. I., Kass, F., and Charles, E. Common mistakes made in group psychotherapy by beginning therapists. Am. J. Psychiatry, *137:* 274, 1980.
Stone, W. N., Blaze, M., and Bozzuto, J. Late dropouts from group psychotherapy. Am. J. Psychother., *34:* 401, 1980.

B.14 Videotape and Group Psychotherapy

ALAN B. WACHTEL, M.D.

Introduction

Electronic media have evolved over the last 3 decades to become a significant therapeutic tool in group and family therapy. The media most frequently used include audiotape, Polaroid snapshot review, film, and videotape. Therapists report various degrees of therapeutic success from media techniques, which objectively demonstrate behavior from the standpoint of a neutral observer (Alger and Hogan, 1969; Sanborn, 1975). Videotape offers the greatest promise because it has instant retrieval and storage potential; technical ease of operation; consumer availability at low cost; and technical potential for multiple sensory input with inserts, split screen, and zoom.

Video playback's combined visual and audio components produce a therapeutic impact which is often more effective than purely verbal intervention. The impartiality of the camera enables the patient to more readily accept the intervention than if it had come from either the therapist or the group. By viewing their own body movements and hearing their own voices, patients' resistance is minimized, the group interaction is maximized (Geertsma and Reivich, 1965), and the patient becomes more available to form a therapeutic alliance.

Effects on the Individual

A primary therapeutic effect of proper use of video is on the individual group member's self-image. In video playback, group members view a television image of a segment, i.e., a few minutes, of their own behavior immediately after it occurred. As opposed to hearing about one's behavior or another's reaction to it, the individual, with his or her own eyes, observes the behavior and the reaction of others to it. Video feedback provides the group member with direct access to viewing his own behavior. This affords an additional level of concentration, and optimally permits a group member to react to his own behavior along with other group members and therapists (Danet, 1968).

Berger (1970) describes how patients discover new views of themselves which previously had been hidden. Group members frequently protect one another because they have protected themselves from seeing undesirable behavioral characteristics.

Video compels a new type of confrontation. Once confrontation occurs, a new level of self-perception may arise, and the group, having shared the feedback experience, can validate the experience for the person. The group becomes more caring, meaningful, and constructive, and is less likely to be experienced as criticizing or attacking.

Initial playback reaction is different from subsequent playback experiences. Patients react in extreme ways—either positively or negatively—to the first video playback experience. The focus of the initial playback experience (as opposed to later playback sessions) is on appearance and sex appeal in women and on masculinity or its absence in men, whereas, in subsequent sessions, the focus moves toward types of interaction and characteristic styles of relating. As sessions progress, patients give up denial as a defense. Furthermore, the playback experience affords immediate observation and reinforcement by the patient of new types of behavior.

In addition to concerns about appearance and sex appeal, the initial self-observation can trigger a significant associative reaction (Wachtel et al., 1979).

One of the woman members said she was aware "I speak more with my hands and with my body than my voice. My initial reaction was one of being very upset, because I recognized my younger sister in an awful lot of my physical gesticulations and my voice . . . which is very, very upsetting, because it wasn't me and in some way, I was her and this bothered me very much."

The observed behavior self-perception sequence can then be generalized to character interpretation:

"I was very uncomfortable in seeing myself, because I started out at the beginning saying something very strongly and it dwindled to nothing. I didn't finish sentences. I didn't say anything really firmly or completely and I left it with expressions like 'you know what I mean.' This is very, very upsetting for me. It has to do with other things in my life where I don't complete things—like getting incompletes on papers."

Playback experiences can stimulate a reliving of the feelings and thoughts of the moment that were not expressed at that time. Alger and Hogan (1969) label this behavior as a second-chance phenomenon. The following are good examples:

"I was really reliving what was happening and all the thoughts that I had at the time that never got expressed. Something had come up in the group. It sounded peculiar to me. I was thinking about it and I went off on that same stream of thought in my head and we argued the case again in my head, but I realize now that I never expressed any of this."

"I knew I was myself and was upset and troubled. There I was moving around and just playing with my beard. I guess that's what I do here every week. And as I was watching it, it seemed incredible that I could keep on doing this without realizing how upset I was. . . ."

The intensity of video confrontation is universally reported to be most effective in the initial session. Its continued use does not produce the same type of high therapeutic impact when compared with the initial video self-image confrontation. Repetitive exposure diminishes the observer role, making the viewer functionally "blind" to his own image.

The difference between initial and subsequent playback sessions may also be understood in terms of video's ability to overwhelm normal defensive structures. The physical nature of video self-image confrontation makes it uniquely effective. Much of its power derives from observations made by the patient focused on body image. The initial session induces a marked diminution in defensive operation which in subsequent sessions reconstitutes to block unpleasant or unacceptable self-images.

It is for this reason that the therapist must take extreme care during the initial session to provide a controlled and limited confrontation. The video self-image confrontation correctly applied has a therapeutic effect on enhancing the functioning of the observing ego.

Effects on Group Interaction

The effects of video playback on group interaction are significant and equally important to that in terms of the group as a whole. The technique fosters cohesion, and depths of emotional expression are more quickly reached. According to Berger:

In the non-demanding silence of the playback they [the patients] could feel deeply and let go of their usual defenses. . . . The presence of the tape for self and others diminishes the pressure (real or fancied) for involvement to exist primarily through words. The lessening of this kind of pressure results in an increased availability to quietly be with and feel with others. This speeds up the process of intimacy and enhances the possibility of change being risked in an atmosphere of mutual trust with close, significant others.

The desire to change is experienced by the person as coming from himself as a result of his own observations and conclusions, rather than these conclusions being imposed upon him by some outside authority. The stimulus of the videotape playback helps the group to focus on the intragroup material; indeed, the effectiveness of the videotape playback in bringing the group forward in its progress to begin to confront each other is unmistakable and most effective. Specifically, videotape playback is useful therapeutically by speeding up and bringing out the following: self-observation and observation of others, the enhanced utilization of the observing ego, the overcoming of resistance, the dealing with the resistive aspects of the transference, and characterological traits in relation to defenses and resistance in the group interaction. The stimulus of the actual presentation of the material does focus on the intragroup process, and enables the group to go into the process of increased confrontation in the group interaction—the most effective therapeutic part of the group therapy (Wachtel et al., 1979).

Effect on Group Attitude towards the Therapist

The third effect of video playback—attitude toward the therapist, including transference—is both the most crucial factor and the most controversial aspect of video playback. In video playback, the image of the group members is displayed for their observation. The therapist, likewise, is displayed on the screen. As the therapist sits and observes the television monitor, he or she, from a process point of view, becomes one of the group. His or her strengths and weaknesses become immediately apparent.

The author has been especially interested on the impact of video playback on the patient's view of the therapist. In an experimental program videotape was used to record group sessions with psychotic patients. Following a 45-minute group session, the group took a 5-minute break and reconvened to view the videotape of the session that had just occurred.

During the taped session, the patients' behavior toward the therapist was similar to that observed in previous non-video sessions. However, in the playback session, there was a marked departure from their previous relationship with the doctor. The doctor, who had been considered with awe and some fear, suddenly become available for comment regarding his picture on the screen. Comments went as follows: "Look, he slouches in his chair." "Boy, he taps his hand, too." "He [the doctor] is a handsome man." All the references were third person to the television image. The video picture permitted a safe triangulation which enabled the expression of previously unacceptable feelings toward the therapist. Following the video session, this doctor—previously held in awe but clearly feared—appeared in the patients' art therapy mural—an extremely unusual phenomenon. The use of video facilitated the development of a therapeutic alliance.

Berger describes the significance of playback in its role clarification of the therapist. The therapist is available to the group member as a person. The group is better able to assess more realistically the therapist's capacity for caring and what the therapist is like as a person. This better understanding of the therapist as a caring and sincere human being may lead to a speeding up of the therapeutic process.

The availability of the objective data as presented on the videotape permits the patient to see behavior for him- or herself independent of the observations of the therapist. But transference and attitudes toward the therapist do not disappear.

The so-called democratizing quality of the playback experience tends to lure therapist and group into the false sense that observation of the tape represents a transference-free interpretation. However, every time the tape is used, it represents a form of interpretation. It is powerful as it goes beyond words to pictorial confrontation, frequently focusing on the basic defenses associated with self and body image. Regardless of the democratic manner in which the tape is introduced, it is obviously in the domain of the therapist, and, as such, its power enhances the real authority of the therapist. Denial of the video's role as this powerful extension of the therapist can lead to a paradoxical heightening of an omnipotent transference and increase the difficulty of analyzing it (Wachtel et al., 1979).

Use of Videotape

PREPARATION OF THE THERAPIST

The therapist should be fully trained in the technical application of video equipment. The therapist must also become comfortable seeing himself or herself on videotape. Optimally, the therapist should have a group experience employing video self-confrontation. Reactions will follow the pattern, seen with patients, of initially focusing on physicalness, then on the nature of the interactions, and, finally, on perception of self. This experience is difficult but should not be minimized.

The absence of appropriate training and experience in self-confrontation leads to inappropriate use of videotape and often to the termination of video experiences.

Finally, the therapeutic goals of the group and the role of media should be carefully defined by the therapist in advance of his utilization of video (Stoller, 1970).

PRELIMINARY PHASE

Video equipment should be in place at the onset of the group. This will avoid the introduction of equipment in an ongoing process.

Informed consent must be obtained before the equipment is used. The process must be fully explained and nonconsenting members requested to leave the group.

Equipment should be demonstrated to all group members. If patients are to operate the equipment, the therapist should be satisfied that every member of the group is able to do so. This technical expertise is required to assure that use or nonuse is a function of factors other than mechanical skill.

Thoughts and feelings relating to the preliminary

stages should be carefully and repeatedly explored. The issue of confidentiality and privacy should be brought up in terms of the playing of the tapes in the future. Failure to resolve resistances to the use of the equipment at the onset will seriously impair future therapeutic potential.

Thereafter, the group should be encouraged to express its thoughts and feelings associated with the anticipated use of the equipment. Fantasy material on how members think they will appear—body image, voice quality, role in group—should be sought.

Particular attention should be paid to the transference feelings associated with the "therapist's camera." Omnipotent and manipulative fantasies associated with the media should be explored.

The equipment, the decision to employ video, and its effect on the group process should be identified as therapeutic issues to be addressed on an ongoing basis as the group evolves.

Absence of therapeutic treatment of the equipment and the playback will result in increased resistance to the use of the media and will hamper the therapeutic goals of the group.

INITIAL PLAYBACK EXPERIENCE

The camera should be turned on by the therapist at the beginning of the session. This serves to normalize video by establishing the video recording as an integral part of the group process.

The therapist should immediately explain the rules, i.e., that video is part of the ongoing group process; that the recording can be stopped and material played back at any time; and that any member of the group, including the therapist, can stop and commence a video playback experience.

The playback process—when the tape is stopped and who initiates the playback—should be explored with the group.

The initial playback experience is extremely significant in terms of group members' self-image. This material should be actively encouraged by the therapist. However, the therapist, aware of the enormous impact on self-image, should be sensitive to any indication of a patient's defenses being overwhelmed. The therapist should intervene supportively during the session and not wait for the next session. Failure to do so will result in future non-compliance with the media.

The therapist should refer back to the initial playback experience in future sessions, since it has great significance for the group.

ONGOING USE OF VIDEO PLAYBACK

The camera should be on during all group sessions, since continued recording will permit the group to become familiar with video as part of the treatment. Likewise, the group should be reminded about the rules for the use of the media.

Playback should be encouraged as part of each group session, and material should be played back when it occurs. Short segments followed by group reaction are the most beneficial. Immediacy is lost after a few minutes, and the process becomes too passive.

Playback of material from previous sessions should be discouraged except for isolated hot segments that become thematically important to the group as a whole. Focusing on past sessions will impede the ongoing group process.

Non-use of the media should be analyzed as resistance to the therapeutic work of the group. Particular attention must be paid to actualization of an omnipotent transference, i.e., camera as extension of the therapist. Correctly handled, this will provide excellent material for analysis of the transference.

Conclusion

Correctly used by a well-trained therapist, video can provide significant therapeutic leverage. But therapists must be careful that they do not slavishly follow a technique or become so used to the tool of electronic gadgetry that their flexibility, empathy, and general awareness become impaired or compromised. With this caveat in mind, the use of the electronic video in the process of psychotherapy can be of enormous benefit to patients and therapists.

References

Alger, I., and Hogan, P. Enduring effects of videotape playback experience on family and marital relationships. Am. J. Orthopsychiatry, *39:* 86, 1969.

Berger, M. M. *Videotape Techniques in Psychiatric Training and Treatment.* Brunner/Mazel, New York, 1970.

Danet, B. M. Self-confrontation in psychotherapy: Video tape playback as a clinical and research tool. Am. J. Psychother., *22:* 245, 1968.

Geertsma, R., and Reivich, R. Repetitive self-observation by videotape playback. J. Nerv. Ment. Dis., *14:* 29, 1965.

Hogan, P., and Alger, I. The impact of videotape recording on insight in group psychotherapy. Int. J. Group Psychother., *19:* 158, 1969.

Sanborn, D. E., III. Video tape playback and psychotherapy: A review. Psychoter. Theory Res. Pract., *12:* 179, 1975.

Stoller, F. H. Videotape feedback in the group setting. J. Nerv. Ment. Dis., *148:* 457, 1970.

Wachtel, A. B., Stein, A., and Baldinger, M. Dynamic implications of videotape recording and playback in analytic group psychotherapy: Paradoxical effect on transference resistance. Int. J. Group Psychother., *29:* 67, 1979.

B.15 Art Therapy in Groups

DORIS J. LUBELL, M.A., A.T.R.

Introduction

"Picture if you will. ..." These four words simply describe the essential nature of artistic creations as a form of communication. Even before Freud spoke about the unconscious, artists knew that their artistic products were a form of communication, employing the language of symbolism and springing from some hidden place within themselves. Creative activity by its nature implies that individuals have the ability to draw upon these inner deeper levels; and created works can thus be considered documents of intense revelation.

The process of creativity, those conscious and unconscious feelings and thoughts that give rise to a finished artistic product, is an essential element of art therapy. The art therapist must be sensitive to the individual's real and symbolic speech. The patient artist is often embarking upon a frightening and risky task. The ability to take a chance and to permit one's self to journey into the symbolic world of imagery is an integral part of the process of creativity. Unlike the professional artist, patient artists are encouraged by an empathic and caring art therapist to help penetrate unconscious areas within themselves. This art-oriented therapeutic relationship has the potential to enable patients to better handle their interpersonal and intrapsychic conflicts, and it lays fertile groundwork for self-expression and self-discovery.

Definition

The contrasting views of the early workers in the field have made a precise definition of art therapy difficult. Many art therapists rely primarily on the healing quality of the use of art materials alone, while others envision the process of creating art as a means of furthering verbal interpretation and insight. These two major approaches within the field consider the use of art as therapy as an aid in fostering self-awareness and personal growth.

The Practice of Art Therapy

Art therapy practitioners involve themselves in the therapeutic process. As advocates of art, they strive for artistic expression from themselves, as well as from their patients. They know how to respond to and work with resisting materials. Their gratification as artists and as therapists comes from accepting and encouraging independent growth. In involving themselves, art therapists are able to temporarily regress and fantasize with control and awareness. The function of their observing egos as artists and as therapists must occasionally be suspended in order to permit them to feel with their patients, share their own imagery in order to journey into unknown territory and return safely. This type of fusion affords the deepest form of empathy.

Art therapists generally share a belief in the transcendent and inherent value of expressive art for the individual, for the group, and for the therapeutic process. Art therapists must be able to trust their own intuition and spontaneous imagery. Listening with a "third ear" and seeing with a "third eye" help art therapists use themselves as instruments of empathic understanding. Art therapists share a belief that the act of creativity is one fundamental way in which human beings grow. Growth arises within the context of having the ability and the freedom to create something new. It is the unique role of the art therapist to help provide opportunities that promote creativity and mental health.

Moreover, art therapists will occasionally use their own artistic ability to further communication with their patient. They may mirror their patients' artistic work by creating images that are similar to those represented by their patients. These mirror images can deepen the emotional impact of their patient's statement, while symbolically showing patients that their communications are shared and understood. Occasionally, therapists may wish to create images that are the opposite of those represented by their patients. This may sensitively enable patients to see that there are other ways of solving problems. Here, opposite representations are operating in complementary ways.

INTERPRETATION OF ART WORK

The fundamental role of art therapists is to be in tune, in a feeling way, with a patient's needs and psychic processes. The use of expressive art created by the patient helps the therapist perform this task. Many art therapists practicing for a few years develop the capacity to recognize a similarity of symbols in patient art work. This capacity can alert therapists to recognize graphic clues which enable them to assess a patient's psychic processes. This interpretive ability is valuable for diagnostic purposes and may be used preventively. It offers quick and accurate responses to the patient.

Graphic clues in art work

Some of the best-kept secrets are revealed through clues seen in the art work of patients unable to

verbalize their feelings of despair, hopelessness, failure, separation, and loss. Harriet Wadeson (1975)
describes the direct suicide messages communicated
by patients:

A number of patients without seeing each other's work
used the same symbol—a spiral—to convey similar feelings.
In every case the symbol appeared without any outside
suggestions.

Schildkraut, Shenker, and Sonnenblick described
the suicidal slash. Many art therapists have seen this
slash, which appears to be a slip of the pencil on a
figure drawing which is inappropriate and inconsistent with the continuity of line (See Figure B.15-1).
Additionally, many art therapists notice the recurring
drawing of blackbirds in deeply depressed patients,
similar to Van Gogh's last painting.

Clara Jo Stember worked extensively with abused children who silently scream their secret terrors out on paper
while their frightened voices remain still. Graphic clues play
an important role in communicating with these children.
Stember (1978) noted that abused children tend to include
darkened skies and suns and frequent heavy shading. They
occasionally leave out that part of their body that has been
hurt when drawing themselves. They omit themselves in
family drawings; show feelings of helplessness by drawing
themselves without hands or feet, while they draw the
abusing parent with well-defined huge hands; frequently
draw half a house coming off the page, as if something
terrible is going on in the other side; and scribble wildly and
paint over an area with white paint, depicting a desire to
undo and cover the turmoil in their lives. Entrapment drawings are also often created, showing feelings of isolation and
alienation. The child-artists place themselves behind a barrier, separating themselves from their family, or portray
themselves in the center of a circle from which there is no
escape. They feel enclosed, encapsulated, and often draw
squared mandalas.

Emanual Hammer (1978) describes in detail the use of
projective drawings as a clinical tool. His research has
proved to be a valuable aid to those therapists who rely on
the use of projective drawing interpretation in diagnosis and
treatment. The powerful symbolism of the House-Tree-Person Test is a highly significant tool for probing into the areas
of personality.

Organicity which can be detected in the art work of
patients facilitates early diagnosis. The most common organic features have been described (Cronin and Werblowsky, 1979) as:

... perseveration, simplification, short picky lines, severe perceptual rotation, figure collisions, errors in proportion, fragmentation, incomplete schemata, marked
concreteness. The problems of form can be so diffuse as
to render the end product unrecognizable.

Jung is well known for his ideas on the collective psychological experience that human beings share. He believed that
our inherited collective unconscious enabled all people to
produce universally similar symbols in art. The mandala
(circle) represents the unconscious center of ourselves and
has been drawn since paleolithic times. Many art therapists
are familiar with spontaneous mandala drawings from some
of their patients, and encourage others to draw them as a
profound symbol of wholeness. They believe, as Jung did,

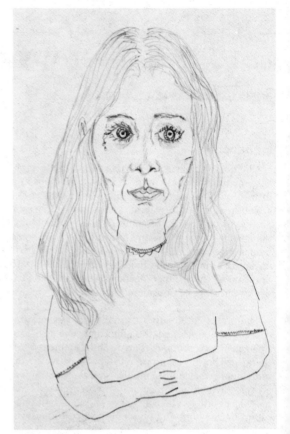

Figure B15-1   Self-portrait by an 18-year-old institutionalized female patient showing a "slip of the pencil" or
"suicidal slash" unconsciously drawn on the left cheek.

that the creation of a mandala is a self-healing process which
satisfies a basic human need for order.

Problems of art interpretation

Art therapists must be cognizant of the limitations
inherent in their ability to read art work. Correct
assessment and diagnosis of art work bear a direct
relationship to all that occurs during the sessions from
the first moment the patient enters the room until the
moment he or she leaves. The patient's affects, body
movements, conversation, use of art materials, ability
to concentrate, and relationship to the art therapist
and others in the room must all be considered as part
of the process. It is during this process that the patient
creates the product. To help clarify the manifest and
latent content of this product, the art therapist must
view it in relationship to the individual patient. The
art therapist must become familiar with the patient's
unique symbolic language and not fall into the dangerous role of making dogmatic generalizations about
the definitive meaning of all colors, shapes, lines,
images, and symbols.

In the subsequent discussion of group art therapy,
it should be noted that art interpretation is used in
conjunction with the individual and group process.

Particular interpretations serve the therapist and the group in providing essential clues as to the psychological make-up of the members.

Art Therapy in Groups

There is a recent trend within the field of art therapy to shift the emphasis from individual psychodynamics to group dynamics. Short-term groups with institutionalized patients and short-term groups with non-institutionalized, well-functioning patients are increasingly becoming the choice of treatment desired by therapists and patients.

Divergent viewpoints predominate in the use of art therapy in groups, not unlike the numerous approaches used generally in group therapy. The means of determining the theory and technique to be used depends on the theoretical orientation of the art therapist and on the needs and goals of the members of the particular group. Art therapists working in hospitals, schools, or community centers rarely have the luxury or opportunity to work with patients individually on a long-term basis. Group art therapy helps fulfill the situational needs of the institution, as well as being the therapeutically effective treatment of choice.

Many groups function best when members are able to interact with each other freely; others require more stringent control. A group of about five or six members enables the therapist to become sensitized to a patient's special problems. This sensitivity, in turn, helps the patient trust the therapist and feel some measure of security within the group. Indeed, the quality of the patient's relationship with an art therapist in a group setting differs from more conventional forms of therapy, where there may be no shared activities. Art activities initially help to reduce anxiety, provide ego support, and speed up the testing out period. However, when not used properly, they can serve negatively to further resistance.

ART MATERIALS

The use of appropriate art materials at the appropriate time helps implement the essential goals of art therapy. The art therapist must be familiar with the special properties of individual art materials, and know how and when these materials should be used. These materials must not be imposed, should be few in number, and should offer optimum opportunity for successful, non-threatening, directive and non-directive self-expression. Certain media may be used to further regression or for the purposes of building up and integration. And materials can be used for exploratory purposes, while still others may provide libidinally gratifying experiences.

Pencil

The use of a #2 drawing pencil with an eraser facilitates fantasy and storytelling. It is usually not used with large groups, where a group goal is to further group synthesis and interaction.

Crayons, cray-pas, pastels, markers

When color is introduced, the therapist is acutely aware of the expressive, as well as the defensive, qualities of different colors. Crayons suggest regressive characteristics and are often preferred by children. When it is desirable to deliberately promote regression, crayons can be used with consenting adults. Markers may be preferred by patients who desire an easily controlled clarity of tone. Children enjoy markers that are manufactured with an olfactory sense.

Paints

Only a few colors need to be available at a time. These are usually the primary colors—red, yellow, and blue—and white and black. The excitement and magic of mixing colors to create other colors enhance the patient's sense of accomplishment and need for control.

Tempera paints

Tempera paints readily mix with other colors and are water soluble. They are easy to control and offer a sense of mastery and confidence.

Water color

Water colors require a willingness to be spontaneous and an ability to go with the flow. The patient must be able to accept possible mistakes, as well as easy accomplishments. Water color is recommended in groups with well-integrated personalities where members have reasonably intact egos.

Acrylic paint

Acrylic paints are water based, dry quickly, are vibrant in hue, and permit optimum success for the talented, fairly well-functioning patient who needs a more advanced ego-oriented art experience.

Finger paints

Finger paints are an excellent medium to use to further regression when this is advised. The use of finger paints can help to relieve stress in some patients and cause anxiety in others. The therapist must be exceedingly sensitive to the needs of the patients so that this paint medium is not misused.

Clay

Clay can be hit, punched, pounded, beaten, smeared, squeezed, caressed, poked, modeled, or molded. It can be thrown, broken, rebuilt, or transposed. It can be rough or smooth, wet or dry, hard or soft, and it responds to the movement and rhythm of the patient. Clay offers an excellent opportunity for regressive activity, as well as a sense of mastery and control. It readily accepts mistakes because the process is subtractive, as well as additive. Clay is an excellent medium in which to take risks, to undo, to rebuild, and to explore.

SELECTION OF PATIENTS

Most child and adult populations are considered suitable for group art therapy. However, when it is felt that a patient may need to defend him- or herself against underlying psychosis, the use of art in group therapy may not be the treatment of choice. Patients must be able to withstand some minimal level of frustration as they struggle with art materials and with their emotions.

Motivation

It is usually not difficult to motivate patients to work with art materials if the art therapist establishes a supportive and trusting rapport. For this reason, a standard therapeutic procedure involves seeing every patient individually for at least two sessions, in order to establish the beginnings of a therapeutic alliance before placing the patient in a group situation. Patients are immediately introduced to art materials during the initial interview. This is often a time of high anxiety for the patient. Using art therapeutically can either add to this anxiety or help alleviate it. Some patients are in serious conflict, and the immediate support that they need is an empathic therapist who shares with them the knowledge of their anxiety.

When necessary, a brief description of the purpose of art therapy follows as soon as the patient can relax sufficiently to listen and participate. Drawing materials, tempera paint, and clay are attractively and conspicuously set out on the table. Adults are usually less secure with art materials than children and will readily admit their fear. "I can't draw," "I haven't done this in years," or "I'm a terrible artist" are common refrains. The art therapist must respond to the feelings expressed.

In a short-range diagnostic center, the art therapist may be more directive and ask for a self-portrait or for the House-Tree-Person Test. Using the images in the drawings as subject, the patient begins to build a rapport with the art therapist, and can often express deep conflicts seen visually in his graphic work. It can be an intense experience for the art therapist steeped in his or her own artistic imagery, and also for the patient who freely paints what comes to mind. The patient may experience an accelerated excitement that is libidinally gratifying. For many patients, the process of creativity is so intense that the art therapist should not try to get the patient to talk and break into this sometimes silent communication. Communication can utilize silence. These freely created artistic creations are often rich in symbolic imagery, reflecting primary-process thinking. An abundance of childhood memories, often traumatic in nature, surges into consciousness.

These two private sessions usually provide adequate knowledge for the art therapist to place patients in group art therapy. The relationship that began to develop with the art therapist continues in a group setting. Patients who are new to the group will often call upon the art therapist to assist with problems of art technique. Sometimes these problems are real, and assistance in solving them helps to build ego boundaries. However, a group member may use this attention to monopolize the art therapist. The desire of some patients to draw correctly may serve as resistance to understanding the feelings that inspired the art work. Art therapists must be aware of all the subtle demands for their attention, and work them through with the group.

ART THERAPY WITH CHILDREN

Children universally and instinctively pursue their need to express themselves graphically. Many children draw before they really speak. Any object or surface will satisfy this need. A pebble and stick in the sand, a piece of black coal on the sidewalk, or even their own saliva on a dry surface will please the creative urge of a 2- or 3-year-old. "Look what I made ...!" they exclaim. Unconsciously, they are making their mark in this world. The child's very first scribble is telling everyone, "I exist, I'm important, and I'm beginning to make sense out of my environment in my own, unique way." Art work is a form of symbolic communication that is a natural and non-threatening vehicle in which children express themselves. The art therapist working with children must, therefore, be knowledgeable about the normal stages of development.

Acting out

At all stages of a child's development, drawings fulfill some of the intense needs to express themselves. Therefore, motivating children is not usually a difficult task. They are often self-motivated and enjoy working with art materials alone or in groups. However, many children test the limits of their art therapy sessions by a variety of disruptive activities. Establishing nonpunitive limits helps to retain the child's ego boundaries by preventing excessive anxiety. Group disruption, destruction of property, including the art work of other members and art materials, or injury to self or others is not permitted. When possible, the therapist tries to interpret the feelings that motivated the acting-out behavior. Some group members will confront those members with poor impulse control, which can be more effective than the interpretations of an adult therapist. Children are usually not resisting treatment when they act out during their sessions. Their drawings provide an ideal opportunity for this type of cathartic communication (see Figure B.15-2).

GROUP ART THERAPY WITH ADOLESCENTS

Self-interpreted symbols in group art therapy permit the adolescent autonomy in his therapy. Adolescents can gain some measure of control as they explore the polarity of their child-like and adult feelings. Dealing with these feelings helps to reduce strong adolescent resistance. Because of an adolescent's extreme narcissism and his or her quest for personal identity and need for peer relationships, he or she finds drawing portraits penetrating and satisfying.

When working with adolescents in a group situation, the art therapist may not always discuss the content of the work. One art therapist asked her patients to do a drawing of their secrets. They were told that they would not have to talk about the content of the drawings. The group could recognize similarities in their drawings. The emotions released by suppressed material often make it unnecessary to discuss the

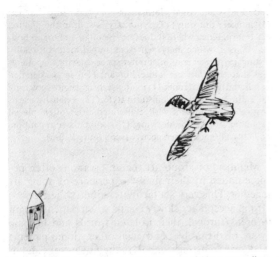

Figure B15-2 Drawing by an 11-year-old boy revealing his intention to escape from the hospital.

specific situation that caused it. In fact, the secrets of the group, as they emerged in their works, appeared to be very similar (see Figure B.15-3).

The art therapist often takes a non-directive role with adolescents and works with suggestions and material that the adolescent brings to each session. An opportunity must be provided which would enable the adolescent to bring some order to his or her life. The adolescent must be able to choose a medium among several that are presented, be able to determine how much and what will be discussed, be encouraged to choose his own topics, and decide how much his parents should be involved in the therapy, if at all. Issues that often appear spontaneously include separation anxiety, identity problems, growing sexual awareness, family problems, and peer relationships. These can be explored in the group as they work on group murals and on shared or individual art work. Affective reactions may be intense. A plea for help is often visible in the art work of adolescents (see Figure B.15-4).

GROUP ART THERAPY WITH SCHIZOPHRENIC PATIENTS

Group art therapy has advantages over individual art therapy for many schizophrenic patients. Art-based socializing experiences tend to reduce excessive anxiety and improve reality testing.

In order for schizophrenic patients to function well in group art therapy, they must have the ability to be motivated and be capable of expressing themselves through the use of art materials. Individual art therapy sessions will help to determine if the patient is able to use art as a medium of expression; if he or she can relate to an art therapist; and if, in fact, art therapy is the correct therapeutic procedure for a particular patient.

The access to primary process—to symbolic im-

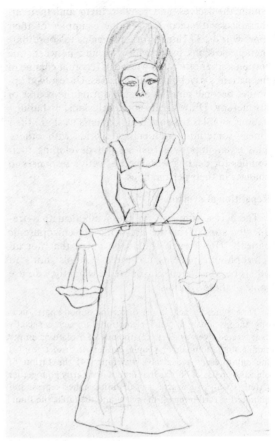

Figure B15-3 Self-portrait drawn by a 14-year-old male patient with problems of sexual identification. He is able to express in his art what he could not express verbally.

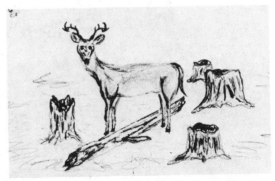

Figure B15-4 This spontaneous drawing was created by a 14-year-old noninstitutionalized boy. Broken trees and lonely, empty landscapes are frequently drawn by adolescents searching for contact and help.

agery in metaphor—helps provide the normal creative person with a desire and a need to create. Many schizophrenic patients need an outlet for their constant bombardment of imagery often unrelieved by the use of secondary process, as it is with the nonschizophrenic person. Art therapy can help schizophrenic patients better understand opposing processes within themselves, and provide them and their art therapists with recorded graphic examples of their inner worlds. Their art work also helps to coordinate therapy sessions by providing a link between one session and another. Art work can record a change in the patient's psychological processes. Unresolved opposites become more integrated during the course of art therapy. Drawing illusions, delusions, or hallucinations enables schizophrenic patients to share their inner—sometimes frightening—worlds with others. This is an important first step in developing their abilities for dealing with their affective responses to changes in their personalities.

Repetition of symbols

There is a similarity in the symbolism that frequently appears in the art work of schizophrenic patients. However, it should be noted that not all schizophrenic patients use these symbols, nor can others be considered schizophrenic when they do use some of these symbols.

These symbols include: (1) distortion of body parts, usually unconsciously drawn for emotional impact, especially exaggerated eyes or ears; (2) themes of isolation: empty chairs, single animals or people, broken or dead trees; (3) the omnipresent eye always watching; (4) the fusion of objects or parts of objects that do not ordinarily go together (Areti, 1976); (5) bizarre lack of unity, cohesiveness, and boundaries; scribbling off the page onto the table, the floor,

and the wall; rigid formalism of geometric shapes; (6) monster drawings; (7) symmetry: a split in the picture; (8) transparency where it does not belong—in human bodies, houses, which may represent impairment of reality testing; (9) perseveration of outer space drawings—patients feel that they are not quite human; (10) large, detailed hands and detailed roofs; (11) intense, bright colors covering the entire page, expressionistic in style; (12) extensive use of writing and numbers with elaborated titles often placed prominently over the drawing; (13) compulsive repetition; and (14) absence of perspective (see Figure B15-5).

Members of group art therapy sessions often become united by their shared experience of doing art together. This very act facilitates group cohesiveness. Group acceptance slowly occurs when patients begin to break through their isolated worlds and become aware of themselves and each other. Some patients recognize recurring symbols in their own work and in the work of other members. In a stable, protected group, many schizophrenic patients are able for the very first time to express their deep emotions in their drawings. Some begin to share these feelings by talking only about the picture and not using the subjective "I." Sharing feelings this way is less threatening for some patients and helps them to break through their isolated emptiness. Their own self-interpreted imagery is a form of controlled communication which also helps to lessen resistance. Themes emerge in their art work that represent powerful opposites: good ver-

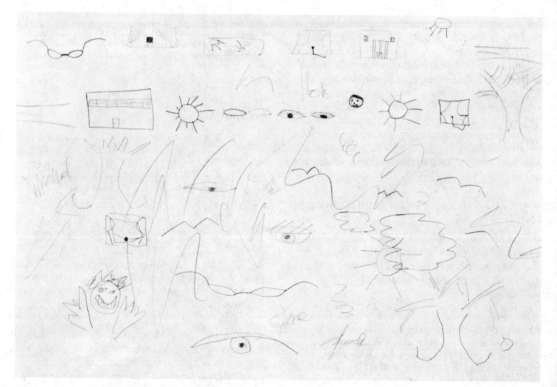

Figure B15-5   A 17-year-old female schizophrenic patient spontaneously created this drawing during the beginning of a group therapy session. Her drawings helped her to communicate her silent thoughts and reestablish contact with her external environment.

sus evil; love versus hate; devil versus angel; life versus death. Many themes express anger, dependency, identity, despondency. These themes are discussed, denied, raised again, and confronted in the group. Success with art materials and acceptance by other members encourages the patients to unburden themselves and to strive toward recompensation. Many patients gain a new respect for their own images as symbols of themselves and, thus, for themselves. Through interaction and communication with others, they become involved in a feeling way with those around them, creating within themselves access to rational, orderly thinking.

An art therapy session with schizophrenic patients

The beginning of most art therapy sessions with schizophrenic patients is often devoted to individual free art productions. Some patients spontaneously draw themselves, their dreams, and their devils. Others create marks at random, not unlike a type of graphic free association. After completion of their work, patients are encouraged to discuss it in a form of go-round. The art therapist interprets only what her patients are emotionally capable of understanding. In the second half of the session, group projects and topics are suggested. These topics focus on the immediate group experience, as well as on the members' inner psychic processes: (1) Draw something about yourself that you would like to share with the group; (2) draw the people in this room; (3) draw feelings that are difficult to talk about; (4) draw what you are feeling right now; (5) non-verbal silent communication drawing with two or three participating members; (6) create the symbol of yourself; (7) draw things that are real, things that are not real; and (8) draw on one side of the paper what you are like on the outside; on the other side, draw how you feel on the inside.

Conclusion

Sharing images in group art therapy encourages perceptions that may be lost in verbal therapy alone. Art therapy enables patients to see things that they often cannot admit are there until their graphic images are dramatically recorded before them. The art-oriented relationship helps them to literally look at themselves, inside and out.

Creative artistic work is a metaphor for communication. Patients and therapists respond to each other, journeying from primary to secondary processes, creating metaphorical dialogues that link fantasy, symbols, dreams, play, and wishes with the real world. This type of contact in the therapeutic relationship is a necessary ingredient for psychological health. Patients and therapists are relating to each other in an empathic, alert, creative, and spontaneous way which, in turn, encourages autonomous growth. The patients' artistic productions are their very own, created from their hearts and minds. Although their artistic products may be different from each other, the feelings that produced them are usually very similar. When patients share these intense feelings with each other and with the art therapist, they are involved in the complex process of building object relationships that are consistent with ego development. To be involved in a therapeutic relationship which involves the use of artistic imagery is, therefore, to be involved in an act of creation.

References

Arieti, S. *Creativity: The Magic Synthesis.* Basic Books, New York, 1976.

Cronin, S. M., and Werblowsky, J. H. Early signs of organicity in art work. Art Psychother. *6:* 103, 1979.

Di Leo, J. *Young Children and Their Drawings.* Brunner/Mazel, New York, 1970.

Garnder, H. *The Arts and Human Development.* John Wiley & Sons, New York, 1973.

Hammer, E. *The Clinical Application of Projective Drawings.* Charles C Thomas, Springfield, IL, 1978.

Janson, H. W. *History of Art.* Harry Abrams, New York, 1971.

Kellog, R. *The Psychology of Children's Art.* Random House, New York, 1967.

Kramer, E. *Art as Therapy in a Children's Community.* Schocken Books, New York, 1977.

Kramer, E. The unity of process and product. Am. J. Art Ther. *14:* 12, 1974.

Naumberg, M. Art therapy: Its scope and function. In: *The clinical Application of Projective Drawings,* E. Hammer editor, p. 511. Charles C Thomas, Springfield, IL, 1978.

Ulman, E. Innovation and aberration. Am. J. Art Ther. *14:* 12, 1974.

Wadeson, H. Suicide: Expression in images. Am. J. Art Ther., *16:* 75, 1975.

B.16 Dance Therapy

VIRGINIA KLEIN, D.T.R.

Introduction

Dance therapy is considered a new modality, having been formally recognized in 1942, with the hiring of pioneer dance therapist Marian Chace at St. Elizabeth's Hospital in Washington, D.C. Although within the profession "dance" and "movement" are used synonomously, each term actually describes a point of view: Movement encompasses the world of physical motion, whereas dance is a specific creative act within that world.

The American Dance Therapy Association defines dance therapy as "the psychotherapeutic use of movement which furthers the emotional and physical integration of the individual."

Dance therapy, as a therapeutic modality, both individual and group, is based on a kinesthetic reality, the idea that there is a logic to movement. Becoming aware of the self physically, combined with executing a dance act, can yield a sense of accomplishment and be a means toward self-understanding: Both these are fundamental to growth via dance therapy. Indeed, the versatility and range of dance enable the patient to express his uniqueness. This expression is a means of communication to both the therapist and other group members. The therapist is then able to interpret these expressions.

Although dance therapy occurs primarily in a hospital setting, and although most dance therapists are working in the mental health field, dance therapy is becoming more accepted as an independent treatment modality in the group form. However, due to the relative newness of the field, dance therapy is most widely used today in conjunction with other forms of therapy.

Dance therapy is particularly suited for group psychotherapy in that the physical activity creates a heightened sense of identification and empathy; the shared movement and rhythm contribute to a cohesiveness that can occur more rapidly than in a traditional group.

Dance therapy has been successfully used with prisoner populations, the learning disabled, the physically handicapped, and the retarded.

History

Dance therapy is considered to begin with Marian Chace (1896–1970), the first acknowledged dance therapist to be hired in the United States. Chace, the first president of the American Dance Therapy Association (ADTA), was hired at St. Elizabeth's Hospital, in Washington, D.C., in 1942. At St. Elizabeth's, Chace introduced programs to meet the needs of backward patients, as well as those of servicemen returning from World War II. In addition to working with patients, she also trained and taught most of the leading dance therapists of the time, many of whom are still practicing. Additionally, Chace's papers, like Freud's papers in psychoanalysis, comprise the bulk of the literature of dance therapy.

Trudy Schoop is another pioneer in dance therapy. Schoop, still practicing, believed that comic pantomimes were the vehicle through which the body revealed its "humorous statements about man's imperfections," and that the expression of these statements, via dance, was the first step toward working through personality disorders.

Mary Sachs Whitehouse is the foremost dance therapy pioneer who worked outside the hospital setting in the dance studio with a normal neurotic population. Whitehouse placed a great deal of emphasis on improvisation, on the idea that dances, prompted by spontaneous feelings and ideas, convey an individual point of view and are especially valid as a means of expressing the inner-subconscious workings of the mind. Whitehouse was a patient of Jung, and her analysis provided her with her approach to dance therapy; she adapted Jung's view that artistic creation (dance) can be the gateway to self-knowledge.

Goals and Aims

Dance therapy, like other therapeutic modalities, is designed to facilitate the growth of the individual's ability to help himself and the ability to interact with others.

All dance therapy sessions, regardless of the type of group and patient, have in common four basic goals: (1) the development of body awareness; (2) the expression of feelings; (3) the fostering of interaction and communication; and (4) the integration of the physical, emotional, and social experiences which result in a sense of increased self-confidence and contentment.

Another factor basic to all kinds of dance therapy groups is that the patient takes an active part in the process, and is not a passive recipient of treatment. The individual uses his body to effect change, and feels a direct and immediate involvement as the reality of his feelings is felt through the reality of his body.

Theoretical Considerations

The theoretical framework of dance therapy is based on a combination of three key concepts: (1) body language and movement behavior are integrally connected to —and reflective of—an individual's psychological state; (2) movement is communication; and (3) there is therapeutic value in the artistic experience.

The first principle reflects the psychoanalytic ideas of Wilhelm Reich and Paul Schilder, as well as the theories of Rudolph Laban's movement language.

Wilhelm Reich focused his attention on the actual behavior of the patient and the meaning of this behavior. He felt that "word language very often functions as a defense" and that these defenses could be observed in the posture, gait, muscular patterns, and muscular tensions of the body. This physical manifestation of psychological conflict and traits Reich called character armor. He felt that this visible manner of resistance was an "armoring against the stimuli of the outer world and against the repressed impulses." He studied various character types and found that there were motoric qualities peculiar to each type, such as the uneven, highly tense, rigid, and restrained motoric qualities of the obsessive and the soft, agile, flowing, and labile motoric qualities of the hysteric.

The body image theories of Paul Schilder are also relevant to dance/movement theory. He believed that "motion influences the body-image and leads from a change in the body-image to a change in the psychic attitude .... body events are feelings."

Additionally, Rudolph Laban devised a system of studying movement language, called effort/shape. This objective method describes and investigates the visible dynamics of movement in terms of how kinetic energy and spatial structure are utilized by the body. This system delineates how the movement is done in terms of the basic motion factors of force, space, time, and flow. Of these motion factors, flow is viewed in a somewhat different light; changes in the quality of flow happen most frequently, and provide a foundation for the other efforts. The body is always in an energized condition, responding to rhythmic changes in breathing and adapting to internal and external stimuli which provide a base of continuous impulses to move. These motion factors are used in infinite combinations and varieties, which Laban believed mirror inner drives and impulses from which movement originates. Effort/shape is used primarily by dance therapists as a tool for research and diagnosis.

Size of group

The optimum size of a group is 7 to 9, plus the leader. This allows for a rich variety of movement styles and for a range of personality types that provides potential for an abundance of interaction, exploration, learning, and discovery. Contagion builds through the group's rhythmic collective movements that wear down feelings of self-consciousness and resistance and increase participation. Moreover, these universal rhythmic gestures enhance feelings of solidarity and stability.

As the session progresses, separate formations occur, such as pairs, trios, lines, and quartets. These formations within the group are useful because they enable the therapist to focus more on the individual, and offer a more intimate socialization experience for the group members.

Some patients move more freely and spontaneously in group sizes of 10 to 14, feeling that this size hides them; their sense of being unnoticed helps them feel less inhibited. The schizoid members may feel safer in a larger group because of this same reason.

Certain types of patients, such as the severely re-gressed and the depressed, may feel overwhelmed by a large group and do better in groups of 3 to 5, which are more individually geared.

Patient selection

Heterogeneous groups, varying in age, sex, and ethnic backgrounds, create an ideal group mix for the dance therapy group. This variety provides many diversified movement styles, which in turn makes possible alternatives of group and therapist interpretation.

Patients are selected because of a specific movement or body image problem, such as visible constriction in the upper body or moving in a frozen or overly rigid manner. Patients are referred for interpersonal problems, such as the inability to clearly express their feelings, or extreme bodily preoccupation. Patients are also referred because they have found dance to be therapeutic for them in the past, such as in the form of a previous leisure time interest.

In the hospital setting, patients particularly suited to this modality are the severely withdrawn, depressed, and psychotic. For the withdrawn, the group provides a socialization experience without verbal communication; for the depressed patient, dance therapy helps to mobilize and reinvolve; and for the psychotic patient, dance therapy helps them to contact reality and become more oriented.

Homogeneous groups

Adolescents and geriatrics seem to function best when worked with in their own groups.

Those issues unique to adolescence, such as identity, separation, individuation, image control, and body image can be focused on in all adolescent groups. Often, it is even more effective when girl adolescents are treated in one group and boys in another.

In a geriatric group, supportive goals—rather than personality change—are focused on, such as the maintenance of physical health, to provide socialization and to enhance self-esteem. The session is geared to their specific needs and is usually a slower paced one, with more conversation about past experiences.

Contraindications

Patients with tenuous impulse control, such as hypomanic types, would be too disruptive and demanding. An extremely paranoid patient would be too frightened.

Process

Every dance therapy session is improvisational in nature, evolving from the needs of the group; however, there is an underlying structure common to all groups. This structure consists of a development and a closure. The major tool of treatment is the movement pattern of the group; all aspects of dance movement are used in the service of self-expression and communication.

Rapport is established on a non-verbal level, as the dance therapist moves with the patient or group in a way that conveys understanding, acceptance, and interest. This is done by adapting her movement patterns to reflect what she sees and feels. This rhythmic synchrony fosters empathy and cohesiveness.

The type of approach used in a session depends on the kind of patient group involved. A direct, focused style is most effective when working with the psychotic, the very depressed, the geriatric, and the adolescent group. Structure reduces idiosyncratic behavior, orients to reality, fosters interaction, and enables those individuals who are either too depressed or threatened to initiate and to function in a productive way. Some examples of structures that are useful in sessions include: martial art exercises, like those found in Tai Chi Chuan; the use of concrete objects, like balls or scarfs; a dance form such as the Virginia reel or the L.A. walk.

An open-ended, more improvisational approach works well with patients who are organized and have good ego functioning. Here the external structure is barely perceptible, and the leader fades into the group as low-key participant and observer. One patient dubbed the improvisational or authentic response part of the session "free lance dance." Overall, however, a session flows between a directive and a nondirective manner, depending on the moment-to-moment needs of the group.

The warm-up

The warm-up is probably the most important part of the session. Rushing this process often results in sessions that lack depth. The purpose of this portion is to spend sufficient time warming up the body physically and to create an environment of trust and exploration that encourages self-expression and interaction.

The session begins the moment the patients enter the room, with the therapist taking in such non-verbal behavior as body posture, facial expression, speed of gestures, and the individual's connection to the environment and to each other. Music is selected to support the level where the majority of the group is at, although the session itself is geared to those individuals who need the most support.

The session usually begins in a circle. This earliest space form is the universal symbol of totality and wholeness; and this containing, protective shape seems to make patients aware of their capacity to both give and receive.

The first movements are designed to activate body parts, gradually beginning with the periphery—such as fingers or toes—and slowly working toward the center of the body; the ultimate aim is to get the movement flowing throughout the body. Work is also done at this time on body alignment, on defining body boundaries, on an increase of breathing, and on reducing muscular tensions.

When this movement starts to flow throughout the body, it is termed postural, rather than gestural. As the trunk becomes involved, the body weight is mobilized, and patients appear more grounded and connected to the environment. In mobilizing an individual's strength and firmness in movement behavior, he is able to counteract feelings of helplessness and lack of control. In addition, greater involvement on the physical level triggers more intense involvement on the emotional and cognitive levels.

At the same time the body is being warmed up, the therapist begins to warm up the group on an interactional level, slowly prompting nonverbal communication through the rhythm and movement patterns.

Development

Most commonly, the middle or core of the session deals with the themes and issues that emerge from the here and now manifest in the movement process. In the following example, the issue of risk stemmed from a simple rocking movement.

A heterogeneous group of young adults was in a circle shifting weight from front leg to back. The leader asked, "What's this movement like?" Someone said, "It's like looking into a wishing well!" Another person said, "Let's make a wish!" So, in pantomime fashion, each group member found a penny and made a wish for themselves as they tossed the coins into the well. Group members began to verbalize wishes for good health, love, inner peace, etc., while underneath the movement provided continuity and cohesion. Ann began to cry and said, "I'm afraid to make a wish!" The leader suggested that perhaps her feeling was related to a fear of being disappointed. The woman nodded in agreement, and several group members verbally identified with Ann. They then explored—on a verbal and movement level—different ways of taking chances and the uncertainty of change.

However, in the case of Zoe, prior knowledge of her suicide provided the opportunity for her group to conduct a funeral rite.

Zoe, a slim, lithe, 43-year-old woman, came into a small Midwestern hospital following the death of her lover of 20 years. On the ward, she was almost mute and kept on the fringe of the community. The only activity she attended was dance therapy, in which she participated twice a week. Her movement style was characterized by a quick, light, impulsive quality. She remained aloof from others by frequently dancing outside the circle or by weaving in and out of the group. She made her presence known through unexpected and often humorous movement patterns. Her indirect, subtle contributions made a solid impact of the group. Then, as she appeared to be improving, she jumped from a window in the hospital.

The next morning, patients and staff used the dance therapy session to memorialize Zoe, and to give each other solace. Through a combination of music, movement, talking, and crying, the group gave vent to their feelings and worked through their fear and helplessness. After a warm-up to soothing music that was characterized by a great deal of comforting through touch and rocking movements, a piece of Greek music was selected by the group. The group improvised a Greek dance, as, passing someone's handkerchief, they made their own movement statement. The handkerchief was the symbol of Zoe, and each individual had a chance to say good-bye to her in his own way.

Dance therapy also helps an individual group member to grow, as illustrated in the following example:

Harry, 37, was a husky, clumsy man. He felt uneasy with others and lived a schizoid life style, both in and out of the hospital. Seven years prior to hospitalization, he was a practicing lawyer but had not functioned in that capacity since.

He walked in a heavy plodding manner, his upper torso rounded forward, giving him a weighted down, tight-as-a-drum appearance.

Harry had been attending dance therapy three times a week for 2 months, where he was a most enthusiastic participant, despite his awkwardness and difficulties with the movement process. His movement patterns were rigid, bound in their flow, and lacking both fluidity and flexibility. This lack of give was evident in his trunk which he used in one piece, unable to make rapid changes of direction. The only movement with which he appeared at ease was a deep bow, which he repeated at least once every session.

Rather than dancing, Harry acted out—in a concrete, formal way similar to pantomime—his ideas, his feelings, and his interactions with others. During a session where the movement sequences had been rapid and complex, Harry struggled but stayed with it. When it was his turn to give the group his movement theme, he mimed a bent-over person with a cane, taking slow tottering steps. When asked who he was, he said, "I'm an old man!" One could surmise that unconsciously he had felt, compared with his peers in the group, like an old man. Another time, at the close of a session, Harry's way of saying good-bye was to mime tears falling from his eyes as he shook hands with everyone. In this symbolic, formal manner, he conveyed his sadness over the group's ending that day.

Although he rarely spontaneously contributed verbal suggestions or contributions that he was there, Harry was, in fact, aware of all that happened, and he functioned best when carried along by the momentum and cohesiveness of the group. At these times, his movements were the most fluid.

Dance therapy helped Harry by providing him with a group experience where he received positive reinforcement of his assets, such as his originality and sense of humor. Thus, his ego in turn was strengthened, and his self-esteem was increased. He participated in an active way and was able to share others' experiences. Indeed, dance therapy finally motivated Harry to begin jogging and to undertake a back-to-work program.

Harry is a typical example of Reich's description of compulsive characters as living machines. This group provided Harry a way to abandon his intellectual controls and to express his emotional self.

Verbal imagery

The dance therapeutic technique of verbal imagery is used to support, maintain, and facilitate the aims of the dance therapy process. The imagery can be reality oriented, such as with phrases that relate to body parts, to the physical environment, or to seasons of the year. The group is encouraged to add their own images. Imagery is used to stimulate the imagination and helps individuals to recall and re-experience. It is phrased in an open-ended way that allows for choice and risk. In addition to words, the dance therapist modulates the sound of her voice to reflect the movement qualities and to serve as a bridge to the patient unable to make eye contact. Whenever possible, sounds are encouraged, and sometimes impromptu singing occurs.

Sometimes, it helps to reveal hitherto concealed spontaneity and creativity.

Michael, an extremely depressed, flat group member, rarely initiated movement phrases or interacted with others. He was part of a group that found themselves moving to the verbal image of being some type of machine, such as an agitator in a washer or a fan. Suddenly, Michael jumped up in a vertical direction, shouting, "I'm a toaster!" This added a surprising and amusing contribution to the session and served to evoke a greater degree of group spontaneity.

Role of the leader

Dance therapy is a process of mutual exchange; the leader assumes a very active role of participation and observation. She must transmit kinesthetic enthusiasm to be a catalyst to the action, as well as having the flexibility to quickly become a background group member.

Since the primary mode of treatment is the interaction between the movement patterns of the patient and the therapist, sensitive, accurate adaptation is necessary, in tandem with a keen kinesthetic awareness to group mood, i.e., the idea of the dance therapist's body as a third ear, listening to the patients. The dance therapist picks up movement cues from the group; these cues are unconsciously expressed needs and reactions which she then mirrors or empathetically imitates in her movement patterns. These movements are then developed more freely on or body level and are interpreted, worked with, and worked through.

The role is a vulnerable one, as the therapist enters the session as a real person and is as physically involved as the patient. It is vital that the therapist know her movement repertoire thoroughly and that she possess a solid dance technique, in order to move in as wide a range of movement as is required to meet a wide variety of patient needs.

Along with all the attributes a qualified verbal therapist needs, the dance therapist additionally must be highly aware on a non-verbal level of her shortcomings, and not use the movement process to satisfy her own exhibitionistic and narcissistic needs, such as imposing her own movement style on the group. Positive countertransference will manifest itself as the leader might pick up a movement that reflects a patient's unconscious movement preferences. And, seeing his movement performed by the leader may give the resistant person permission to move. On the negative side, the leader may not see the movement of someone or may subtly change it due to her unconscious hostile feelings toward the individual.

Use of music

Music is the dance therapist's major tool, and is an invaluable aid in creating a therapeutic environment. It creates this environment by providing, through rhythm and melody, a structure that induces self-expression, communication, empathy, and cohesiveness. Further, music cuts through hallucinations and language barriers, and can illicit memories and associations.

Music is carefully selected for the dance therapy session. It should have a consistent beat and reflect the needs of the group. For example, lively music is used to support an extroverted, high-energy group and soft music to support a subdued, low-energy group.

In a geriatric group, one 70-year-old depressed women was a very active member. She had been attending the group on a weekly basis for 6 weeks, and she had displayed considerable flexibility, strength, and humor. Prior to admission to the hospital, she had cared for her dying husband for over a year. Three weeks after her admission, he died. Mrs. L. had been unable to cry or talk about the event. The staff was quite concerned about her denial and potential for suicide. In the middle of the session, as she was dancing to a polka, she began to cry, saying, "The music reminds me of dancing with my husband at weddings." Afterward, in the verbal discussion that followed the movement part, she received feedback and support from other widows in the group. During subsequent sessions with her psychiatrist and on the ward, she was able to weep and talk about her complex feelings toward her husband. The combination of music and movement process brought about emotional change and growth more quickly than the use of words alone would have.

Closure

With a return to the circle formation, ending of the session begins. This process is a gradual winding down, leveling off, and tying together of everything that has preceded. This centering happens on a kinesthetic level, as the movements tend to get smaller and closer to the body.

The feeling of group intimacy is at its most intense during closure; and this is augmented by touch—a holding of hands or arms around the shoulders. Also, there is more ease with eye contact.

Often, the preparation to separate precipitates tears, and issues about separation are discussed. This is a timely place for a group member to say good-bye. Patients come up with many innovative ways of doing this, frequently moving in their own characteristic or favorite movement phrase.

Resistance

Resistance shows itself in obvious verbal ways, like excessive talking or giggling. It can be observed on the movement level in effort-shape parameters, and in rhythmic factors. Resistance can also be seen in excessively rapid movement changes, which indicate a flight from feeling in the same way a person might continually change the subject in resisting entering into an issue. The dance therapist helps the patient stick with a movement repeatedly so that he can feel it and work it through. Group rhythm often breaks through resistance, and repetition decreases self-consciousness.

Training

In the last 40 years, dance therapy training has moved from an apprentice system to formal study on the graduate level. Before 1971, dancers coming from performing-teaching careers learned the dance therapy craft from practicing dance therapists, such as Marian Chace, Trudy Schoop, and Mary Whitehouse. The next step was to volunteer in a clinical setting, usually working from 6 months to a year before being hired. Today, there are 11 Masters programs, all of which are ADTA approved, offering a Masters in dance therapy. Additionally one dance therapist is usually part of the therapeutic team in psychiatric and rehabilitative settings.

In 1966, the ADTA was founded to set standards for professional competency, ethics, and education of dance therapists. Marian Chace was the first president. Today the membership is 1,100 (50 of these foreign), and there are presently 265 registered dance therapists.

In 1968, the ADTA formed the Registry, to further standardize and assure for professional competency. To be a registered dance therapist (D.T.R.), applicants must meet registry criteria, which include 3,640 dance therapy hours in a clinical setting and a Masters degree in dance therapy or a related field, such as dance, social work, expressive therapies, or psychology.

References

Bartenieff, I. Dance therapy: A new profession or a rediscovery of an ancient role of the dance. Dance Scope, 7: 1, 1972.
Bernstein, P. L., editor. *Eight Theoretical Approaches in Dance-Movement Therapy.* Kendall/Hunt, Dubuque, IA, 1979.
Chaiklin, H., editor. *Marian Chace: Her Papers.* American Dance Therapy Association, New York, 1975.
Davis, M. Movement characteristics of hospitalized psychiatric patients. Am. J. Dance Ther., 4: 1, 1981.
Laban, R., and Lawrence, F. C. *Effort.* Macdonald and Evans, Boston, 1947.
North, M. *Personality Assessment through Movement.* Macdonald and Evans, London, 1972.

B.17 Overview of Family and Network Therapy

C. CHRISTIAN BEELS, M.D., M.S.

Introduction

There is an essential difference between group therapy and family therapy. A therapy group is a special group of individuals who come together for the purpose of the therapy; a family is a natural group with many purposes and functions more important to its members than the hopefully temporary one of being in therapy. Consequently, the relationship of the group to the therapist, the contract governing the meeting, and the time between meetings, is different.

The contract in group therapy is similar to that in individual therapy: Each person is there to further his own development and self-discovery. A family, on the other hand, is a strong and well-organized group which has hired a therapist for purposes that are hidden in the tangle of its own politics and processes. These purposes are influenced by considerations outside the boundary of the treatment situation. Examples of such influence include culture, locality, stage of family life cycle, and extended family. Establishing and changing this boundary, such as the inclusion of grandparents or seeing only the parents without the children, is an important question of therapeutic strategy. Going beyond the household and convening or consulting with an entire network of friends, relatives, and neighbors is carrying the strategy of changing the boundary several steps further. In family and network therapy, then, the expert is a consultant to a natural group which he must in some way invade and influence, perhaps enlarge and reorganize. This kind of infiltration from the periphery of an organized group requires considerable diplomacy and other social skills not necessarily involved in group therapy.

Family therapy is a distinctively American phenomenon whose origins are deep in our culture. The author will trace only two of its intellectual roots, one in anthropology and one in psychoanalysis.

Alliance with Anthropology

The idea that meaning arises most significantly from present sequences of behavior in natural human groups goes back at least to G. H. Mead's earliest lectures (ca. 1910) about the conversation of gestures which in man and animals is the basis of the evolution of language, and indeed of mind, self, and society. Mead's colleague at Chicago, the linguist Edward Sapir, wrote about the analysis of language and gesture, emphasizing the existence of unconscious structure in communication, an elaborate and secret code that is written nowhere, known by none, and understood by all.

Sapir was the first of several anthropologists who understood well the interdependence of three different social determinants—the individual's personal history of experience, the cultural background, and the immediate organization of the communicating group. The first was the province of psychiatry, the second of cultural anthropology, and the third of a new science of communication which drew upon an understanding of sequence and structure at many levels of description. The mutual influence between anthropology and psychiatry, then, began in the 1920's, with the behavior of people in natural groups as their common meeting ground.

The collaboration flourished under the influence of Margaret Mead's work on culture and personality and her contributions to the new science of semiotics, to which the psychiatrist Harley Shands brought one of the most important syntheses. It reached a high state of technical development when Ray Birdwhistell and Albert Scheflen together published their method of context analysis.

In this tradition of anthropologists and psychiatrists working together, anthropology contributed the discipline of exact observation of the social process, often retrievable for detailed analysis by film and sound recording. It also contributed the idea that communication as social structure might have its own regularities and laws independent of a psychology rooted in individual experience and interpretation. Family therapists were part of all this research; Don Jackson and Jay Haley are two prominent examples.

Bateson's group proposed the double bind as a hypothesis of the etiology of schizophrenia. It was the high point of the collaboration with anthropology, and it was in many ways the model for the investigation of communication pathology.

Bateson was one of the principal philosophers of science of our time. When he died in 1980, he had just published *Mind and Nature: A Necessary Unity*, which is not only the summation of his own researches but a general model for the integration of mind in the social and biological world.

In 1956, when Bateson's group in Palo Alto published "Towards A Theory of Schizophrenia," his extraordinary ability to find profound unities among seemingly discordant social phenomena was already apparent. With his former wife, Margaret Mead, he had made a very innovative study of Balinese personality and culture, using film and still photography. In his monograph *Naven* he had shown how contradictions in sex roles and age grades in a South Sea culture were integrated by the group's major rituals. In Palo Alto, he had gathered together a group to study communication in the families of schizophrenics at the Veterans Hospital. The question was how to explain the thought disorder of the patient—a puzzling and central feature of the disorder. The theory, based on observation of family interaction, was that taking leave of rational discourse could be an adaptive response to a communication dilemma; if a person experiences a primary negative communication (such as a criticism) and a command concerning it on another level (such as "Do not notice this criticism") from a person of importance to him (such as a parent) in a situation from which there is no escape (such as the family of such a vulnerable person), then a psychotic response could be adaptive because it preserves the relationship by being a response (to the criticism) which at the same time is not a response (does not point out the conflict exactly). It is thus a contribution to the homeostasis of the family system, an avoidance of differentiation from the parent. In the original paper, the authors made parallels to hypnosis, humor, poetry, and other resolutions of contradictions between levels of communication.

Because it addressed the problem of the disorder of thinking and related it to problems of epistomology in other fields, the theory immediately appealed to many investigators of schizophrenia and drew approval from writers as diverse as Ronald Laing and Harold Searles. The words "double bind" passed quickly into common speech as a general term for what Laing called "mystification." It became one of the prototypes of interpersonal psychopathology.

Family Therapy and Psychoanalysis

Many originators of the family therapy movement were psychoanalytically trained or had enough personal analysis to be strongly influenced by the method and theory. This was certainly true of Ackerman, Bowen, Jackson, Whitaker, Lidz, and Wynne. On the whole, the separate traditions of family therapy and psychoanalysis have enriched each other in practice.

Most people learn to speak the language of both modalities, so that they practice in effect what Gurman and Kniskern (1981) call "pragmatic, psychodynamic therapy." Wynne, in his introduction to their volume, says that this is the most widespread form of family therapy. It implies, he says, that "dynamic principles are acknowledged and accepted, but are conceptualized within a general system rather than a psychoanalytic framework, and that this framework is used in selecting whatever varieties of techniques and strategies appear most likely to resolve rapidly the presenting problems of the family." In other words, good therapists use psychodynamic ideas, among others, to devise good strategies. This point is particularly evident in marital therapy. For example, we use psychodynamic formulations in treating marital trouble between a hysterical wife and an obsessive husband. Marital therapy is the part of the field whose literature is most informed by psychoanalytic insights. There is an elegant, mostly British, tradition of marital treatment, drawing on object relations theory, beginning with Main's paper on mutual projection in a marriage and including the writings of Dicks, Howells, and Martin, among many others. The conjoint treatment of middle-class couples whose marriages are in trouble is a particularly good place to introduce ideas of this sort.

However eclectic the sources of family therapy general practice may be, it has not been eclectic in some areas of its training, research, and development. One stream of family therapy development especially has diverged from psychoanalytic training and epistomology; that divergence is described in the next sections.

The model of training and development

The teaching of psychoanalytic technique requires the establishment of two analyst-patient relationships: the trainee's own training analysis and the analysis the trainee does with the patient (three, counting the trainee's supervision insofar as it is similar in technique). In each of these confidential compartments, what is transpiring is the detailed examination of a verbal report of one person's memories, thoughts, fantasies, and associations. The report is a text which is subjected to (mostly private) explication by the listener, using the key of the speaker's past life, resistances, and distortions; from this mosaic, the listener selects some pieces of the explication to offer as interpretation or intervention. The ultimate subject of each analysis is a kaleidoscope of transferences, in which characters who originate in one story appear disguised in another. The essence of the method is privacy, confidentiality, and historical and textual accuracy (as opposed to distortion); the esthetic technique is literary.

The teaching and development of family therapy, on the other hand, is theater. It is filmed, videotaped, and observed from behind the one-way screen. As Lynn Hoffman has observed, this has led to a bicameral treatment, with one room where the interview happens and another on the dark side of the one-way mirror, where the observers and teachers are watching the sequences and refining the strategies. This was indeed, as Hoffman says, the microscope of the new method, revealing levels of understanding not suspected before.

The therapist in the room with the family and the teacher with the audience behind the mirror are directors who are trying to understand the movement and blocking of the scene. They are trying to get it to play differently and will give stage directions, recast, and reorganize the scene. If the director behind the mirror wants to change something, he will go into the other room and give directions. Ritual and exercise are important here, as in the theater. The therapist will retire behind the mirror to watch and consult with those who have been observing, assuming they have been able to see what he could not because he was too much part of the action. And changing the action to get the right ensemble effect is the purpose of the interview. Control over timing, sequence, and the structure of relationships is what the therapist is after. Analysis of transference and of distortions of report is absent. In their place are enactments of scenes with metaphors supplied by the director-therapists.

This dramaturgy has taken a number of forms quite beyond the training of novice therapists. Charles Fulweiler spent most of his time behind the mirror, emerging only to give the family directions. Minuchin split the family into groups, asking one group to observe the other, sometimes from behind the mirror where he could comment as the action was going on. The Palozzoli group uses consultants behind the mirror as the source of a final written instruction to the family. Ian Alger uses immediate video playback of the interview as an intervention. Norman Paul plays video clips from other families to stimulate the responses of the family he is seeing.

Epistomology

The two methods differ also in how they come to know the truth. Psychoanalysis searches out as evidence the innermost accessible—and, therefore, ultimate individual—structure. The less the therapist appears to direct the process, the more genuinely will the evidence of the interview appear to proceed only from the patient's interior. Family therapy, on the other hand, is concerned with what Laing called "the politics of the family," and the therapist must somehow get the members to behave differently toward each other in order to learn the truth. He has no other choice. The family's political organization, from which their present ideas and thoughts proceed, is very strong; the therapist must get something different going in the session and, beyond that, in the life between sessions. Understanding or insight is a by-product, perhaps not even a necessary by-product, of a difference in action or process.

Structure, Behavior, Strategy, and Paradox

There are several groups of family therapists of whom the above description is especially true. Their approaches may be grouped under the headings of some of the key concepts which have been used in the field. It should be kept in mind, however, that this is only a device for exposition; many kinds of therapists do these things at different times in the practice of good eclectic therapy.

This description refers to exponents of particular techniques who have developed them to a special degree. If there is anything these specialists have in common, it might be the following tendencies: (1) they take the family's complaint as the problem to work on in its own terms; (2) they do not have a set of ideals about how healthy families ought to be; (3) they tend to invent new metaphors for each family and keep their own philosophy and personality in the background; and (4) they are interested in brief treatment and outcome research.

Structure

The structures which the family therapist is interested in are for the most part quite visible or, at least, diagrammable from data in the session. There are natural divisions between the generations, between the sexes, between age grades of children, and between life stages of adults. There are coalitions, both open and covert. A favorite family structure is the triangle, in which any pair may be close to the expense of the distant third. Haley has explicated a theory of

the perverse triangle, in which the close pair is a covert coalition of two people on opposite sides of a gradient, such as a generation boundary, and the outsider is one who, according to rule, should be the partner of one of the pair. The oedipal triangle of parent and child, covertly united against the other parent, is an example. Another kind of structure is the characteristic quality of dyadic relationships, which may, for example, be either symmetrical (equal and potentially competitive) or complementary (unequal and reciprocally reinforcing), as in the parent-child caretaking dyad.

The evidence for these structures is in the behavior of the family. It may be manifested by seating arrangements, ordering of speech and topics, interruption patterns, silencing strategies, agreements and disagreements, disqualifying and undermining gestures, or symmetry and synchrony of movement. The group that has developed the use of such observations technically to the greatest extent and has labeled their approach "structural family therapy" is Salvador Minuchin's group at the Philadelphia Child Guidance Center. This approach contains the clearest picture of the therapist working on the structure of the family—organizing them into subgroupings, inducing enactments between specific members, joining with those who need support, and giving tasks to be carried out between sessions to change relationships or reframe the meaning of symptomatic behavior. The therapist is always a moving force in the organization of the family.

Behavior

This interest in control of the process and giving tasks for the life outside the session is very close to behavior therapy. Indeed, there are whole behavioral schools of family therapy—behavioral parent training, behavioral marital therapy, and sex therapy—which have in common family members coming with the expectation of resolving a particular problem or changing symptomatic behavior within the family. The contract to promote change is made explicitly, the methods discussed openly, the learning program arranged, and the treatment finished when the behavior has been changed. Most family therapists would recognize some of this in what they do, and are happy to find favorable cases or problems which will yield to this straightforward approach. There is not much reluctance in this field about giving advice, education, and training exercises wherever they work.

Strategy

Often straight behavior change does not work. On the contrary, the family may be faced with and agree to very reasonable programs of self-reform, clear communication, and so on, and repeatedly find itself unable to make these changes. In these situations, the therapist must recognize that he is dealing with an organization of considerable stability and strength—stronger even than their own individual wills to change—and a strategy is called for which will deal with this group resistance, or homeostasis. The people who have written the most about this call themselves strategic therapists; among them are Jay Haley, Duncan Stanton, Gerald Zuk, and a series of people at the Mental Research Institute in Palo Alto.

These strategic therapists have been specifically concerned with the most effective way for the therapist to enter into the politics of the family. Some strategies are fairly straightforward. Zuk, for example, employs a go-between strategy, alternately siding with one faction and then the other in order to shape the form of the negotiation. Haley, when working with very difficult two-generation problems, tries to throw all the control to the parents in order to interrupt the subtle alternations of the struggle.

Paradox

Another group of more indirect strategies are called paradoxical, since the therapist moves in such a way as to go with, rather than against, the force of the resistance. This approach, with both individuals and families, has been advocated by Milton Erickson and Richard Rabkin. It is significant that Haley, Erickson, and Rabkin have all been interested in hypnotism as a basic model of therapy. In hypnotism, as in strategic treatment, the objective is to overcome the subject's resistance by redefining the relationship as a cooperative (complementary) one, rather than an antagonistic (symmetrical) one. This is spelled out in Haley's seminal early book, *Strategies of Psychotherapy.* There are three basic forms of paradoxical maneuver (Fisher et al., 1981): (1) reframing, in which a new metaphor or meaning of the symptom is supplied, which alters its function within the family; (2) escalation or crisis induction (called a runaway), in which the redefined symptom is prescribed, reinforced, and amplified until the family moves to alter the relationships which sustain it; and (3) redirection, a kind of active reframing in which the symptom is ritualistically recast as part of the family's routine and, therefore, under control. In all three cases, when the family responds to the move, their reassertion of control will be in a different form from the original homeostasis.

This kind of therapy consists of phenomena that are ancient. Invented metaphors, crisis induction, and ritual prescription have roots in magic, shamanism, spiritism, and other practices widely dispersed in history and other cultures. Like the phenomenon of the individual unconscious, their validity as the basis of healing practices in the human group is suggested by their constant rediscovery.

Recent interest in paradox comes from two sources: a compelling book, *Paradox and Counterparadox* by Palazzoli and his associates (1978), and the reports, from many groups practicing paradoxical therapy, of rapid and dramatic effectiveness in difficult cases.

The Founders' Schools

In the early 1960's, family therapy was presided over by a group of charismatic personalities, each of whom was connected with a training program and a distinct approach. Many of the people described above can be grouped together as contributors to several system schools.

At the same time, several other leaders of the field developed schools which use the methods and ideas already described where they are felt to be indicated, but which have a different or additional emphasis. What these so-called founders' schools have in common are the following:

(1) A central teacher with a major theoretical and personal commitment concerning the nature of human relations, which goes outside the here and now of social systems theory to include something else. In this something else, the founder's background in psychodynamic therapy often shows through with the language somewhat altered. The language also radiates the founder's vision of a healthy family; (2) An interest in the past (uncharacteristic of the system purists), which shows in a tendency to explore early relationships, bring grandparents into the therapy, send people on journeys home to talk to relatives and visit graveyards—generally, an interest in the resolution of separation, loss, and the claims of buried loyalties; (3) Less concern with brevity as a virtue by itself and more with growth—the idea that change involves some personal acceptance by individuals in the family of things in life which they can best integrate sometimes only gradually, from experience with each other and with the therapist; and (4) Very little evaluation research.

Since the founders' personal philosophy and style is such an important aspect of each of these schools, it warrants brief discussion.

Nathan Ackerman

The founder of the Ackerman Family Institute in New York City, believed that the experience of honest feelings in the session—sexual, aggressive, dependent—is a liberating experience. To this end, he challenged the family's defenses against such feelings, using himself and his own openness of response as a catalyst. He was everyone's knowing, joking, giving, feeling grandfather. Indeed, so personal and ingenious was his method that today, in the matter of style, he has very few followers.

Carl Whitaker

Whitaker has taught countless students through a special form of co-therapy apprenticeship. He believes, like Ackerman, in the value of candor and emotional challenge, and in the importance of the therapists' personal response to the family members. He carries this further to include the emotional system of the co-therapists, each of whom, like auxiliary parents in a family, should gain something for their own growth from the experience of going through the family crucible.

Murray Bowen

The founder of the Family Institute of Georgetown in Washington, D.C., he propounded that the path to maturity is working at the life-long task of differentiating one's self from the triangular and sometimes multigenerational entanglements with others: family, intimates, associates. His is a philosophy of subduing the emotions and delaying hasty action by using the intellect to analyze emotional systems. The therapist's emotions and his own family of origin are kept in mind as model systems, but are not intruded into the therapy.

Ivan Boszormenyi-Nagy

One of the founders of the Eastern Pennsylvania Psychiatric Institute school of family therapy, he has developed over the years a unique theory of intergenerational and interpersonal family dynamics which is based on the concept of exchange. A balance of indebtedness or obligation builds up between family members over time, and one of the principal purposes of the therapy is to clarify and resolve these obligations, especially those that are unexpressed or unacknowledged.

Family Approaches to Schizophrenia

In the 1960's, the family therapy of schizophrenia had prestige because the principal figures in the field, such as Bateson's group, were interested in it. There were other theories of the family contribution to schizophrenia: Lidz's theory that it was associated with a subtly skewed—rather than openly schizmatic—relationship between the parents; Bowen's theory that it came from three generations of immaturity with failure of intergenerational differentiation; and Wynne and Singer's work that thought disorder could be transmitted through the medium of parental communication deviance. In this climate, a family therapy aimed at straightening out communication patterns seemed a logical approach to schizophrenia.

Parents of schizophrenics had for some time been getting the message that they were responsible for the illness. They received this message from popular scientific writing on the subject, from the way they were interviewed when their children were hospitalized (a general overview of all the things they had done wrong), and from their children's own accusations. The staff of hospital and clinic were usually in a not-so-subtle competition with parents, trying to give the patient a "corrective" experience which would be better than the home. Added to all this was an indefinite series of family therapy meetings, designed to straighten out the parents' pathogenic communication patterns so that they would not drive the patient crazy again. The results of these efforts, for the parents, was a paralyzing sense of stigmatization, guilt, and helplessness.

Under these institutional circumstances, the family therapy of schizophrenia was much written about, widely practiced, and of doubtful effect. In recent years, however, several developments have changed both the theory and the practice.

Genetic theories of the illness were supported by several studies, suggesting a less guilt-provoking means of transmission.

Subgroups of schizophrenia were identified with special courses, heredities, and medication responses, supporting the idea that schizophrenia is primarily a medical syndrome with a variety of possible causes, and only secondarily an existential dilemma of modern man imprisoned in the contradictions of family life.

Some parents of schizophrenics were getting organized. The middle-class suburban parents of chronic but still young schizophrenics (who lived with them at home between hospitalizations) were beginning to realize that nobody was doing anything for them. These parents realized that what they really needed was scientific and practical information, mutual support, and a sense of not being alone with the problem. They also began to suggest that, if their communication patterns were peculiar, it might be the result of living in a crazy situation. By 1978, several such groups had coalesced to form the National Alliance for the Mentally Ill, now a self-help group and lobby of 5,000 members.

There was also increased attention to identifying factors in successful course and treatment, including factors that had to do with the family. Brown et al. (1972), for example, found that a particular attitude on the part of parents of patients discharged home hastened relapse. This attitude was a mixture of negativity, intensity, intrusiveness, and intolerance. Noting that it was more frequent in isolated families, Julian Leff (1979) tried to modify it by putting these parents into support groups with other parents who faced the same problems but had a more accepting attitude toward them. Leff's program involved lectures on the nature of the illness and the offer of membership in the British Schizophrenia Fellowship, an organization which disseminates information about the illness to patients and families. These elements were the same ones which the Alliance for the Mentally Ill was advocating in this country: education, membership in the medical enterprise, and peer support. These are the essential ingredients of any good program of rehabilitative medicine for the management of chronic illness. This approach, while not so much a new treatment, represented a change of context for the treatment.

A number of programs in this country have demonstrated the effectiveness of these elements in various formats. Many aftercare facilities use multifamily groups as a form of social support and education for families of chronic patients. The program of Anderson et al. (1980) in Pittsburgh, for example, utilizes an all-day survival skills workshop for relatives of the schizophrenic patients, which forms the base for a mutual support group. In this context, brief, practical family therapy at times of crisis is quite well accepted.

Other effective family approaches to schizophrenia have been reported. One important technique is the leaving-home approach of Haley and Madanes. This approach is strategic, treating the problem as one of insufficient parental authority in helping the offspring get ready to leave home. It is also antimedical, in that it avoids the chronic disease model. This approach may work best with resistant families.

Network Therapy

There are times when the family is not the natural group—when the only way to make an effective approach to a problem is to include a number of people connected with the family. Various systematic ways of doing this are called network therapy.

As with family therapy, the practice of network therapy goes back to social work, and the theory goes back to anthropology. The connection with social work will be obvious. The connection with anthropology begins with the work of Elizabeth Bott, who investigated the kin and friendship relations of London working-class couples and who related emotional and other characteristics of the marriage with characteristics of the spouse's peripheral ties to others outside the home. A natural history of urban social relationships (family, friends, neighbors, co-workers, professonial helpers, and others) began to be worked out, as anthropologists emphasized that the nature of urban life was different from that of the village life on which their field had previously concentrated. City dwellers opportunistically shape their social networks through a variety of informal and formal exchanges of obligation and favor, outside the rules of kinship and organizational hierarchies. Migration and class mobility in the city create both opportunities and challenges to one's ability to form new networks of friends and neighbors.

Therapists such as Speck, Rueveni, and Attneave, experienced in both family therapy and network studies, noted that some patients in crisis—such as the acutely ill, depressed, suicidal, or psychotic—seemed to be cut off from the usual resources of their networks. Recalling that in tribal societies these crises would often be handled by an official healer who could call the tribe together for a healing ceremony, they began to experiment with assemblies of extended family, friends, and other important people. These would be selected and called in by the patient and family to help deal with the crisis. The meetings would last for hours, with the therapists acting as the facilitators of a rather free agenda, which often strayed far from the precipitating crisis and dealt with many relationships in the group. The ideal number of people is between 50 and 80, and a team of several experienced therapists is needed to handle the dramatic shifting of mood and the emergence of subgroups of more active participants who offer help with the different problems which arise. Energies released by such a meeting or series of meetings are often strikingly successful in breaking the deadlock of the crisis, and more conventional treatment can follow with good effect.

Other networkers do not convene full-scale assemblies, but work with small groups recruited after studying the family's resources. These are strategic, focused meetings designed to re-establish the family's neglected social context. Such methods resemble Langlsley's crisis intervention methods and, more re-

cently, the function of the case manager in the care of the chronic patient, a collection of techniques which have been advocated by the National Institute of Mental Health's Community Support Program.

Conclusion

Family therapy, multiple family therapy, educational rehabilitative programs, network therapy, and the Community Support Program are a series of increasingly outward-looking criticisms and interventions aimed at successively larger contexts in which individual suffering takes place. They lead inevitably to criticism and reform of the professions and establishments which have tried to deal with this suffering as a problem facing the individual alone. To the question of what the individual's natural group is, they have posed a series of answers in action which have required moving against the grain of a society that celebrates the individual career. These answers have successively declared the individual's natural group to be the family, the network, and now (in the case of the schizophrenia programs) the whole institutional and professional context in which treatment takes place.

References

Anderson, C. M., Hogarty, G. E., and Reiss, D. J. Family treatment of adult schizophrenic patients. Schizophrenia Bull., *6:* 490, 1980.
Brown, G. W., Birley, J. L. T., and Wing, J. K. The influence of family life on schizophrenic disorder: a replication. Br. J. Psychiatry, *121:* 241, 1972.
Fisher, L., Anderson, A., and Jones, J. E. Types of paradoxical intervention and indications/contraindications for use in clinical practice Fam. Proc., *20:* 25, 1981.
Gurman, A. S., and Kniskern, D. P. *Handbook of Family Therapy.* Brunner/Mazel, New York, 1981.
Leff, J. P. Developments in family treatment of schizophrenia Psychiatr. Q., *51:* 216, 1979.
Massie, H. N., and Beels, C. C. The outcome of the family treatmen of schizophrenia. Schizophrenia Bull., *6:* 24, 1972.
Napier, A. Y., and Whitaker, C. A. *The Family Crucible.* Harper & Row, New York, 1978.
Rabkin, R. *Strategic Psychotherapy.* Basic Books, New York, 1977.
Selvini Palazzoli, M., Boscolo, L., Cecchin, G. F., and Prata, G *Paradox and Counterparadox: A New Model in the Therapy of the Family in Schizophrenic Transaction,* Jason Aronson, New York 1978.

B.18 Psychopharmacology and Group Psychotherapy

NORMAN SUSSMAN, M.D.

Introduction

As part of the general trend toward the simultaneous use of psychological and pharmacological treatment modalities, there has been an increase in the concurrent use of group psychotherapy and drug therapy. This combined approach derives from the observation that individuals with drug-responsive disorders frequently demonstrate greater improvement when medication is used along with some form of psychotherapy. It is believed that medication, by reducing the frequency, duration, and cognitive dysfunctions of psychiatric disorders, permits greater efforts toward using insight, improving social functions, and developing living skills. One goal of psychiatric pharmacotherapy is thus to help the patient participate in other treatment modalities.

Although precise figures are not available, it is estimated that about 50 per cent of all psychiatric patients are now treated with a combined approach. According to one report, 60 per cent of psychoanalysts surveyed reported prescribing medication for some of their patients (Pulver, 1978).

The following discussion focuses on some basic issues in the clinical use of psychoactive drugs. In keeping with current practice, the drugs are classified according to their treatment effect: anti-psychotic, anti-depressant, anti-manic, and anti-anxiety (sedative-hypnotic) agents. Accompanying tables present more detailed information about the specific drugs. This discussion is intended as a brief, convenient reference and should be supplemented by a more detailed review of psychopharmacology, such as the review by Davis (1980) in *Comprehensive Textbook of Psychiatry*.

Pharmacotherapy and Group Processes

The act of prescribing medication is invariably accompanied by complex phenomena that transcend the direct biological actions of the given drug. The placebo effect—a phenomenon in which a person exhibits a significant clinical response to a compound that is therapeutically inert—is a vivid testimonial to this fact. Other psychological responses to medication might be manifested by failure to comply with drug regimen or histrionic reactions to minor side effects.

In the treatment of most medical disorders, there is minimal concern with psychological responses to drug treatment. For psychiatrists the situation is reversed.

Behavioral and dynamic issues that arise may, therefore, become of importance in the treatment process. Behavior toward pharmacotherapy can provide an opportunity to further understand the patient and may serve as a tool in the service of therapeutic change.

When pharmacological agents are used in a group setting, several areas need special consideration. These areas include the dynamics of the group member to be medicated, the dynamics of other group members, the current status of group processes, and the maturity of the group. Reactions in the group that surround pharmacotherapy are best conceptualized in such traditional terms as transference, countertransference, resistance, and identification. For example, medication may become the focus of resistance and thus facilitate the analysis of resistance, removing an obstacle to the general therapy.

As a rule, transference reactions occur earlier in the course of treatment during group psychotherapy than they do in the individual setting. Medication often augments or precipitates these reactions. This can allow observation of characteristic behaviors. It may be possible to discern in a patient's negotiations about medication certain traits or behavior patterns that are present in other life situations (Beitman, 1981). Baldessarini (1977) has outlined reactions to medication as they might appear in persons with specific personality traits. For example, the obsessive patient may show excessive concern and rumination about the details of treatment and provoke antagonism as a result of debates over treatment; the histrionic or impulsive patient may overreact to side effects or impulsively misuse medication; narcissistic or hypomanic patients may rebel at the thought of drugs reducing their creativity or physical abilities; the depressed patient may be reluctant to take medication; the schizophrenic patient may refuse to cooperate fully as a result of suspicions or delusions; and the antisocial personality may abuse drugs with euphoria-like effects and provoke stormy encounters over the issue of control.

A negative transference issue should be suspected whenever there is a seemingly irrational refusal to comply with prescribing instructions. Conversely, overly compliant reactions to a medication regimen may reflect a positive transference reaction. Unusual timidity in the face of medication may indicate needs for acceptance and nurturing.

The group setting tends to provoke manifestations of unresolved sibling rivalry. This dynamic process may be seen as a competition for the affection of the leader. The request for medication by a patient may

Table B.18-1
Phenothiazine Anti-psychotic Agents (Major Tranquilizers)

Class	Name		Manufacturer	Adult Dose Range		Adult Single Dose Range
	Generic	Trade		*mg./day*		
				Acute	Maintenance	
Aliphatic	Chlorpromazine	Thorazine	Smith, Kline & French	25–800 Oral 25–2,000 IM	40–100 Oral	10–25 Oral 10–400 IM
	Triflupromazine	Vesprin	Squibb	100–150 Oral 25–150 IM	50–100 Oral	10–50 Oral 10–50 IM
Piperazine	Prochlorperazine	Compazine	Smith, Kline & French	30–150 Oral 30–100 IM	15–75 Oral	5–25 Oral 10–20 IM
	Perphenazine	Trilafon	Schering	16–64 Oral 10–20 IM	8–16 Oral	2–16 Oral 5 IM
	Trifluoperazine	Stelazine	Smith, Kline & French	10–60 Oral 1–6 IM	5–15 Oral	1–10 Oral 1–2 IM

Class	Generic	Brand	Manufacturer			
Piperazine	Fluphenazine	Prolixin Permitil	Squibb Schering	5–20 Oral 5–20 IM (HCl)	1.0–5.0 Oral 25–50 IM (deca- noate or enan- thate, weekly or biweekly)	0.5–10 Oral 1.0–5.0 Oral
	Acetophenazine	Tindal	Schering	40–120 Oral	20–40 Oral	20–40
	Butaperazine	Repoise	Robins	15–100 Oral	5–50 Oral	5–30
	Carphenazine	Proketazine	Wyeth	100–200	50–150	12.5–50
Piperidine	Thioridazine	Mellaril	Sandoz	300–800 Oral	100–300 Oral	20–200
	Mesoridazine	Serentil	Boehringer	100–400 Oral 25–200 IM	30–150 Oral	10–100 Oral 25 IM
	Piperacetazine	Quide	Merrell Dow	40–160 Oral	40–80 Oral	10–60

Table B.18-1—Continued

| | Oral | | | | | | Injection | | | |
	Tablet	Capsule	Syrup	Elixir	Concentrate	Ampul	Vial	Syringe	Suppository	Equivalence*
Chlorpromazine	10, 25, 50, 100, 200	Sustained release: 30, 75, 150, 200, 300	10 mg./ml.		30 mg./ml. 100 mg./ml.	25 mg./ml.	25 mg./ml.		25, 100	100
Triflupromazine	10, 25, 50		50 mg./5 ml.		30 mg./ml.	25 mg./ml.	10 mg./ml.	10 mg./ml.		25
Promazine	10, 25, 50, 100, 200		10 mg./5 ml.		100 mg./ml.	25 mg./ml.				100
Prochlorperazine	5, 10, 25	Sustained release: 10, 15, 30, 75	5 mg./5 ml.		10 mg./ml.	5 mg./ml.	5 mg./ml.		2.5, 5, 25	15
Perphenazine	2, 4, 8, 16				16 mg./5 ml.	5 mg./inj.				10
Trifluoperazine	1, 2, 5, 10				10 mg./ml.					5
Fluphenazine	1, 2, 5, 5, 10, sustained release: 1			0.5 mg./ml.	5 mg./ml.		2.5 mg./ml. HCl (decanoate or enanthate)			2
							25 mg./ml. (decanoate or enanthate)			7
Acetophenazine	20									25
Butaperazine	10, 25				30 mg./ml.					10
Carphenazine	12.5, 25, 50				100 mg./ml.					25
Thioridazine	10, 15, 25, 50, 100, 150, 200									100
Mesoridazine	10, 25, 50, 100				25 mg./ml.	25 mg./ml.				50
Piperacetazine	10, 25									10

* Dose required to achieve therapeutic efficacy of 100 mg of chlorpromazine. All drug enforcement control level "0".

Side Effects

Dry mouth and throat
Blurred vision
Cutaneous flushing
Constipation
Urinary retention
Paralytic ileus
Mental confusion
Miosis
Mydriasis
Postural hypotension
Broadened, flattened, or clove T-waves and increased Q-R intervals on electrocardiogram
Parkinsonian syndrome
Mask-like face
Tremor at rest
Rigidity
Shuffling gait
Motor retardation
Drooling
Dyskinesias
Bizarre movements of tongue, face, and neck
Buccofacial movements
Salivation
Torticollis
Oculogyric crisis
Opisthotonos
Akathisia

Lowered seizure threshold
Convulsive seizures
Sedation
Insomnia
Bizarre dreams
Impaired psychomotor activity
Somnambulism
Confusion
Paradoxical aggravation of psychotic symptoms
Skin eruptions (urticarial, maculopapular, petechial, or edematous)
Contact dermatitis
Photosensitivity reaction
Blue-gray metallic discoloration of the skin over areas exposed to sunlight
Deposits in the anterior lens and posterior cornea (visible only by slit-lens examination)
Retinitis pigmentosa
Abnormal glucose tolerance curve
Breast engorgement and lactation in female patients
Weight gain
Delayed ejaculation
Loss of erectile ability
Agranulocytosis
Eosinophilia
Leukopenia
Hemolytic anemia
Thrombocytic purpura
Pancytopenia
Jaundice

Table B.18-2
Nonphenothiazine Anti-psychotic Agents (Major Tranquilizers)

| Class | Name | | Manufacturer | Adult Dose Range *mg./day* | | Adult Single Dose Range *mg.* |
	Generic	Trade		Acute	Maintenance	
Butyrophen-ones	Haloperidol	Haldol	McNeil	1–15 Oral 2–15 IM	1–15	0.5–5 Oral 2–5 IM
Thioxanthenes	Chlorprothixene	Taractan	Roche	75–600 Oral 75–200 IM	75	25–150 Oral 25–50 IM
	Thiothixene	Navane	Roerig	6–60 Oral 8–30 IM	6–60	2–20 Oral 4–5 IM
Dibenzoxaze-pines	Loxapine	Loxitane	Lederle	20–100	60–100	10–60
Dihydroindo-lones	Molindone	Moban Lidone	Endo Abbott	15–225	15–225	5–75

Class	Available Preparations						Drug Enforcement Administration Control Level	Dose Equivalent†	Side Effects
	Oral				Injection				
	Tablet *mg.*	Capsule *mg.*	Elixer	Concentrate	Ampul	Vial			
Rauwolfia alka-loid Reserpine* Serpasil Rau-sed Sandril Raurine Reserpoid Vio-serpine — Ciba Squibb Lilly Westerfield Upjohn Rowell							0.1–5 2.5–10.0 IM (after a small initial dose to test patient responsiveness)	0.1–5	0.1–5 Oral
Haloperidol	0.5, 1, 2, 5, 10			2 mg./ml.	5 mg./ml.		0	1.6	Same as for phenothiazine anti-psychotic agents
Chlorprothixene	10, 25, 50, 100			20 mg./ml.	12.5 mg./ml.		0	50	
Thiothixene				5 mg./ml.		2 mg./ml.	0	5	
Loxapine		5, 10, 25, 50		25 mg./ml.			0	10	
Molindone	5, 10, 25						0	6–10	
Reserpine	0.1, 0.25, 1, 2, 5	0.25, 0.5	0.05 mg./ml.		2.5 mg./ml.	2.5 g./ml.	0		Reserpine is associated with many of the same side effects as the phenothiazine anti-psychotic agents. However, in addition, it frequently produces depression. Approximately 6 per cent of all patients on reserpine require hospitalization or electroconvulsive therapy for depression caused by the drug.

* Rarely prescribed for psychosis.
† Dose equivalent, 100 mg. of chlorpromazine.

Table B.18-3
Tricyclic, Tetracyclic, Dibenzoxapine Triazolopyridine, and Monoamine Oxidase Inhibitor Anti-depressant Agents

Name			Manufacturer	Dose Range Adult			Available Preparations					D.E.A. Control Level
Class	Generic	Trade		Initial week	After second week	Single Dose Range	Oral			Injection		
							Tablet	Capsule	Concentrate	Ampul	Vial	
				mg./day	mg./day	mg.	mg.					
Tricyclic	Imipramine	Presamine Tofranil SK-Pramine Imavate Antipress	USV Geigy Smith, Kline & French Robins Uemmon	30-100	75-300	10-200	10, 25, 50	75, 100, 125, 150		25 mg./2 cc. (IM)		0
	Desipramine	Norpramin Pertofrane	Merrell National USV	25-150	75-300	25-150	25, 50, 75, 100, 150	25, 50				0
	Amitriptyline	Elavil Endep Amitril SK-Amitriptyline	Merck, Sharp & Dohme Roche Warner-Chilcott Smith, Kline & French	50-150	40-300	10-200	10, 25, 50, 75, 100, 150				10 mg./ml.	0
	Nortriptyline	Aventyl Pamelor	Lilly Sandoz	25-50	50-100	10-100		10, 25	10 mg./5 ml.			0
	Protriptyline	Vivactil	Merck, Sharp & Dohme	10-30	10-60	5-30	5, 10					0

Class	Generic	Trade	Manufacturer						
	Doxepin	Sinequan, Adapin	Pfizer, Pennwalt	50–100	75–300	10–100	10, 25, 50, 75, 100, 150	10 mg./ml.	0
	Trimipramine	Surmontil	Ives	75–150	75–200	25–300	25–50		0
Tetracyclic	Maprotiline	Ludiomil	Ciba	75–125	125–150	25–150	25, 50		0
Dibenzoxapine	Amoxapine	Asendin	Lederle	150–300	200–300	50–300	50, 100, 150		0
Triazolopyridine	Trazodone	Desyrel	Mead Johnson	150–250	250–400		50, 100		
Monoamine oxidase inhibitor	Isocarboxazid	Marplan	Roche	10–30	10–20	10–30	10		0
	Phenelzine	Nardil	Warner-Chilcott	30–45	45–75	15–90	15		0
	Tranylcypromine	Parnate	Smith, Kline & French	20	20–30	10–30	10		0

Side Effects

Dry mouth
Palpitations
Tachycardia
Heart block
Myocardial infarction
Loss of accommodation
Orthostatic hypotension
Fainting
Dizziness
Nausea
Vomiting
Constipation
Sedation
Agitation
Hallucinations and delusions (in latent psychotics)
Diarrhea
Black tongue
Edema
Aggravation of narrow-angle glaucoma (not chronic simple glaucoma)
Urinary retention (caution in benign prostatic hypertrophy)
Paralytic ileus
Peculiar taste
Skin rash
Galactorrhea
Gynecomastia (in males)
Bone marrow depression

**Table B.18-4
Benzodiazepines**

| Name | | | Adult Dose Range | Adult Single Dose Range | Available Preparations | | | | | | Addictive | |
| Generic | Trade | Manufacturer | | | Oral | | Injection | | | | Psychological dependence | Physiological dependence |
					Tablet	Capsule	Ampul	Vial	Syringe			
			mg./day	mg.	mg.							
Chlordiazepoxide	Librium Libritabs	Roche Roche	15–100	5–25	5, 10, 25	5, 10, 25	Duplex pkg., 100 mg./5 ml. + 2 ml. diluent				+	+
Diazepam	Valium	Roche	2–40	2–10	2, 5, 10		2 ml.	10 ml. 5 mg./ml.			+	+
Oxazepam	Serax	Wyeth	30–120	10–30	15	10, 15, 30					±	+
Clorazepate	Tranxene Azene†	Abbott Endo	7.5–60	3.25–22.5	22.5, 11.25 3.25	3.25, 3.75, 6.5, 7.5, 13.0					+	+
Alprazolan	Xanax	Upjohn		0.75–4	0.25–2	0.25, 0.5, 1.0					+	+
Halazepam	Paxipam	Schering	60–160		20–40	20, 40					+	+

Generic	Trade	Manufacturer							
Flurazepam	Dalmane	Roche	15–30	15–30		15, 30	?	?	IV
Temazepam	Restoril	Sandoz	15–30	15–30		15, 30	?	?	IV
Prazepam	Centrax (Verstran)	Parke-Davis	20–60	5–60	10	5, 10	±	+	IV
Clonaze-pam*	Clonopin	Roche	1.5–20	0.5–15		0.5, 1, 2	+	+	IV

* Unlike the other benzodiazepines available for clinical use, clonazepam is not indicated for use as a sedative or a hypnotic. It is classified as an anti-epileptic agent, useful alone or as an adjunct in the treatment of the Lennox-Gastaut syndrome (petit mal variant), akinetic and myoclonic seizures. Clonopin may also be useful in patients with absence seizures (petit mal) who have failed to respond to succinimides.

Side effects: Paradoxical excitement; hypnagogic hallucination; phlebitis; fatigue; drowsiness; somnolence; muscle weakness; nystagmus; ataxia; dysarthria; impaired reaction time, motor coordination, and intellectual function; and central nervous system depression.
† Clorazepate monopotassium.

Table B.18-5
Nonbarbiturate, Nonbenzodiazepine Sedatives, Hypnotics, and Anti-anxiety Agents

Name		Manu-facturer	Adult Dose Range	Adult Single Dose Range		Available Preparations									Addictive		D.E.A.‡ Control Level
Generic	Trade			Sedative*	Hypnotic†	Oral					Injection			Suppository	Psychological dependence	Physiological dependence	
						Tablet	Capsule	Syrup	Elixir	Ampul	Ampul	Vial	Syringe				
			mg./day	mg.	mg.	mg.	mg.						mg.				
Meprobamate	Equanil Miltown	Wyeth Wallace	1,200–1,600	200–400		200, 400, 600									+	+	IV
Tybamate	Tybatran	Robins	250–2000	250–500			250, 350								–	–	0
Ethinamate	Valmid	Dista	500–1000		500–1000		500								+	+	IV
Glutethimide	Doriden	USV	250–500	250–500	500	125, 250, 500									+	+	III
Methyprylon	Noludar	Roche	50–400	50–100	200–400	150, 200	300								+	+	III
Ethchlorvynol	Placidyl	Abbott	500–750		500–750		100, 200, 500, 750								+	+	IV

Methaqualone	Mequin, Sopor	Lemmon, Arnar-Stone	75-300	75	150-300	150-300				+	+	II
Diphenhydramine	Benadryl	Parke, Davis	10-400	50	150-300	25, 50	12.5 mg./5 ml.	50 mg./ml. 10 mg./ml. 50 mg./ml.		−	−	0
Hydroxyzine	Vistaril, Atarax	Pfizer, Roerig	25-400	25-100	10, 25, 50, 100	10, 25, 50, 100	10 mg./5 ml. 25 mg./5 ml.			−	−	0
Chloral hydrate	Noctec, Kesso-drate, Felsules, Aqua-chloral	Squibb, McKesson, Fellows, Webcon	250-750	250	500-2000	250, 500	500 mg./5 ml.	100 mg./2 ml.	325 650 975 1,300	+	+	IV
Promethazine	Phenergan	Wyeth	12.5-50	12.5-50	12.5, 25, 50	12.5, 25, 50	6.25 mg./5 cc. 25 mg./5 cc.	25 mg./cc. 50 mg./cc.	12.5 mg. 25 mg. 50 mg.	−	−	0
Paraldehyde	Paral	O'Neal, Jones, Feldman	4-10 ml.	4-10 ml.	4-10 ml.	1000 (1000 mg./ = 1 ml.)	30 ml.	5 ml. 10 ml.		+	+	IV

* Sedative dose is that amount given at one time sufficient to reduce anxiety without inducing sleep.
† Hypnotic dose is that amount given at one time sufficient to induce sleep.
Side effects: Impaired judgment and performance; drowsiness; lethargy; residual sedation ("hangover"); skin eruptions; nausea; vomiting; paradoxical restlessness or excitement; exacerbation of symptoms of organic brain syndrome; ataxia; atropine psychosis with hypnotic doses of diphenhydramine or hydroxyzine; unpredictable clinical course after glutethimide overdose; high addictive potential and low margin of safety in suicide attempts with glutethimide; and with promethazine, a phenothiazine without anti-psychotic activity, side effects of the phenothiazine class may be observed.
‡ D.E.A., Drug Enforcement Administration.

have as its basis the fact that another group member has been started on medication.

The phase of group formation may influence medication patterns. An immature group—one that is in an early stage of development—experiences greater collective and individual stress, causing a rise in symptomatic behavior. Subsequent requests for medication or the recommendation that a patient take medication might be more appropriately managed by interpretation than pharmacological agents.

Beitman (1981) has summarized some of the more obvious benefits of combined treatment approach: involvement of the patient in the therapeutic process, strengthening of the therapeutic alliance, reduction of symptom-engendered interference with effective psychotherapeutic communication, initiation of change, and acceleration of the working-through process.

Being in a psychotherapy group can alter a member's expectation of drug effect, and subsequently predispose the individual toward a specific type of drug response. This phenomenon has been reported in social groups where many effects of alcohol are often more dependent on factors such as the anticipation of drug effect than the pharmacological properties of the drug. In a therapeutic setting, this manifestation might be related to identification with other members who had taken or are taking medication for a specific disorder.

A specific application of group procedures to the process of psychopharmacology is the medication or drug group. Such groups are homogeneous in that all members are being treated with the same or similar class of medication. In contrast to the more generalized therapeutic objective of psychotherapy groups, the primary aim of the drug group is to maximize the therapeutic response to medication and to enhance compliance with the drug regimen. Since rates of non-compliance with psychotropic drugs are reported to be between 30 and 80 per cent, depending on the specific survey, this is a major application of the group process.

Successful use of medication in groups has also been reported with anti-psychotic agents and lithium. Because of the severe pathology generally present in the disorders these drugs treat and the unpleasant side effects these drugs may cause, obtaining treatment compliance is often difficult. Payn (1965, 1974) successfully used the group approach to improve adherence to drug treatment among chronic schizophrenic patients; all prescribing was done during the group meetings. Davenport and his associates (1977) reported greater acceptance of medication and an improved treatment outcome when couples group therapy was used as an adjunct to lithium maintenance in manic patients.

Anti-psychotic Agents

Five classes of anti-psychotic drugs are currently available for clinical use in the United States. Tables B.18-1 and B.18-2 contain lists of these drugs, as well as subgroups within each class. The anti-psychotic drugs, sometimes termed "neuroleptics" or "major tranquilizers," have produced their greatest impact in the treatment of schizophrenia. These agents ameliorate many fundamental signs and symptoms of schizophrenia, prevent relapse, and arrest progression of the disease.

All the present medications are of equal efficacy, i.e., they produce the same quality of change. Individual drugs may produce superior improvements in a given patient, but statistically these medications all produce the same improvement in a random patient population.

All currently marketed anti-psychotic agents cause mild to severe autonomic and extrapyramidal symptoms. Many patients terminate drug treatment because they are unable to tolerate these side effects, even if there has been good clinical response. Autonomic symptoms include blurred vision, constipation, dry mouth, and urinary retention. These symptoms persist during the course of treatment and disappear completely when the anti-psychotic medication is discontinued.

The most distressing and sometimes most persistent of the side effects are the extrapyramidal reactions. These are the parkinsonian syndrome and the dyskinesias. Haloperidol (Haldol), thiothixene (Navane), and fluphenazine (Prolixin) produce the most extrapyramidal effects. Thioridazine (Mellaril) produces the fewest extrapyramidal effects. Advantages to the use of thioridazine are the general absence of the need to use concurrent anti-parkinsonian medication and the possibility that thioridazine is associated with a lower incidence of tardive dyskinesia.

Clozapine (Leponex) is an effective anti-psychotic agent that has been available in Europe for many years. The incidence of extrapyramidal reactions associated with clozapine has been extremely low and there have been no reports of tardive dyskinesia resulting from its use.

Anti-depressant Agents

The tricyclic anti-depressants are the dominant drugs in the treatment of depression. Several newer drugs, the dibenzoxapines, tetracyclics, and triazolopyridines are similar to the tricyclic agents in their clinical effects. The monoamine oxidase inhibitors (MAOI's) represent another group of drugs that is useful in treating depression. Table B.18-3 summarizes these compounds.

The tricyclic drugs are effective in the treatment of many forms of depression. They are most effective in acute endogenous depressive illness. They are not consistently effective in alleviating reactive, neurotic, or atypical depressions.

All the tricyclic drugs appear to be equally effective in the treatment of depression. Nevertheless, some patients who do not respond to one drug show a positive response to another.

Dosage and length of treatment are important to the success of tricyclic therapy. Some of the drugs are known to be effective only when they fall within a narrow range of blood serum levels. Inadequate or excessive blood levels are associated with treatment failure.

Nortriptyline (Pamelor) is the only anti-depressant with such a defined and clearly documented therapeutic range of activity. Steady state plasma levels of nortriptyline correspond highly with therapeutic effects.

MAOI's are useful in cases of neurotic and atypical depression, as well as in some cases of refractory depression. They are not as effective as tricyclic drugs in cases of severe depression. The MAOI's are used with caution because of their potential for interacting with drugs or foods to produce severe hypertension.

Anti-manic Agents

Lithium carbonate is indicated for the treatment of acute mania and for the prophylaxis of affective swings in patients with bipolar (manic-depressive) disorders. Reports that lithium may be of value in treating other disorders, most notably recurrent episodes of unipolar depression, remain contradictory. Although lithium has a dramatic impact when it does work, it often has only a partial effect or no effect in some patients.

Anti-anxiety and Hypnotic Agents

A wide variety of drugs is included in the group of anti-anxiety agents. The most widely prescribed class of these drugs is the benzodiazepines (see Table B.18-4). A once popular but now less frequently utilized class of drugs is the barbiturates. Other substances of diverse molecular structure are available (see Table B.18-5), but these lag far behind in terms of general clinical value. Collectively, the anti-anxiety agents are the drugs most often used today.

The anti-anxiety agents are also termed sedatives or hypnotics because of their ability to reduce agitation, produce a sense of calmness, and induce sleep.

The hypnotic agent of choice, based on currently available drugs, is temazepam (Restoril). This benzodiazepine has a half-life of 10 hours, which parallels normal sleep time, so most patients do not experience drug hangover during the next day. Also REM sleep remains essentially unchanged.

Anti-anxiety drugs should be limited to short-term treatment. Because tolerance develops to all the compounds, they probably lose all clinical effects after 3 to 4 months. Although patients may continue to take medication, mainly for reasons of dependence, any perceived therapeutic value is probably derived from the placebo effect. Nevertheless, the danger of mild to severe withdrawal syndromes remains. Both diazepam (Valium) and lorazepam (Ativan) are excellent anxiolytic agents. The latter drug is reported to have a shorter half-life which is a desirable property.

References

Arieti, S. Psychotherapy of severe depression. Am. J. Psychiatry, *134:* 864, 1977.

Baldessarini, R. J. *Chemotherapy in Psychiatry.* Harvard University Press, Cambridge, MA, 1977.

Beitman, B. D. Pharmacotherapy as an intervention during the stages of psychotherapy. Am. J. Psychother, *35:* 206, 1981.

Blackwell, B. Adverse effects of anti-depressant drugs. Part 1. Monoamine oxidase inhibitors and tricyclics. Drugs, *21:* 201, 1981.

Blackwell, B. Adverse effects of anti-depressant drugs. Part 2. "Second generation" anti-depressants and rational decision making in antidepressant therapy. Drugs, *21:* 273, 1981b.

Berg, G., Laberg, V. C., Skuttle, A., and Arne, O. Instructed versus pharmacological effects of alcohol in alcoholics and social drinkers. Behav. Res. Ther., *19:* 55, 1981.

Berger, F. The use of anti-anxiety drugs. Clin. Pharmacol. Ther., *29:* 291, 1981.

Davenport, Y. B., Ebert, M. H., Adland, M. L., and Goodwin, F. K. Couples therapy as an adjunct to lithium maintenance of the manic patient. Am. J. Orthopsychiatry, *47:* 495, 1977.

Davis, J. M. Anti-psychotic drugs; anti-depressant drugs; and minor tranquilizers, sedatives, and hypnotics. In *Comprehensive Textbook of Psychiatry,* ed. 3, H. I. Kaplan, A. M. Freedman, and B. J. Sadock, editors, p. 2257. Williams & Wilkins, Baltimore, 1980.

Desmond, P. V., Patwardham, R. V., Schenker, S., and Speeg, K. V., Jr. Cimetidine impairs elimination of chlordiazepoxide (Librium) in man. Ann. Intern. Med., *93:* 266, 1980.

Jankovic, J. Drug-induced and other orofacial-cervical dyskinesias. Ann. Intern. Med., *94:* 788, 1981.

Johnson, D. A. W. Drug induced psychiatric disorders. Drugs, *22:* 57, 1981.

Payn, S. B. Group methods in the pharmacotherapy of chronic psychotic patients. Psychiatr. Q., *39:* 258, 1965.

Payn, S. B. Treating chronic schizophrenic patients. Int. J. Group Psychother., *24:* 25, 1974.

Pulver, S. Survey of psychoanalytic practice, 1976: Some trends and implications. J. Am. Psychoanal. Assoc., *26:* 615, 1978.

Simpson, G. M., Edmond, H. P., and Sramek, J. J., Jr. Adverse effects of anti-psychotic agents. Drugs, *21:* 138, 1981.

B.19 Gestalt and Other Types of Group Psychotherapy

BENNETT E. ROTH, Ph.D.

Introduction

It is not a simple task to explain the proliferation of the group psychotherapy movement within the last 20 years, for there are many contributing forces. It can be assumed that certain elements within the fabric of our society have changed as group psychotherapy has grown, and that these changes have generated a need for people to do something in a group setting. Changes in the quality of life and within the structure of the family have contributed to an increased need for people to belong somewhere and to something. Anthony (1971) asserted that World War I and World War II provided the impetus for the development and propagation of the study of groups and group behavior because "individual man was forced into groups of all sizes and structures for reason of survival"; if this is true, then the current movement into groups has to be generated by a different form of anxiety. This anxiety seems to be spawned from the growing sense that the groups upon which we have historically depended have proven unreliable; consequently, other groups are being used for the original psychological purposes. Jacques (1955) has proposed that social institutions derive from attempted solutions to basic anxieties in a complex evolutionary process. When these social institutions fail in their psychological task, the people who sought anxiety relief from these institutions must then seek remedy elsewhere.

While many group psychotherapists react with alarm to group techniques that fall outside of the legitimate canons of psychotherapy, there is a hybrid vigor to these techniques. Time will tell if it is the hybrid or the vigor that engenders the changes ascribed to the techniques. When new orientations are presented, it is necessary to appeal to the good reader and the good psychotherapist. Care should be exercised not to confuse understanding with acceptance. Today, there is hardly a patient who comes to treatment who has not been exposed to some sort of group experience, psychotherapy or otherwise. From another perspective, aspects or essences of group dynamics are often strikingly revealed in nontraditional group techniques.

Most readers, when evaluating a new technique or a new therapeutic orientation, are concerned with the basic criteria of effectiveness in ameliorating disease or discomfort. Or they are concerned about the fit between the type of group leader they are, their particular groups, and the fit between the theory, their identity, and group role. This will not be the case here. For in most of these situations we are and will likely remain outsiders, nonparticipants, and objective observers. No doubt conclusions will be reached from the vantage of being other than a patient; therefore, our expectancies, beliefs, values, and mood are substantially different from those who participate in these groups as patients.

For current purposes, a group is defined as being a meeting of three or more people, and will not refer to a specific theoretical orientation. The group orientations under consideration are non-psychoanalytic. Two specific criteria must be met in order for an orientation to be considered psychoanalytic: The theory must have a developmental perspective, as well as one that explains behavior in the here and now. In addition, change must be explained in both the developmental and contemporary mode. Using such a definition, the new types of group psychotherapy are not psychoanalytic, but many are based on psychological theories. Some new types may not be psychotherapy at all but may be experiences which occur in a group, or for which people have paid a fee.

Gestalt Theory

As a psychological theory, Gestalt psychology addressed the problems of unity, continuity, and organization of and in the perceptual field. While much of the theory was not new, what was new was the importance which was placed upon the concept of organization of events. For example, while listening to a tune, the tune is inseparable from the various notes which make it up. The tune is the arrangement or organization of the notes.

A wealth of experiments were produced demonstrating the organization of the perceptual field. Specific modes of organization were described as principles. Among the principles are nearness (groupings of things qualitatively similar), closure (groupings of things enclosing a space), common destiny (groupings of things moving in the same direction), good whole gestalt or pregnance (groupings of things as good as conditions permit), isomorphism (a correspondence between the perceptual field and the physiological field of the brain), and insight (novel solutions, provided the problem situation could be seen as an organized whole and not in isolated elements). Many of these issues are still the clinical concern of group therapists and group psychotherapists.

Early in the development of this theory, the issue of motivation was ignored. Lewin (1935) attempted a correction by systematically applying the concept of field to motivation. In Lewin's system, the mind is viewed as a dynamic tension system, and behavior is regarded as a purposive attempt to relieve tension and re-establish equilibrium. An individual is also understood as belonging to a wider field, his or her physical and social environment. Lewin succeeded in organizing a more complete theory that brought personality and motivated behavior into an interactive mode: interaction between inside and outside the person and his life field.

It would seem natural that many concepts that are based upon groupings and organization would naturally find their way into theories of group psychology and group psychotherapy, and this has happened. System theory itself seems a logical extention of gestalt principles, and Bion's (1959) notation of basic assumptions and group-as-a-whole may be understood as organization of quality or elements in common.

GESTALT GROUP THERAPY

As derived from Perls's interpretation of Gestalt theory, Gestalt techniques are designed to promote increased awareness in the present. The techniques expressed as rules or games are designed to remove perceptual blocks, and to force attention to neglected psychological and physical stimuli. Forcing attention completes the patient's awareness and permits an immediate and more whole response. Within this system, intellectual understanding inhibits insight or novel solutions and serves to maintain repressions. Only sensory motor discharge, activity as a wholly natural response, allows discovery and awareness. Explicit in this model—and perhaps part of its appeal—is the assertion that self-control and social inhibition can only lead to neurotic and stereotyped behavior. Fundamentally, what is expressed is that man is healthy, and civilization and other agents of repression make for neurosis.

Understanding this perspective, one can see that the group is cast as an alternate social system in which it is permitted, encouraged, or required not only to feel the repressed but to feel the repressed in the here-and-now. The group therapist is active in directing or demonstrating full awareness, and the group members are encouraged toward exchanges (games) that will allow expression of their true feelings and become aware of forces influencing their behavior.

There is more to the influence of Gestalt psychology in group therapy than Perls. If Perls remained true to the earlier Gestalt cognitive theorists and researchers, many group therapists owe their origin to Lewin's attempts to form a holistic theory. For Lewin, the group was a unit or field of action and, therefore, is a legitimate and comprehensive unit of study. Whitaker and Lieberman (1964) in this country and Bion and Foulkes in England have added to our understanding of whole-group dynamics. These additions of preconscious or unconscious conflicts seem divergent with the original cognitive underpinning of Gestalt psychology, yet the idea of group focal conflict embodies much of Lewin's description of conflicts. In a focal-conflict model, the group interaction, regardless of the manifest

levels of conversation, flows from one conflict situation to another, from focal conflicts to partial solutions. A solution may adequately solve one group conflict while generating the appearance of another conflict.

In understanding the impact of Gestalt theory and therapy, it may be concluded that nothing radically new has been advanced; rather, a corrective has been inserted into existing group theories. Gestalt theory seems specifically to lack a developmental perspective, unless the work of Piaget can eventually be integrated into its organizational structure. By stressing the wholeness of the individual mind or of tension systems and the inseparability that Lewin (1935) emphasized of the individual from his life space, this theory is a correction of theories of atomistic instincts and isolated individuals.

As a clinical enterprise, Gestalt theory seems to make little use of group dynamics, since the focus is usually on one person. Perls's idea of a simple defensive organization built around repression and splitting ignores the significance of the adaptational history of the individual. Those who have followed Lewin's theoretical orientation continue the tradition of exploring and quantifying the emerging stages and conflicts within the group as a field or as a unit. Their work holds the promise of simplifying and quantifying much of what goes on in a group. Yet while Lewin castigated instinct theorists for neglecting social environmental forces and variations in drive states, at the same time he used some of these assumptions in his account of needs and tensions systems.

Among group theorists, there has been a clear distinction between the English and American school representatives of the group-as-a-whole orientation or group dynamicists. The English school—represented by Bion, Foulkes, and Ezreil—seems to view Gestalt principles as inherently part of a psychoanalytic orientation. The American representatives—Whitaker, Stock, Leiberman, and Simkin, among others—have remained unaffected by psychoanalytic constructs and maintain their practical, here-and-now perspective.

Bioenergetic Therapy

If Gestalt theory and therapy focused on the organization of the mind, then Lowen's correction is to focus on the body. In this situation, it is not possible to present a comprehensive theory of therapy, nor can a series of assertions of principles be presented. What can be offered is a description of rationale.

In bioenergetic group therapy, the body is involved in three ways: It is sufficiently exposed and available (men wear trunks and leotards), energy is mobilized by physical movement and breathing in a setting that is provided for activity, and there is physical contact between patient and therapist. At the core of the therapy is the idea that body expression is analyzed and interpreted as a function of mental activity. The body and all physical functioning are viewed as a depository of both feeling and memory.

While contemporary therapists may now be comfortable referring to body language or nonverbal communication, the historical referent point can be found in Reich's (1945) character armoring. As with Reich, aspects of physical tension, structure, body flexibility, and rigidity are directly interpreted not only as having unconscious meaning but as having direct unconscious expression. The group members and the therapist are able to see each others' body language and body stance more or less directly, where the individual is usually not aware of this level of communication. Individual unawareness is assumed to be generated by an internal image of the self that exerts direct influence over the structure of the body. Tension in the body is understood as a form of protest which requires rhythmic or muscular expression to be released.

Members of the group function to encourage active and direct expressions of feelings, or to pick up disparity between actions and feelings or actions and verbalizations. As in all groups, activity by one member builds up tensions in the observers that then seek expression and offer a comparative basis.

Negative as well as positive feelings are expressed, but repressed negative feelings are believed to precede positive ones. Calls for help and reassurance are encouraged and are met with physical contact by the therapist, as well as the group members, until brought under the individual's control.

The basis for this method seems rooted in the need for activity and physical discharge to accomplish a healing of the mind-body split. Physical activity in the presence of a group seems to occur quite rapidly, which may allow for a sense of immediate relief and good feelings toward the group and its members. No doubt physical activity and emotional discharge have beneficial effects and rapidly produce good feeling. Whether or not this kind of activity in a group can produce long-term changes seems unclear. Inhibitions, particularly of a physical nature, can easily be overcome in a group setting, under group pressure, and through permission to act. And there are gains that can accrue from the intimacy afforded by physical contact within a group setting. Whether or not there are ways to transfer the learning to situations outside the group is not clear. Nor is there a satisfactory explanation for the manner in which physical discharge can result in emotional understanding.

If one allows that both Gestalt and bioenergetic approaches have something in common, it may be that they both assume that a repression or a splitting off has occurred. They assume that there is in each person a residue of deficits that seek expression and are blocked off from full expression. One result is the build-up of tension and the restriction of activity. In the case of bioenergetic group therapy, the group becomes a situation in which a fuller expression is encouraged, if not required. Both approaches may be seen as correctives on differing sides of the coin to the atomistic mental approaches to viewing personality or to social inhibitions. Whether or not a group psychotherapy situation can be wholly constructed as a corrective emotional experience is not the present question; rather, it is to understand the appeal and usefulness of these approaches.

Groups in Which to Learn

Among the new group approaches are those that are small, carefully composed, and homogenous and that meet for a short period of time. A patient must fit specific criteria in order to belong, and it is usually these criteria that form the basis of the treatment. While the form and method of these groups may be variable, their intent is straightforward: To increase the adaptive behavior of an individual and to unlearn maladaptive behavior. The theoretical underpinning of these groups comes from the psychological study of learning and may be seen to form two distinct clusters: desensitization and assertiveness learning. Stated another way, the core of this approach is to learn new methods of dealing with anxiety, to learn new habits or to break bad habits. Originally employed to master phobias, this form of treatment within a group is commonly used for a wide range of inhibitory behaviors: Common phobias, on the one hand, and compulsive behaviors, on the other. Among the compulsive behaviors are overeating and overspending. Most recently, this learning or adaptational approach has been applied to people who share a similar condition—for example, children of divorced parents, cardiac patients, and those with other physical disabilities.

While theories of learning have become more sophisticated, much of the underpinning of these groups can be found in the work of Wolpe (1958) on reciprocal inhibition and Pratt in his work with tubercular patients. Wolpe's techniques involve causing a response that is incompatible with anxiety to occur in the presence of an anxiety-evoking stimulus. What happens is that the anxiety is then lessened, and the bond between the stimulus and the anxiety is weakened. Through explanation and suggestion, Pratt was able to teach breathing and relaxation to tubercular patients in a ward setting. Both Pratt and Wolpe made use of the idea that muscular relaxation inhibits anxiety and that relaxation and anxiety are concurrently impossible.

Learning therapy in groups is conducted mostly by the therapist, although the group situation serves an important contribution. This is particularly so when there are differing degrees of disability among the group participants. Public exposure of maladaption and competition and being in a shared environment with people who suffer similar problems set up psychological dimensions within the group, based upon its near homogeneity. Clearly, encouragement for gains made serves both to reinforce and to be a model for change, while forming a possibility of shared learning. Another benefit of this form of treatment is the short-term nature of the groups. Patients are not expected to make long-term commitments and may focus singularly on their shared problems.

The therapist's main goal, one that he or she shares with the patient, is the removal of maladaptive behavior, symptomatic improvement, or greater adaptive flexibility. The therapist willingly takes on the role of empathic teacher; he or she is learned, helpful, and non-punitive. This therapeutic atmosphere may in itself serve some of the therapeutic outcome.

Within the rubric of desensitization, the group takes on a different structure. In individual desensitization, graded lists of anxiety-evoking stimuli are constructed from the patient's history and remarks. In the group situation, a group hierarchy is constructed by the therapist. It is stressed that the hierarchical situations are imaginary ones and are presented symbolically to the patient. The early groups are devoted to learning relaxation techniques, which are also practiced at home. When the group hierarchy is presented, with the least disturbing items first, the patients are asked to imagine the scene and report on their level of disturbance. Relaxation techniques immediately follow each presentation. The groups follow the same pattern: A level of deep relaxation is achieved, and items are presented successively from the group hierarchy. The procedure is conducted at the rate of the most anxious patient.

Biofeedback Groups

Advances in technological apparatus have resulted in the development of apparatus that permit monitoring of certain vital functions, such as blood pressure. Following some of the same principles as advocated by learning theorists, there will soon emerge sufficient technology to permit biofeedback to occur in groups. While there is precious little in the literature at present, this is included as a prelude to the future relationships of people, machines, and groups. Perhaps the greatest impact in the future will be in sophisticated monitoring devices that will bring another technological entity into the treatment room.

Early on, there was an expectancy that learning to remove symptoms would only generate a displacement of anxiety and the formation of additional symptoms. This seems not to have been the result. Clearly, learning therapy does work for some persons who are more amenable to short-term, focused groups. Leaning therapists make no claim to be dealing with the entire personality, and for some the positive effects of learning new behaviors may serve as a bridge to seek help with less well-defined problems.

There seems to remain a bias against learning to cope or learning to adapt as being either simple-minded or simply away from the source of a person's conflict. However, persons who suffer debilitating fears or compulsions have benefited from straightforward solutions. If the learning approach does not work, there is nothing in these techniques that impedes further or other treatment.

Secular Conversion Groups

One trend present in contemporary society might be called a crisis of belief or a sense of unsureness, with companion feelings of helplessness and depression. Whether this sort of crisis is explained as adolescent-like, such a pervasive feeling among a large number of people created a stage set for certain kinds of group events and group leaders to emerge.

In group experiences, a number of events can be understood in terms of conversion experiences to either the group or its leader. This is different from brainwashing, in which the subjects are under another's total control. Christ (1975) asserts that leaders of conversion experiences are charismatic, engender loyalty in their followers, and bring to their followers a sense of being supported. Liff (1975) adds that such leadership is one that promises with absolute certainty deliverance from all disasters and distress. Weber (1947) describes part of the appeal of the charismatic as being the open defiance of rules, routine, and tradition, while being scornful of old ideas or alternative explanations.

In contemporary society, forms of secular conversion are witnessed in a number of proselytizing groups and in est (Erhard sensitivity training). Est here serves as an example, for it is the largest and best known of the group experiences of this sort. Est has over 100,000 graduates who have paid at least $250 each to be a part of the experience. Each person has paid this money to get "it." "It," according to Erhard, is to experience the world as it is without the interference of human understanding.

During the est procedure, the people are told that some of them will retch, faint, flip out, be hungry, ache, be bored, want their money back, etc. Later, as people have these feelings, it is used as verification of the leader's insight and authority. Psychological humiliation also plays a part in the establishment of the leader's authority—being told you are stupid, ignorant, and have not got "it." At the same time that the leader becomes an authority, he becomes an external guilt- and shame-inducing authority, who may then show the way to salvation.

The processes by which human beings can easily and readily be overcome in a group were described by Freud when he referred to the group's ability to influence and profoundly alter a person's belief system and mental activity through suggestion from the leader, multiple identification processes, and the loss of physical restraint. James (1958), in his classic lectures, offers insight into the conversion experience. In crises of self-despair and inner doubt, salvation, either religious or secular, offers a process of remedying inner incompleteness and discord. Revivalism, either secular or religious, has always assumed that only its own type of experience can be perfect and that before salvation comes mortification. Goffman (1961) describes mortification or curtailment of the self as likely to involve acute psychological stress. But for an individual sick with his world or guilt ridden in it, mortification may bring psychological relief. Both James and Goffman elucidate part of the dynamic of conversion and mortification used to modify thinking and behavior in such total institutions as prisons, monasteries, mental hospitals, orphanages, armed forces training, and certain educational institutions. From the perspective of psychological therapy, the staff that manages the mortification process, as well as those who promise relief, become the objects of powerful transference assumptions.

The positive tie that follows mortification procedures is complex and yet follows certain proscriptions. Following the painful experience and the relief from expiation of guilt, there is usually permission to express physical feelings—anger, love, affection—in a festival of triumph over what in other situations would be viewed as transgressions. One end product of the mortification and salvation experience is a special form of immunity from self-criticism, a reduction in inhibitions, coupled with increased consideration for others. Although the intensity of these feelings may vary among members, they usually require intermittent refueling or reinforcement.

References

Anthony, E. J. The history of group psychotherapy. In *Comprehensive Group Psychotherapy*, H. I. Kaplan and B. J. Sadock, editors, p. 4. Williams & Williams, Baltimore, 1971.

Bion W. *Experiences in Groups*. Basic Books, New York, 1959.

Christ, J. Contrasting the charismatic and reflective leader. In *The Leader in the Group*, Z. Liff, editor, p. 104. Jason Aronson, New York, 1975.

Goffman, E. *Asylums: Essays on the Social Situation of Mental Patients and Other Inmates*. Anchor Press, New York, 1961.

Jacques, E. Social systems as a defense against persecutory and depressive anxiety. In *New Directions in Psychoanalysis*, M. Klein, P. Heimann, and R. E. Money-Kyrle, editors, p. 478. Basic Books, New York, 1955.

James, W. *The Varieties of Religious Experience*. Mentor Books, New York, 1958.

Lewin, K. *A Dynamic Theory of Personality*. McGraw-Hill, New York, 1935.

Liff, Z. The charismatic leader. In *The Leader in the Group*, Z. Liff, editor, p. 114. Jason Aronson, New York, 1975.

Reich, W. *Character Analysis*. Farrar, Straus & Giroux, New York, 1945.

Weber, M. *The Theory of Social and Economic Organization*. Oxford University Press, New York, 1947.

Whitaker, D. S., and Lieberman, M. *Psychotherapy through the Group Process*, Atherton Press, New York, 1964.

Wolpe, J. *Psychotherapy by Reciprocal Inhibition*. Standford University Press, Palo Alto, CA, 1958.

AREA C

Psychotherapy with Groups in Special Categories

C.1 Group Psychotherapy with Gender-dysphoric Patients

STANLEY E. ALTHOF, Ph.D.
ANN KELLER HILLMAN, M.S.W.

Introduction

The wish to change one's biological sex is a phenomenon which has persisted throughout the ages. Although Green (1974) has unearthed fascinating examples of cross-gender identification over the last 2,000 years, Christine Jorgenson's surgery in Denmark in 1952 was the first example of the sensationalism of the transsexual phenomenon in the United States. Since Harry Benjamin's pioneer work in the 1950's, a number of clinics have been established for the investigation or treatment of gender identity disorders. Clinical reports from these clinics and analytic case studies have given rise to several major theories on the etiology of transsexualism, including the most basic question as to whether the disorder(s) are of biological or psychological origin.

Definitions and Diagnostic Dilemmas

Gender identity disorders are defined in DSM-III as being "characterized by the individual's feelings of discomfort and inappropriateness about his or her anatomic sex and by persistent behaviors generally associated with the other sex. Gender identity is the sense of knowing to which sex one belongs ... (it) is the private experience of gender role and gender role is the public expression of gender identity." The gender identity disorders are divided into three diagnoses: transsexualism, gender identity disorder of childhood, and atypical gender identity disorder.

The diagnostic criteria for transsexualism in DSM-III are: "(A) Sense of discomfort and inappropriateness about one's anatomic sex; (B) Wish to be rid of one's own genitals and to live as a member of the opposite sex; (C) The disturbance has been continuous (not limited to periods of stress) for at least two years; (D) Absence of physical intersex or genetic abnormality; (E) Not due to another mental disorder, such as schizophrenia."

Gender identity disorders seem best viewed as fluid developmental adaptational processes, whose forms change according to the individual's intrapsychic balances, biological events, and interpersonal milieu. At different points in time, the same individual may be labeled as transsexual, asexual, homosexual, bisexual, transvestitic, or any combination.

Although transsexualism has been officially incorporated into the diagnostic nomenclature, it has been attacked for suggesting a similarity among individuals with vast differences (Fisk, 1973). In an attempt to acknowledge a broader spectrum of gender disorders, Fisk (1973) introduced the term gender dysphoria syndrome. One inconsistency with the DSM-III diagnosis of transsexualism is that not all patients requesting sex reassignment surgery (SRS) fit the aforementioned diagnostic criteria. Similarly, when Meyer (1974) attempted to demonstrate the narrowness of the diagnosis transsexualism, he divided SRS candidates into the following clinical variants: aging transvestites, younger transvestites, sadists and masochists, stigmatized homosexuals, polymorphous perverse, schizoid, and eonists, a term designating individuals who "with constant and persistent conviction, [have] the desire to live as a member of the opposite sex, and progressively takes steps to live in the opposite sex role full time (Money and Gaskin (1970))."

Biological Theories of Transsexualism

A number of researchers believe that biological forces underlie the development of transsexualism. Neuroendocrine abnormalities, brain pathology, and chromosomal defects have all been examined in association with atypical gender identity development.

Neuroendocrine abnormalities

The basic biological predisposition of the mammalian embryo is female. The fetus will develop as male if sufficient male sex hormones are introduced at the critical periods. Natural and experimental research in animals and humans demonstrates that subjects exposed prenatally to opposite-sex hormones show some opposite-sex behaviors, i.e., boys whose mothers took estrogen compounds during pregnancy exhibited lower ratings on several variables related to general masculinity, assertiveness, and athletic ability. Although most studies show that the plasma testosterone levels of adult male and female transsexuals are within the normal range (Jones and Samimig, 1973; Kolodny et al., 1979), Meyer-Bahlburg has reviewed three studies reporting increased testosterone levels in female-to-male transsexuals. The effects of prenatal sex hormones on anatomical sexual differentiation and childhood behaviors lead to the intriguing yet unproven hypothesis that prenatal hormones result in a sexual differentiation of the brain, thereby influencing the foundation of core gender identity.

The following case report by Robert Stoller (1979) highlights the relationship between neuroendocrine abnormalities and gender identity formation.

At birth, Mary appeared to be a normal female. From infancy on, she rebelled against the trappings of femininity, despite her parents' encouragement to be feminine. Mary was medically evaluated at age 14 because of a voice defect, hirsutism of the extremities, and the absence of secondary sex characteristics. The evaluation revealed that Mary was a male hermaphrodite with cryptorchid testes, a recently enlarged phallus, small prostate, no internal female organs, and a rudimentary vagina. Upon Stoller's recommendation, Mary began to live as a male and underwent surgical procedures to masculinize his genitals. Some years after the initial evaluation, it was determined that the patient suffered from a rare enzyme deficiency (17: beta hydroxysteroid dehydrogenase), which Stoller hypothesized had masculinized his brain.

Brain pathology

Transsexualism has been related to various brain pathologies. Randell reported that more than 50 per cent of his sample showed some degree of electroencephalogram abnormality. The same phenomenon has been described by others, although the frequency of the findings is significantly less. Gender identity disorders have also been associated to a very small degree with brain tumors and asymmetric enlargement of the sella turcica (Lundberg et al., 1975).

Chromosomal defects

There are few reports of chromosomal defects associated with the transsexual population. These rare accounts include individuals with both 47, XYY (Buhrich et al., 1978) and 47, XXY karyotypes (Davidson, 1966), and one report of mosaicism (James et al., 1972). The most intriguing report (Imperato-McGinley et al., 1974), however, is from the Dominican Republic. Thirty-seven newborns who appeared to be essentially female were reared accordingly. At puberty their vaginas healed over, testes descended, and they developed normal penises. They adapted to the traditional male roles and vocations with no apparent difficulty; some even married and had children. Investigators attribute this phenomenon to a rare mutant gene which prevents the fetus from processing testosterone into another male hormone responsible for shaping the external male genitalia.

Psychological Theories

Theories about biological males

Person and Ovesey (1974b) theorize that the transsexual wish "originates from unresolved separation anxiety during the separation-individuation phase of infantile development. To counter this separation anxiety, the child resorts to a reparation fantasy of symbolic fusion with the mother ... the final transsexual resolution is an attempt to get rid of the anxiety through sex reassignment." These authors speak of a "developmental gradient" of effeminate homosexuality, transvestism, and transsexualism; the individual's ability to deal with the separation anxiety determines his position.

Stoller differs from Person and Ovesey in that he believes the female core gender identity of the male transsexual is conflict free. Stoller delineates a number of psychological factors about the parents of male transsexuals: a blissful physical and emotional closeness between a depressed mother and an exceptionally pretty infant, which is uninterrupted by siblings and goes on for years; mothers have strong bisexual components and are married to effeminate or passive fathers who are rarely at home; and the marriage is empty and angry but does not move toward separation or divorce.

Theories about biological females

Stoller (1975) views the following constellation of psychological variables as being responsible for female transsexuals: At birth, the infant is perceived as vigorous and strong, not pretty or cuddly. The mother is unavailable to nurture the child, due to a depression or physical illness. The father is unable or unwilling to take over the parenting functions and is unsupportive of the mother's depression or illness. The child is then shackled with the burden of relieving the mother's depressions. Finally, the father encourages and admires his daughter's acquisition of masculine identifications and behaviors.

In contrast to Stoller's non-conflictual theory of female transsexualism, Person and Ovesey (1974a, 1974b) maintain that there is no female equivalent to primary male transsexualism—asexual individuals constantly progressing toward the transsexual solution.

Theory encompassing both sexes

Dorothy Block believes that the threat of parental infanticide underlies a person's belief that he is a member of the opposite sex. The assumption of the opposite gender identity is seen as an acted-out defensive fantasy, in which the child simultaneously guards against being killed and maintains the illusion of being loved.

Developmental theories

John Money writes about a "critical developmental period of gender identity differentiation and the effect of any detrimental social experience during this critical period. It is possible for detrimental social experiences to become imprinted and produce the indelibility that a genetic trait has once it has expressed itself." Thus, he explains transsexualism as "an extremely tenacious critical-period effect in the gender identity differentiation of a child with a particular, that is yet unspecifiable, vulnerability."

Green (1974) reviews social learning theory in relation to transsexuals. This theory views the child's identification with the appropriate sex role model as crucial to gender identity development.

Diagnostic Considerations

There are a number of reports on the psychiatric diagnoses of individuals with transsexual wishes. Levine's 4-year study indicates that 84 per cent of SRS applicants received psychiatric diagnoses; various types of character pathology were diagnosed in 66 per cent, and 18 per cent were psychotic.

Person and Ovesey (1974b) suggest that all transsexuals have borderline character organizations. Person and Ovesey describe these patients as having

uniformly displayed the clinical manifestation typically found in the borderline syndrome: chronic anxiety, empty depression, sense of void, oral dependency, defective self-identity and impaired object relationships with absence of trust and withdrawal from intimacy. These manifestations reflect not only unresolved separation anxiety but also primitive defenses and defective ego functions developmentally associated with it.

As a group, the biological females are generally considered healthier than the biological males. This is borne out by Levine's study, where only 58 per cent of the females requesting SRS were given psychiatric diagnoses, compared with 92 per cent of the males.

Interventions

As increasing numbers of patients present to gender clinics requesting SRS, clinicians must develop sophisticated techniques for evaluation and treatment. The treatment of gender-dysphoric patients is a highly controversial, emotionally charged topic. The possible range of interventions includes various forms of psychotherapy, hormone therapy, and sex reassignment surgery. Stoller captures the therapeutic dilemma in his statement that "the general rule that applies to the treatment of transsexuals is that no matter what one does—including nothing—it will be wrong."

The proponents of SRS as the treatment of choice tend to favor a biological etiology of the disorder, are pessimistic about the outcome of psychotherapy, or believe that surgery would provide patients with better social and psychological adjustments.

The following are quotes from a surgeon, a physician, and a psychologist, respectively, in the field. "The only open avenue of therapy if one wishes to do anything to help these unfortunate people seems to be that of the surgical route." "Psychiatry in its presently available form cannot cure grown-up transsexuals, cannot even give them sufficient relief. Not even years of psychoanalysis did any good. Help has to be found elsewhere." "Clinical evidence indicates the surgical reassignment for transsexual patients is a justifiable, ameliorative therapy and the majority of patients make an adequate social adjustment."

At the other extreme are those who believe that (1) providing patients with SRS violates the physician's dictum, "above all do no harm"; (2) the removal of healthy tissue is immoral and unethical; (3) surgery represents collusion with the patient's delusion; and (4) surgery provides patients with an environmental (alloplastic) remedy for an intrapsychic conflict. Moreover, the follow-up studies of patients receiving SRS are methodologically weak, inconclusive, and contradictory.

Although the treatment approach to adult transsexuals remains confusing and controversial, there is a strong consensus that early psychotherapeutic intervention in children or adolescents is appropriate. The reports on analytic, behavioral, and group psychotherapy are very encouraging.

With few exceptions, the literature describes the inability of individual psychotherapy to change adult transsexuals into masculine men or feminine women, free of transsexual, transvestic, or homosexual wishes. The exceptions include one case of exorcism (Barlow et al., 1977), one description of intensive behavioral psychotherapy (Barlow et al., 1973), and a psychotherapeutic work with aging transvestites (Lothstein, 1979b; Wise, 1979).

Regardless of whether the patient will eventually receive SRS, it appears that psychotherapy is the treatment of choice. These patients have multiple profound psychological problems that cannot be ameliorated with SRS alone, some of which may be helped by individual psychotherapy. Treatment also provides an ongoing diagnostic evaluation of the patient's changing gender wishes and adaptations over time. Although patients may feel guilty, ostracized, and stigmatized by their transsexual wishes, they feel empty, depressed, false, and cheated if they do not pursue them. Psychotherapy may help patients cope with the trauma of announcing transsexual wishes to family, friends, and employers, beginning to cross-dress in public, and working in the opposite-sex role. Patients can compare the reality of living in a cross-gender role with their long-held private fantasies. The therapist's knowledge about the limitations of surgery enables the discussion of hormones and SRS decisions in a neutral atmosphere. Psychotherapy may also assist in the patient's postsurgical adjustment.

Educational Groups

Most educational groups for gender-dysphoric patients provide advice about personal grooming. For example, Fisk (1973) writes about a charm school or grooming clinic formed to assist biological males in appearing more feminine. Eventually the group became a monthly forum for members "to exchange information, opinions, experiences, and to mutually share feelings, successes, and failures."

These educational groups are often led by postsurgical patients. By answering questions, they can dispel unrealistic concerns or exaggerated expectations about surgery. Legal advice and vocational guidance are also common topics.

Support groups

Support groups are integral parts of some gender programs. Laub suggested a halfway house for patients who are "completely down and out and in need of advice and support." The Seattle Gender Identity Clinic's main function is to organize support groups so "cross-dressers could come to discuss their problems." These groups usually emphasize support, advice, and guidance; they do not promote insight into the etiology and persistence of a patient's gender problems.

Group psychotherapy

At best, the majority of clinicians have questioned the use of individual psychotherapy with gender patients; at worst, it has been deemed futile. Treatment difficulties are intensified by the frequency of associated character pathologies. The problems encountered in treating individuals with serious character pathologies are well documented in the literature. The use of therapy with borderline patients is supported by Horwitz. The group milieu protects the patient from personal criticism, since interpretations are made to the group as a whole.

Similarly, Guttmacher and Fisk (1971) found groups to be effective for patients with homogeneous personality disorders with ego-syntonic problems. They write:

It is almost a truism that group psychotherapy is especially helpful in terms of relief from isolation, realization that others share the same problems, and relief from unrealistic shame.

These characteristics are typical of patients presenting to gender programs across the country.

Forester and Swiller (1972) believe that group psychotherapy is an effective treatment modality with gender patients due to their fear of authority figures which results in massive resistance to individual psychotherapy. They have found that peer support decreases fear, thus allowing the patient to become involved in the group process. Various group approaches have been used with gender patients and their families. Heterogeneous psychotherapy groups are composed of both male and female and both pre- and postsurgical gender-dysphoric patients (Lothstein, 1979a; Althof and Keller, 1980). Green and Fuller (1973) describe three groups—one for feminine boys, one for their mothers, and one for their fathers. Forester and Swiller (1972) described a group with one gender patient, in which the other group members without gender problems were generally supportive of the patient.

The therapeutic goals for these groups ranged from helping the person to become himself (Sadoughi et al., 1973), to orienting the patient back to his anatomically congruent gender role and identity (Forester and Swiller, 1972), to decreasing effeminate behavior in a group of latency-aged boys (Green and Fuller, 1973).

Althof and Keller's group psychotherapy at Case Western Reserve University's Department of Psychiatry (CWRU) has multiple goals, including preparation for surgery and consolidation in a postsurgical gender role, and stabilization in a homosexual or transvestic adaptation (Lothstein, 1979a). This group did not strive for profound characterological changes; patients were, however, made aware of how their self-presentations affected others. They increased their reality testing and judgment, and learned to delay impulse expression (Althof and Keller, 1980).

Given the diverse psychological, biological, and social problems of gender-dysphoric patients, groups have successfully fulfilled a number of functions. In addition to providing general support and education, the group process promotes interpersonal and intrapsychic changes.

Special Issues

The Case Western Reserve University (CWRU) Experience

A multidisciplinary clinic at CWRU Department of Psychiatry began evaluating, treating, and studying patients with gender identity disturbances in 1975. The patients are psychiatrically evaluated by two clinicians and given a battery of psychometric tests. The evaluation results are presented to the clinic staff and used as the basis for treatment recommendations. Group psychotherapy is one possible treatment option.

The decision to treat patients in group psychotherapy is based on several factors, including patients' rigid characterological defenses that would likely impede the progress of individual psychotherapy, a wish to dilute the transference relationships, improving impoverished object relationships, lending support, decreasing social isolation and ostracism, and a sense that individual treatment alone would not be successful.

The majority of patients referred to the group had severe character pathology, predominantly borderline and narcissistic disturbances. While group therapy served as their primary treatment modality, patients were also seen in individual therapy; frequency of the latter ranged from weekly to once every 3 months.

Concomitant individual and group treatment

Clinicians generally recommend a combination of individual (concomitantly or prior to group) and group psychotherapy for the majority of patients with borderline personality disorders and narcissistic disturbances. While group therapy was the primary treatment, individual sessions facilitated the group progress made by the patients. Specifically, the concomitant individual sessions served to emotionally refuel members after trying group meetings, clarify distortions about the ongoing group process (Wong, 1980), and allow for the working through of particularly sensitive issues.

The literature is divided as to whether the individual and group treatments should be conducted by the same therapist. In one group, some patients were seen individually by either therapist; others were seen by various other therapists. This proved to be an undesirable situation because of the co-therapists' special relationships with certain patients. This resulted in unnecessary rivalry, petty jealousies, increased tendencies to split the therapists, and subgrouping. Patients who were not seen by either therapist could temporarily avoid talking about certain important topics because "they had already discussed it with their private doctors."

Beginning Group Treatment

Gender identity patients have markedly ambivalent feelings at the beginning of their group therapy, more so than patients beginning other groups. On the one hand, they over-idealize the powers of the therapists, believing they are in the hands of world-famous experts who will magically remove any vestiges of their unwanted gender and unconditionally support their driven desire for SRS. They feel they have finally arrived at a place where someone will understand their suffering and unique life experiences. They sense a chance to achieve their lifelong goal of sex change, if they can just make it through the 2-year waiting period and be good in group. They look forward to learning the secrets of the subculture from other patients, e.g., the transsexual hangouts, who will perform electrolysis without hassling them, where to buy clothes, cosmetic tricks, and where underground hormones can be obtained. They hope to make friends and enlarge their social networks.

The negative side of patients' ambivalence about beginning group psychotherapy often has a paranoid quality to it. They fear that the therapists will magically remove their transsexual wishes against their will, leaving them empty and hopeless. They believe they will be tricked, deceived, and misunderstood. Moreover, they are disappointed when the experts fail to see that immediate surgery will surely be their salvation, even though they are completely aware of the minimum 2-year waiting period. Patients resent having others make important life decisions for them, such as whether they will receive hormone therapy or SRS.

Initially, new members view the group as an arena where others will judge and confront the nature of their transsexual wishes. This often leads to carefully orchestrated and rehearsed self-presentations during the initial visits to the group. Patients complain about the group being an obstacle to the fulfillment of their dreams. Their initial responses are guarded, expressing the belief that, "What I say will be held against me later."

Patients do not believe they need psychotherapy. They sense themselves as normal apart from their gender dysphoria. One patient jokingly compared her condition to going to the "tailor for a minor alteration." Initially, patients have little interest in understanding how they arrived at their transsexual solutions. They are reluctant to talk about the past, vociferously stating that it has no relevance to their current situation. They prefer to focus upon issues of surgery, cross-dressing, hormones, and the perceived coldness and distance of the gender program staff who fail to understand their dilemma. Finally, there are constant threats to leave the program and seek immediate solutions elsewhere.

The universality of the patients' desires to obtain SRS, their current unhappiness, and their disappointment and anger at the therapists and gender program serve as cohesive group factors. Their resistances to discussing the past decrease as patients become more interested in each other and their similar life experiences. Competition between members often engenders confrontation as well as self-revelations.

Group composition

The use of a heterogeneous group population (that is, both pre- and post-surgical patients of both sexes) has proved valuable in group psychotherapy with gender patients. Post-surgical patients are able to pierce the rigid defenses of the pre-surgical candidates, which results in the emergence of repressed and denied anxiety. This in turn allows for meaningful interpretations, which can lead to a rearrangement of the ego's defensive organization, as well as behavioral change.

For example, one male-to-female group patient revealed the loneliness and isolation of her post-surgical experience. She recounted the painful separation from family and friends, the loss of a high-level administrative position, and her multiple surgical complications. She dramatically described two desperate suicide attempts and her current uncertainty about the future. Her vivid presentation generated enough anxiety to break down the group's intensive and extensive denial. For the first time, pre-surgical patients began to discuss current and past hurts, losses, and frustrations.

The post-surgical patients seemed anxious to share their surgical and post-operative experiences with other members. This represents not only an interest in sharing information but also an attempt to master a traumatic experience. The patients focused on the pain, the unexpected surgical complications, and the alienation from significant others. One post-surgical patient described the intense pain of daily dilations over a 6-month period. Her confession broke through many of the pre-surgical patients' fantasies about surgery being free of pain and emotionally uncomplicated. As a result, pre-surgical patients' desires for immediate surgery were refocused. New concerns included pain, i.e., losing control due to prolonged suffering, fear of death, fantasized surgical complications (e.g., cancer), and realistic worries about genital malfunction.

All of the post-surgical patients reported going through mild to severe depressions after the loss or rupture of at least one supportive relationship—spouse, parents, or children. These accounts allowed the therapists to reinforce the fact that SRS would not magically remove long-standing interpersonal or intrapsychic problems.

The second advantage of a heterogeneous group composition is that the post-surgical patients are forced to reconsider dormant issues. One post-surgical patient was horrified by a pre-surgical patient's cross-dressing, especially when she realized that she, too, must have looked freakish at one time. Although initially idealized as gurus with special knowledge, it soon became apparent that the post-surgical patients still had significant problems. In fact, two post-surgical patients left the group to avoid dealing with painful issues and to protect their brittle sense of being special. Questions about the quality of post-surgical patients' relationships with their children brought about interesting responses. One female-to-male patient said his children had really flipped about his surgery and "thought it was just great because I'd always been more of a father than a mother to them anyway." Unfortunately, his children made extremely poor adjustments. After becoming psychotic, his son spent several years at an adolescent treatment center (Althof and Keller, 1980).

There are no reports of gender identity groups composed entirely of males or entirely of females. Although an all-male or all-female group might hasten the development of universality and cohesion, it could also promote a negatively reinforced one-sided view of their own gender experience. Without a blend of males and females, such a homogeneous group might well foster the overidealization of the opposite gender identity.

Advantages of opposite-sexed co-therapists

The predominant borderline and narcissistic pathology of the CWRU group members and their defenses of splitting and projection were the rationale for employing opposite-sexed co-therapists. The development of patients' gender-specific transference is enhanced by using opposite-sexed co-therapists (Lothstein, 1979a). They also serve flexible role models, allowing the patients to learn by a process of imitation. The patients' perceptions of masculinity and femininity are often projected as good and bad male and female images. When intense transference prevents the patient from accepting one therapist's interpretations, the opposite-sexed therapist may be able to intervene therapeutically.

Mr. J. was a 40-year-old white male whose father suffered from an organic brain syndrome. The father would dress the patient in girls' clothes and stand him in the corner for punishment. The patient had always been plagued by feelings that he should have been a girl. The understandable anger toward his father was later manifested through the loss of numerous jobs, and it interfered with his interpersonal relationships. The group experience became a transferential microcosm of Mr. J.'s earlier family interactions, as clearly demonstrated in his angry reactions to the male therapist. When the female therapist suggested that the patient's anger toward Dr. A. stemmed from past experiences with his father, the response was an intellectualized, "I see what you mean, but I doubt it." When the male therapist had previously offered the same interpretation, it produced a brief, psychotic transference reaction; the patient accused the therapist of being sadistically cruel and unfair. He blamed Dr. A. because he had "almost been attacked by a pack of vicious dogs" on the way to the group therapy session. When another male group member revealed that Mr. J. had made overt sexual advances toward him, Mr. J. accused the male therapist of pushing him into homosexuality. After this session, Mr. J.'s guilt and depression over his behavior caused him to seek help from the female therapist.

The volume of highly charged, sexual material in group meetings makes an open, supportive relationship between co-therapists essential. It is not uncommon for group sessions to include probing questions, confrontations, and remarks ranging from innuendos about the therapists' gender identities to hostile verbal attacks. Co-therapists deflect the intensity of these episodes without interfering with the therapeutic process. Lothstein (1979a) reports that a single group therapist is more easily manipulated and overwhelmed by these attacks (Althof and Keller, 1980).

Expression of hostility

It was unusual for a group session to proceed without anger and hostility being discharged, either by the patients toward the therapists or among the group members themselves. Although it was not surprising in light of the patients' character structures, it was often difficult therapeutically to manage the primitiveness, intensity, and frequency of the anger.

Sadoughi et al. suggest that the attitude of the group therapists treating gender identity patients should be nonjudgmental and empathic, thus enabling patients to examine their adjustment patterns. The literature reports that intense anger was often nonproductive and refractory to usual therapeutic interventions, i.e. interpretation or reflection. Episodes of hostility forced the therapists temporarily to assume a more active, limit-setting stance. In addition, it sometimes became necessary for the therapists to protect patients who were being scapegoated by the other group members.

In addition to the typical demands and questions regarding therapists' personal lives by group members, there would be angry accusations made, such as, "You've trapped us into this group; you're only the therapists of a group like this for the money; you talk about us behind our backs." Or, there would be degrading remarks about the therapists' personal lives, e.g. speculation about how the therapists would look in drag, or the nature of their sexual hang-ups. When the male therapist announced that he was taking a week off because his wife was having a baby, one biological male responded, "I wonder whose baby it really is."

On another occasion, the therapists told the group they would both be gone for a week. Two patients thought the female therapist, "who usually has a halo around her head," would probably "cut loose, get drunk and dance wildly on barroom tables." They fantasized about the male therapist sitting at home with his feet up by his swimming pool. He would be with his wife, the fantasy continued, picking his teeth and thinking that he had it made.

The more degrading nature of the group members' remarks was exemplified by a biological female patient's offer to slam the female therapist on the back while she was coughing and then laughingly saying, "I was going to ask you what his name was." This transparent sexual reference typified the jealousy, anger, cruelty, crudeness of expression, and curiosity about the therapist's sexual life. Exploration into remarks such as these proved difficult because of the group's high level of excitement. Subsequently, any motivation other than friendly humor was negated or denied.

Group members' interactions can be constructively oriented, as in encouraging insight and lending support. However, as was more frequently the case, they can also be quite hostile. This was exhibited in relation to differences between the group members, such as age and race, and around the issue of competition between members and the introduction of new members into the group.

Although new members are not welcomed into any

group with open arms, those entering the gender group were usually drilled by the more hostile members. These attacks were defended on the grounds that they were just preparing the new members for what lay ahead. The more unusual or bizarre a new member appeared, the more abusively he was treated.

For example, Daniel (a biological female) resisted having her male name made legal. This 41-year-old patient had lived and worked in the male role for 5 years; she still had a female name on her checks, however, which caused quite a stir at the bank. She also refused to correct or challenge family members who continued to use her given name. Needless to say, the patient's tales of woe about family members calling her Denise met with little to no sympathy from group members. In fact, three group members implied she was not much of a transsexual if she did not get the legal name change. The patient became more and more uncomfortable and finally shouted, "It would kill my mother if I were to go ahead with this." The therapist suggested that perhaps Daniel's feelings about the name change were related to his feelings about his mother. The therapist also felt that he was not ready to change his name at this time, even though the group was trying to push him into it. The patient was visibly relieved at being protected by the therapist.

Subgrouping and cliques among the members were based on outside contacts and issues of race. At various times, all the blacks or all the whites would engage in private group conversations, accompanied by whispering, giggling, and the use of slang expressions unique to their subculture. This type of interaction was clearly meant to exclude outsiders; since it was amenable to interpretation, it eventually ceased to be a resistance.

Group members were often fiercely competitive, especially in regard to who was the "best transsexual." During one session, two members had a prolonged, heated argument. A biological male claimed to have tucked his penis between his legs since the age of 10. Another patient angrily retorted that this patient was merely attempting to impress the other group members, for if she had really been tucking since age 10 she would have had SRS by now.

Passive-aggressive remarks were frequently made in an offhand manner, "You wore that to group therapy? ... You don't plan to keep working in that grocery store, do you? ... Your hair looks nice now, but it's too bad you don't wear it the way you used to." More direct remarks often stirred up angry feelings, such as one biological female remarking to another, "I really feel you don't pass well; I don't think you should come to my house, because people might start to suspect me."

The emotional deprivation, social isolation, and severe ego defects of many gender identity patients make it inevitable for their rage to surface. Therapists undertaking the treatment of gender patients should realize that the seemingly limitless anger may impede the progress of treatment. The therapists need to be prepared to set limits, interpret and defuse anger, and protect other patients.

Therapists' reactions

Imagine yourself sitting down among eight other people who at first glance look and act like normal men and women. Yet all the time you are aware that the women are really men, and the men are really women. You may wonder how some manage to look so convincing or how others have the nerve to go out in public looking so unconvincing. You may even find yourself looking for telltale signs of their biological sex. It is not unusual to find yourself confused and struggling to call patients by their new names, misusing male and female pronouns, and briefly wondering about your own sexual orientation and gender identity. You may imagine what it would be like to be a member of the opposite sex, rethink your evaluation of the efficacy of psychotherapy or surgery, and, in general, begin to wonder whether you are the one with a problem.

Two therapists experienced all the above countertransferential reactions to leading the group, reactions that stem from the negation of one of the basic assumptions of life—masculinity/femininity. The equation of biological sex and gender identity is generally automatic. In this group therapy, however, this basic assumption no longer applies.

Although the therapists were aware that patients often develop erotic transferences, this phenomenon caused them more discomfort than was apparent in their work with non-gender patients. At the core of their discomfort lay their reawakened concerns about homosexuality and bisexuality. Were the therapists responding to the patients as men to men, men to women, women to men, or women to women?

The close bond between the co-therapists was based on a mutual caring and admiration; it was also a defense against the countertransference anxieties elicited by the group experience. It became clear that for the other, the co-therapist was the only real man or woman in the room. The therapists found themselves using the rehash time to affirm their masculinity/femininity via the other. In addition to discussing group process, the therapists found themselves talking about social relationships, marriage, and children. This type of exchange helped the therapists to consolidate and recover from the group process.

While most initial countertransferential anxieties diminished with time, reactions to patients' borderline pathologies remained a problem. The therapists' concerns include a fear that the group is getting out of control, difficulty in listening to the primitive aggressive and sexual material, anger at the lack of mutual concern among group members, and a desire to desert the group.

Another source of anxiety was the reaction of colleagues and ancillary staff to the therapists' work with gender patients. For instance, secretaries who were exceptionally skilled at dealing with demanding, acutely suicidal and psychotic patients were sometimes unable to effectively interact with gender patients. Their anxieties escalated when a cross-dressed patient entered a bathroom occupied by a secretary. Although the patient did not say or do anything unusual, the female staff secretaries demanded that a departmental meeting be held to discuss whether gender patients should be allowed to use the bathroom; no questions had ever been raised about other patients. Another member of the gender team had to help the secretaries work through some of their anxieties.

The reactions of professional colleagues ranged from genuine interest and support to vociferous criticism of their professionalism, competence, and morality. These criticisms did cause some concern about whether they were hurting their reputations as clinicians, teachers, and researchers by working in this area.

Finally, the therapists had reactions to being involved in the decision-making process to grant patients SRS. Each decision about surgery reawakened their ambivalence toward the procedure and their work in general. The therapists questioned the efficacy of their clinical skills, wondered if there was something they missed or if surgery could be considered a successful outcome.

Other Applications

Group psychotherapy facilitates the gathering of clinical research data, in addition to providing psychological treatment. Careful process notes and individual summaries of patients' progress become tools for research and extended patient evaluation. Additionally, the therapeutic setting provokes a reconsideration of traditional concepts, and stimulates the generation of new perspectives into the development of gender identity.

In addition to research, two other applications of groups are for those involved both personally and medically with gender identity patients. Short-term groups for the hospital staff who care for postsurgical patients serve a dual function. They provide an avenue for the staff to vent their anxieties, fears, and anger around caring for such individuals; and the nurses and nurses aides can be educated about gender dysphoria and sensitized to the patients for whom they care.

The spouses or significant others in gender patients' lives might well benefit from group therapy, as might children who are faced with the devastating dilemma of adjusting to a parent's gender dysphoria.

Conclusion

The course and treatment of gender patients cannot be predicted on the basis of the initial evaluation or brief psychometric testing. Long-term evaluation and intensive individual or group psychotherapy are important for several reasons: It is extremely difficult to make accurate diagnostic predictions of the course of gender dysphoria; SRS is irreversible; there are no adequate criteria for determining which patients make the best surgical candidates; and there are many unanswered bioethical questions surrounding SRS.

References

Althof, S., and Keller, A. Group therapy with gender identity patients. Int. J. Group Psychother., 30: 481, 1980.

Barlow, D. H., Abel, G. A., and Blanchard, E. G. Gender identity change in a transsexual: An exorcism. Arch. Sex. Behav., 6: 387, 1977.
Barlow, D. H., Reynolds, E. J., and Agras, W. S. Gender identity change in a transsexual. Arch. Gen. Psychiatry, 28: 569, 1973.
Benjamin, H. Should surgery be performed on transsexuals. Am. J. Psychother., 25: 74, 1971.
Buhrich, N., Barr, R., and Lam-Po-Tang, P. R. Two transsexuals with 47-XYY karyotype. Br. J. Psychiatry, 133: 77, 1978.
Davidson, P. W. Transsexualism in Kleinfelters syndrome. Psychosomatics, 7: 94, 1966.
Fisk, N. Gender dysphoria syndrome. In Proceedings of the Second Interdisciplinary Symposium on Gender Dysphoria Syndrome, D. R. Laub and P. Gandy, editors, p. 223. Stanford University Medical Center, Stanford, CA, 1973.
Forester, B., and Swiller, H. Transsexualism: Review of syndrome and presentation of possible successful therapeutic approach. Int. J. Group Psychother., 22: 343, 1972.
Green, R. Sexual Identity Conflict in Children and Adults. Basic Books, New York, 1974.
Green, R., and Fuller, M. Group therapy and feminine boys and their parents. Int. J. Group Psychother., 23: 54, 1973.
Guttmacher, J., and Fisk, L. Group therapy: What specific advantages? Comp. Psychiatry, 12: 546, 1971.
Imperato-McGinley, J., Guenero, L., Gauther, T., and Peterson, R. Steroid 5-alpha reductase deficiency in man: An inherited form of male pseudohermaphrodism. Science, 186: 1213, 1974.
James, S., Orwin, A. Davies, and D. W. Sex chromosome abnormality in a patient with transsexualism. Br. Med. J., 3: 29, 1972.
Jones, J. R., and Samimig, J. Plasma testosterone levels and female transsexualism. Arch. Sex. Behav., 7: 370, 1973.
Kolodny, R. C., Masters, W. H., and Johnson, V. E. Textbook of Sexual Medicine. Little, Brown, and Co., Boston, 1979.
Levine, S. B. Psychiatric diagnosis of patients requesting sex reassignment surgery. J. Sex Marital Ther., 6: 164, 1980.
Lothstein, L. M. Group therapy with gender dysphoric patients. Am. J. Psychother., 33: 67, 1979a.
Lothstein, L. M. The aging gender dysphoria (transsexual) patient. Arch. Sex. Behav., 8: 431, 1979b.
Lundberg, P. O., Sjovall, A., and Walender, J. Sella turcica in male-to-female transsexuals. Arch. Sex. Behav., 4: 657, 1975.
Meyer, J. K. Clinical variants among applicants for sex reassignment. Arch. Sex. Behav., 3: 527, 1974.
Money, J., and Gaskin, R. Sex reassignment. Int. J. Psychiatry, 9: 249, 1970.
Person, E., and Ovesey, L. The transsexual syndrome in males. I. Primary transsexualism. Am. J. Psychother., 28: 4, 1974a.
Person, E., and Ovesey, L. The transsexual syndrome in males. II. Secondary transsexualism. Am. J. Psychother., 28: 174, 1974b.
Posler, K. Combined individual and group psychotherapy: A review of the literature. Int. J. Group Psychother., 30: 107, 1980.
Sadoughi, W., Overman, C., and Bush, J. Group therapy as an integral part of surgical experience. In Proceedings of the Second Interdisciplinary Symposium on Gender Dysphoria Syndrome, D. R. Laub and P. Gandy, editors, p. 223. Stanford University Medical Center, Stanford, 1973.
Stoller, R. Gender identity. In Comprehensive Textbook of Psychiatry A. M. Freedman, H. I. Kaplan and B. J. Sadock, editors, ed.2, p. 1400. Williams & Wilkins, Baltimore, 1975.
Stoller, R. J. A contribution to the study of gender identity: Follow-up. Int. J. Psychoanal., 60: 433, 1979.
Wise, T. N. Psychotherapy of an aging transvestite. J. Sex Marital Ther., 5: 368, 1979.
Wong, N. Combined group and individual treatment of borderline and narcissistic patients: Heterogeneous versus homogeneous. Int. J. Group Psychother., 30: 389, 1980.

C.2 Child and Adolescent Group Psychotherapy

IRVIN A. KRAFT, M.D.

Introduction

Group psychotherapy of children sets up goals of education and control of the emotions which the children accomplish in various ways. These accomplishments are centered on the acceptance of both feelings and specific types of behavior that are pertinent to the child's developmental progress. The therapist, in his role as leader of the group, furnishes situations that encourage behavior containing messages, the emotional content of which lends itself to interaction and intellectual translation.

Experiential insight arises from the verbalization of feelings and from interactions with other group members, which utilize such defense mechanisms as identification, rationalization, denial, catharsis, and identification with the aggressor in an atmosphere of impunity and safety.

As the child proceeds in treatment, his response can be measured in terms of his verbal and nonverbal behavior, his activity level, and his interrelationship with other group members and the leader. These responses correlate roughly with alterations in his behavior at home and in school. Group learning experiences translate into the less contrived, more natural occurrences in the outside world.

Since the child's mind differs in its synthetic capacities and ability to control both emergency and welfare emotions, methods and techniques commonly used in adult group psychotherapy cannot be applied to children without significant alterations. In a treatment situation the child requires freedom to emote and to speak what crosses his mind—but all within limits set by the leader, consistent with his view of himself and the setting. Generally, the therapist allows motoric expressions by small children (less so with adolescents in a group) knowing he can and must intervene at times.

The group provides a matrix of peer relationships in a context of authority and security different from what the child or adolescent experienced previously. Peer groups provide experiences in interpersonal relations, in new loyalties, in the identity consolidation process, and in leaving one's family for a peer world.

Treatment Theories

Theoretical formulation beleaguers beginning therapists, who often want a settled, directed statement of theory to guide them. The therapist should be exposed to a number of theories from which he evolves both a practical self fit for work and a vocabulary to describe what transpires.

Age of child

Over the decades that group psychotherapy has been used with children and adolescents, most workers followed age and developmental considerations. Generally speaking, several classifications became available.

One such grouping bases itself on psychoanalytic approaches: (1) psychodrama, which is based on techniques for the symbolic expression of conflicts; (2) nondirective therapy, in which structure and the active interference of the therapist are kept to a minimum; (3) psychoanalytic therapy, which relies on psychoanalytic concepts and seeks to impart these concepts to the patients to some degree; and (4) transactional analysis, another educative type of therapy that imparts to the child some understanding of his actions and that encourages him to apply this knowledge. Therapists differ in their reliance on verbalization and conceptualization in therapy, as opposed to the symbolic expression of conflicts, in the degree to which group interaction is spontaneous or structured, in their view of the role of the therapist, and in their understanding of how group therapy actually works.

These approaches, however, fail to describe adequately techniques which have been devised over the years for children. The traits of developmental stages influenced the growth of group psychotherapy techniques more than perhaps any other factor. Because the standard diagnostic nomenclature, prior to DSM-III, failed to describe adequately the disorders in children, investigators grouped children by age and by the characteristics of the presenting difficulties. They also assumed that children's verbalizations would not be extensively used much before puberty or adolescence; thus, play activity dominated their approaches. Exclusive of psychotic children and sexual deviates, the following categories were established and tended to maintain themselves as experience accumulated: (1) preschool and early school age; (2) late latency, ages 9 to 11; (3) pubertal, ages 12 and 13; (4) early adolescence, ages 13 and 14; and (5) middle adolescence through late adolescence, ages 14 to 17.

Setting of treatment

Just as developmental patterns lead to age divisions of group members, so the setting in which therapists operate greatly influences their procedures and work patterns. Group psychotherapy of children, including adolescents, occurs wherever they are treated or confined. The outpatient clinic or child guidance center, except with delinquents, tends to be the arena most described in the literature.

Settings vary widely, yet must be consistent with the practicalities of the therapist's working arrangements. Often, this requires a room whose primary purpose is to service group functions, with durable furnishings and an unencumbered carpeted and undercushioned area of a minimal size of 8 feet by 10 feet. Some therapists use sturdy chairs and perhaps a strong, low, central table, whereas others prefer a rather bare room. They may have tools, models, games, or other artifacts available to the group. As with the basic rule that the therapist does not permit injuries to self or to others in the group and does not allow destruction of furniture, lights, or windows, he also clearly delineates what will be permitted and what will not be allowed in the use of tools, furniture, food, audiovisual instruments, and the like.

Clinics. During the past decade or so, group psychotherapy of children, independently or concomitantly with treatment of the parents, has taken place in most orthodox child guidance centers. These units—and in many cases the current community mental health centers—found their traditional divisions of labor, notwithstanding the crossover propensities of group therapy, so that social workers, as well as psychiatrists and psychologists, began seeing themselves as therapists.

Outpatient Departments. Several therapists have described the diagnostic use of groups in outpatient settings. Field described two activity groups as providing an exploring, role-taking, and testing medium whose main contribution may be the accumulation of behavioral data for the psychiatric social worker who guides the therapeutic effort at home and at school.

In such a setting, an unusual use was made of a mixed adolescent and adult group in an evaluation process. A content analysis revealed that most of their transactions fell into the areas of authority, dependency, and identity conflict. Smolen demonstrated diagnostic as well as therapeutic group work with severely disturbed young children preparatory to their total hospitalization. In these circumstances, several of the children improved, and the clinical diagnosis altered.

An additional approach to pretreatment commitments by both clinic and family involves group sessions for adolescents and parents already recommended for therapy. Gartner points out the seasonal fluctuations in the flow of patients and also in the availability of staff time. For example, intakes fall to a very low point between June and October, owing to the scarcity of school referrals.

An interesting commentary on the roles of group psychotherapy in outpatient clinics derives from the work of Haizlip et al. They sampled 10 randomly selected clinics and discovered that only one offered group psychotherapy for preschool children. Resist-ance by administration and staff members hindered the institution and development of this modality.

Hospitals. In a hospital setting for chronic diseases of children, Ghory, as did Weisfield and Laser, worked with the parents of the children by group methods, primarily groups with both mothers and fathers. The children, presumably, did not receive much psychotherapy. In contrast, Andre and his coworkers dealt with difficulties in the social functioning of the children. They brought children together to be a group in beds, in wheelchairs, and on foot, and they sought verbalization of concerns. One worry the children expressed was a sense of difference from their non-hospitalized peers.

Anderson described his treatment of 4 boys, ages 10 through 13, in a state hospital. They demonstrated brain damage and retardation with severe behavior problems and I.Q. levels ranging from 61 to 75. They showed poor peer relationships, inadequate self-control, faulty judgment, fire-setting habits, disobedience, hyperactivity, and impulsivity. The therapist took a passive role, using the group as a catalytic agent. He used gestures and facial expressions to stimulate or control the group. No props—such as coats, toys, and magazines—were permitted. Short-term group therapy proved valuable for the patients, judging by their hospital behavior and home-visit patterns.

Other reports describe the pattern of group therapy in mental institutions as tailor-made to the problems constantly besetting adolescent patients. Struggle against authority, often enhanced and intensified by the setting, requires the construction of rules for sensible limits to provide the children with another opportunity to work through and to live through their conflicts with the therapist, the representative of the institutional authority. Therapists in these circumstances face the question of control each time the group meets, such as in the regulation of the motor apparatus, the restraint of destructiveness, the restriction of fighting and bodily harm, and the distribution of pleasurable variations, such as parties, outside the group meetings.

Schools. Another place in which the children can undergo group psychotherapy is within their schools, where they often have their first and most sustained extra-familial social contacts. Exploratory usage of group therapy naturally raises the ancient question of how to use schools as sites for early detection of emotional problems and how to manage these problems. Ample opportunity for subject population exists, since most surveys demonstrate a 10 per cent incidence of emotional problems. Any attempt to find and to treat patients involves many basic problems, a major one being selection of patients. Teachers identify as problem children anyone who interrupts educational procedural flow and interferes with classroom management at whatever level the teacher personally finds comfortable. The quietly schizoid or the compulsively achieving child may escape the designation of being troubled.

Some school systems provide a continuous spectrum of care for their emotionally disturbed children.

Services range from the enlightened approach of an individual teacher in a regular classroom through activities of the school counselor or social worker, to referral for day hospital or other forms of intensive care. Group therapeutic work occurs at several points along the continuum.

Day Hospitals. Another setting, which resembles the school, is the day hospital or day care center devoted to a psychoeducational goal. Specifically, psychoeducation represents a combination of psychiatric and educational sources that are used in special settings to remedy learning deficiencies and emotional disturbances. Two working models have evolved. The first, a clinical model, encompasses traditional diagnostic and treatment patterns for deviant personalities. The second is a competence model emphasizing the development of various social, physical, and cognitive skills. This approach helps to modify and prevent developmental problems in children at various age levels.

Patient selection

Sex of child. Many vectors influence the kind of group psychotherapy performed. Certainly, the sex of the children and adolescents becomes a significant variable, partially influencing the considerations for therapist selection. Guidance centers usually have a three-to-one boy-girl ratio, making it hard to form groups with girls. Some attention has been given the question at various age and developmental levels, but the literature emphasizes separate-sex groups.

Psychotherapists of groups made up of one sex usually believe the choice is self-evident, as in an institution or in a successful program of group treatment with older boys (15 to 17 years old) in a family agency. A clear statement of preference for one-sex groups emerges in Teicher's discussion of his hospital-centered outpatient work in which mixed groups tend to be too stimulating, probably as a result of his population's usual history of early sexual experience.

The basis of gender involvement seems at this writing to be rather well settled. Ultimately, external factors, such as the setting, patient availability, and the proclivities of the therapist, decide the issue, perhaps more than theoretical considerations.

Diagnosis of child. Patient composition of a children's group is determined to a significant extent more easily than the theoretical conceptions of the therapist may indicate. The setting, the availability of patients, and the therapeutic bent of the therapist override a particular theoretical position. Some investigators in state hospital settings find that, even with a large number of children available, the group membership follows the critera of accessibility to insight and to group interaction. Psychotic children tend to be treated in like-membership groups, although Coffey and Wiener used non-psychotic children as catalyzers to influence autistic children by promoting communication and interaction. They termed this behavioral contagion.

Homogeneity versus heterogeneity with reference to sex, diagnostic category, age, and other criteria still

besets the therapist, unless he has made up his mind firmly. The composition of the group, however, can be almost any kind, if the therapist is flexible enough in his outlook. Generally speaking, the degree of ego strength is a major factor in patient selection, especially when combined with an estimate of the degree of hyperactivity and the possible disruptions created by impulse-ridden youngsters. Hyperkinesis, which may be thought of as a function of ego strength, since it is often more relative to the situation than to aberrant brain impulses, could exclude some children who are too disruptive to the group. This holds true particularly for late-latency children being treated primarily for school performance problems.

The therapist and the over-all structure of the group constitute the overriding considerations of patient selection, for if the group, especially a latency-age one, already contains several withdrawn and taciturn members, it behooves the leader not to include another similar child at that time. Patient choice, although hopefully not too limited by availability factors, can also be based on intuitive ideas and a spirit of experimentation. Personal contact between a prospective group member and the therapist before entry into the group makes it easier for all. One meeting often proves sufficient to establish the patient-therapist relationship so that the child can enter the group.

Size of group

In group play therapy of preschool children, a group includes four to six children. Activity group therapy uses a larger number of children, not exceeding eight. Latency and preadolescent groups, mixed-sex or not, accommodate up to eight children well. When groups of early, middle, or late adolescents are being formed, however, getting enough group members is sometimes difficult. The adolescents, although 12 to 15 may be immediately available on a waiting list, develop obstacles, such as participation in important school events, jobs, or transportation difficulties. The therapist must screen 20 or 30 adolescents to wind up with a group of 15. Absenteeism resolves the group to about six or eight regular members, a secondary ring of three or four, and three who may be absent more than they appear. The larger size of groups reflects wider ranges of patient types and diagnoses, with a mixture of the taciturn, the loquacious, the dull, and the bright.

Schedule of meetings

Once the therapist forms his group, he confronts the questions of where, how often, and when the group should meet. Usually, the circumstances of time, as a scheduled matter, determine how long the group meets. The range goes from 45 to 90 minutes, rarely longer. Once again, as with so many aspects of group psychotherapy of children, age levels create the variations of time. An hour with a latency-age group just about covers their attention span and tension accumulation. With longer periods, they become restless, interruptive, and too tangential. Adolescents, especially in the middle and late strata, tolerate 90 minutes well and sometimes extend the period spontaneously to 2 hours, either with the therapist present or by other devices, such as gathering in the waiting room 15 to 30 minutes early.

The day of the week assumes importance and relevance. For example a previously withdrawn 16-year-old youth now goes out for basketball. Should the therapist insist that he join the group or consider the ramification of the sport as possibly being of equal therapeutic value? Friday afternoon usually provides many more events competitive to the group than does Monday. The therapist also keeps in mind his own schedule for, if he is active in professional societies, his absences for meetings occur more often during the latter days of the week.

The time of the day for the group to meet confronts the therapist, parents, and school authorities with the basic questions of group values versus school and social ones. Should the latency-age child attend his group during or after school hours? Generally speaking, for all ages it is preferable that the patient not miss school for the group. Leaving early every week on the same day and with the same patients sets him apart and acts negatively as a deterrent to progress. In urban areas with safe, adequate public transportation, adolescents find their way to the group without difficulty, but, if the group terminates too late in the day, traveling home, especially for the girls, may have unfavorable consequences. The time of the year also presents problems. The summer school recess produces conflicts with camp, family trips, and, for adolescents, work hours.

Attendance

Attendance at the group meetings presents certain unique problems. Usually, the therapist believes regular involvement helps the child more than irregularities. This feature carries certain basic implications in outpatient settings of parental cooperation in situations where often the adolescent's symptoms complexly signal pathological family turmoil. When the adolescent starts to become healthier, the family patterns cannot stand the strain, the parents withdraw the youth prematurely or find excessive barriers to transporting him to the group meetings.

Another consideration about attendance confronts the therapist. If the child misses several sessions in sequence, does the therapist drop him? When is absenteeism too much for the group's own integration and when does it go too far for the child's own good? In general, it seems that absences reflect resistance at some level, usually in more than the child alone, and a family conference confronts the parents and the child with this resistance for resolution. Otherwise, rigid rules for attendance simply challenge the family, especially the adolescent, to violations and angry encounters.

Selection of therapist

The question of therapist selection is a large and pressing one. The traditionally passive role of the therapist has come under attack, especially from the pressure of the new techniques which have developed during the past decade.

Stein describes an extensive set of training experiences with psychologists and social workers in a social agency, with beginnng psychiatric residents, and with a third group made up of graduate psychiatrists in the psychiatric outpatient department of a general hospital—all in New York City. He found each group of trainees undergoing discernible degrees of anxiety. In each of the three groups, anxiety emerged from different causes—inexperience with any psychotherapy for the first group, and the conflicts of the third group in shifting from years of practicing intensive, individual psychotherapy to doing group therapy. He summarizes his experiences:

> The group psychotherapist needs to know something of mental and emotional illness and its treatment, especially the type of treatment that utilizes a group and a group method to facilitate communication in the groups, both verbal and nonverbal, through the establishment of relationships and interaction to the therapist and between the patients.

Additional facets of therapist selection were scrutinized by Spruiell, who describes the countertransference in a situation of crisis for an adolescent group wherein the therapist's adolescent yearnings supplemented the group's transference, leading to a riot.

Generally, the literature on outpatient group psychotherapy of adolescents and younger children focuses on sex and number of therapists, as do Solomon and Axelrod, who strongly suggest that the leader be of the same sex as members of one-sex groups. Speaking from the psychoanalytic model of the basically triangular configurations of mother, father, and child, Boenheim believes that the use of male and female therapists works well by simulating a father figure and a mother figure. Some theorists might argue that one treats the group, and the group processes induce pairing as a main dynamic of the patient in the group with the leader, thus probably negating the need for a male-female leader duality. Whether this notion— based on group psychotherapy with adults— applies to children's work remains untested experimentally.

Adler et al. and Westman et al. consider dual, mixed-sex leadership valuable. Other authors indicate the value of a woman therapist for an all-girl group, especially for the adoelscent ages, as a person with whom they can identify. In 1964 and 1965, Godenne discussed this point, coming to the conclusion that the identity of leadership proves valuable, but that the male leader should assume the dominant role.

Clinical Aspects

Jobless adolescents

Jobless, aimless adolescents need more than vocational testing or aptitude delineation. Group psychotherapy has been effective in helping these youths find ego-syntonic pathways. MacLennan and Kline extensively used groups in their work of focusing on and learning occupational roles and associated behavioral patterns, and they found groups to be the technique that was the most useful, productive, and congruent with the demands of the system. Similarly, Gavales combined individual and group counseling and vocational training for an aggregation of 85 adolescents, the majority of whom were high school dropouts. Using the Manson Evaluation Test and counselor ratings, he found 72 per cent improved after 6 months.

Unwed mothers

Adolescents in another sociomedical difficulty showed significant responses to group therapy. Kaufmann and Deutsch worked with pregnant, unwed adolescents, ages 12 to 16, in a milieu approach using group psychotherapy as an integral part. The staff of the clinic and the parents of the patients were involved in a combination of group psychotherapy and counseling, orientation, and education. The therapist, a woman who was flexible, refrained from imposing her middle-class standards, and she fed the girls symbolically and emotionally.

Twenty unwed adolescent primiparas were assigned randomly to an experimental group of eight and to a control group of 12. A 12-month follow-up, after termination of the 18-month treatment period, showed that none of the eight girls in the treatment group repeated the pregnancy; in the control group, nine of the 12 girls had become pregnant for the second time.

Delinquents

Almost uniformly excluded from routine outpatient treatment groups, delinquents are treated in homogeneous groups. There is little mention in the literature of group psychotherapy with delinquent, latency-age boys and girls; the focus rests on the adolescents. Sex considerations in patient selection become finalized at once, for no one discusses mixing the sexes in groups of delinquents.

Work with delinquents concerns their sociopathic behavioral patterns and related themes, such as reading disabilities and deprivations. Most therapists work with adolescents in institutional settings, rather than in clinics. The therapists encounter conflicts of institutional rules with their traditional impartiality, passivity, and authority roles. Perl described the delinquent's view of reality, pointing out that authority is the one theme really grappled with in the institution.

Grouping by Ages

Preschool and early school-age groups

Work with the preschool group is usually structured by the therapist through the use of a particular technique, such as puppets or artwork, or it is couched in terms of a permissive play atmosphere. In therapy with puppets, the children project onto the puppets their fantasies in a way not unlike ordinary play. The main value lies in the catharsis afforded the child, especially if he shows difficulty in expressing his feelings. Here the group aids the child less by interaction with other members than by action with the puppets.

Nielsen worked with preschool children, infancy to age 3, in a family living project in which the mothers sat with a therapist in a group or as a group, able to observe their children interacting with one another and with child care personnel. The leisurely, informal sessions focused on play and its importance in a child's development. This indirect form of group therapy of children, modified to fit varying conditions, may help in the preventive mental health aspects for children in the extensive day care programs for working mothers.

Similarly, Hoffman et al. sought to determine if elements of already acceptable forms of group treatment could be combined to increase their effectiveness while minimizing their separate disadvantages. They put the boys and mothers in the same room at the same time with a line of chairs and a rope between them. The obvious opening in this barricade channeled the physical moves of the children to go to their mothers' side of the room. They encountered many intriguing byplays of the two groups. In the main, after experimenting with different formats, they concluded the two groups did maintain individual integrity, and each developed along a path of a definite initial phase, a middle or work phase, and a concluding one.

In play group therapy, the emphasis rests on the interactional qualities of the children with each other and with the therapist in the permissive playroom setting. Slavson stated that the therapist should be a woman who can allow the children to produce fantasies verbally and in play but who also can use active restraint when the children undergo excessive tension. The toys are the traditional ones used in individual play therapy, such as water, plasticine, a doll's house, and toy guns. The children use the toys to act out aggressive impulses and to relive with the group members and with the therapist their home difficulties. The children catalyze each other and obtain libido-activating stimulation from this catalysis and from their play materials. The therapist interprets a child to the group in the context of the transference to her and to other group members.

Ginott aimed in group play therapy to effect basic changes in the child's intrapsychic equilibrium through relationship, catharsis, insight, reality testing, and sublimation. The mechanism of identification affords the child major opportunities for therapeutic gain as he identifies himself with the other group members and with the therapist. Because the individual child constitutes the focus of the treatment, little attention is given to the group as an entity in itself. As in the ordinary play relationships of children, attachments to peers and toys and the formations of subgroups shift for each child.

The children selected for group treatment show in common a social hunger, the need to be like their peers and to be accepted by them. Usually, the therapist excludes the child who has never realized a primary relationship, as with his mother, inasmuch as individual psychotherapy can better help this child. Ginott also rejected children with murderous attitudes toward siblings, sociopathic children, those with perverse sexual experiences, habitual thieves, and extremely aggressive children. Usually the children selected include those with phobic reactions, effeminate boys, shy and withdrawn children, and children with primary behavior disorders.

A modification of group therapy was used for physically

handicapped toddlers who showed speech and language delays. This experience of twice-a-week group activities involved the mothers and their children in a mutual teaching-learning setting. The experience proved effective to the mothers, who received supportive psychotherapy in this group experience; their formerly hidden fantasies about the children emerged to be dealt with therapeutically.

Latency-age groups

Essentially, most forms of group psychotherapy for latency-age and pubertal children follow some modification of the two basic designs formulated by Slavson and developed significantly by Schiffer and others. Activity group therapy assumes that poor and divergent experiences have led to deficits in appropriate personality development in the behavior of children; therefore, corrective experiences in a therapeutically conditioned environment will modify them. Because some latency-age children present deep disturbances, involving neurotic traits (fears, high anxiety levels, and guilt), an activity-interview group psychotherapy modification evolved. This format uses interview techniques, verbal explanations of fantasies, group play, work, and other communications.

In this type of group therapy, as with pubertal and adolescent groups, the children verbalize in a problem-oriented manner, with the awareness that problems brought them together and that the group aims to change them. They report dreams, fantasies, and daydreams, as well as traumatic and unpleasant experiences. Both these experiences and their group behavior undergo open discussion. Therapists vary in their use of time, of co-therapists, and of food and materials. Most groups are after school and last at least 1 hour, although some leaders prefer 90 minutes. Some therapists serve food in the last 10 minutes, and others prefer serving times when the children are more together for talking. Food, however, does not become a major feature, central to the group's activities.

Once involved in doing group psychotherapy of this age group, a majority of the therapists believe in it, as if it were a natural environment for the child to retrieve himself from his developmental detour. One study demonstrated the mechanisms of projection in such groups. Dupont and de Wasongarz (1979) spent 2 years with a group of children of both sexes and of various ages. They established initially a rule of no rules, no pre-established limits, and no restrictive procedures; the children responded with regression, enabling the therapists to draw closer to the patients. They called this a natural group, because the structure simulated a basic family. By not having any toys, the children fastened onto real objects in the transference. The children slowly arrived at the same basic rules for themselves as other therapists tend to use at the outset of a group's existence.

Composition of the group. In some clinic and private practice situations in which an activity therapy setting may not be feasible, the emphasis in the group treatment of latency-age children can be shifted to an interview type, with little toy play and no use made of tools or arts and crafts. Late latency-age children (ages 9 to 11), who usually constitute the majority of referrals to a child psychiatric clinic, use this procedure well. The children can be of both sexes, and their selection depends more on the over-all structure

of the group than on the individual patient's characteristics. The optimum size of the group is six children. The leader, of either sex, uses psychodynamic generalizations in verbalizing with and for the children as they relate daily experiences and comments about their parents and discuss their interactions with other group members. Here, as in other forms of group psychotherapy of children, the professional discipline of the therapist may be any of the traditional ones in the mental health field. A co-therapist of the same or the opposite sex can be useful in these groups.

The patients not usually taken into these groups include the incorrigible or psychopathic child, the homicidal child, and the overt sexually deviant child. The severely threatened, ritualistic, socially peculiar children who cannot establish effective communication at any useful level with the group members fail to do well in these groups. Developmental phases serve as signposts in this exclusion process.

Intellectual ability should be well distributed, for too many retardates in the group impede interaction and tend to enhance motoric patterns of all the group members. Children with physical deformities, tics, protruding teeth, or behavior based on maturational brain dysfunction find the group situation helpful. Vehement interactions or taunts about their disabilities produce in time a group response of support as the members perceive the victim's sensitivities and feelings.

Because the sex ratio inherent in child psychiatric work with latency-age children runs three to one of boys to girls, finding enough girls becomes a problem for these groups. If possible, equal numbers of each sex should be sought. The girls act as a modulating influence and diminish extremes of behavior.

Freedom of expression and activity instigates responses among the members so that a number of roles emerge. There are the instigators, who enable the group to stay alive dynamically; the neutralizers, who, by greater superegos, keep impulsive acts down and help regulate behavior; the social neuters, who seem impotent to accelerate or impede the flow of group activity; and the isolates, who are so neurotically constricted that they initially find the group too frightening to join in its activities.

Psychodynamics. During exposures to the group, the child demonstrates his customary and usual adaptational patterns. If, for example, he has used his helplessness to elicit dependency fostering and psychological feeding responses from adults and peers, he finds the group and the therapist failing him. The neutrality and the passivity of the therapist impede these patterns and create enough frustration to initiate different behavior in time. Similarly, the provocative, extremely aggressive child finds no rejection or punishment for his behavioral distortions. In time, he begins to react differently toward the therapist and his fellow group members.

The therapist needs to be consistently aware of himself and the individuality of each patient. He sees himself as a catalyst for each child in special situations at appropriately timed moments. All these demands confront the therapist with an intense need for appropriate use of himself and non-exploitation of the children. He makes use of himself in detecting and working with resistances in the group, as seen in silences, stereotyped or repetitive talk or play, and absences. Such behavior can assail the therapist's self-esteem, trigger his anger, and seduce him to respond as other adults have responded to these well-practiced techniques, when he should be using joining techniques with humor, interpretations, and reflections.

This therapeutic medium helps children with deficient and distorted self-images, inadequate role identifications, habit and conduct problems, and mild neuroses. Neurotic traits that may be present in behavior disorders diminish in this type of group. Characterological disorders—as shown by the passive, dependent, infantilized child—tend to alter as these personality traits persistently fail to achieve satisfaction and as other behaviors become possible.

Milieu therapy is a related technique in that it involves structured activities and projects, but it sees itself as constituting a therapeutic home or milieu, and the primary emphasis is on the associative element, rather than on the activities involved. The central technique is the formation of a club, which is formed by the children themselves. The members name the club themselves, determine its goals, and elect its leadership. The very fact that the club is chosen, not imposed, generates enthusiasm and enables members to participate actively in the therapeutic process itself—as agents, rather than as patients. The club forms a therapeutic milieu that allows members to face competitors and to dramatize conflicts that, without the support of an integrated group, might have destroyed them. Parental participation is sometimes encouraged. Therapeutic clubs have been successful with disadvantaged children of minority groups, psychotic children, and severely disturbed pubertal boys, resulting in reported strengthening of impulse control, reality testing, and self-esteem and in the improvement of object relations.

Functions. The latency-age grouping centers on the child's attuning himself to peers, teachers, leaders, community groups, ideals, and sublimated interests. Conscience formation, deriving from the resolution of oedipal strivings, involves both behavioral and cognitive vectors. Grinder found that maturity of moral judgment increased significantly for both sexes with age; however, behavioral and cognitive dimensions develop independently, almost as if there are several consciences and not a singular unitary one.

Most therapists agree that the function of group psychotherapy in this age band is to aid the organization of drives into socially acceptable behavior modes. The child gains in coping patterns and in understanding certain levels of psychological material more difficult to deal with. He gains experiential insight as he seeks his place in the group by modifying his behavior. Thus, beyond certain fundamental rules established by the therapist, children set their own group behavioral standards openly and explicitly, as well as the usual covert ones any group constructs automatically.

Rules. The therapist usually states that none of the children's verbalizations will undergo censure and that he will not permit behavior destructive to persons or the building. Beginning about 1968, therapists added the injunction of not allowing drug use (marijuana, alcohol, acid, and so on) in the sessions. The therapist also reserves the responsibility and attendant right to notify parents if a serious matter significantly affecting health emerges. Also, he notifies the children of telephone and other contacts that their parents make with him about them. In the process of trying to get their parents to understand them better and change the situation, the therapist feels free to tell parents of the general concerns of the patient without quoting his words. Although some children test the therapist on these regulations, no one seriously bothers to defy them.

Pubertal groups

Similar group therapy methods can be used with pubertal children, who are often grouped monosexually, rather than mixed. Their problems resemble those of late latency-age children, but they are also beginning, especially the girls, to feel the impact and pressures of early adolescence. In a way, these groups offer help during a transitional period. The group appears to satisfy the social appetite of preadolescents, who compensate for feelings of inferiority and self-doubt by the formation of groups. This form of therapy puts to advantage the influence of the process of socialization during these years. Because children of this age experience difficulties in conceptualizing, pubertal therapy groups tend to use play, drawing, psychodrama, and other nonverbal modes of expression. The therapist's role is active and directive, as opposed to the older, more passive role assigned him.

Activity group psychotherapy has been the recommended type of group therapy for latency-age and pubertal children who do not have significantly neurotic personality patterns. The children, usually of the same sex and in groups of not more than eight, freely act out in a setting especially designed and planned for its physical and milieu characteristics. Slavson pictured the group as a substitute family in which the passive, neutral therapist becomes the surrogate for parents. The therapist assumes different roles, mostly in a nonverbal manner, as each child interacts with him and with other group members. Recent therapists, however, tend to see the group as a form of peer group, with its attendant socializing processes, rather than as a re-enactment of the family.

Activity therapy involves games, structured activities, and projects that must be planned and carried out. For children with neurotic-type difficulties, equipment is minimal in order to reduce the potential for frustration and failure, the goal being the maximal elicitation of fantasies and the expression of feelings about others. Anxiety, however, is allowed to develop, and the therapist works to help the group members cope with it. In the ego-impaired group, the sessions are highly structured, and anxiety is reduced to a minimum, although the structure is progressively loosened as their frustration tolerance rises. In the neurotic-type groups, limit setting is maintained only to protect personal safety and to prevent property damage, whereas in the ego-impairment group all destructive behavior is actively discouraged.

Egan suggested a modification in the form of activity

discussion group therapy. Certain dynamisms occur in the groups: (1) identification with the therapist, with group members, and with the group as a family; (2) reinforcement and other behavioral techniques that modify behavioral patterns; (3) development of direct (verbal) or indirect or derivative insight. The physical characteristics of the room, as with routine activity group therapy, discourage practitioners in cramped quarters.

In general, latency activity groups, when the physical situation permits, provide an emotionally corrective experience by using a highly permissive setting to encourage freedom of expression of pent-up feelings, along with regression. Interview activity and other variants along the spectrum of therapeutic techniques also provide effective experiential insight opportunities. The consistency, warmth, flexibility, and empathic qualities of the therapist, coupled with adequate knowledge of personality theory and therapeutic techniques, provide the ingredients for good group therapy in this and other age bands.

Adolescent groups

Boys and girls tend to be divergent in social awareness and responsivity in early and middle adolescence. However, the mainstreams of emotional striving run throughout these two periods, being met and handled somewhat differently as the youth acquires more social tools within his peer group and with adults. Adolescent deviancy sounds its own commonalities, as if, of ordainment, they must occur and be gone through. Each observer attaches significance to an element that compels his attention. Goldberg, for example, suggests that, in the search for identity, some adolescents lack the ability to love adequately, thereby feeling they are missing out on something. Such an adolescent uses other people primarily as specific psychological structures out of his own narcissism, rather than loving them for their own qualities.

Techniques of group therapy with adolescents vary rather widely, usually correlating well with the therapist's background and present outlook. Ackerman readily placed both genders, ranging in age from 15 to 23, in the same group. Each patient had previously undergone individual psychotherapy, and his group therapy experience supplemented it. Ackerman suggested that the group functioned to "provide a social testing ground for the perceptions of self and of relations to others." He emphasized the importance of nonverbal behavioral patterns as material for the group.

Subsequent reports tended to agree that group therapy dealt more with conscious and preconscious levels than did an intensive, deeply introspective approach. Hulse listed clarification, mutual support, facilitation of catharsis, reality testing, superego relaxation, and group integration as ego-supportive techniques.

Composition of the group. Adolescent patients can be treated in an outpatient clinic, a private office, a hospital, or a special setting, such as a detention home, with modifications appropriate to the setting. The setting itself strongly influences the total group process. The group format is that of an open-ended, interview-interaction, activity organization. The preferred number of adolescents for these groups is 8 to 10, but often circumstances require the screening of 30 or more to produce a group of 15. Of these, about six form a core group with constant attendance and effort, another three or four constitute an intermediate group who attend more than they miss, and the remainder make up a peripheral group who attend occasionally. Attendance and therapeutic output are difficult to predict for the individual patient, because they do not seem to be related to age, to presenting problem, or to diagnosis. Some therapists suggest separation of patients in early adolescence (ages 13 and 14) from older patients, because boys of 13 and 14 find 17-year-old girls difficult to deal with in these groups. Otherwise, therapy procedures remain the same.

In working with two groups of adolescent girls, Schechter also discovered a significant difference in topics, ways of discussion, and the ability to examine problems in an analytic way between 13- and 14-year-olds and the 15- to 17-year-old girls.

Attendance, especially beyond 10 sessions, correlates roughly with graduation from the group and with the achievement of treatment goals. The pre-10 session dropouts tend to have character and behavior disorders. The post-10 dropouts are more often borderline or psychotic teenagers.

The diagnostic categories fail to distinguish sufficiently among patients to serve as guideposts to patient selection. Certain behavioral patterns—such as overt homosexuality, a flagrant sociopathic history, drug addiction, and psychosis—contraindicate inclusion in these groups. Group methods for these patients can be used, particularly with homosexuality and drug addiction, but they require special considerations. Depressed adolescents need to be evaluated extremely carefully, for this presenting picture may be a facade for extensive substance abuse and for a brooding, preoccupied schizophrenic configuration.

With the recent emphasis on borderline and narcissistic personalities, more attention has been attracted to this feature of the adolescent, both normal and disturbed. The therapeutic dust still hovers over the scene, and more time and much work will have to ensue before the picture appears clear. A basic consideration rests on diagnosis, and this still contains elusive elements. Adolescent suicide attempts and borderline personality disorders play a major role in this ever-increasing problem.

Scott addressed the issue of the narcissistic personality disorder in adolescent group therapy from the viewpoint that narcissistic behavior developmentally increases in this period. Kohut suggests that aberrant and delinquent behavior may be based on achievements of the ego more than a deficit in superego. When such a patient, especially in these days of widespread substance abuse, can learn to identify with and to share the parental figures of the leader with the others of the group, then his narcissistic features blend with his total structure and diminish his drug usage and acting out.

Aims and techniques. Interview mixed-group psychotherapy offers an opportunity for the adolescent to relearn peer-relating techniques in a protective and supportive situation. Diminution of anxiety about sexual feelings and consolidation of sexual identification occur. The adolescent participates in group interaction in time and feels the pull of group cohesiveness. He also goes through relationship, catharsis, insight, reality testing, and sublimation as he reacts to the group's pace and to its changes, as when the group shifts its content level, a phenomenon that occurs frequently, often within a single session. The mechanism of identification affords the adolescent major opportunities for therapeutic gain as he identifies himself with other group members and the therapist. The individual adolescent constitutes the focus of treatment, but he and the therapist are continually involved with the group as a sounding board and testing ground.

The adolescents use diversionary tactics to avoid discussing threatening subjects. A favorite maneuver is to change the focus by a question or a comment about an unrelated topic. Sometimes diversion masks itself behind physical activity, such as throwing a gum wrapper at the wastebasket or showing a picture in a textbook to others. These and other behaviors frequently receive comments by group members; if not, the therapist calls attention to them.

Schulman and Kraft each commented that the therapist must be active, ego supportive, and in control of the group situation at all times. He interprets with caution in order to avoid the patient's misconstruing interpretation as personal criticism. Interpretations also focus on reality, rather than on symbolisms. They are couched in simple direct references to basic feelings and to unconscious intent of behavior when it lies quite close to awareness. Transactional analysis has the advantage of a simple, easily understood terminology of interpretations that allows the individual patient or the group to analyze behavior as well as the therapist. This analysis is encouraged in the transactional analysis type of therapy. These cognitive conceptualizations and techniques go along with an appropriate use of an active, directive, and guiding role for the severely depressed patients.

The content of the discussions varies enormously, ranging over school examinations, sibling competition, parental attitudes, difficulties with self-concepts, and sexual concerns. Sexual acting out and impulse eruption rarely occur. Brief group responses to significant experiences narrated by a patient fulfill his needs, for he can return to the subject later if necessary. The group often prefers short discussions, because the anxiety is too high to dwell at length on a topic.

One valuable type of therapy is the encounter group, which uses psychodrama, role playing, and other active forms of interaction. The raw material offers opportunities from which insight develops. The group becomes the vehicle for heightened emotional interaction between therapist and patient and between patient and patient. The group is expected to experience and share the feelings of a member, rather than merely attending to them, in order to increase group interaction. A key concept is free role experimenta-tion, which facilitates the resolution of the adolescent ego identity crisis by allowing the adolescent to experiment with a wide variety of feelings, thoughts, and behaviors in a group setting. Group cohesion is fostered, however, by common emotional experiences in which all share, by field trips undertaken together, and by other group activities. One of the most useful of these activities is the camping trip, which is popular with adolescents and serves to bond them together. Popular music can be used as a catalyst in the initial stage of the group.

Minithons (small marathons) have been tried with a mixed group of adolescents. The minithon consists of a meeting at the regular or at another place for 4 to 6 consecutive hours. After about 2 hours of the usual group session, a break for food and a stretch interrupts for about 30 to 45 minutes. The group then resumes for several hours more. Essentially, the longer time allows for greater exploration of a number of topics without malaise and fatigue overcoming all. Greater depth and more intensity to themes seem to develop.

Transactional analysis, increasingly being used among adolescent therapy groups, emphasizes treatment with specific goals defined in terms of observable changes in behavior and in attitudes. The concepts of transactional analysis provide a common vocabulary and a frame of reference readily intelligible to adolescents and preadolescents for group discussions and analysis. Group members learn to detect games in their own behavior and in that of others, to analyze transactions, and to put into practice various techniques that enable them to solve crossed transactions and to acquire strokes. Behavior is changed primarily by increasing the group members' understanding of themselves and of each other. Transactional analysis uses role play, gestalts, psychodrama, and other group therapy techniques that involve verbalization and analysis. It also uses verbal contracting, in which the patient defines specific goals he plans to work toward and the length of time in which he expects to achieve them.

The theory of modeling has shown that adolescents respond to new stimulus situations in a manner consistent with the model's dispositions, even if the adolescents had never observed the models responding to these particular stimuli. Modeling influences thus produce not only specific mimicry, but also generative and innovative behavior. Group therapists working with disadvantaged children have been successful when they introduce star students into the group and encourage the members to model some aspects of their behavior on that of the stars. Peers have also been used as agents who dispense social reinforcers, resulting in significant changes in the behavior of group members, especially when reinforced by friends, rather than by non-preferred peers. Modeling and peer reinforcement are part of a trend to recognize the group itself as an active therapeutic factor, in addition to being something acted on by the therapist, a trend also visible in transactional analysis and encounter therapy.

Other Groupings

Retardates

The intellectual level of a child often signifies his functioning in a therapy group, depending on the age and I.Q. level of the other children in the group.

Generally, therapists believe that children with average or above-average intelligence function adequately in a group. Major problems occur with children who have I.Q. levels below 85 and, oddly enough, often with children who are extremely brilliant. Difficulties arise for the less intelligent children when they do not understand what is going on and are the butt of jokes injected by the brighter group members. It proves unrealistic in most cases to expect a group of bright neurotic children to accommodate the slow pace and often grossly immature development of a retardate, despite the frequency of emotional immaturity in disturbed children.

Most investigators prefer to place retardates in groups that are homogeneous without reference to intellectual ability. Some therapists, assuming a type of intellectual insight as the *sine qua non* of successful group therapy, disparage retardates as group members. Sternlicht opposes this notion in his strong support of group therapy for retardates. The group process tends to be ego supportive, often focusing on social reinforcement as a major goal. Cowen stresses group play techniques in working with the exceptional child. Even children with limited imagination find outlets and strength in the group.

Underachievers

Underachievement occurs in any age bracket. Some parents look for it in preschool nurseries. In its broadest definition, the term applies to any failure to achieve expected biopsychological, age-adequate performance. Thus, most disturbed children show development as a major criterion for improvement.

Gurman examined the literature on the effectiveness of group counseling and the multiplicity of methodological problems and found a lack of work using behavioral modification techniques. He noted that leader-structured groups seem to be the most effective group method and, consequently, insight, "as it is defined by psychoanalytically oriented counselors and therapists, is not essential to the successful treatment of underachievers."

Drug users

Linked to underachievement in ever-increasing frequency among mid- and preadolescents is the use of mind-altering drugs—marijuana, methadone, LSD and mescaline—and other drugs. The majority of the adolescents seen in private practice consultation use these drugs to varying degrees. And, as the availability increases, younger children, such as those in late latency, begin to speak of marijuana as a precursor to new adventures.

Little in the literature on group psychotherapy deals with adolescents and hard drugs; no article discusses preadolescents and younger children. Eliasoph worked with drug addicts, some of whom apparently were adolescents, and said that psychodrama techniques proved helpful "in eliciting feelings about treatment and in bringing the patients into fuller participation in the therapy sessions." He found these patients ineffectual in coping with interpersonal relationships. For example, a patient in role playing would enact his inability to say "No" to a user of drugs for fear that the other person would be antagonized and no longer friendly to him.

Galbis, who became interested in the hippie population of Georgetown in the District of Columbia, founded the Washington Free Clinic, which rapidly grew into a busy psychiatric service utilizing crisis intervention and individual and group therapies. Narcotics usage among his adolescent patients increased, but LSD intake seemed to decline. These alienated youths, living in a drug-controlled world, worked in his groups, but some of his patients required methadone treatment after intensive individual and group psychotherapy failed.

Peer orientation dominates throughout the therapeutic communities which have grown greatly as having a special, useful therapeutic function in the treatment of addicts. Rachman and Heller (1976) believe the key foundation for this rests in identity formation, and they define several significant concepts involved: peers are the helping agents in the healing relationship; peer modeling is fostered; group identity emerges from this therapeutic subculture; a sense of community and family life is provided; and absence of purpose and direction becomes evident and enhanced. The goal is to have the addict replace a negative, peer group-based identity with a positive one.

Children with physical problems

In 1948 Cruikshank and Cowen described their group work with physically handicapped children. Several years later, Dubo reported a study of 25 hospitalized tuberculous children treated in both individual interviews and groups. They preoccupied themselves with thoughts of death and other morbid content, as they were menaced by an introjected malignancy and needed to flee. Their motoric patterns reflected these fantasies, despite the medical injunctions against activity that would aggravate their illness. In the group work, identification was established easily, as children who found the verbal expression of anxiety quite difficult in individual sessions emphathized with fellow patients. They could then verbalize their feelings. Dubo commented that the group discussions proved far more effective than the traditional explanatory movies commonly shown to tuberculosis patients.

Foster children

These children number more than 300,000 in a given year. The difficulties they encounter in their frequent shifts from one foster setting to another are notorious, and almost any treatment procedure that diminishes the trauma and alienates the distress is valuable. Watson and Boverman used group discussions to explore and to resolve the foster child's particular problems. They chose children in the late-latency age range, ages 8 to 12, who were of the same sex and without symptoms of emotional illness. The children, strangers to one another at the start, met once a week for 90 minutes for five to seven sessions. Self-worth, dependency, and identity themes continually recurred in the substrates of such questions as: "What will I grow up to be?" "Why aren't my parents raising me?" "Who will care for me tomorrow?"

Psychotic children

Psychiatry has been challenged for decades by both the diagnosis and the treatment of psychotic children. With etiologies unknown in either the area of psychogenicity or organicity, relationships have been adduced that, according to psychoanalytic or other theories, produce the deep psychopathology observed in these children. Individual psychotherapy to instill correct object relations, sensory deprivation to reduce input to a minimum, LSD treatment, behavioral modification, and group psychotherapy—these and other procedures have been used in attempts to heal these aggrieved children.

During the past 10 years, psychotherapy has been used in a few units. Since psychosis in children does not occur so frequently that a private practitioner could have enough patients to treat, most group therapy studies have been in treatment centers at universities or in agencies. Speers and Lansing placed four psychotic children in a group treatment plan; later they added another preschool psychotic and traveled a treatment path for more than 4 years and 828 hours. Their consultant, E. James Anthony, originally predicted that therapeutic developments would be slow and sparse in providing satisfaction to the therapists, and that the patients would not be kept in the place for long by their parents. Both surmises were wrong, and Anthony concluded:

I was left with the feeling that a major contributing factor lay in the metamorphosis that led gradually and most inevitably to the emergence of a communicative, conscious, cooperative self and of something impersonal and anonymous.

Anthony further noted that the group techniques were deeply involved in the children's improvement. The investigator's theoretical position was based on the development of group ego, which then sustained the defective egos of the individuals in the group. This theory seemed especially applicable to symbiotic psychotic children, offering them a therapeutic symbiosis. Results included enhanced or achieved communicative speech, some degree of self-identity, and movement upward in the developmental scale.

The Family

Implicit in this discussion is the group's relationship to the child's family of origin, for that biosocial structure remains a powerful influence on his performance and production within a group. Peer orientation overcomes the immediate, directly discernible family background, especially in the older age groupings, and it dominates the interactions when the group member must confront his fellow family members in full view. Few studies describe the results of this therapy in children, although the multiple-impact therapists report favorable results in 75 per cent after 18 months.

In family therapy, more than two people are involved, and the interaction to that extent is not confidential, in contrast to the usual patient-therapist dyad. Nonverbal interaction assumes a primary importance along with the verbal. And family therapy is often briefer than individual therapy, although length of treatment is enormously variable. The aims are changes in the family system of interaction, not changes in the behavior of individuals.

The family should function better as a family; this is the goal of family therapy. Family therapy that involves the children in group interaction—whether it be regularly, such as weekly, or intermittently—should be considered as a form of group psychotherapy for children.

Kraft has found multiple-impact therapy an excellent therapeutic device for opening a family. He has used the original format described by MacGregor and also a number of modifications, depending on the circumstances. Using a full-scale multiple-impact therapy proved valuable for teaching family dynamics and children-parent interactions to first-year psychiatry residents and to other professionals.

The multiple-impact therapy format has proved quite alterable and still productive. The team interactions among themselves receive less emphasis, especially since the number of student observers has increased via closed-circuit television and one-way mirrors. The basic intent of opening the family to itself and to the staff is accomplished in varying degrees in each of the variations employed.

Conclusion

The results of group therapy with children are difficult to evaluate. Several reports using control groups show favorable results in non-directive play therapy and in specific intervention group therapy with underachievers and delinquents. Milieu therapy has resulted in striking improvements in ghetto children and even in child psychotics. Evaluating the results of group psychotherapy of children is as difficult as assessing individual psychotherapy of children. Few studies have been controlled for time, as well as for other factors, particularly follow-up evaluations (a point that critics emphasize), but one can say that group therapy does not supplant or replace individual psychotherapy. Group therapy is, rather, another tool that the therapist can become familiar with by using it under supervision.

Impressionistically, certain results can be indicated. Group psychotherapy helps children feel unconditionally accepted by the therapist and by the group members; failures become seen as part of each child's development; complexes of feeling and ideation gain expression; feelings of guilt, anxiety, inferiority, and insecurity find relief; and affection and aggression are evidenced without retaliation and danger.

References

Abramowitz, C. W. The effectiveness of group psychotherapy with children. Arch. Gen. Psychiatry, *33:* 320, 1976.

Burgess, A. W., Groth, A. N., and McCausland, M. P. Child sex initiation rings. Am. J. Orthopsychiatry, *51:* 110, 1981.

Chiles, J. A., Miller, M., and Cox, G. B. Depression in an adolescent delinquent population. Arch. Gen. Psychiatry, *37:* 1179, 1980.

Corder, B. F., Haizlip, T. M., and Walker, P. A. Critical areas of therapist's functioning in adolescent group psychotherapy: A comparison with self-perception of functioning in adult groups by experienced therapists. Adolescence, *15:* 127, 1980.

Dube, B. D., Mitchell, C. A., and Bergman, L. A. Use of the self-run group in a child-guidance setting. Int. J. Group Psychother., *30:* 461, 1980.

Dupont, M. A., and de Wasongarz, A. J. The natural children's group: A psychoanalytic experience. In *Group Therapy 1979: An Overview,* L. R. Wolberg and M. L. Aronson, editors, p. 159. Stratton Intercontinental, New York, 1979.

Fluet, N. R., Holmes, G. R., and Gordon, L. C. Adolescent group psychotherapy: A modified fishbowl format. Adolescence, *15:* 75, 1980.

Grunebaum, H., and Solomon, L. Toward peer theory of group psychotherapy. I. On the developmental significance of peers and play. Int. J. Group Psychother., *30:* 23, 1980.

Harris, F. C. The behavioral approach to group therapy. Int. J. Group Psychother., *29:* 453, 1979.

Higgins, J. P., and Thies, A.P. Problem solving and social position among emotionally disturbed boys. Am. J. Orthopsychiatry, *51:* 356, 1981.

Hurst, A., and Gladieux, J. Guidelines for heading an adolescent therapy group. In *Group and Family Therapy.* L. R. Wolberg and M. L. Aronson, editors, p. 151. Brunner/Mazel, New York, 1980.

Julian, A., III, and Kilmann, P. R. Group treatment of juvenile delinquents: A review of the outcome literature. Int. J. Group Psychother., *29:* 3, 1979.

Knittle, B. J., and Tuana, S. J. Group therapy as primary treatment for adolescent victims of intrafamilial sexual abuse. Clin. Soc. Work J., *8:* 236, 1980.

Lewis, D. O., and Shanok, S. S. The use of a correctional setting for follow-up care of psychiatrically disturbed adolescents. Am. J. Psychiatry, *137:* 953, 1980.

Malone, C. A. Child psychiatry and family therapy: An overview. J. Am. Acad. Child Psychiatry, *18:* 4, 1979.

Minuchin, S., and Fishman, H. C. The psychosomatic family in child psychiatry. J. Am. Acad. Child Psychiatry, *18:* 76, 1979.

Rachman, A. W., and Heller, M. E. Peer group psychotherapy with adolescent drug abusers. Int. J. Group Psychother., *26:* 373, 1976.

Rosenberg, J., and Cherbutiez, T. Inpatient group therapy for older children and pre-adolescents. Int. J. Group Psychother., *29:* 393, 1979.

Ruger, U. Various regressive processes and their prognostic value in inpatient group psychotherapy. Int. J. Group Psychother., *30:* 95, 1980.

Schoettle, U. C., and Cantwell, D. P. Children of divorce. J. Am. Acad. Child Psychiatry, *19:* 453, 1980.

Slavson, S. R., and Schiffer, M. Selection and grouping. In *Group Psychotherapies for Children,* S. R. Slavson and M. Schiffer, editors, p. 427. International Universities Press, New York, 1975.

Suda, W., and Fouts, G. Effects of peer presence on helping introverted and extroverted children. Child Dev., *51:* 1272, 1980.

Trafimow, E., and Pattak, S. J. Group psychotherapy and objectal development in children. Int. J. Group Psychother., *31:* 193, 1981.

Weinstock, A. A group treatment of characterologically damaged developmentally disabled adolescents in a residential treatment center. Int. J. Group Psychother., *23:* 369, 1979.

C.3 Group Psychotherapy with Neurotic Disorders

HOWARD D. KIBEL, M.D.

Introduction

Ever since the term "neurosis" was introduced into the medical literature by William Cullen of Edinburgh, the word has tended to be used in an etiological sense. For example, Freud originally classified the neuroses according to their hypothesized origins, dividing them into actual neuroses and psychoneuroses (later to be called the transference neuroses). In the actual neuroses, symptoms were assumed to be caused by toxic substances that accumulated as the result of sexual frustrations. In the psychoneuroses, psychological conflict was deemed causative, and the symptoms were viewed as symbolic expressions of forbidden unconscious wishes. Subsequently, Freud—and Fenichel after him—expanded the term

"neurosis" to include myriad functional and presumably psychogenic disturbances. Thus, the early psychoanalytic literature speaks of the transference neuroses, narcissistic neuroses (schizophrenia and manic-depressive disorders), traumatic neuroses, organ neuroses, impulse neuroses, etc. Such a broad application of the term did not find favor, and has since been dropped. Currently, the term "neurosis" is used to refer to a disturbance of feeling or functioning, which is ego dystonic, and a disturbance in the presence of both intact reality testing and generally appropriate behavior.

More often than not, the term "neurosis" is used to indicate the degree of disturbance, rather than to define a circumscribed disorder. Kubie spoke of the neurotic process, rather than neurosis as a discrete entity. The same process, he noted, may produce discrete symptoms in some individuals, or pervade the personality of others. This view—that symptom neurosis and character neurosis are variants of the same pathological stimulus—is endemic to clinical theory. As a consequence, the literature on the group psychotherapy of neurotic disorders and that of personality disorders has been confluent. While this does limit evaluation of treatment results, it is not without merit.

Kuiper states that a good diagnosis consists of a description of the symptoms, a delineation of the syndrome, an investigation of the dynamics involved in the symptoms, and the exploration of the etiology. He notes that while neurotic symptoms, which are ego alien, usually first bring the patient to treatment the sustained neurotic, but ego-syntonic, character pathology also requires attention. He further states that "the neurotic relationship represents an expression of the neurosis on the level of interpersonal relationships." Thus, treatment of neurotic symptoms cannot be undertaken without consideration of the underlying personality formation or disorder, as the case may be; hence, there is value to multiaxial diagnosis.

The current *Diagnostic and Statistical Manual of Mental Disorders* (DSM-III, American Psychiatric Association, 1980) attempts to be atheoretical with regard to etiology. Its approach is descriptive. Particularly for the neurotic disorders, the definitions consist of descriptions of their clinical features, as opposed to their dynamic origins. A relatively low order of inference is used to describe the characteristic features of these disorders. The purpose here is to standardize diagnosis, in order to improve communication among clinicians and to provide a data base for research. Prior to DSM-III, diagnostic reliability had been poor, as similar terms had been used differently by clinicians (Spitzer and Fleiss, 1974).

Multiaxial Diagnosis and Treatment Planning

Multiaxial diagnosis may prove particularly useful for consideration of group treatment. Taken together, the five axes permit the clinician to formulate a comprehensive, descriptive diagnosis.

DSM-III is a multiaxial system for evaluation that includes the following five axes: axis I, clinical syndromes and conditions not attributable to a mental disorder that are a focus of attention or treatment; axis II, personality disorders and specific developmental disorders; axis III, physical disorders or conditions; axis IV, severity of psychosocial stressors; and axis V, highest level of adaptive functioning in the past year.

In the case of neurotic disorders, such a diagnosis is far more meaningful than merely a narrow definition of the presenting problem. This is because an individual with an obsessive-compulsive disorder will respond to, for example, a psychodynamic psychotherapy group differently, depending upon whether or not the underlying personality is compulsive or histrionic, whether or not the individual is coping with a serious or chronic physical illness, and whether psychosocial stressors have been minimal or extreme; the given of the premorbid level of functioning must be considered.

For referral to a psychodynamic group, a diagnosis on axis II will be telling, since this often assumes a major role in the etiology of a disability from the presenting neurotic disorder. A psychodynamic view of etiology presumes that both neurotic and personality disorders spring from a common pool of unconscious conflicts. When the neurotic symptoms emanate from a pre-existing personality disorder, the two disorders may be termed concordant, implying that they evolve in tandem. In such an instance, ongoing treatment ought to be directed toward the underlying character pathology. Psychodynamic group psychotherapy is particularly useful here. On the other hand, when axes I and II disorders evolve independently of each other, they bear little etiological relationship; these are said to be evolutionally discordant. Likewise, when only personality traits are recorded on axis II, these bear less upon the origin of the neurotic condition. When the diagnoses on these axes are discordant, a psychodynamic group may prove unworkable. The group, by its very nature, will encourage unfolding of the personality disorder, while the patient's presenting symptoms will be neglected.

GROUP COMPOSITION

Therapy groups, by virtue of their social interactive nature, encourage an unfolding of personality in the treatment setting. When groups are composed of heterogeneous personality types, expressive or uncovering psychotherapy is possible. Patients suitable for such a group include those who show character pathology reflecting a high level of psychostructural organization. Examples include compulsive personalities, passive-aggressive personalities, and some of the better functioning dependent, borderline, histrionic, and narcissistic personalities. In contrast, those with lower levels of structural pathology—such as paranoid, schizoid, schizotypal, antisocial, and the poorer functioning borderline and avoidant personalities—are notably poor candidates for expressive group psychotherapy.

Different considerations are needed when one plans treatment of a focal neurotic disturbance. Here, a specialized group of like-symptom patients (homogeneous) may be particularly effective in alleviating the neurotic disorder. These groups should be considered whenever axes I and II diagnoses are discordant. In these instances, one may treat only the neurotic disorder, while leaving untouched or even reinforcing adaptive personality defenses.

Homogeneity of groups may be defined by diagnostic or psychodynamic criteria, or by any one of several characteristics of its members (e.g., gender, age, culture). When a dominant aspect of psychopathology is central to the formation and life of the group, it is not only homogeneous in composition but will be functionally specialized. In such groups, members readily identify with one another, and soon identify with the group entity. Because group identification takes place fairly rapidly, cohesion will be an important instrument for treatment. The sense of belonging enhances the neurotic's sense of well-being, often lessening the cause for symptoms. Group norms and pressure can motivate individuals to improve. On the other hand, members tend to reinforce mutual personality defenses, so that collective resistances are relatively impermeable. Consequently, specialized groups tend to be supportive (e.g., through universality) but superficial; they reinforce defenses, rather than promote change. However, this is precisely what is wanted in certain instances, especially when symptom relief takes precedence over exposure of deeper levels of personality. The supportive effects of these groups nurture adaptive defenses, thereby liberating those aspects of personality that have been bound up in focal neurotic symptoms.

OTHER AXES

When an axis III diagnosis has been important in the etiology of a neurotic disorder, a specialized group for the physically ill may be of value. Patients with serious or chronic illness derive much support in such groups. On the other hand, when a primary neurotic disorder complicates the management of an organic condition, a group for medically ill individuals would be of little value. In fact, it might even be counterproductive, because such patients can, through identification, reinforce a concept of themselves as physically disabled, rather than adhere to their regime of medical treatment.

Anxiety Disorders

In this group of disorders, anxiety is experienced either predominantly or as a consequence of the attempt to master symptoms. Included here are the anxiety states, obsessive-compulsive neurosis, post-traumatic stress disorder, and the phobias.

ANXIETY STATES

According to classic psychoanalytic theory, anxiety is the basis of all neuroses. It is intimately associated with the neurotic symptoms of hysteria, phobia, and obsessive-compulsive disorder. In these instances, with partial failure of repression, the ego uses auxiliary defenses—such as conversion, displacement, and regression—to achieve a partial, though disguised, expression of unconscious wishes. Should the failure of repression be more extensive and auxiliary defenses not present, anxiety is found as the only symptom. In DMS-III, the diagnosis of anxiety (state) neurosis itself is limited to those situations where anxiety is found as the only symptom. It may occur in a recurrent, episodic form as panic disorder, or in a pervasive, persistent form as generalized anxiety disorder.

Panic attacks are manifested by the sudden onset of intense apprehension, fear, or terror, often with a sense of impending doom. In its chronic form, anticipatory fears of helplessness or loss of control may lead to agoraphobia. Generalized anxiety is characterized by motor tension, autonomic hyperactivity, apprehensive expectation, vigilance, and scanning. These patients may be irritable, distractible or suffer insomnia, and they often worry that something bad will happen to themselves or loved ones.

In contrast to classic psychoanalytic theory, modern theories suggest "a hierarchy of levels of clinical anxiety in which the degree of pathology of the clinical manifestations is determined by the phase of development from which it is derived—the earlier the phase, the more serious its diagnostic and prognostic import" (Nemiah, 1980). In other words, anxiety states may result from affective flooding of the pristine ego, failure of primitive splitting mechanisms, castration fears of the phallic phase, or an oedipal conflict of the genital phase. Hence, the existence of an anxiety state may not reflect a neurotic level of conflict. For appropriate treatment planning, the clinician must go beyond a diagnosis of anxiety state, since the method of therapy will depend upon the nature of the underlying problem. It must be determined from what the anxiety emanates, the underlying character structure, the presence or absence of other mental disorders, the individual's defensive structure, personality traits, temperament, psychological-mindedness, and motivation. From this, standard criteria of suitability for group psychotherapy can be applied, and the kind of group required can be determined.

Consider the case of a patient with a generalized anxiety disorder but with an underlying paranoid personality disorder. For such a patient, group therapy would be contraindicated. Paranoid patients are far too distrustful of others to tolerate the free-flowing interaction of a group. Thus, for the anxiety states, more than any other of the neurotic disorders (with the exception of certain post-traumatic stress reactions), the symptomatic neurosis must be seen as a nonspecific, final common pathway of an underlying disturbance.

OBSESSIVE-COMPULSIVE DISORDER

This classic neurotic condition is characterized by the presence either of ego-dystonic, recurrent, and persistent thoughts or impulses, or of repetitive behaviors that are performed in either stereotyped fashion or according to one's private rules. Its clinical course is variable. It may cause differing degrees of impairment, even leading the patient to the brink of psychosis.

Freud classified this disorder as a transference neurosis. Yet he and, especially, Abraham believed that its characteristics derive from the anal-sadistic phase. This traditional psychoanalytic view maintains that in this neurosis, there is a defensive regression of the intrapsychic structures from an oedipal to a preoedipal phase of development. Viewing this disorder as a transference neurosis, Slavson (1972) argued against the use of group psychotherapy and favored individual psychoanalytic treatment. In contrast, Salzman advised against the use of free association and genetic reconstruction, since these techniques encourage greater obsessionalism.

Gutheil argued that therapy cannot follow traditional psychoanalytic lines. He noted that these patients show an inability to distinguish the self from the non-self, have little observing ego, suffer great separation anxiety, have fantasies of omnipotent control, fear loss of control, and struggle against feelings of impotence.

Schwartz (1972) recommended psychoanalytic group treatment as preferable to a dyadic approach, precisely because it is more ego oriented, realistic, less penetrating into unconscious processes, and focused in the here and now. Stein also preferred group psychotherapy, noting that it lessens guilt-laden transferences associated with these patients' archaic-harsh superegos. Anger and rage, a consequence of anal fixations, can be worked through more easily in a psychotherapy group. The patient, in early stages of treatment, vicariously identifies with both aggressor and victim during hostile interchanges between others. Later, with the support of the group, the patient may permit himself to express anger toward others and, within the collective transference, toward the therapist. The presence of multiple targets for aggression can dilute the experience when needed, while collective leader transference reactions can intensify catharsis, but with support.

Salzman and Thaler note that these patients require considerable support, encouragement, guidance, and sometimes even pressure in order to change. Groups are well suited to this effort. They also note that the central dynamics of this disorder revolve around issues of autonomy that originated in the early mother-child relationship. Analytically oriented groups are well suited for working through these issues by serving as transitional objects between the omnipotently invested image of the therapist and the external world. And, groups are well suited to the expression of emotions, in general, which these patients find difficult, particularly tender feelings that have been long suppressed. Therefore, it would seem that for many, if not for most, obsessive-compulsive patients, psychodynamic group therapy offers the most promise.

POST-TRAUMATIC STRESS DISORDER

This disorder follows a psychologically traumatic event, which is unusual and outside the range of most people's experience and would cause distress in anyone. Its characteristic symptoms include some form of re-experiencing the traumatic event, psychic numbing or reduced involvement with the external world, and a variety of autonomic, dysphoric, or cognitive symptoms. The syndrome may have various associated features and a broad range of complications. This disorder may occur in the presence or absence of pre-existing psychopathology and in association with almost any personality type. Therefore, treatment is usually focused on the syndrome itself and on its dynamic components.

Fenichel noted that in traumatic neurosis the intensity and unexpectedness of incoming stimuli overwhelm the ego, causing dedifferentiation of its higher functions. Primitivation of the ego produces attitudes of helplessness and passive dependency. Indeed, excessive dependency and secondary gain may complicate the treatment of this disorder. As the ego regresses, the aggressive drives, often stimulated by the trauma itself, assume ascendancy. The emergence of aggression in the face of poor ego control accounts for the typical symptoms of insomnia, impaired concentration, irritability, hypersensitivity, and depressive features. Additionally, feelings of guilt may be present and associated with the relief in having survived the disaster when others did not.

Whenever the ego is overwhelmed, it tries to recuperate spontaneously. Psychic numbing serves both to get distance from the trauma and to rest, collecting energy for the task of belated mastery. The latter is attempted by the reliving or re-experiencing phenomena that are so characteristic of this disorder.

The phenomena of dependency, weakening of the ego, impaired control of aggressive impulses, guilt, and the need for mastery must be the object of treatment. Experience has shown that treatment should be supportive and short term, with quick reentry to a normal living environment. Catharsis and abreaction help to develop conscious verbal mastery in place of the symptomatic re-experiencing. While several treatment modalities can accomplish these tasks, homogeneous groups are ideally suited because of their ego orientation, the support members can give one another, mutual stimulation by members for ventilation, and the opportunity for sharing of conscious and unconscious guilt. These groups tend to counter regression and help to contain impulses, both through the socialization process and members' mutual reassurances.

Moses and co-workers almost by chance, developed a systematic approach refining group methods used for the so-called combat neuroses during World War II. They devised an intensive 14-day inpatient experience, which was devoted exclusively to the treatment of combat reactions. They used milieu techniques and daily individual and group psychotherapy sessions. The structure of a therapeutic community and the therapy groups seemed supportive because they adhered closely to the framework of a military unit. Cohesion crystallized early in all psychotherapy groups. Members gave each other support and encouragement, particularly to counteract passive trends toward inertia and withdrawal. As some members left, the rest did not want to stay behind without their buddies. This served to counteract the dependent wish to remain in the army and avoid reentry to civilian life. Thus, antiregressive forces existed in the group.

The group provided many opportunities for relief—from survivor guilt and expression of aggressive-laden content—through a sharing of experiences. The expression of direct aggression within the transference proved to be an essential feature of the therapeutic process. In a broad sense, this was contained in rebellious attitudes that reflected projection of blame for the breakdown onto the Establishment and its representatives in the treatment team. More specifically, the group facilitated collective expressions of negative transference during the usual phase of group development.

When dealing with combat reactions, treatment considerations must extend well beyond the psychotherapy group; the goals of the treatment unit must foster autonomy and discourage dependent helplessness. Ben-Yahar et al. demonstrated that therapy groups progress through successive phases of development in accordance with the expectations of the milieu. When chemically induced narcosis is relied upon, the group remains stagnated in the earliest phase of development, that of helpless dependency.

PHOBIC DISORDERS

These neurotic conditions are characterized by one or more persistent and irrational fears of a specific object, activity, or situation, producing avoidant behavior. Even though the individual recognizes that the fear is excessive or unreasonable, the phobic stimulus remains a source of considerable anxiety. To be considered a disorder, the condition must impair functioning. In contrast, many specific phobic reactions, such as those to insects or snakes, or social fears, such as one of public speaking, do not cause impairment and, therefore, should not be given a diagnostic label.

This disorder is divided into three major types: agoraphobia, social phobia, and simple phobia. Their treatment will be discussed collectively, since past efforts have not been aimed toward identifying differential approaches. Yet, these disorders seem to constitute a spectrum with simple phobia on one side and agoraphobia on the other. Simple phobics often modify their life style to avoid anxiety and are, therefore, less likely to seek treatment. Social phobics and agoraphobics may fear similar public situations. Agoraphobia causes the most impairment, sometimes leading to a housebound existence, and is often associated with excessive dependency upon loved ones, to such a point where their lives may suffer major effects. Agoraphobia is the most common form among those seeking treatment. The psychodynamics of these conditions also suggest a continuum which may prove useful for future application. Etiological theories have focused on the role of repressed sexual and aggressive impulses (for simple phobia) but in recent years increasingly (particularly for agoraphobia) on the role of separation anxiety. The roots of these disorders may span from oedipal to preoedipal conflicts.

Freud postulated that these patients ward off incestuous genital strivings and castration anxiety through displacement onto the phobic object. Fenichel additionally noted the tension between aggressive, as well as sexual, impulses and the superego. The conflict is held in abeyance by means of repression so that psychic equilibrium is maintained. Anxieties are displaced onto some aspect of an external object or situation, which is seemingly far removed from the original target of the impulses but is somehow symbolically connected to it. As the individual approaches the phobic situation, repression is weakened and anxiety increases; removal from the same abates anxiety and restores psychic equilibrium. Thus, there is a powerful motivation in these patients to seek solutions through compromises in life style. Even Freud recognized that the patient must confront the phobic situation in order to make progress in treatment. These observations account for the difficulties in treating such patients using dynamic psychotherapies and the appeal of behavioral approaches (even in groups).

Increased attention to the role of separation anxiety in these patients has paralleled an increasing aware-ness of preoedipal influences. Many of these patients recoil from intimate relationships in which mutual autonomy is demanded; they retreat to hostile dependency. Unable to achieve individuation, passive dependency is preferred. Such patients readily find gratification in dyadic therapies, resisting change. This suggests a suitability for group therapy, in that transference dependency is decreased in favor of a turning to the group entity and the other members. However, initially an increase in dependency upon the leader may be required to serve as a buffer to such an alteration of the focus for need gratification (Al-Salih, 1969).

It has long been noted that phobic patients bear some resemblance to obsessive-compulsives. They use similar defense mechanisms. In obsessive-compulsive disorder, patients employ symptoms to actively overcome anxiety; in phobia the patient is passive. Some symptoms, such as a fear of knives, lie midway between the two disorders. Character types range from hysterical to obsessional, with either showing passive-dependent features. These factors are important for treatment planning to alert the clinician to the pressure of a concordant personality disorder, since the desire for personality change provides the motivation to work in a psychodynamic group.

Every clinician has successfully treated some phobics in heterogeneous, psychodynamic groups. Yet, the literature on this subject focuses on homogeneous groups. Al-Salih (1969) treated a time-limited, homogeneous group of basically agoraphobic women. While attempting an unstructured approach, he found it necessary to modify treatment as follows: During the initial phase the therapist needed to structure the discussions, and later on he needed to encourage the members to confront their respective phobic situations. He found that sibling rivalry to win the leader's attention spurred the members toward health, that the group was both supportive and pressuring for change, and that it gave each member a sense of belonging and identity which helped them to separate from pathologically dependent family relationships. Once cohesion and solidarity were established, the members were able to discuss sexual frustrations and repressed hostility in ways they had never been able to in individual sessions.

Except for this one report of a psychodynamic approach, others in the literature have relied upon behavioral methods. Lazarus was the first to use systematic desensitization in a therapy group for phobic individuals. Aronson claimed 90 percent success in the treatment of the fear of flying with a program using short-term, homogeneous, task-oriented groups which were based upon both psychoanalytic and behavioral modification principles. Harris (1979) summarized the literature on the successful treatment of a variety of phobias—examination anxiety, speech anxiety, and snake phobia—with behavioral group therapy. Practically all the reports use volunteers as subjects; thus, these subjects are individuals who do not see themselves as patients, who lack the corresponding social role, and who usually do not show sufficient impairment to warrant the diagnosis of a disorder. In contrast, Gelder and Marks treated identified psychiatric patients, most of whom had agoraphobia. They found group desensitization to be superior to traditional group therapy in alleviating specific phobic symptoms. However, those patients with widespread symptoms, complicated social problems, and marked personality disorder did less well with desensitization unless it was preceded by more traditional treatment (a finding previously noted by Lazarus). They concluded that, only when the phobias remained as relatively isolated disorders, were they amenable to desensitization. A 4-year follow-up revealed that symptom substitution, in general, did not occur, except in the most severe phobic cases. These patients were prone to depression, requiring further psychiatric treatment. This finding prevailed regardless of the type of phobia present. Therefore, while behavioral methods are very effective in treating many phobic conditions, when widespread symptoms and disabilities are present, comprehensive treatment is required, of which dynamic group psychotherapy may be an invaluable component.

Somatoform Disorders

This group of disorders is characterized by physical symptoms suggestive of physical illness, but for which there are no organic findings and at least a strong presumption of psychological causes. Included here are somatization disorder, conversion and psychogenic pain (the group of hysterias), and hypochondriasis.

SOMATIZATION DISORDER

Somatization disorder (also known as Briquet's syndrome) is a chronic condition characterized by recurrent and multiple functional somatic complaints for which persistent medical attention has been sought. It must be distinguished from hypochondriasis. Patients with somatization disorder have more insidious complaints related to multiple organ symptoms, usually producing actual functional disturbances, such as urinary retention, vomiting or diarrhea, and dysmenorrhea. These patients believe that they have been sick for a good part of their lives.

Unfortunately, most of these patients do not come to the attention of the psychotherapist until they have developed some complication of this disorder, such as substance abuse of prescription medications or suicide attempts as a consequence of secondary depression. As a result of constantly seeking doctors, these patients often unwittingly submit to unnecessary surgery (Brody, 1959). Most of the time, attention to these secondary complications takes precedence over treatment of the primary disorder.

Individually, these patients rarely seek psychological help and respond angrily to any suggestion that they need it. Typically, in medical centers, "they circulate through the specialty clinics asking for remedies to cure their many ills, but any relief they obtain is not successful for long. These patients become frustrated by the physicians and are frustrating to them" (Mally and Ogston, 1964). Even when such patients make it to the psychiatrist's office, they are apt to be poor group referrals. Kotov found that these patients have a high group dropout rate; they are poorly motivated for treatment. Many of them have depressive-masochistic

trends and rigid character patterns, making them poor candidates for any psychotherapy.

Despite these considerations, certain aspects of their pathology suggest a potential to do well in a heterogeneous group. Many unpsychologically minded individuals whose anxieties are somatized—so-called emotional illiterates—learn from a group how to communicate at a feeling level. Group may be suitable for many strain-inducing patients, liberating both patient and therapist from the latter's demanding and manipulative behavior. Many of these patients are relatively isolated and could benefit from the social stimulation of a mixed diagnostic group. Additionally, a group could provide a format for re-enactment and resolution of highly pathological family relationships. Certainly, the presence of severe character pathology and underlying borderline personality organization are prime indications for group psychotherapy.

Further work is needed to determine which of these patients can be treated in a heterogeneous psychotherapy group. Most reports in the literature generally fail to distinguish patients with somatization disorder per se from other forms of somatizing (Brody, 1959). Clinical experience suggests that, when the disorder is still in the subacute phase, patients may respond well to an explorative approach. Once the illness has entered the chronic phase, supportive treatment is required. At this point, clinical attention is needed for the secondary complications, rather than for the primary disturbance. Furthermore, these patients feel too different from others to tolerate a mixed group. A homogeneous group is suited to their needs.

Two reports in the literature (Mally and Ogston, 1964; Valko, 1976) describe the successful use of homogeneous group therapy only for patients with somatization disorder. Both drew from large medical treatment centers. The patients were supportive to one another and benefited from the universalization process in group. They were less of a strain both on the therapist, if seen individually, and on one another, as might be in a heterogeneous group. Most notably, their use of medication and the frequency of visits to physicians decreased; their over-all functioning, in terms of work or household chores, improved.

Valko claimed that the patients felt relieved when told they had an identifiable disorder, Briquet's syndrome. This seemed to diminish their sense of fault, thereby raising self-esteem and improving family relationships. He also claimed that patients could eventually find the psychological link between external stress and their physical symptoms. In contrast, Mally and Ogston noted that mutual support increased certain resistances; namely, the patients justified, for one another, their social withdrawal and their belief that others had failed them. This finding is consistent with the usual experience that homogeneous groups support defenses and members tend to project blame onto the out-group.

Both studies demonstrate the need for maintenance therapy of these patients. This is reasonable for such chronically handicapped people who require management, rather than cure. Valid goals include decreased use of medication, less misuse of physican time, and avoidance of secondary complications, such as substance abuse, unnecessary surgery, depression, and even suicide.

CONVERSION DISORDER

Conversion disorder, as defined in DSM-III, is relatively uncommon. Yet, conversion symptoms may be associated with many other conditions. The classic conversion symptoms are those that suggest neurological disease, but any area of physical function may be affected. Usually, the symptom develops under conditions of extreme psychological stress. Its clinical course may be of short duration, with abrupt onset and resolution. Thus, the disorder is usually treated supportively in a one-to-one relationship. Only under conditions of collective stress, such as might occur on a battlefield, would patients be treated in groups. Here, the relationship to post-traumatic stress disorder is obvious, and the reader is referred to that section of this chapter.

The classic hysteric suffers from fixation of psychosexual development at the level of the Oedipus complex. Psychoanalysis or individual, expressive, analytically oriented psychotherapy are the treatments of choice. However, such patients with genital conflicts are rare. The battlefield experience demonstrates that conversion disorder need not arise from sexual conflict; rather, fear and aggressive conflicts may lie at its root. It is usually the preoedipal sexual and aggressive drives that are processed by the mechanism of conversion and expressed symbolically in physical symptoms. Thus, conversion disorder may be associated with a variety of personality types. In the presence of a pre-existing histrionic, passive-aggressive, or dependent personality disorder, the conversion symptom expresses related areas of conflict; the neurotic and personality disorders are concordant. Consequently, treatment of both conditions through a psychotherapy group may be warranted. In contrast, in the presence of a personality disorder which is discordant to the hysterical symptoms—such as can be found in paranoid, schizoid, or compulsive personalities—a group would be unproductive.

Reckless treated two patients with hysterical blepharospasm in a heterogeneous group. Both had rather rigid personality styles. Treatment was supportive and directive and used desensitization techniques. The results were fairly good. Whenever these patients became symptomatic during sessions, "they were requested to identify the affect that they were experiencing plus the theme of the group discussion preceding the eye closing and the specific connection to their own situation." This interesting use of a group could be applied to others, regardless of the personality disorder diagnosis, whenever there are conversion symptoms which vary in intensity.

PSYCHOGENIC PAIN DISORDER

This is a sharply delineated disorder in which functional pain is associated with clear evidence of a psychogenic precipitant. Unlike somatization disorder, physiological mechanisms are not involved in the production of the symptom. Thus, tension headache from muscle spasm is not included in this disorder. If organic pathology is present, the pain reported cannot be accounted for by the physical findings; it is exaggerated pain. Like patients with somatization disorder, these individuals doctor-shop in attempting to seek relief, are antagonistic to psychological help, and are prone to invalidism and all its complications. They, too, can develop the secondary complications of substance abuse of prescribed medications or repeated unnecessary surgery.

These patients are strikingly, unpsychologically minded and appear almost naive. Typically, they remain adamantly unaware of obvious causative factors. Thus, Nemiah (1978) has postulated that symptom formation "is related to major defects in the ego functions underlying the experience and expression of feelings." This deficit has been labeled "alexithymia." According to this view, emotional illiteracy is not so much the product of intrapsychic conflict as much as it represents a maturational deficiency, perhaps constitutional in origin. Such patients need to be educated about emotions. A heterogeneous, psychodynamic group can be used for this. Many patients who cannot verbalize inner thoughts and feelings learn how from others. However, given these patients' downright antagonism to traditional psychological techniques, there remains the question of their perseverance with a therapy group long enough to benefit.

In contrast to an ego-deficiency theory of this disorder, Blumer and Heilbronn (1981) view intrapsychic conflict as etiological. They state that "the pain-prone disorder may be appropriately characterized as a 'depressive spectrum disease,'" since these patients show typically associated clinical symptoms and some response to low doses of antidepressant medication. Premorbidly, a pattern of relentless work serves to deny pressing infantile needs and binds unacceptable hostility. Once symptomatic, long-denied dependent and passive needs are aroused, but hostility remains well masked and turned inward. These aspects of psychopathology should respond well to group treatment.

Two studies in the literature report the use of homogeneous group therapy for chronic pain patients. In both studies, patients with objective pain were mixed with those with psychogenic pain. In both, patients had excessive preoccupation with bodily functions, disruptive social relationships, and excessive use of prescription medications, all of which were alleviated through treatment. Pinsky (1978) conducted a 7-week inpatient program with almost exclusive use of group as the psychotherapeutic modality. Recognizing these patients' shame with being identified as having a mental disorder, he found the medical orientation of the psychotherapist to be invaluable; patients felt their pain was taken seriously. During the course of treatment, their bias against psychotherapy withered. This was true whether or not there was any change in their pain complaint. Benefits were measured not in terms of pain reduction but in improvement in their quality of life.

Hendler et al. (1981) conducted an inpatient group therapy program with outpatient group therapy follow-up of 1 to 2 years. They examined the thematic content of these sessions. These pain patients complained bitterly about their pain making them dependent. Mutual support of the members for one another attenuated shame and thereby permitted some acceptance of help for their psychological needs. Anger at the medical community was readily evident. As the group progressed, the psychiatrist began to function as a model for physicians in general, especially as patients discovered that their level of pain did not appreciably change. The group therapist became a focal point for the discharge of unacceptable, internalized hostility. Collective expression afforded each member protection of the group theme and facilitated the development of group cohesion, which was generally slow for these patients because of the narcissism attendant to chronic pain. This study suggests how specific areas of confict—namely, anger, dependency, and fear of passivity (specifically in the role of psychotherapy patient)—can be alleviated but not eliminated through group therapy. Specific aspects of group dynamics accounted for the benefit these patients received.

HYPOCHONDRIASIS

Patients with this disorder are preoccupied with bodily functions. Unrealistic interpretation of physical signs or sensations as abnormal leads them to fear or believe they have a serious disease. Their clinical course is chronic, with waxing and waning of symptoms. They are frequently seen in the general practice of medicine and are known to doctor-shop for diagnoses or remedies. They are generally resistant to referral for psychological help.

Freud noted a withdrawal of object cathexes, so that libido becomes transferred to ideas concerning one's own organs. This process he identified as "narcissistic withdrawal." Indeed, many of these patients appear narcissistic; they are egocentric and unduly sensitive to minor criticisms or slight. They treat their bodies as libidinal objects and are excessively concerned with themselves, to the exclusion of concern for others. Additionally, they may use physical complaints to exert control over others. Although narcissism is frequently seen in these patients, it is not pathognomonic for this condition.

Kernberg lists hypochondriasis as one of the presumptive diagnostic elements of borderline personality organization. He states that this constellation is probably more related to character pathology than to symptomatic neurosis. Kohut mentions hypochondriacal preoccupations as a frequent finding in narcissistic disturbances, and describes symptomatic hypochondriasis as a specific neurotic feature in his analysis of Mr. W. (Kohut, 1977). Thus, it would appear that treatment for hypochondriacal patients should be considered in the light of the treatment for borderline and narcissistic conditions, with these terms used in their structural sense, not descriptively. Indeed, group therapy has proven successful with many of these patients when they are carefully selected.

Group therapy can be beneficial for several reasons. Dilution of transference and countertransference can be a welcome relief, given these patients'

histories of deteriorated relationships with physicians. Some may be weaned from egocentricity through carefully titrated doses of social interaction. A group provides many opportunities for systematic exploration of interpersonal relatedness and character armor, as these patients gradually move from organ cathexis to object cathexis. Given their feelings of sensitivity to criticism by authority, these patients might accept confrontation from peers in a group more easily than from a therapist. The supportive and nurturing effects of a group may be helpful for these lonely, sensitive, and frightened people.

The question remains as to whether these patients respond better in a group of homogeneous or heterogeneous composition. Schoenberg and Senescu successfully conducted group therapy for patients with a variety of somatoform disorders, including hypochondriasis. Despite these patients' envy, feelings of competition, and intense need for individual attention from the leader, they responded to an analytic approach in which somatic symptoms were interpreted as resistance to getting close to one another. In contrast, Slavson believes that "hypochondriacal patients have to be excluded [from a heterogeneous group] because of their compulsive need to speak repeatedly, and sometimes continually, about their symptoms without any constructive focus or direction"; that is, they are overly demanding of exclusive attention. While this represents the view of most group therapists today, newer structural and multiaxial descriptive diagnoses may change this.

Dissociative Disorders

This group of disorders is characterized by sudden and temporary alterations in the normal integrative functions of consciousness, producing dramatic disturbances of memory or identity, sometimes accompanied by complex motor behavior. This group includes depersonalization disorder, which is generally discussed separately from the other three syndromes.

Psychogenic amnesia and psychogenic fugue are rare, while multiple personality is extremely rare. Freud believed that for all three disorders, symptoms were produced by selective, dynamically determined repression. This view still holds sway with many clinicians today. With multiple personality the use of group therapy is untried and most probably of no value. Psychogenic amnesia and fugue typically are precipitated by severe psychological stress, often in wartime or in the wake of a natural disorder. Therefore, except when memory recall is urgently required, these conditions may be treated as one would treat most post-traumatic stress disorders. In fact, this has been the case for combat reactions with dissociative components. However, the specific response of this variant to group therapy has not been reported.

Depersonalization disorder as a pure syndrome—being ego dystonic and with gross reality testing intact—occurs infrequently. Yet, as a symptom, it is commonly seen in anxiety states and borderline conditions. Little is known about the treatment of this disorder. When precipitated by severe stress, it, too, may be treated as one would treat a post-traumatic stress disorder. At other times, treatment should be directed to the underlying condition, for which group therapy may or may not be indicated.

Conclusion

Current nomenclature applies the term "neurosis" in a narrow descriptive sense. In planning treatment, consideration of the suitability for group therapy usually requires additional diagnoses, specifically of the underlying personality traits or disorder, and often of the associated structural pathology. Neurotic disorders have been found to span the realm of oedipal and preoedipal pathology. A comprehensive diagnosis, which includes all these elements, is needed for the clinician to consider which type of therapy group holds the most promise for a particular patient.

References

Al-Salih, H. A. Phobics in group psychotherapy. Int. J. Group Psychother., *19:* 79, 1969.

American Psychiatric Association. *Diagnostic and Statistical Manual of Mental Disorders,* ed. 3. American Psychiatric Association, Washington, D.C., 1980.

Blumer, D., and Heilbronn, M. The pain-prone disorder: A clinical and psychological profile. Psychosomatics, *22:* 395, 1981.

Brody, S. Value of group psychotherapy in patients with poly-surgery addiction. Psychiatr. Q., *33:* 260, 1959.

Harris, F. C. The behavioral approach of group psychotherapy. Int. J. Group Psychother., *29:* 453, 1979.

Hendler, N., Viernstein, M., Shallenberger, C., and Long, D. Group therapy with chronic pain patients. Psychosomatics, *22:* 333, 1981.

Kohut, H. *The Restoration of the Self.* International Universities Press, New York, 1977.

Mally, M., and Ogston, W. Treatment of the "untreatables." Int. J. Group Psychother., *14:* 369, 1964.

Moses, R., et al. A real unit for the treatment of combat reactions in the wake of the Yom Kippur War. Psychiatry, *39:* 153, 1976.

Nemiah, J. C. Alexithymia and psychosomatic illness. J. Cont. Educ. Psychiatry, *39:* 25, 1978.

Nemiah, J. C. Anxiety state. In *Comprehensive Textbook of Psychiatry,* H. I. Kaplan, A. M. Freedman, and B. J. Sadock, editors, ed. 3., p. 1483. Williams & Wilkins, Baltimore, 1980.

Parloff, M. B., and Dies, R. R. Group psychotherapy outcome research. Int. J. Group Psychother., *27:* 281, 1977.

Pinsky, J. D. Chronic, intractable benign pain: A syndrome and its treatment with intensive short-term group psychotherapy. J. Hum. Stress, *4:* 17, 1978.

Schoenberg, B., and Senescu, R. Group psychotherapy for patients with chronic multiple somatic complaints. J. Chronic Dis., *19:* 649, 1966.

Schwartz, E. K. The treatment of the obsessive patient in the group therapy setting. Am. J. Psychother., *26:* 352, 1972.

Slavson, S. R. Group psychotherapy and the transference neurosis. Int. J. Group Psychother., *22:* 433, 1972.

Spitzer, R. L., Endicott, J., and Robbins, E. Research diagnostic criteria: Rationale and reliability. Arch. Gen. Psychiatry, *35:* 773, 1978.

Spitzer, R. L., and Fleiss, J. L. A re-analysis of the reliability of psychiatric diagnosis. Br. J. Psychiatry, *125:* 341, 1974.

Valko, R. J. Group therapy for patients with hysteria (Briquet's disorder). Dis. Nerv. Sys., *37:* 484, 1976.

C.4 Group Psychotherapy with Schizophrenia and Affective Disorders

CHARLES P. O'BRIEN, M.D., Ph.D.

Introduction

Seriously disturbed patients can benefit from group therapy even if pharmacotherapy is the primary modality. Perhaps the best evidence for the effectiveness of group therapy comes from the schizophrenia literature. The group technique has been used in the treatment of schizophrenia for more than 60 years. Various advantages for group over individual therapy have been cited on the basis of clinical experience. Payn (1974), for example, noted that the group provides socializing experiences for patients, and this tends to diminish anxiety, improve reality testing, increase self-esteem, and reduce necessity for hospitalization. Schizophrenics can learn to overcome some of their basic mistrust in other people while in a protected group setting. Striking improvement in social functioning has been reported by several authors. A consistent finding from many studies is that therapists, even those who had initial misgivings about group therapy for schizophrenics, reported spontaneously that the group experience increased their enthusiasm for psychotherapy with schizophrenics. Working in a group was less draining on the therapist than individual psychotherapy with a chronic schizophrenic.

Data suggest that group treatment is more effective than individual therapy with schizophrenics. Most of the studies of effectiveness have been in outpatient settings where long-term follow-up is feasible. Medication is continued, but the type of psychotherapy—group or individual—is experimentally manipulated. Shatton et al. compared outcome in 45 schizophrenic patients randomly assigned to an experimental team using group therapy with outcome of 45 matched controls who received only individual therapy; both groups received neuroleptic medication. After 1 year, the group patients had a significantly lower rehospitalization rate and a higher rate of absolute discharge from the clinic. While this finding might be attributed to the increased attention and clinic contact coincident with being the experimental group, this would not explain the results of a random assignment study.

One hundred consecutive schizophrenic patients recently discharged from a state mental hospital were rated by an independent research team and then randomly assigned to either group or individual treatment (O'Brien et al., 1972). No special groups were formed, and no special attention was given. At 1- and 2-year follow-ups, the group patients had fewer rehospitalizations (12 per cent group versus 24 per cent individual at 1 year), but the difference was not statistically significant. On social function rating scales, however, there was a significant advantage for group patients at both 1 and 2-year assessments. Subsequently, Prince et al., in a similar study, found a significant reduction in rehospitalization rates for group-treated chronic schizophrenics. Claghorn et al. (1974), in still another controlled study, noted significant improvement for group patients on an interpersonal test battery, suggesting a "healthier orientation toward relationships with others." The controls for their study consisted of patients seen by a psychiatrist for medication checks only. Herz et al. (1974) compared group and individual aftercare for 108 patients, 66 per cent of them with a diagnosis of schizophrenia. In this mixed but predominantly schizophrenic population, the patients assigned to group therapy had a lower rehospitalization rate (16 per cent versus 24 per cent), but this difference disappeared when early dropouts were excluded. Herz and his associates did note a dramatic shift in therapists' attitudes in favor of group therapy, and they observed that group patients seemed "more lively and enthusiastic."

In contrast, Levene et al. found no significant differences in the results of group and individual therapy after 1 year of treatment. The Levene study, although well controlled, suffered from a small initial population (N = 30), so that at the 1 year follow-up only 8 group and 7 individual patients remained in therapy. More recently, Alden et al. (1979) reported a longitudinal study of 15 schizophrenic patients had reported a dramatic improvement after group therapy was introduced.

At least two reviewers of these studies interpret them as showing an advantage for group, while one review concludes that group contributes a useful but not unique therapeutic benefit (Parloff and Dies, 1977). It is significant that no report of group therapy for schizophrenia has concluded that group treatment is less effective than individual therapy.

Group Therapy in a Comprehensive Treatment Program

INPATIENT TREATMENT

In the acute phase of schizophrenia, treatment is usually conducted in a hospital, and neuroleptic medication is generally considered to be the mainstay of treatment. Group therapy has been advocated for

inpatient schizophrenics, but this has usually been in long-stay institutions. Now that inpatient care for acute schizophrenics is relatively brief, there is insufficient time for the group process to fully develop. Moreover, some therapists have the impression that acute psychotics may become further fragmented in a therapy group. Prince, Ackerman, and Barksdale collected data showing that schizophrenics benefit from outpatient but not from inpatient group therapy. This does not mean that acute schizophrenics should not take part in large ward meetings; rather, a group always exists on an inpatient ward, and the staff should try to give it some structure by holding ward meetings attended by all the patients and staff of a given unit. Practical problems of living on the ward can be the focus of such meetings.

During the inpatient phase, the patient can also be involved in family therapy—a special form of group therapy that is important for diagnosis, disposition, and treatment. These sessions can be used to elucidate the dynamics of the patient's family situation. Excessive dependence is a common problem that can be worked on in family sessions during the inpatient phase. Extricating the patient from his family may be a useful—although often unrealistic—goal, and to this end, discharge to a halfway house or independent living is desirable when possible. During outpatient treatment, the frequency of family sessions depends on whether or not the patient is living with the family and how well he transfers dependency from his family to the group. Periodic outpatient family sessions are almost always helpful.

OUTPATIENT TREATMENT

In the outpatient phase of treatment, group therapy can be the primary modality. Medication should, of course, be continued as long as necessary. Maintenance neuroleptic medication does not interfere with group therapy, and, in fact, the two treatments may facilitate each other. There are no published studies to support this impression, but patients doing well in a group seem able to be maintained on less medication, possibly because of the effects of group support. Certainly, each group session enables the therapist to see the patient express a greater variety of behaviors over a longer period of time than in individual sessions, and he may, therefore, feel more comfortable about trials of reduced medication or no medication. If group behavior shows beginning symptoms of deterioration, medication can be reinstituted or increased at the therapist's discretion. The risk of long-term neuroleptic side effects, such as tardive dyskinesia, is, therefore, kept to a minimum.

SELECTION OF PATIENTS

Plans for aftercare should begin before the patient's discharge from the hospital. Continuity of care is very important. Since it is usually not possible for the patient to have the same therapist during both inpatient and outpatient care, his hospital therapist should acquaint him with what to expect after discharge. The patient should be given a specific appointment within 2 weeks of his release from the hospital.

In the controlled studies referred to above, patients were assigned to outpatient groups at random. This was simply a method to determine what the results would be in the extreme case, that of putting unselected patients into group therapy. It resulted in a high initial dropout rate, since not all patients are ready for groups at the time of hospital discharge.

Patients who have had no previous group experience and patients who have had prior upsetting experience, perhaps with an inpatient group, require a thorough explanation of outpatient groups. This explanation may entail several visits, and should be presented by a therapist who is himself fully acquainted with the value of the group approach. If the patient or his family is resistant, the group should not be forced on them. Too often, in a busy clinic with a low staff-patient ratio, the patient and his family gain the impression that group therapy is stressed because there are not enough therapists to go around. The fact that group treatment is a unique experience—one that seems to provide some things that individual therapy does not—is the aspect that should be emphasized.

For purposes of this discussion, ambulatory schizophrenic patients will be divided into two categories: withdrawn and activated. Acutely ill patients will not be considered here because they are usually hospitalized.

Withdrawn patients include the familiar chronic, poor prognosis, or process patients who never fully recover between hospitalizations. Affect remains blunted, and spontaneous speech is limited. Delusions may still be present, but the patient has learned not to talk about them, so that he can be released from the hospital. This type of patient usually requires maintenance neuroleptic medication.

Activated patients speak spontaneously and show affect; they may have had repeated psychotic episodes, but these are likely to have been reactive or associated with a precipitating event. Activated patients are less likely than withdrawn patients to require maintenance neuroleptics, but they may do well if neuroleptics are resumed at times of stress. The term "activated" also includes the borderline, pseudoneurotic, or latent schizophrenic (schizotypal personality disorder).

ORGANIZING SCHIZOPHRENIC GROUPS

In a community mental health center, separate groups for withdrawn and activated schizophrenics can usually be organized, although mixing is occasionally necessary because of scheduling problems. Mixing is more often done in private practice because the population from which groups are drawn is more limited. Research indicates that one or two withdrawn patients may do well in a group of activated patients, but that one or two activated patients will fit poorly into a predominantly withdrawn group. Similarly, a few activated schizophrenics may do nicely in a group of patients with psychoneurotic or personality disorders. Astrup (1961) feels that neurotic patients themselves may benefit in groups composed mainly of schizophrenics.

The distinction between withdrawn and activated patients is made on the basis of ability to function in a group, rather than on a diagnostic label. A withdrawn patient will often become activated during the course of group therapy. This, of course, is one of the treatment goals. He could then be transferred to another group, but in most instances it is best to leave him with his original group, where he can exert a positive effect on the other patients. On the other hand, putting an already activated patient into a predominantly withdrawn group can lead to difficulties. The activated patient may become bored or impatient with the slow pace and meager participation of the withdrawn members.

Another issue to be considered in the selection of patients is that of group balance. This is achieved by considering age, sex, race, education, assertiveness, expressiveness, and overt symptoms. A blend of different qualities among the group members is desirable. Good results can be achieved with an age spread of 15 to 20 years; however, adolescents should be considered in a separate category. Balance is easier to achieve in a group of activated patients or in a mixed neurotic-schizophrenic group. A withdrawn group, by its very nature, may be out of balance because most of the patients begin as passive, nonspontaneous people. This makes the therapist's job more difficult, especially when a group is beginning. After a group is doing well, it can absorb a quiet, withdrawn patient more successfully. Symptom considerations are also important. A group can usually deal with one or two paranoid individuals, but including more of them creates a difficult situation.

THE THERAPISTS

A group composed mainly of patients on medication (usually a predominantly withdrawn group) may function well at the beginning with the subject of medication as the major focus. In such a group, it is convenient to have a physician as a co-therapist. If a psychiatrist or other physician is not a co-therapist, then the patients receiving neuroleptic medication will have to be seen separately by the responsible physician at least once every 3 months.

In groups of activated schizophrenics or mixed groups of neurotics and activated schizophrenics, the focus on medication is much less common, and the need for physician involvement is thus less. An activated schizophrenic group may function much as a neurotic group does. Effective treatment teams for activated groups can come from a variety of disciplines; they can be psychologists, social workers, nurses, students, and other professionals or apprentices.

It is always important that supervision or consultation be available for treatment teams. Subtle aspects of group dynamics may not become apparent until the sessions are discussed with a supervisor or consultant. The supervisor should be an experienced group therapist from any of the several disciplines. If a majority of the patients are on medication, it is convenient to have a psychiatrist as supervisor.

The co-therapy team approach has several advantages. The therapists may interact with one another and thus provide a model of interpersonal relations for the patients. They provide useful support for one another during discouraging phases of the group's development; this is especially true when groups are just getting started. The team approach also provides a valuable opportunity for an inexperienced therapist to work with a more experienced one. But the therapists may, of course, be equals in experience.

A male-female team has the unique advantage of re-creating aspects of the parental roles in the group. Patients may exhibit patterns of relating to each therapist that can be interpreted or used as information during therapy.

There are no published studies comparing the effectiveness of single group therapists versus co-therapy teams, but good results can certainly be obtained by either approach. Teams are recommended if staffing permits, however, because of the advantages already cited.

The best training for group therapy with schizophrenics is supervised experience with individual schizophrenic patients and a period of apprenticeship as a co-therapist. Of course, the therapist or apprentice should be a mature, stable individual who can tolerate the stress of having to deal with chaotic thinking from all directions. Even relatively inexperienced therapists can get good results with schizophrenic patients in group therapy. What they lack in experience, they may make up in enthusiasm and optimism. The period of apprenticeship with an experienced group therapist and the availability of regular supervisory sessions are important, however. In evaluating the results of group therapy with predominantly withdrawn schizophrenics, supervised medical students (doing a prolonged elective in psychiatry) obtained results—i.e., improvement on ratings of their patients by independent observers—not significantly different from those of psychiatrists and psychiatric social workers.

An opposite finding regarding experience, however, was observed by Karon (1972). He found that experienced therapists generally used less medication and obtained better results. In Karon's study, comparing three different individual treatment approaches, there seemed to be a correlation between therapist experience and use of medication. When inexperienced trainees did not use medication, they obtained better results than their supervisors on some measures. Overall, the supervisors tended to produce more balanced improvement. Studies in the literature on the relationship between outcome of treatment with schizoprenics and the length of therapist experience are not in agreement, and more work on this issue is needed.

Practical Issues

SIZE OF GROUP

Various recommendations have been made regarding group size (Herschelman and Freundlich, 1970).

Clinical research indicates that withdrawn schizophrenics do well in groups of 8 to 12 persons. Activated patients seem to tolerate the stress of smaller groups, but this is more difficult for the withdrawn patients. Individual group members feel more pressure to speak up in smaller groups, and thus a withdrawn patient who cannot respond may simply drop out. Giant groups consisting of 20 to 40 patients and multiple therapists have been described (Herschelman and Freundlich, 1970), but these have generally been sessions with ward-meeting formats and with little evidence of group process.

FREQUENCY OF SESSIONS

Group sessions are usually held once a week, but good results with withdrawn patients have been obtained with sessions as infrequent as once a month. More frequent sessions are desirable but not always possible, due to staffing limitations. The less frequent the sessions, the more likely the sessions are to be focused on drugs and side effects. For withdrawn patients this may be useful (Isenberg et al., 1974; Payn, 1974), but with activated groups, the time is better spent on non-medication issues.

LENGTH OF SESSIONS

The duration of sessions is usually 60 minutes for withdrawn groups and 60 to 90 minutes for activated ones. It may be very difficult at first for therapists to spend a full 60 minutes with a withdrawn group. Having a co-therapist helps, and having structured activities, such as coffee making and cake baking, provides the patients with concrete topics of conversation (Masnik et al, 1971).

OPEN AND CLOSED GROUPS

It is usually convenient to have groups open ended. New members can be admitted as openings occur. The admitting process can be structured to meet the requirements of both mental health clinics and private practice situations. New patients can be interviewed at the time of referral, and a determination made as to whether any of the existing groups has an opening suitable for a particular patient.

Openings may occur because of termination due to graduation or dropout. In either case, the group should have time to deal with its feelings of separation from the former member before the new member is introduced. When a termination is known in advance, the group should have several sessions to discuss it with the departing member. The process of termination and of accepting new members is a vital one. It often evokes feelings from individuals previously thought to be flat.

An alternative system would be closed groups in which members start and terminate together. This enables the patients to experience termination simultaneously and to share their feelings. A problem in using this system for schizophrenics is the chronicity of the illness. It is likely that at least some of the group members will need continuing care after the group's termination. Even if the group disbands, therefore, some of the patients tend to remain attached to the therapist or clinic.

An interesting variant of the closed group was described by Melzer (1979). Hospitalized patients in a state mental hospital were started in a group together and, after 4 to 6 months of sessions, the entire group was discharged to the community together. In other words, the inpatient group became an outpatient group. Their living quarters were arranged to be in the same neighborhood, and the group continued to meet regularly after discharge. Results for the initial patients treated this way were good, but long-term follow-ups and comparison with control populations are not yet available. While this method presents many practical difficulties, it has much theoretical appeal. It would enable patients to develop a sense of trust and stability in the group prior to discharge and then maintain the same relationships after discharge. Chronic mental patients in the community are known to be quite vulnerable, particularly during the period immediately after leaving the hospital. It is difficult for them to start in a new group at this time, but continuity with the hospital group would be ideal.

Therapeutic Goals and Stages

A common-sense psychodynamic approach is recommended. Schizophrenics tend to have a basic mistrust of people. Problems in relationships produce increased stress for schizophrenic patients. Many have never learned the fundamentals of interpersonal relationships. If the therapist is an aloof, nondirective person, this will only frustrate the patient further. A down-to-earth approach with simple goals can eventually lead to a very complex objective: the development of trust.

The specific techniques employed in group therapy with schizophrenics depend in large measure on the background of the therapist, the setting, and the level of functioning of the group at that moment. Many of the techniques are identical to those employed in neurotic groups. Group process develops in stages (Forer, 1961), but there seems to be no generally agreed-upon sequence of group development. The common elements in the various schemes proposed seem to be: the development of communication; the development of trust; behavior changes within the group; and, finally, changes in the members' behavior outside the group.

PROMOTING INTERACTION

In general, the job of the therapist is to promote interaction among patients, who look to him for wisdom, guidance, and medication. Although various techniques may be used to encourage interaction, sensitivity techniques featuring touching and confrontation are generally not recommended; they may be too frightening for the average schizophrenic outpatient.

Bowers et al. (1974), however, have described the use of some nonverbal exercises that are not excessively provocative when used in a group whose members have begun to develop some trust in the therapist and in each other. Exercises that are focused on a here-and-now situation are selected. They are frequently designed to help a group member who is having difficulty in becoming aware of his feelings, even though they seem apparent to other members and therapists.

An example of nonverbal techniques for promoting interaction would be the rearrangement of chairs so that the members do not sit in the same pattern each week; a break in the pattern often causes a shift in communication and helps to get the group out of a rut. When two members are angry with one another but are not expressing their hostility, the following exercise may be employed (Bowers et al., 1974): The two members are instructed to face each other and clasp both hands palm to palm. At a signal from the therapist, both begin pushing. This often facilitates the verbal expression of anger in individuals who have had great trouble in even becoming aware of emotion.

Food is often an excellent means of stimulating interaction among withdrawn patients. Masnik et al. (1971) have described a technique called "Coffee and ..." that uses coffee and cookies to promote conversation. The clinic may supply the coffee, but the patients should be encouraged to bring in their own cakes and cookies. Something similar was independently described by Parras (1974). The "Coffee and ..." technique can be enlarged upon to provide an experience of sharing and pride. One group composed of withdrawn members who could not interact verbally was prompted to begin sharing a communal meal at the clinic. Each member was given responsibility for a different part of the meal: punch, fried chicken, salad, bread, dessert, coffee. At first, the therapist had to organize the patients, but later they did this themselves. They rotated the responsibilities, took pride in their own contribution of food, and began to show feeling for one another. Eventually, they were able to contribute verbally and discuss problems, instead of just food.

One can speculate theoretically about the need to gratify exaggerated oral-dependent strivings in regressed schizophrenics. But from a practical point of view, the concern is for a healthy social experience. When people interact in a group, whether verbally or through the sharing of food, they find the process easier the next time. One social interaction leads to another in a progressive fashion.

Medication can be another important focus for withdrawn patients. If one of the therapists is a physician, prescription writing may be an important part of a withdrawn group session (Payn, 1974). The medication ritual, including the discussion of side effects, may actually facilitate group interaction. Medication is something the patients share in common. It is a concrete, here-and-now subject. In turn, the group process may facilitate the taking of medication by exerting pressure on a reluctant member to take his medicine regularly. Occasionally, several patients at once rebel against medication. Usually, however, in a group of chronic withdrawn patients, one of the members points out what happened when he abruptly stopped medication in the past; the patients seem to develop a feeling of responsibility for one another. In most instances, the reluctant patient is convinced that he should continue with the treatment.

In groups that have been functioning for 6 months or more, there may be patients who have had their medication decreased or stopped because of clinical improvement. This may cause a problem because of competition among group members who think they, too, should be able to discontinue medication. Such issues should be dealt with openly in the group. The therapist may be tempted to give an intellectual explanation about such things as different rates of progress, but this approach would avert the opportunity to deal with the member's feelings about having to remain on daily medication. Discussion of feelings in this area is of dual importance. It provides the experience of appropriate emotional expression, something badly needed by schizophrenics, and, by providing a forum for ventilation, it also lessens the likelihood that the patient will abruptly discontinue his medication.

It should be emphasized that groups are not designed simply as a convenient mechanism to keep patients medicated. Actually, group therapy permits a lower dose of medication and perhaps a shorter period of neuroleptic treatment. This is a readily testable observation and should be the object of further research.

Medication is not often the main focus of activated schizophrenic groups, because fewer activated patients require maintenance medication, and because they are not restricted to such concrete items of discussion. Activated patients are capable of expressing emotion and gaining insight. Still, the therapist should not, as a rule, deliberately provoke anxiety. A therapist who is totally nondirective or almost completely silent during a session may create unnecessary tension and may lose the opportunity to actively direct the group in important areas. The manner of ending a session is also important. In a strict analytic group, the therapist may wish to stop at precisely the contracted minute. In a schizophrenic or mixed neurotic-schizophrenic group, however, he should be aware of the momentum of the session and not cut the members off abruptly. Going a few minutes overtime may be a good idea if it permits an important interaction to develop.

Verbal interaction

The importance of patient-to-patient interaction cannot be overemphasized; it is the immediate objective of group treatment. While nonverbal techniques, as described above, have their place, most of the therapist's efforts center upon verbal methods.

The go-around is a simple but time-tested method to get people to talk. The therapist asks each member to give his opinion on a particular subject. The subject may be something that has just occurred in the session, or it may relate to something in the members' personal lives. Schizophrenic patients and even some nonschizophrenics feel excessive pressure when their turn comes around. When a group is just beginning or when a new member enters an established group, the therapist must be aware of this pressure and try steering the go-arounds to noncontroversial matters. The easiest subjects are the most concrete: "How does the brand of coffee compare with the one we had last week?" More difficult are issues dealing with emotional or abstract matters: "How would you feel if you had just been disappointed the way John was?"

Often the go-around stimulates interaction among group members, who comment on each other's comments. Withdrawn patients, however, may refuse to respond at all or may simply say, "I don't know." Pressuring a withdrawn patient to commit himself usually fails. The therapist should move on to the next member without calling undue attention to the fact that the previous patient failed to contribute anything.

Not all therapists would approach withdrawn patients as actively as is suggested here. Ward (1974), for example, tells of letting a group sit in total silence for 50 minutes in order for the members to feel responsibility to be active on their own. Although this was described as a successful technique, most therapists would probably consider it extreme. On the other hand, when the therapist is too active, the responsibility to interact may be taken from the group members. All this touches on one of the differences of opinion when clinical experience, rather than research, must be used. Actual outcome studies comparing very active therapists with very passive ones are not available. Presumably, extremes in either direction are counterproductive.

Another technique to stimulate expression in schizophrenic groups is to organize a simplified form of psychodrama, a structured dialogue. The patients are first given a story in the form of a dialogue that they act out under the direction of the co-therapists. Later, they are given themes and asked to make up their own dialogue. The structured dialogue takes up only the first 15 minutes or so of the session. The group can then discuss the dialogue and the feelings expressed by the actors. Once warmed up, the group finds it easier to start discussion problems.

Role playing is another technique that can be borrowed from psychodrama. A patient may be asked to rehearse a difficult task, such as a job interview, during a group session. Another member will play the role of interviewer. The interview may be repeated with a third member playing the role of applicant, so the first patient can see how someone else might handle the situation. Similarly, other members can be asked to play the role of parents, siblings, spouse, or landlord, to name a few, and to aid in working out other problems. Role reversal, in which group members play one another, is usually difficult in predominantly withdrawn groups. Schizophrenics tend to be self-centered, and it is difficult for them to show interest in other people. It may be possible, however, if the therapist is sufficiently enthusiastic, particularly if a therapist models the behavior first. This technique may help greatly in working out angry conflicts within the group by enabling patients to see things from each other's point of view.

The above techniques require no special equipment or meeting room. Rearranging chairs may be helpful not only during role playing but at any time the group seems to be stuck in a set pattern. If special equipment, such as a tape recorder or a videotape system, is available, it can be quite useful in loosening up withdrawn members in a gentle way. Playing back segments of a meeting is a great stimulus for expression.

Group activities

Usually a predominantly activated schizophrenic group or a mixed group will acquire some group cohesion within 3 to 5 sessions and begin sharing feelings and dealing effectively with problems. In contrast, a withdrawn group may require much more of the therapist's efforts at promoting interaction. The use of a communal meal has been mentioned. Sometimes the group can be formed as part of a day hospital program, with interaction initial centering on games, workshops, parties, etc. Activities such as writing a card to a sick member or a constructive letter to the editor of a newspaper may help develop a sense of working together. Members may offer each other rides to group meetings and exchange telephone numbers for the purposes of supportive phone calls. Although there are potential problems with such out-of-group contact, these can be dealt with if members do not keep secrets from the rest or form subgroups within the main group.

PROMOTING AND MAINTAINING BEHAVIORAL CHANGES

In a sense, much of what has already been presented here constitutes behavior therapy. It has been predicated on the behaviorist notion that the experience of interaction can be reinforced in a protected group setting and that this will generalize to the outside world, facilitating social functioning. Formal behavior therapy utilizing token economies and food reinforcement has been shown to be useful for hospitalized patients. However, little has been written about the use of behavioral methods for outpatient schizophrenics.

Role-playing techniques can be a form of behavioral training. Bloomfield (1974), for example, has described their use in assertive training for schizophrenic outpatients. He notes that such patients—who tend to be excessively compliant, submissive, and socially inhibited—can be taught socially appropriate assertiveness in a group setting with the consequent release of pent-up hostility. Bloomfield finds chronic schizophrenic patients fully capable of behavior rehearsal, role playing, and role reversal with no negative effects.

Other behavior therapy principles may be used in group therapy. The therapist should always keep in mind the power of reinforcement and make a conscious effort to reward desirable behavior. Any show of emotion from a previously flat patient should be given much positive attention. When a patient begins to interact with other members for the first time, the therapist should always give reinforcement. This need not be a direct comment to the patient, praising him for the interaction. Rather, it can ostensibly be directed to another: "Ellen, John's comment to you really makes sense; have you ever looked at it that way before?" Such a response makes it more likely that John will repeat the behavior soon.

Reward is only one of the therapist's techniques for altering behavior. He can selectively ignore behavior that is regressive—e.g., inappropriate laughter, grossly loose associations, or obvious hallucinations. When the patient makes an appropriate comment, it should be promptly reinforced.

An exception to the nonreinforcement of inappropriate behavior would be the case of a patient who has been a rational member of the group for a number of sessions and whose behavior is suddenly and severely out of context. The therapist should try ot determine the factors that might be responsible for the regression. Are there stresses at home, on the job, in the group? Or is it a need for resumption or increase in medication?

Psychotic Deterioration

It is a psychiatric truism that the relapse rate for outpatient schizophrenics is quite high. Even with the best of aftercare, some patients will have repeated psychotic episodes. If the deterioration is a gradual process, it can be dealt with by group support, supplementary individual sessions, and increased medication. Sometimes a member who is doing poorly will simply drop out and turn up later in the hospital. If a member misses a few sessions and then comes to a group meeting in a grossly psychotic state, it requires a real effort on the part of the therapist to deal with the situation.

Psychotic behavior is a threat to the other members because of the frightening recollections it raises in them. It is also quite threatening to therapists, who worry that their entire group may suddenly become uncontrollably psychotic. However, this almost never happens. It upsets the group, though, and it may have to be discussed for several sessions thereafter. A therapist may feel guilty because of his own sense of failure in the treatment. The group members may share this guilty feeling at having failed to help the individual. If the therapist first recognizes his own feelings in the situation, he will be more successful in reassuring the disturbed patients.

Theoretical Considerations

That neuroleptic medications are effective in ameliorating the symptoms of schizophrenia, and that the quality of the treatment can be improved, at least in some patients, by psychosocial intervention (Hogarty et al., 1974) seem unarguable. If group psychotherapy does nothing more than permit a greater proportion of schizophrenic patients to remain drug free or on a low dosage, this achievement is worthwhile. The hypothesis of a group-neuroleptic drug synergism, however, is as yet unsupported by evidence from controlled studies.

Several theoretical reports have dealt with the psychodynamic theory of schizophrenic groups. Wolman, Slavson, and Alikakos discussed multiple transference, so to speak, among the group members spread the transference, so to speak, among the therapists and the other members of the group. Slavson further emphasizes the importance of confrontation, rather than exploration. One need not try to uncover unconscious drives in treating schizophrenics. The therapy should be oriented to the present reality. When schizophrenic patients are given a healthy group social experience, the therapist is fulfilling this goal.

Therapists with different backgrounds in psychodynamic theory may interpret group behavior in different ways. Thus, some of them emphasize the manifestations of ego weakness, some stress the transactions, and some are strict behaviorists. Good results have been obtained by therapists using vastly different theoretical rationales and even by therapists with little theoretical training beyond their supervised experience.

In using group therapy with schizophrenics, it is important to remember that the process of interaction is more important than the content, however rich the content may seem in material for analysis.

Prior to the discovery of effective pharmacological agents, seriously disturbed patients could disrupt a group. The stress of group interaction might have even precipitated deterioration in a fragile schizophrenic or manic-depressive patient. In recent years, however, group therapy and pharmacotherapy have been found to be a very effective combination. They appear to work synergistically, although data quantifying this interaction are difficult to obtain. Medication appears to permit patients to participate in group therapy. In turn, the group method promotes adherence to the medication regimen. The therapist is also able to titrate the dose more effectively, because the patient is observed during a variety of social interactions. Moreover, the group provides the patient with a social learning experience that can generalize to many other situations, and this aids in rehabilitation.

Affective Disorders

The use of lithium over the past decade has had a major impact on the rehabilitation of manic-depressive patients. Pharmacological leveling of their dramatic mood swings has enabled these people to have the potential to lead normal lives. However, lithium alone may not be enough.

Problems in living occur during the course of lithium maintenance, and patients may need to learn new adaptive patterns. Some patients remember certain aspects of their prelithium days with fondness, and idealize their previous ability to get charged up. Drug side effects, the nuisance of blood tests, fears of toxicity, fears of what family and friends think, fears of passing a defect on to children, and the identity crisis which may come with the realization that "my brain has a chemical imbalance"—all these thoughts and fears require ventilation, discussion, and sorting out.

Often, a busy lithium clinic is run on a strict medical model. Five to 15 minutes per visit may allow just enough time to check for side effects, dosage, and serum levels. Recently, it has been found that group therapy appears to be a helpful technique for dealing with the problems of bipolar patients. Homogeneous groups which consist only of lithium maintenance patients have been found to improve clinic efficiency, increase patient compliance, and enhance the rehabilitation of manic-depressive patients (Shakir et al., 1979; Ellenberg et al., 1980). Lithium patients can also participate successfully in heterogeneous groups. After mood swings are controlled, psychodynamic issues can be addressed in a group consisting primarily of neutrotics (Hawkins, 1978).

Controlled outcome studies of group therapy for affective disorders are not yet available. The use of group therapy for monopolar depressed patients has generally not been conducted in homogeneous groups.

References

Alden, A. R., Weddington, Jr., W. W., Jacobson, C., and Gianturco, D. T. Group aftercare for chronic schizophrenia. J. Clin. Psychiatry, *6:* 249, 1979.

Astrup, C. A note on clinical and experimental observations of the application of group therapy. Int. J. Group Psychother., *11:* 74, 1961.

Bloomfield, H. H. Assertive training in an outpatient group of chronic schizophrenics: A preliminary report. In *Annual Review of Behavioral Therapy, Theory and Practice.* C. M. Frank and G. T. Wilson, editors, vol. 2, p. 745. Brunner/Mazel, New York, 1974.

Bowers, P. F., Banquer, M., and Bloomfield, H. H. Utilization of nonverbal exercises in the group therapy of outpatient chronic schizophrenics. Int. J. Group Psychother., *24:* 13, 1974.

Claghorn, J. L., Johnston, E. E., Cook, T. H., and Itschner, L. Group therapy and maintenance treatment of schizophrenics. Arch. Gen. Psychiatry, *31:* 361, 1974.

Ellenberg, J., Salamon, I., and Meany, C. A lithium clinic in a community mental health center. Hosp. Community Psychiatry, *31:* 834, 1980.

Forer, B. R. Group psychotherapy with outpatient schizophrenics. Int. J. Psychother., *11:* 188, 1961.

Hawkins, D. M. Reactive affective cycles and lithium. J. Clin Psychiatry, *39:* 667, 1978.

Herschelman, P., and Freundlich, D. Group therapy with multiple therapists in a large group. Am. J. Psychiatry, *127:* 457, 1970.

Herz, M. I., Spitzerr, R. L., Gibbon, M., Greenspan, K., and Reibel, S. Individual versus group aftercare treatment. Am J. Psychiatry, *131:* 808, 1974.

Hogarty, G. E., Goldberg, S. C., Schooler, N. R., and Ulrich, R. F. Drug and sociotherapy in the aftercare of schizophrenic patients: Adjustment of non-relapsed patients. Arch. Gen. Psychiatry, *31:* 609, 1974.

Isenberg, P. L., Mahnke, M. W., and Shields, W. E. Medication groups for continuing care. Hosp. Community Psychiatry, *25:* 517, 1974.

Karon, B. P. The consequences of psychotherapy for schizophrenic patients. Psychother. Theory Res. Pract., *9:* 111, 1972.

Masnik, R., Bucci, L., Isenberg, D., and Normand, W. "Coffee and . . .": A way to treat the untreatable. Am. J. Psychiatry, *128:* 164, 1971.

Melzer, M. Group treatment to combat loneliness and mistrust in chronic schizophrenics. Hosp. Community Psychiatry, *30:* 19, 1979.

O'Brien, C. P., Hamm, K. B., Ray, B. A., Pierce, J. F., Luborsky, L., and Mintz, J. Group vs. individual psychotherapy with schizophrenics. Arch. Gen. Psychiatry, *27:* 474, 1972.

Parloff, M. B., and Dies, R. R. Group psychotherapy outcome research. Int. J. Group Psychother., *27:* 281, 1977.

Parras, A. The lounge: Treatment for chronic schizophrenics. Schizophrenia Bull., *10:* 93, 1974.

Payn, S. B. Reaching chronic schizophrenic patients. Int. J. Group Psychother., *24:* 25, 1974.

Prince, R. M., Ackerman, R. E., and Barksdale, B. S. Collaborative provision of aftercare services. Am. J. Psychiatry, *122:* 798, 1966.

Shakir, S. A., Volkmar, F. R., Bacon, S., and Pfefferbaum, A. Group psychotherapy as an adjunct to lithium maintenance. Am. J. Psychiatry, *136:* 4A, 1979.

Ward, J. T. The sounds of silence: Group psychotherapy with nonverbal patients. Perspect. Psychiatr. Care, *12:* 13, 1974.

C.5 Group Psychotherapy with Psychosomatically Ill Patients

AARON STEIN, M.D.

Introduction

Many conditions are usually designated as psychosomatic:

Duodenal ulcer, anorexia nervosa, obesity, certain types of ileitis and colitis, especially mucous colitis and ulcerative colitis, are commonly considered psychosomatic syndromes of the gastrointestinal system. In the cardiovascular system, the anginal syndrome, essential hypertension, coronary thrombosis or myocardial infarction, and certain cases of cerebral hemorrhage are considered to be psychosomatic. Other syndromes designated as psychosomatic are rheumatoid arthritis, hyperthyroidism, diabetes mellitus, obesity, myxedma, migraine, certain cases of anemia, many skin conditions (especially alopecia areata, pruritus, urticaria, and neurodermatitis), certain cases of conjunctivitis and blepharitis, certain types of rhinitis, some cases of bronchitis, and most cases of bronchial asthma. Most infections, many neoplasms, and many metabolic disorders should also be included in the category of psychosomatic illness.

This list, which includes all sorts of conditions affecting every system of the body, could be extended, but these are the disorders in which it is generally recognized at the present time that the psychic reaction of the individual, including the factors noted above, play a major etiological role.

While there has not been a very large number of papers describing the use of group therapy with psychosomatically ill patients, the literature has maintained a steady flow of papers related to this. In addition, the number of papers about the use of group therapy for physically ill patients—for example, cancer patients, cardiac patients, and renal dialysis patients—has increased in the past 10 years.

However, the most important development in the past 10 years has been a growth of literature describing clinical and laboratory research on conditions considered to be psychosomatic. The findings of these research reports confirm a basic theoretical concept stated in the original article on group therapy with psychosomatically ill patients. This is the concept that abnormal closeness to—and traumatic separation from—significant figures in the early development of the individual and the associated maturational difficulties lead to the development of both physical illness and psychosomatic illness, as well as significant psychopathological changes in individuals exposed to these maturational and developmental relationship traumas.

Developmental Factors

A reading of both the laboratory and the clinical research indicates that disturbances in the early relationship to the mother and the associated maturational difficulties lead to changes mediated through the brain and the central nervous system in all organ systems of the newly developing organism, whether animal or human. In addition, while acknowledging that a multiplicity of factors is involved in each traumatic incident to the newly developing organism, the literature also clearly states that, as a result of the early trauma, a pathological predisposition to abnormal types of reaction responses to internal and external environmental changes and stress does occur, including an organism's predisposition to the development of physical illness, psychosomatic illness, and psychological illness.

It is useful here to summarize the current views on the development of early object relations in the individual or organism. The same stages and processes that have been described for the human infant have also been described for various types of laboratory animals during their early developmental stages. An excellent summary of the present-day views in early object relationships has been given by Horner (1979).

At birth, the first stage, which has been designated the stage of normal autism, begins; it is a process of attachment to the mother and develops during the next 4 to 5 months into what is called the stage of normal symbiosis. In this early stage of development, failure of attachment to the mother leads to serious psychiatric illness in the human infant and a predisposition to the psychopathic type of personality. A secondary type of autism occurs in the autistic child as a result of failure of attachment to the mother and the organization of the symbiotic phase. (These early failures of attachment and development of normal symbiosis to the mother predispose the infant to psychosis—both schizophrenic and affective–in later life.)

After the developing infant has attached himself to the mother and entered the stage of normal symbiosis, which occurs about the age of 4 to 5 months and lasts for a year or more, a gradual process of developing differentiation from the mother occurs. During the period of a year or so, the process Mahler calls separation-individuation proceeds in the usual type of infant development. During this period, the infant begins to differentiate himself from his mother, tries out various perceptions and behavior to establish the difference between himself and his mother, prepares for the development of self and ego boundaries and completes separation from his mother in terms of establishing his own identity as an individual. Failure of this separation-individuation process leads to severe pathological predispositions and psychopathological difficulties.

The crucial time for the completion of the process of separation from the mother and the beginning of the establishment of the infant's own individuality—the separation-individuation phase of Mahler—is between 18 months and 3 years. During this time, the infant has accomplished developing cognitive abilities and increased skill at perception, learning, and the awareness of objects other than himself, beginning with the mother. He has also begun the process of being free to run about by himself and has learned to walk alone and upright, an accomplishment which brings much elation and a feeling of having some magic power. At this point, the infant begins to internalize some of his perceptive and cognitive functions in object differentiation and, if supported by the mother, he begins to function through an identification with the cognitive rationalizing abilities of the mother. At this point, in about 3 years, he should be able to be aware of himself and self-representation, both cognitively and affectively, and be aware of his own abilities as a person. He should also have the feeling of reliability and the awareness of others as objects—the so-called stage of object constancy of Mahler—beginning with the mother and going to other people. This phase—from 18 months to 3 years—during which the infant establishes identity and object constancy has been called the stage of rapprochement.

The period between 6 months and 18 months is the period when failure of the maturational development leads to pathological predispositions being set up, which result in various types of severe character disorder and personality impairment.

After 3 years, the difficulties that arise in the development of individuality have to do with failures in the attachment of satisfaction of object relationship, with resultant fixation of—or regression to—the various earlier phases of object relationship. These can be described in terms of drive satisfaction, such as fixation or regression.

All of this is connected with the development of the ego and the ability to master and control the tensions and frustrations associated with failure to satisfy certain drives or needs in relation to the object. When such deprivations and frustrations occur in the development of the individual, the greater the predisposition to severe psychopathology and, as noted above, the predisposition also for development of physical illness and psychosomatic illness.

Theoretical Considerations

Stemming from the faulty maturational development, the failure to establish effective object relationships and the persistence of the symbiotic relationship to a mother figure, there are resultant disturbed reactions and personality characteristics which make any form of therapy most difficult, especially psychotherapy. These disturbances may be summarized as follows:

First, and foremost, as a result of the persistence of an intense symbiotic relation to the mother figure, there is intense separation anxiety and depression, with, at times, overwhelming reactions to object loss. There are intense emotional needs and conflicts that are largely uncontrolled and are particularly related to all oral craving and anal-aggressive tendencies. Any type of deprivation or frustration results in tensions which are poorly tolerated; at times, these tensions are overwhelming, resulting in the mobilization of destructive drives and necessitating specific defense reactions to an extreme degree. Because of the failure of the self-differentiation and the weakness of the ego that occur in most of these patients, they have an inability to master and control these emotional reactions. Similarly, because of the intensely felt oral and aggressive drives and the splitting of objects and affects, a punitive archaic superego persists; this results in excessive unconscious guilt and marked ambivalence, with a fear of retaliation and punishment. The failure of separation-individuation leads further to a defective self-image, so that patients do not know their own identity, either sexually or as a person. They see themselves in an incomplete and distorted fashion. Defensive reactions are of the primitive type—denial, isolation, projection, and splitting of affect, object and self-image. Many of these patients develop reaction formations, such as submissiveness, obedience, and pseudoself-sufficiency, leading to rigid characterological and social roles in interaction and relationships. These patients also have little knowledge or awareness of their emotional reactions: They are emotional illiterates.

It is important to emphasize that the type of reactions and difficulties in object relations described above stem from predispositions that originated in some type of traumatic interference with the early development of these patients, specifically in their relationship to the mother figure or her surrogate. Various types of stress, internal and external, including psychosocial and environmental difficulties, result in the development of not only faulty behavior and reactions of the type described above, but also various types of illness.

This last point cannot be too strongly emphasized, since there is some beginning understanding of the fact that disturbances in early development lead to predispositions which, under environmental and psychosocial stress later in life, lead to illness. This illness may be physical illness—cardiovascular, renal, or cancer—or it may be psychosomatic—colitis, hypertension, asthma, or obesity—or it may be psychological or psychopathological—psychosis, character disorder, or neurosis.

The literature suggests that the use of psychotherapy with psychosomatically ill patients is extremely difficult (Karush et al., 1977). One of the major reasons for difficulty in treating such patients is the block to affective therapeutic contact with them, particularly in individual treatment. This stems from the nature of the transference they develop to the therapist, which tends to be a primitive regressive type, particularly in individual treatment. There is an intense drive to establish a symbiotic fusion with the individual therapist, and there is also a need for excessive dependency and a wish to control the therapist, the object of their dependency.

These same factors—the primitive regressive symbiotic type of transference to the therapist and the excessive emotional reactions accompanying this—which make individual psychotherapy with such patients difficult, constitute specific indications for the use of group psychotherapy with these patients. Of primary importance, is the fact that group therapy is useful in helping these patients enter into a psychotherapeutic relationship. This results from the nature of the relationships of the members of the group to the therapist and the relationships among the members themselves. These relationships are different in group therapy from those in individual therapy, and, as a result, they facilitate the establishment of the psychotherapeutic relationship and interaction.

The basic nature of the relationship to the therapist in group psychotherapy differs from that in individual therapy. It is lessened in intensity because the leader—the therapist—is shared by all the members of the group. The emotional ties among the members of the group consist largely of a number of identifications, the most important of which is their sharing of the same object—the therapist. This diffuses the intensity of the transference drives directed toward the therapist, making these less threatening and becoming experienced by the members of the group in a much more realistic fashion. Another important way in which the transference to the therapist in the group differs from that in individual therapy is that the need for gratification from the therapist as an object is made less intense by the presence of others, but also because, as a regression in the service of the ego, the therapist becomes less an object for gratification and more of an idealized figure with whom the members can identify.

A second important factor is a change in the relationship of the members to the therapist in the fact that the intensity of the drive toward the therapist for gratification of transference needs is deflected onto the other members of the group. This factor is extremely helpful in the treatment.

The importance of this change in the intensity and direction of the transference to the therapist in group therapy relates to its usefulness in dealing with the primitive symbiotic relationship that this type of patient tends to develop with all figures, especially the therapist, in any kind of treatment. The change in transference by a deflection of the transference drives onto other members of the group, and the regressive change from object relationship to identification with the therapist, enable the patient to begin the therapeutic work. The phase of separation-individuation is entered into, and the excessive, primitive, and ineffective ways of reacting and interacting begin to be dealt with, so as to establish more mature and effective relationships and reactions. In other words, the basic regressive difficulty—the persistence of a symbiotic relationship to the therapist as a dependency figure—is immediately dealt with as soon as the patient enters the group, with the change in relationship and the transference described above.

Dynamics

In the development of any group, particularly a therapy group, certain phases of development occur. Many writers have described these developmental phases which the group goes through in different ways. The relationship of these phases of development of the group are related to the regressive type of reaction previously noted, and to ambivalent deflection of the transference needs onto others that occur at the beginning of the group.

Essentially, the phases of group development are as follows:

First, there is an initial phase of dependency on the therapist in which each member tries to establish a special relationship with the group leader in order to satisfy and gratify his dependency needs. The members then seek gratification of their dependency needs, and the sicker type of patient may even seek some type of symbiotic-like fusion with the leader. In groups composed of severely ill patients, the development of the group does not go past its first initial dependency stage. This is true with groups of psychotic patients and groups of severely ill psychosomatic patients—severely ill not only from the standpoint of their illness, but in terms of their regressive personality make-up. In groups of severely ill patients who remain in this dependency stage of group development, the therapist has to assume certain roles and handle the therapeutic relationship in a specific way which will be described later.

In groups of less severely ill patients who have some ability to establish their own identity and maintain some independence in dealing with their life's situations and their illness, the group goes on to other phases. The ambivalence to the therapist is increased as he, by maintaining a group-centered attitude, frustrates the dependency needs of the members of the group. A rebellious anger then becomes clear toward the therapist, and is manifested by interaction among the patients. They turn away from the therapist and toward each other, using roles based on unconscious fantasies—transference fantasies—to interact with each other. They try to get each other to act out these roles. The presence of the other members of the group represents to them the availability of multiple transference objects who are realistically present, and who actually respond at first to each other in terms of the multiple transference role. The result is a here-and-now interaction that actually constitutes the therapeutic interaction of the group session and makes it readily available for the therapeutic work. The interactions frequently take the form of group-as-a-whole interactions in which the members cooperate with each other as acting out various transference conflicts and demands.

When the group-as-a-whole interaction occurs, each member contributes in his characteristic fashion. This is particularly true of pathological character traits and pathological defensive attitudes which become apparent very quickly. All these then become available for therapeutic scrutiny and discussion. A rigid patient with psychosomatic illness or physical illness, who is not aware of the nature and significance of his characteristic style of emotional reaction and interaction, is confronted by the others in the therapeutic discussion and is helped in this way to become aware of his reactions and to understand their significance. Pathological character traits such as masochistic attitudes, passive-aggressive attitudes, and excessively hysterical or aggressive attitudes are readily demonstrated and can be pointed out by other members of the group. Projection, denial, isolation, and other primitive types of defenses—including splitting of objects and affects in self-representation—can readily be seen in these interactions with the group and pointed out to them. This is an insight that is of special value to these emotionally illiterate patients.

It is in phase one, the dependency phase of the group, that the presence of a number of patients in the group and the need to share the therapist tend to lessen the intensity of this type of transference. Since the transference needs are also directed toward other members of the group and are shared by them, these intense transference dependency needs are directed toward many individuals, instead of just one. This provides an opportunity for the members to enter into psychotherapeutic relationships to examine the nature of these relationships, and gives them an opportunity to develop new relationships.

Several factors in group therapy help these regressed patients deal with their primitive, harsh, archaic superegos. One very important factor is the identification with the therapist as an idealized figure, even if there is ambivalence about this, and the identification with him during group psychotherapy enables the patients to substitute him as an ego ideal, instead of their own primitive, harsh superego. The patients' have increased awareness of emotional reactions and know that others also have intense forbidden feelings. The use of various kinds of spokesmen to express guilt-laden material enables the group members to deal with certain rigid superego attitudes much more readily in the group. The feeling that others share forbidden erotic and aggressive wishes and conflicts lessens the fear of retaliation, and, as one member acknowledges these conflicts, others are helped to speak of their own. When they can observe that the therapist and the other patients in the group will accept competitive, aggressive, demanding, envious, and generally dependent feelings, they can speak about them much more clearly and express them much more directly and effectively in the therapy than they were previously able to do, except through somatic symptoms.

The presence of a number of patients in the group, plus the fact that the patients themselves—through their identification with the therapist—assume the role of therapist in discussing each other's reactions, helps provide many stimuli for participation. The opportunity for increased interpersonal contact and the group's realistic nature and atmosphere help to lessen isolation and to strengthen contact with reality. The nature of the ties in the group, especially the identifications with each other, helps the members supply each other with a great deal of emotional support, and lessens their feeling of being different and alienated.

The majority of such patients also suffer identity disorders, often to an extreme degree and frequently with a great distortion of their masculine or feminine self-image. An example is the dread of colitis patients about having the operation of a colectomy and colostomy which may be lifesaving. Losing one's body integrity, to these patients, represents a castration fear more dreaded than death (Karush et al., 1977).

Of special importance in group therapy is the help and support that the patients give each other, resulting in an increased sense of self-esteem: They find that their opinions are valued by the others in the group. The amount of support helps them to develop more effective and more realistic ego functioning. This is also greatly helped by the members' acceptance of each other's suggestions on dealing effectively with the emotional and situational difficulties associated with the illness. These points are of particular importance in helping patients manage their illness (Stein and Weiner, 1978).

This last point is of particular importance, not only because the patients help each other in terms of developing more self-esteem and feelings of self-worth, but also because they help each other in more effective ego functioning, in dealing with the realities of their situation and their illness. In addition, by exposing pathological and ineffective character traits, they help each other to lessen pathological defenses which lead to unrealistic and ineffective coping with their situations and illness. This is a point which is of great value to patients who have to struggle with chronic or progressive illness, such as arthritis patients, hypertensives, and, particularly, cancer patients.

Finally, because of the presence of the group, the nature of the object relationships to the therapist and the other members changes, and enables the patients to go forward from the symbiotic type of relationship to a more mature type of relationship in both the therapy and their life situation. And, in the group, the interaction makes clear much more rapidly and effectively the pathological defenses and character traits that prevent the patients from dealing realistically with the difficulties in their situations, whether these difficulties stem from physical illness, psychosomatic illness or psychological illness. Helping each other to deal more effectively and realistically with the needs of their lives and their situations is the greatest help that group therapy can give to these patients. As noted before, this often makes group therapy the treatment of choice for many psychosomatically ill patients.

Case History

A clinical example of the use of group psychotherapy with a patient with somatic illness is presented below. This patient did not have a clear-cut psychosomatic disorder, such as peptic ulcer but, instead, showed a mixture of psychosomatic and psychological symptoms and physical illness.

The patient described cardiac and phobic symptoms. She was a 55-year-old woman who was referred for group therapy by her individual therapist after many years of individual therapy. She was referred because of symptoms of palpitations, anxiety, depression and a fear of speaking in groups, which interfered with some of her teaching and training activities as a health professional. She had been a stutterer, and the stuttering would recur during periods of anxiety.

The patient was the only child of a Viennese couple who had been put into a concentration camp and killed during the time of Hitler. She was about 15 at the time of the German occupation of Vienna and, at her parents' urging, she obtained a visa, after some 2 years delay, which enabled her to go to the United States. About a year after she came to America, her parents were killed in the concentration camp. She felt full of guilt about having left them, and blamed herself for their deaths.

Her father had been a traveling salesman in Europe and was away from home for long periods of time. He was a cripple, having one deformed foot. Her mother was an extremely anxious woman, overly concerned about the patient's health, and had periods of anxiety and depression whenever the father was away. These were so clearly evident that the patient remembered as a child her mother being terrified at being alone. The mother showed great anxiety while the father was away and would cling to the patient because of her anxiety. She projected fears of illness onto the child and took her frequently to doctors and clinics for various illnesses. The great anxiety of the mother during the periods of separation from the father made a deep impression upon the patient as a child, and the separation from the parents at the age of 16—which she tried to delay for two years—also left her with great anxiety.

When she was about 18, a few years before her marriage, she had an episode of rheumatic fever. While her heart did not seem to be affected then, she was under the care of a physician who was at great pains to see that she had adequate bed rest.

She entered professional training school and successfully completed her training course. She was considered an excellent worker and worked until she married a distant relative of her family, a man whom she considered somewhat inferior to her own intellectual capabilities. She continued her work until she became pregnant with her first child, who turned out to be deformed and who was transferred to another hospital shortly after his birth. In the other hospital, the child died, allegedly of pneumonia. But the patient always felt that, by consenting to have the child transferred and not taken home, she was responsible for the child's death. Several years later she had another child, a son, who grew up to be quite normal. However, from the very first, she was overly anxious about her son and repeated the pattern of her mother: she projected her extreme anxiety and guilt onto him.

Like her father, her husband was a salesman who frequently was away for weeks at a time on trips. During this time she repeated the anxiety and depression of her mother. In addition, she had periods of intense metrorrhagia and periods of extreme gastrointestinal upsets, marked by cramps and diarrhea. Again, all these symptoms made it difficult for her to leave the house.

She similarly repeated the pattern of her mother in that she would keep the son home and cling to him. Also, she would be overwhelmed by fears that she would bleed to death from excessive menstrual bleeding or have uncontrollable diarrhea and get sick and there would be nobody to take care of her. In addition, she had the usual phobic symptoms—a fear that, if she went to places where there were crowds or large open spaces, the people who could see her would lead to her being overwhelmed by an uncontrollable panic, and she would then have some kind of a physical or mental breakdown.

She continued under the care of the doctor who had treated her for rheumatic heart disease and was constantly fearful that she would have a heart attack or a stroke; as a result, she kept constantly running to doctors to check her cardiac status. She was constantly fearful that her own son would develop rheumatic fever and a heart condition.

As already noted, she had been in individual treatment with another therapist for many years. He had a deformed foot just like her father, and she had developed an attachment to him both as a father figure and as an erotic attachment. Despite this, he was able to help her pursue her work, overcome her guilt about the death of her first child,

and go on to get a postgraduate degree. However, for many years she was not making a great deal of progress, and the difficult transference—the ambivalent clinging attachment to him as a combined father and mother figure—made it clear that she needed another form of therapy. Consequently, she was referred for group therapy.

The patient was very fearful of entering the group, largely because she was afraid that she would stutter. From the first, her stuttering was minimal or absent. After a period when she was hesitant to participate in the group, she began to participate, at first hesitantly but then fairly actively. She was helped to participate because of the presence in the group of a man who had intense anxiety about having a heart attack; she was able to identify with him, share his anxiety, and express her own. A long period then followed, where she spoke only of her physical and psychosomatic symptoms in the group. The group at first was sympathetic and listened, but after awhile they began to express impatience and pointed out to her that all she talked about was her physical symptoms, and that she said very little or nothing about her emotional reactions. They pointed out how her anxiety when her husband was away was similar to what her mother had experienced when her father was away. Very slowly, the patient began to acknowledge some of her underlying anxiety, guilt, fear, rage, and depression in relation to the separation from the husband, who was, like her parents, someone whom she was afraid would leave and abandon her. At first, she was hesitant to speak in the group, because of her expressed fear of stuttering; however, the group confronted her repeatedly with the fact that she did not stutter. While at first she angrily denied this, gradually she began to speak more clearly and more aggressively in the group. She then went into a period where she actively participated and took leadership in the volunteer activities of a child guidance clinic in which she was interested. This event foreshadowed her taking a position of leadership in the group a year or so later.

The group also began to confront her with the fact that her physical complaints and her running to doctors were ways to avoid dealing with certain emotional conflicts in relationship to her ambivalent feelings about her husband, her son, and her own unresolved guilt and anger toward her parents and her previous therapist. She began to react to members of the group in terms of deflected transference, seeing one man as her husband, an anxious woman as her mother, and a somewhat aggressive exhibitionistic man as her father. Her attitude toward the therapist also began to change. For some time, she was very compliant, acting toward him as a father figure whom she was trying to please. Gradually, she began to complain about her lack of progress, the fact that he did not seem to treat her with special care and consideration, and that he did not seem to be concerned about her physical fears and complaints. After she had been in the group for some time, her complaints about her physical illnesses and her concern about having a heart condition lessened to a considerable degree. She then went for a physical examination, as part of her phobic complaints had been palpitations. When she explained this to the examining doctor, he did a sonogram, and it was found that she did have a defect in one of the cardiac valves a defect consistent with someone who had an episode of rheumatic fever. This frightened her, but she returned triumphantly to the group and to the therapist to point out that her complaints were based on something real, not something imaginary, as she felt the group and therapist had claimed.

At this point, she became much more aggressive and outspoken in the group and in her outside activities, despite her fear of something being wrong with her heart. In the midst of this, she had an episode of blindness in part of her right eye, which was attributed to a small stroke. Again, one of her fears was confirmed in reality. Again, her reaction was a triumphant one.

The group and the therapist acknowledged the validity of her fears, but they also continued to point out to her that she knew how to handle these things and that she could make a good adjustment and go ahead with whatever she wanted to do. The result was that, at first, she was very angry and argued with the group, but finally, she quite clearly accepted the idea that she could handle things, and went ahead to do exactly that. She worked out an excellent system of medical care with several doctors for her eye and for her cardiac conditions. She went ahead with her work in the clinic and became a chairman of one of the divisions. She was then able to go ahead and do something which she had not been able to do for many years—namely, begin to get some things for herself. Her husband had become prosperous in his business, so she was able to buy a vacation home for the summer. Also, she began to take some trips. Her projections of anxiety and ambivalence toward her son lessened, and she established a better relationship with him. She was also able to establish a better social life in relation to the people whom she met in the course of her volunteer work and was able to point with satisfaction to how well she had done the work, to her ability to speak publicly and clearly on various issues, and to the positive acknowledgment of others and her capability and the warmth and respect they had for her.

The group slowly but steadily enabled the patient to stop displacing her intense emotional conflicts onto physical complaints, and to become aware of her feelings and to begin to acknowledge them. The change in the relationship with the therapist enabled her to bring out the ambivalence and aggression that she had felt toward her previous therapist and her parents. When real physical illness appeared, her personality traits and her characterological approach to dealing with these things were so much improved that she was able to handle them in an adult, realistic and effective fashion.

All this stemmed from the group's confronting her with her excessive defenses against anger, anxiety, guilt, fear and depression, which in turn grew out of the fear of separation and illness which had occurred during her childhood. The group therapy—because of the identification with other people, a changed relationship with the therapist, the lessening of superego guilt and the stimulation to express feelings—enabled this patient to work out her conflicts to a very considerable extent.

Conclusion

The nature of psychosomatically ill patients' reactions and regressive behavior in individual relationships makes any kind of psychotherapy difficult. In group psychotherapy, from the very first, specific relationships are established that enable these patients to begin to deal with the traumatic effects of the early maturational difficulties. They are able to overcome their regressive fixation at the passive-symbiotic level and to enter into relationships with the leader of the group and the other patients that make the psychotherapy possible and effective. All this has been described above. It is useful, however, to repeat that the change in the nature of the relationship that occurs

as soon as the group is formed is the most important and useful factor that enables these patients to begin to overcome their regressive reactions and object relationships, and to move on to continue their development. They seem to establish new and more realistic relationships, become aware of the primitive nature of their emotional reactions, and correct these. They become able to see and correct their pathological traits. As was said many times by some of the pioneers of group psychotherapy, they find in the group the relationships and the support that was painfully interrupted in the early stage of their development.

Finally, it is clear that not only patients with so-called psychosomatic conditions but patients with physical illness and certainly patients with psychological illness as well, all tend to regress toward the primitive level of behavior and emotional difficulties and object relationship difficulties that are shown in the passive-symbiotic phase. This has been demonstrated through experience with group discussions and group therapy of patients, such as cancer patients, myocardial infarction patients, and patients with other physical illness. It has also become evident that group discussions are useful in the management of patients with physical illness, and that staff discussion groups that are carefully set up and utilized help the staff to more effectively manage patients with chronic and serious physical illness. This extension of the use of group therapeutic approaches has begun to be proven to be a rapid and effective way of dealing with regressive emotional and psychological symptoms resulting from physical illness. The usefulness of group psychotherapy and group therapeutic approaches with patients with psychosomatic illness and psychological illness has now been established. The specific features of group psychotherapy that help in the treatment and management of these three types of illness are the nature of the relationships in the group and the interactions that occur as a result of the establishment of these new relationships.

References

Ackerman, S. A., Manaker, B. A., and Cohen, M. I. Recent separation and the onset of peptic ulcer disease in older children and adolescents. Psychosom. Med., *43:* 305, 1981.

Banik, S. N., and Mendelson, M. A. Group psychotherapy with a paraplegic group, with an emphasis on specific problems of sexuality. Int. J. Group Psychother., *28:* 123, 1978.

Ford, C. Y., and Long, K. D. Group psychotherapy of somatizing patients. Psychother. Psychosom., *28:* 294, 1977.

Friedman, W. H., Jelly, E., and Jelly, P. Group therapy for psychosomatic patients. Psychosomatics, *20:* 674, 1979.

Hackett, T. P. Group therapy in cardiac rehabilitation. Cardiology, *62:* 75, 1977.

Horner, A. J. *Object Relations and the Developing Ego in Therapy.* Jason Aronson, New York, 1979.

Karush, A., Daniels, G. E., Flood, C., and O'Connor, J. F. *Chronic Ulcerative Colitis.* W. B. Saunders, Philadelphia, 1977.

Lindgren, L. F. Educative psychotherapeutic rehabilitation groups following myocardial infarction: A study of denial and depression in the post infarct patient. Diss. Abs. Int., *39:* 5566, 1979.

Lipowski, Z. J., Lipsitt, D. R., and Whybrow, D. C., editors. *Psychosomatic Medicine: Current Trends and Clinical Applications.* Oxford University Press, New York, 1977.

Mascia, A. Y., and Reiter, S. R. Group therapy in the rehabilitation of the severe chronic asthmatic child. J. Asthma. Res., *9:* 81, 1981.

Pinsky, J. J. Chronic intractable, benign pain: A syndrome and its treatment with intensive short-term group psychotherapy. J. Hum. Stress, *4:* 17, 1978.

Pohl, J. The clinic as an interpersonal field of dynamic psychiatric treatment of psychosomatic diseases. Am. J. Psychiatry, *31:* 190, 1979.

Rahe, R. H., Ward, H. W., and Hayes, V. Brief group therapy in myocardial infarction rehabilitation: Three-to-four-year follow-up of a controlled trial. Psychosom. Med., *41:* 229, 1979.

Roberts, J. P. The problems of group psychotherapy for psychosomatic patients. Psychother. Psychosom., *19:* 135, 1978.

Schwartz, L. H., Marcus, R., and Condon, R. Multidisciplinary group therapy for rheumatoid arthritis. Psychosomatics, *19:* 289, 1978.

Stein, A., and Wiener, S. Group therapy with medically ill patients. In *Psychotherapeutic Approaches in Medicine*, T. B. Karasu and R. I. Stenguller editors, p. 223. Grune & Stratton, New York, 1978.

Wollersheim, J. P. Effectiveness of group therapy based upon learning principles in the treatment of overweight women. J. Abnorm. Psychol., *76:* 462, 1970.

C.6 Group Psychotherapy with Substance Abusers and Alcoholics

JOYCE H. LOWINSON, M.D.

Introduction

In the 1960's, as heroin addiction was escalating, classical psychotherapeutic approaches to its treatment were recognized as being of limited value in controlling the problem, and new methods were sought. Therapists such as Nyswander attributed modest success in controlling actual drug use to psychoanalytic techniques, but these techniques failed to help the vast majority of patients alleviate their persistent narcotic craving. Along with the development of the new modalities, such as methadone maintenance and therapeutic communities, group therapy was and still is widely employed in certain treatment settings. It is also used widely in the treatment of alcoholism. In fact, Alcoholics Anonymous was a stimulus for the development of group approaches to the treatment of drug abuse.

Definition

The philosophical orientation of programs using group therapy may range from analytically oriented therapy—where the therapist, psychiatrist, or other trained professional plays a central role—to encounters directed by trained ex-addicts who reject the central role of professionals.

Group therapy may take place in an intramural setting, such as a hospital, rehabilitation center, therapeutic community, or prison; or in a community setting, such as a doctor's office, an ambulatory drug treatment program, counseling clinic, induction center for a therapeutic community, probation or parole center, hospital aftercare center; or in self-help groups such as Alcoholics Anonymous. According to Korn-

blith and Kaplan (1981), the rationale for using group therapy is "to utilize the constructive influence of positive peer group relations to improve the member's realistic capacity for adaptation."

Circumstances

The reasons for an addict's participation in group therapy and the degree to which this participation is voluntary are varied. Some addicts enter treatment because of the cumulative effect produced by social, family, legal, and financial pressures. Other addicts feel that their drug addiction stems from a psychological disorder for which they need treatment. Still others participate in group therapy because it is one of the conditions for being accepted into—or remaining in—a voluntary treatment program such as Synanon, Daytop Village, Odyssey House, or Phoenix House—and some methadone maintenance treatment programs.

Some patients in hospital situations attend group therapy because of boredom or the desire to ventilate complaints about the treatment facility or both. Readiness for ending treatment in some programs is based to a large degree on the extent of participation in group therapy and on the insight and growth that the patient has derived from this experience.

Abstinence-oriented Treatment Programs

Most abstinence-oriented treatment programs view heroin addiction as a manifestation of underlying character disorder. One of their principal goals is to effect the cessation of heroin use. Most group therapy programs are equally concerned with other types of behavioral change. A problem, related but separate, faced by practitioners of group therapy concerns the extent to which demands can be made of participants in groups. If the abstinence requirements for group participants are too lax, the unmotivated patient may thwart the therapeutic goal by using such defense mechanisms as superficial discussions or by complaining about the agency's regulations about drugs. If, on the other hand, the requirements are too stringent, a smaller number of addicts will remain in therapy.

The practitioners of classical group therapy hold that the addict seeks immediate gratification and demonstrates a low threshold of pain, frustration, depression, and anxiety. In 1961, Zucker noted that, in a group setting, peers may be more successful that the professional therapist in making the addict aware of his self-defeating, regressive behavior. This finding influenced the development of groups directed by ex-addicts. These groups are more concerned with the modification of present behavior and attitudes than with analysis of the patients' histories and the unconscious factors in their addiction.

Therapeutic Communities

Although therapeutic communites acknowledge that the movement developed from principles devised by Alcoholics Anonymous (its own roots going back to the Oxford Movement), a humanistic orientation toward treatment in psychiatric institutions that appeared—or reappeared—in the 1940's, and the work of Maxwell Jones in the early 1950's, it is generally agreed that this modality originated in 1958 with the founding of Synanon. Numerous programs based on the Synanon model have since been developed. A characteristic feature of the best of these programs is the provision of a sense of an extended family within which the patient, who in many cases has experienced an impaired family life, can grow emotionally. Many of these programs postulate that the addict is an immature person, a baby, who tends to blame others for his problems. Therefore, when the patient begins treatment, he starts at the lowest level, washing floors and dishes, because that is all the responsibility a child is capable of handling. He is constantly confronted about his behavior, and he takes instructions from a senior resident, who acts as a role model and as living proof that the new resident can succeed. In encounter therapy sessions, the patient's defenses are stripped away by heavy attack and ridicule, forcing him to be honest and more aware of his actions.

Because the residents do most of the work in a therapeutic community, the job structure takes the form of a sharply differentiated hierarchy in which each resident can theoretically work his way to the top. The structure is divided into separate departments, ranging from the kitchen and maintenance staff at the lowest level to the policy-making administrative position at the top. Each resident begins his career at the bottom, and his job performance is rated periodically If a resident wants a different job, he is expected to assert himself and make his wishes known to the community leaders.

Being shifted from job to job and having to wait for promotions are viewed as training designed to increase the patient's acceptance of change and frustration, which is considered as a sign of maturity and growth.

In addition to job promotions, rewards are given in the form of passes to leave the facility for short periods of time. In some programs, the possibility of becoming sexually involved with another resident or with a non-resident spouse is also construed as a reward.

Punishment may take the form of verbal reprimand, loss of pass privilege, job demotion, and such ridicule as having to wear diapers and a sign stating, "I am a baby." The ultimate punishment, short of expulsion from the community, is shaving of a resident's hair. This punishment is usually reserved for residents who steal or who leave the program and then return. Punishment must be accepted in good grace, as its acceptance by the resident is taken as a sign of maturity. Sometimes residents who are unfairly or severely punished leave the program.

DAYTOP VILLAGE

Daytop Village serves as a prototype for all other therapeutic communities, although many therapeutic communities have digressed in certain areas of philosophy or implementation of goals. Daytop was founded in 1963, financed by a National Institute of Mental Health grant given to the Brooklyn Supreme Court Probation Department. Originally called Daytop Lodge, it was founded by three men who had extensively studied the Synanon experience: Daniel Casriel, a psychiatrist; Monsignor William O'Brien, who still serves as Daytop's president; and David Deitch, a former director of Synanon. Later, the name of the program was changed from Daytop Lodge to Daytop Village, and entry requirements were modified to include heroin addicts who were not on probation but who wished to enter voluntarily. This program has widely proliferated and serves as a prototype for therapeutic communities throughout the Western world and in the Pacific. Daytop, like other therapeutic communities, accepts only the highly motivated addict who has demonstrated his desire for treatment. The addict must convince the intake worker, himself a former heroin addict, of his sincere desire to give up drugs. If necessary, the applicant is sent to a detoxification center prior to his admission to be detoxified.

Daytop, as well as many other therapeutic communities, receives public funds and is committed to returning the patient to the community. In actual fact, most therapeutic community programs like to retain some successful graduates with leadership potential as staff members to serve as role models and therapists for the new patients.

However, Daytop's philosophy is based on the necessity for successful re-entry into the community, a signal deviation from Dederich's goals at Synanon. Daytop has recently opened an ambulatory program in response to the needs of younger drug abusers who are able to remain in their homes and communities during treatment. Associated with this aspect of the program are weekly family therapy sessions, which appear to play a significant role in successful treatment outcome.

USE OF THERAPY

Encounter therapy

The universal therapeutic tool in these programs is the group encounter. Although some programs vary their approach in small details, a basic format for encounters remains standard.

A typical encounter group consists of 8 to 15 residents who may or may not be representative of the make-up of the program. Some groups are composed of residents who are within the same age range or at the same level of job responsibility or who have been in the program for about the same length of time. Other encounter groups are designed to deal with specific grievances between residents. If a resident has complained about another resident by placing a grievance slip in a special box, the person in charge of setting up the encounter groups will schedule the complainants and the accused for the same group. Participants in encounter groups may also be selected at random by picking out names from a shuffled card deck. Still other groups represent a cross-section of the population of the community.

The composition of an encounter group may vary from session to session, subjecting a resident to different experiences, attitudes, and viewpoints at each session. Or the population of a group may remain constant over a period of time. The needs of the participants determine the method used. Residents usually attend three encounter groups a week, and the length of a session generally ranges from 2 to 4 hours.

Unlike groups led by a psychiatrist or some other qualified professional who observes, guides, and interprets the behavior of the patient group, the therapeutic community encounter group does not have a fixed, formal leader. Usually, the group is loosely directed by a more experienced resident who is himself in treatment and who participates both as an equal in treatment and as a group leader. Often, encounter leaders emerge during the course of a session, and leadership may shift from person to person, depending on the nature of the problems discussed.

Physical violence is not tolerated. However, extreme verbal hostility involving screaming and cursing is permitted and may even be encouraged as a form of catharsis, since such behavior is prohibited outside of the encounter sessions. Screaming, crying, and cursing are also viewed as indicators of the degree to which feelings are being aroused, feelings that had previously been encapsulated by the use of drugs.

All group members are expected to participate during an encounter session. Those who do not participate voluntarily are challenged. The session leader or facilitator seeks maximal participation and tries to focus on problems that the group is not dealing with adequately.

Each participant is confronted individually for at least some part of a session and he is, in turn, expected to confront others. Members of an encounter group are confronted about their negative attitudes toward others and themselves, poor job performance, sloppiness, pro-drug attitudes, irresponsible behavior, immature sexual acting out, and general appearance. The group does not encourage rationalizing of negative behavior and probing of a psychoanalytic nature. The emphasis is on each member's responsibility for his daily behavior, which in the beginning is usually described as stupid, self-destructive, and immature but never as sick. The group helps the resident view himself and the consequences of his behavior with greater objectivity. The focus of the group is on day-to-day problems and interactions within the group. Secondary importance is assigned to past experiences, because they themselves were consequences of attitudes still currently held that need to be attacked and changed.

The participant is presented with a standard of behavior and is expected to act as if he were a mature adult. The fact that he may not feel mature is immaterial; he must act as if he were responsible, and he must obey without question the more experienced residents and staff members. At the start of treatment, it is not important for the resident to understand the rationale of the rules, since, like a young child, he would be unable to comprehend the rationale.

During encounter sessions, all participants are expected to make a commitment to change their behavior. This commitment must be carried over from the encounter group to everyday life within the community.

Techniques used to elicit responses during an encounter session may range from a simple questioning about what is bothering a participant to abrasive accusations and ridicule. The participant who is being confronted is expected to be completely honest in his responses about himself and his behavior. An effort is made to strip the patient of his defenses. Discussion of repressed or denied material may be particularly traumatic. As a result, the patients are frequently reduced to tears during the confrontation.

At the end of the encounter a conscious effort is made to build up the participants. Affection may be shown to an individual member as a sign of responsible concern, love, and acceptance. Friendly interaction is sought by serving coffee and snacks to the group.

One complaint often heard about professionals is that they are easily conned and made to feel sorry for their addict patients. It is assumed that ex-addicts, having been through the experience, are not fooled by the actions of their peers. Admission about one's faults and negative attitudes are usually not held against a person; instead, they are mainly regarded as indications of growth and maturity.

Tacit agreements known as contracts between participants to rationalize each other's behavior or attitudes in order to avoid the full impact of confrontation or assumption of responsibility for one's behavior are severely chastised. To grow, the participant must cope honestly with his behavior and attitudes.

Techniques to build verbal skills

Participation in encounter groups requires the possession of verbal skills, as does membership in therapeutic communities in general; those lacking such skills are at a disadvantage. The following are among the techniques used to assist the resident in acquiring these skills.

Morning meetings. Because the encounter sessions tend to be critical, the morning meeting is intended to start the day off in a friendly fashion. The residents give talks, sing, and recite poetry. A resident presents a thought for the day derived from literature, the classics, or religious texts. The group then analyzes the phrase or poem, searching out its meaning and application to life.

Word for the day. Each day a new word goes up on the bulletin board, and residents are required to learn its meaning and its message.

Speaking engagements. Residents go out into the community to explain the program and to solicit funds.

Grab-Bag Seminars. The residents pick topics out of a hat and give ad lib speeches on the topics selected.

Debates. Residents are arbitrarily assigned opposite sides in debates about controversial subjects. At the end of the debate, the participants are forced to switch sides and argue the other point of view.

Open House. Once a week the residents hold open house, when they are expected to communicate and interact socially with non-addicted visitors.

Extended encounter techniques

Another type of group technique is the probe. This extended encounter session may last from 12 to 18 hours. At Daytop Village, the probe is designed to deal with deep-rooted fears and anxieties that may not be resolved in shorter encounter sessions. An example would be anxiety resulting from repressed homosexual impulses. Probes are often more emotional than regular encounter sessions, and the participating group is smaller, with 2 staff members in charge.

At Odyssey House, probes are used for the purpose of judging whether an applicant can be fully accepted as a member of the community. The applicant has to assure the residents and the staff that he is fully committed to the philosophy of the program. The probes take place after the applicant has been in the therapeutic community for about 6 weeks.

Group meetings called "cop-outs" at Daytop Village and "house encounters" at Phoenix House are group sessions that involve all residents and staff members. Problems affecting the entire community are dealt with. Examples are failure to keep the community clean, extensive sexual acting out, secretive use of drugs within the community, and general misbehavior of cliques within the house. These problems are exposed and dealt with by the entire group. If these sessions fail, smaller motivation groups for those persons presenting serious problems may be established.

The most extended encounter group technique is the marathon, which can last for 30 or more continuous hours. The marathon is designed to enhance group solidarity and break down defenses that do not yield in regular encounters. Sears found that marathons have, indeed, enhanced lagging group solidarity and improved participation in groups. But marathons have been eliminated at Daytop Village, because the results obtained were minimal in relation to the time spent. Furthermore, since 15 or more people may participate in a marathon, the group can become unmanageable in a prolonged session.

Classical group therapy

Groups used in the treatment of addicts have varied in size and composition. Therapy groups at Central Islip State Hospital in New York have been composed exclusively of male patients. At New York's Baird House, a voluntary residential facility for female addicts, groups are made up exclusively of women. Groups at New York's Riverside Hospital (now closed) were composed of adolescents of both sexes. The Riverside patients were mixed with non-drug-using college students to determine whether the non-addicts would accept the addicts during the course of therapy.

Although a majority of the addicts relapsed into drug use after leaving therapy, they did form friendships with non-addicts as a result of contact within the groups. Laskowitz et al. describe a group composed of both male and female addicts at New York's Greenwich House, a community-based counseling center. Most of the group members were using drugs while in therapy, and the attrition rate of the group during a 6-month period was about 50 per cent due to re-arrests and hospitalizations. The Greenwich House group was directed by a team of male and female co-therapists, with a view toward the enhancement of transference relationships. In a variation of co-therapy developed at New York's Lincoln Hospital, each co-therapy team is composed of a professional and a nonprofessional.

Results

On the basis of current information, it appears that the group therapy and abstention-oriented therapeutic communities are unable to halt persistent heroin craving for a substantial number of addicts. Except for the information received from the aftercare division of the California Civil Commitment program, no discharges were followed up by the respective agencies. Until thorough research and impartial evaluations are completed, the effectiveness of therapeutic communities and group therapy per se remains in doubt as to successful treatment for the majority of hard-core heroin addicts. However, Winick observed that all therapeutic communities in a recent study which had a high success rate offered more individualized therapy than group therapy, and group was not valued very highly by patients in these programs.

Methadone Maintenance

The methadone maintenance treatment program has as its primary goal the productive social functioning of the addict in the community. This goal includes the voluntary retention of the patient in treatment; the increase in his socially productive behavior (employment and schooling); the cessation of criminal activity; and the curtailment of narcotic and other drug abuse, whether with heroin, amphetamine, sedatives, cocaine, or alcohol.

Acceptable social functioning as the principal goal of addiction treatment constituted a radical departure from the predominant abstinence orientation of other treatment programs.

Treatment success can be measured by comparing the patient's behavior before and after admission to the methadone program. In general, methadone patients reflect the wide spectrum of activities of the non-addicted population within the respective communities. Patients are assisted in coping with problems of everyday living, such as finding a job or a place to live. Some patients require assistance in reestablishing family ties that were broken as a result of addiction. Total dependence on the program for social relationships is not encouraged, and the patient is assisted in developing a life of his own.

Although methadone maintenance treatment relieves the craving for narcotics, some patients have personality problems that require intervention of a psychotherapeutic nature. Patients manifest their psychopathology in one or more of the following ways: (1) a continuing need for an altered state of consciousness achieved by the abuse of alcohol and other drugs; (2) an inability to adhere to a medical program, which manifests itself in multiple-drug abuse designed to obtain relief from anxiety or depression; (3) deviant behavior or drug abuse resulting from an inability to give up addict friends or criminal associations or both; (4) continuing antisocial or drug-using behavior as a result of conditioning acquired through years of drug abuse; and (5) the emergence of problems that were formerly masked by the narcotizing effects of heroin, particularly problems related to marriage, work, and other interpersonal relationships.

In rare cases, psychotic patients who used heroin as a tranquilizing agent may have a recurrence of symptoms when they give up heroin. These patients should be the target group for psychotherapy in the methadone program. How well they respond depends on the applicability of the treatment given and on the patient's motivation for entering the methadone program. Therapists who have worked with methadone patients in groups and in dyads report that the medication does not blunt or otherwise alter affect or anxiety level, perception, or mood. Furthermore, the resolution of the patient's psychiatric problems does not mean that his narcotic hunger will be abated if he is withdrawn from methadone.

Group Therapy and Treatment of Alcoholism

Alcoholism or alcohol abuse reportedly afflicts approximately 10 million Americans. The majority of these are not dropouts from society but, rather, people who consider themselves socially well adjusted, with normal family and work situations; their behavior thus creates a burden for those around them who depend on—and work with—them.

Many deny dependence on alcohol until the destructive effects of compulsive drinking have taken their toll in terms of serious disturbances in family relationships, trouble on the job, highway or other accidents, homicide, suicide, or a number of life-threatening health problems.

Indeed, we are only now beginning to recognize the seriousness of some of the medical problems caused by the chronic consumption of alcohol. Cirrhosis of the liver was, at one time, thought to result mainly from the malnutrition inevitably associated with alcoholism. Recent research indicates that the toxic action of alcohol itself causes this disease, the sixth most common cause of death in the United States (Lieber, 1981). Alcoholic pancreatitis, heart disease, and neurological disease are also common consequences of compulsive drinking. Since alcohol freely passes the placental barrier, alcohol consumption during pregnancy can have profound effects on the fetus. The fetal alcohol syndrome involves a number of major abnormalities, some of which are usually present and others which appear only sporadically.

Alcoholism is a chronic illness; thus, Alcoholics Anonymous, the organization which has had the most experience with its treatment, uses the term "recovering alcoholic," rather than "recovered alcoholic," for one who has successfully maintained abstinence, thereby acknowledging the ever-present possibility of relapse. It is a complex illness and involves psychological, physiological, and sociological components.

Psychological factors have been considered to be of primary importance in treating this illness. While no single personality structure can be said to characterize alcoholics, certain types of personality and character disorders are frequently seen in this population (Stein and Friedman, 1971). According to Knight, there are two classes of alcoholic patients: primary alcoholics, those with a severe character or even psychotic type of disorder, and secondary (symptomatic or reactive) alcoholics, who have developed a more integrated personality and character but who regress, under the impact of emotional conflicts, to earlier levels of development, especially when drinking heavily (Stein and Friedman, 1971). This distinction has important implications for treatment.

The alcoholic patient very often has experienced inconsistent parenting in infancy and childhood, has developed a rigid and harsh superego, and has turned aggressive, destructive drives inward. The primary alcoholic, as described by Feibel, is fixated at an "early infantile level with primitive and unstable defenses and inadequate reality-testing. There is an inability to withstand tensions associated with the lack of fulfillment, particularly of oral needs . . .. [These patients] show an inability to withstand frustration of any type of need" and are markedly narcissistic (Feibel, 1960).

Because it has been found that most alcoholics do not respond well to individual psychotherapy (Stein and Friedman, 1971) and because of the success of group approaches such as Alcoholics Anonymous, group therapy has been increasingly used in the treatment of alcoholics. Group therapy and, more recently, family therapy have become the treatments of choice for alcoholics.

There are many types of group approaches to the problems of the alcoholic; which are used depends on the needs of the patient and the type of facility in which he is being treated. Usually, a combination of approaches is used.

ANALYTIC GROUP PSYCHOTHERAPY

The purpose of this type of group therapy is the development of insight into personality problems by uncovering and dealing with the psychopathology of each group member. This is done through verbal communication and group interaction. Interpretations and analysis of resistance and unconscious conflicts are not as intensive as in individual therapy. Although group therapy has certain limitations when compared with individual therapy, it also has certain advantages. Some of its characteristics which facilitate the therapeutic process are listed by Slavson as "identification, mutual support, catalysis, dilution of transference, a multiplicity of targets for aggression, and the liberating recognition by patients that other people have problems similar to their own."

The alcoholic patient needs group confrontation and support in dealing with disturbances in interpersonal relationships. He or she is less threatened by transference that is more diffuse than is the case in a one-to-one relationship. Defense mechanisms—typically denial and projection—are recognized in other group members and, consequently, acknowledged in the patient's own behavior. The group setting also offers greater opportunity for reality testing.

The group can provide support and help in withstanding frustrations and stress and in maintaining sobriety. The most telling argument for use of group therapy over individual therapy with the alcoholic patient is the relative acceptability of this form of treatment to the patient. To be in treatment, the alcoholic must acknowledge his need for help, and he must refrain from drinking. Alcoholism, perhaps more than any other disease system, involves denial of the presence of the disease because the alcohol itself momentarily reduces tensions and anxieties, even though there is a rebound effect. In individual therapy, confrontation of the denial process may be more difficult than in a situation of group interaction with other alcoholics. Abstaining from alcohol may be reinforced by Antabuse, but the support and understanding of the other alcoholics in the group cannot be overestimated.

GROUP COUNSELING

This centers on issues and problems of a practical nature, and the counselor is actively involved in finding solutions. Attitudes and feelings may be explored, but underlying psychopathology is not exposed. An example of this kind of group is the coping skills group, employed as one of several group approaches to alcoholism and drug addiction at Ridgeview Institute in Atlanta, Georgia. The coping skills element focuses on developing non-chemical means of coping with life's problems that previously made the addict vulnerable to repeated chemical use. Coping skills covered in this element include basic communication skills, stress management, leisure planning, and goal setting.

ACTIVITY GROUPS

An activity group is organized around such activities as work, dance, music, crafts, or sports in order to develop social and leisure skills. Physical activity may be emphasized as a means of coping with stress, anxiety, and tension. Withdrawn, isolated patients can be activated and resocialized through activity groups, and the risks of unstructured time for the alcoholic are lessened.

FAMILY THERAPY

Recognition of the family's involvement in the alcoholic's drinking problem has only recently developed, possibly because of the persistent perception of alcoholism as a disease, the focus of which was the individual and for which the individual held no responsibility. Nevertheless, most treatment centers for alcoholism now include family therapy.

In this mode of treatment, the family system is the focus of therapy, rather than simply the achievement of sobriety for the alcoholic. Family therapy involves a variety of approaches, including concurrent therapy for alcoholics and spouses, conjoint family therapy, multiple couples group therapy, and multiple family therapy, but all family therapists believe that there is a relationship between individual and family psychopathology and that there are therapeutic benefits in seeing the family together.

Kaufman (1981) finds there are many parallels between the families of drug abusers and those of younger alcoholics;

in fact, many younger alcoholics are polydrug abusers. He had adapted Minuchin's structural theory (Minuchin, 1975) to the specific family problems of substance abusers, including elements of the systems, psychodynamic, communication, behavioral, and existential approaches. The therapeutic procedure he follows consists of joining, i.e., establishing rapport with each member of the family, and restructuring, which involves the changing of dysfunctional relationships. In joining, the therapist supports the family structures and follows their rules, adopting the family's own communication systems and style. In restructuring, the family's homeostasis is challenged through changes in the family's bonding and power alignments. Minuchin suggests several techniques for producing change, including "the contract, probing, actualization, marking boundaries, assigning tasks, utilizing symptoms, manipulating mood, and, lastly, support, education, and guidance." In practice, the therapist frequently moves between joining and restructuring.

The approach of family therapy to the problem of alcoholism offers the advantage of reaching the alcoholic and his family early, before irreparable damage is done and when the chance for recovery is greatest; and, since the entire family is changing together, recovery will be lasting (Hindman, 1976).

Reports based on clinical impressions generally indicate satisfaction with the effectiveness of family therapy in the treatment of alcoholic families. There have been few studies to determine the outcome of family therapy treatment, but those reviewed by Steinglass show positive results. However, control groups were usually absent, very few female alcoholics were included, and some outcome measures were highly subjective, so that basing conclusions as to the effectiveness of family therapy with alcoholics on these studies must be done with caution. It should be noted also that these studies were done with intact families from the middle and upper classes.

Alcoholics Anonymous and Al-anon

These two self-help organizations are frequently recommended by therapists as adjuncts to individual therapy or group therapy of other kinds. Alcoholics Anonymous (AA) may be the single most effective means of helping alcoholics to achieve and maintain sobriety. It is unfortunate that there has been little scientific evaluation of its effectiveness in treating alcoholics to support the impression of its efficacy. It is estimated that there are, in the United States alone, 1½ million individuals associated with AA.

Both AA and Al-Anon adhere to the concept of alcoholism as a disease and perceive the alcoholic as the helpless victim. Despite this focus on the individual, however, Al-Anon appears to be guided by at least some of the principles upon which family therapy is based.

The goal of the alcoholic as he or she enters an AA group is to achieve and maintain abstinence from drinking through support of a sponsor and the group—which shares its "hope, strength and experience"—and a "higher power—God, as we understand Him." By admitting one is powerless over alcohol, strength from external sources and from the unconscious apparently become operative.

The new member learns new ways of coping; for example, he or she deals with problems "one day at a time," this being one of many slogans available as aids in times of weakness. The new member is encouraged to attend as many meetings as possible—one a day is not unusual initially—and to communicate by telephone with one's sponsor and other members at least once a day and in times of stress. Meetings offer the structure necessary for individuals whose lives are out of control. They begin and end on time. Cross-talk is not permitted, so that the entire group remains involved, and everyone has a chance to contribute. The 12 steps, an important part of AA's operational philosophy, are often the basis of discussion. And, as the individual begins to recover, more and more of his or her time is devoted to helping other members in their recovery efforts. This is held to be of special therapeutic value to oneself, as well as to the recipient.

Al-Anon family groups are composed of spouses, children, and close relatives of alcoholics who are usually, but not necessarily, AA members. The meetings follow the AA format, and the program has much the same structure and function as that of AA. Family members are expected to adopt a position of loving detachment with respect to the alcoholic family member. With this emotional disengagement, each individual is free to deal with his or her own problems.

AA is viewed as the first major self-help recovery program for alcoholism. The program has been expanded to include other addictions as well. It has been considered to be the prototype of the self-help movements that have proliferated in the form of therapeutic communities for drug abusers. A basic tenet is that, while professional therapies are not rejected, nothing can substitute for the understanding and help of others who have suffered the same problems.

References

Collier, W. V. *An Evaluation Report on the Therapeutic Program of Daytop Village, Inc.* Daytop Village, New York, 1970.

Davis, D. I., Berenson, D., Steinglass, P., and Davis, S. The adaptive consequences of drinking. Psychiatry, *37:* 209, 1974.

Feibel, C. The archaic personality structure of alcoholics and its indications for group therapy. Int. J. Group Psychother., *10:* 39, 1960.

Finnegan, L. P. The effects of narcotics and alcohol on pregnancy and the newborn. Ann. N. Y. Acad. Sci., *362:* 136, 1981.

Hindman, M. Family therapy in alcoholism. Alcohol Health Res. World, Fall 1976.

Kaufman, E. Family therapy; a treatment approach with substance abusers. In *Substance Abuse: Clinical Problems and Perspectives,* J. Lowinson and P. Ruiz, editors. Williams & Wilkins, Baltimore, 1981.

Kornblith, A. B., and Kaplan, S. R. Group approaches in drug treatment programs. In *Substance Abuse: Clinical Problems and Perspectives,* J. Lowinson and P. Ruiz, editors, p. 449. Williams & Wilkins, Baltimore, 1981.

Lieber, C. S., Alcoholism: Medical complications. Ann. N. Y. Acad. Sci., *362:* 132, 1981.

Minuchin, S. *Families and Family Therapy,* Harvard University Press, Cambridge, MA, 1975.

Rosenthal, M. S., and Blase, D. V. Phoenix Houses: Therapeutic communities for drug addicts. Hosp. Community Psychiatry, *20:* 27, 1969.

Slavson, S. R. *Analytic Group Psychotherapy with Children, Adolescents and Adults.* Columbia University Press, New York, 1950.

Stein, A., and Friedman, E. Group therapy with alcoholics. In *Comprehensive Group Psychotherapy,* H. I., Kaplan and B. J. Sadock, editors, p. 499. Williams & Wilkins, Baltimore, 1971.

Stuart, R. B. Behavioral contracting within the families of delinquents. J. Behav. Ther. Exp. Psychiatry, *2:* 1, 1971.

Zucker, A. H. Group psychotherapy and the nature of drug addiction. Int. J. Psychother., *11:* 209, 1961.

C.7 Group Psychotherapy with Personality Disorders

FERN J. CRAMER AZIMA, Ph.D.

Definition

As outlined in the American Psychiatric Association's *Diagnostic and Statistical Manual of Mental Disorders* (1980), personality disorders are diagnosed only when personality traits become significantly maladaptive as to impair social or occupational functioning and constitute subjective distress. The roots of the personality disorder commence in early childhood and are usually first acknowledged in adolescence and young adulthood, and they appear to wane in middle and old age. The individual with repetitive ego-syntonic personality patterns rarely seeks treatment or becomes hospitalized until he becomes acutely anxious or depressed. The complications that bring such an individual into treatment include a neurotic or psychotic reaction to a catastrophic loss, a significant failure, abandonment, involvement with the law, alcoholism, or drug abuse. The DSM-III (1980) classification method permits the parallel coding of possible neurotic or psychotic disorders on axis I and the presence of personality disorder on axis II.

The clinician may now diagnose one or more specific personality disorders if the criteria are sufficient for separate codings. DSM-III presently subdivides personality disorders into three clusters—cluster 1: paranoid, schizoid, and schizotypal; cluster 2: histrionic, narcissistic, antisocial, and borderline; and cluster 3: avoidance, dependent, compulsive, and passive-aggressive.

Efficacy

Group psychotherapy appears to be the treatment of choice for most personality disorders, especially when the individual is oblivious to his maladaptive behavior and the degree to which it irritates or distances others. Alone, he is usually content, and in a dyadic relationship he is more able to evade, rationalize, or project. In the ongoing group context, the individual is actively confronted, and his character pattern is unfolded in the myriad interactions with other personalities who may recognize and identify with similar behavior patterns. Unlike the two-person therapy, where the introjects are slowly brought into consciousness, in the group each member—or parts of each member—become the projected introjects, and the ensuing communications may be symbolically to the father, mother, sister, brother, lover, etc. The intensive verbal and nonverbal interchange quickly unmasks the repetitive maladaptive personality traits. Frequently, it is the peers and not the therapist who are able to confront and retaliate against the narcissistic exhibitionist, the dramatic histrionic, the overclinging complainer, or the manipulator. Ego styles alter quickly in the presence of others, and the therapist is alert to spotting the disparity between private and public selves of the patient and of himself. Only when self-disclosure is acknowledged by the individual has the actual therapy begun, and this process is accelerated in the group, since denial, evasion, and rationalization are more difficult. Group pressure and conformity are powerful weapons to institute change, especially in the presence of a therapist who can be both an empathic ally for one's hurt and an active confronter of long-held deviant pathological patterns.

HETEROGENEOUS VERSUS HOMOGENEOUS GROUP

In most instances there is general agreement that heterogeneous groups are preferrable and that personality disorders should be intermingled with other neurotic and psychosomatic disorders. There are exceptions to this rule, as in treatment of delinquents and prisoners.

Under close examination, the concept of homogeneity is of less importance than the actual personality style and ego strength of the individuals who participate in the group. For example, two antisocial or two paranoid persons are never exactly alike in terms of level of ego impairment, degree of maturity, and individual ability to accept a therapeutic commitment.

Further, within the group matrix the alliances and support for some members and not others reposition the member into more powerful or more vulnerable positions. Two

equally talkative or silent members outside of the group, when faced with each other in the group, reciprocate and compete in unexpected ways, and one member must lower his talking rate. When his rival is absent, the member likely becomes more dominant and returns to his more usual personality style.

THERAPEUTIC ALLIANCE

Since individuals with personality disorders often have little motivation or understanding of their need for change, the problem of promoting a therapeutic alliance is of paramount importance. Glatzer (1978) utilized the concept of the working alliance to refer to "the healthy, realistic collaboration between the patient and his therapist and between the patient and other group patients in working therapeutically." Glatzer also postulated that the group process accelerated the working alliance of all members and was especially useful to borderline, narcissistic, and impulse-ridden patients whose fragile ego resources were supported to form the necessary kind of object relationships to establish and continue a working alliance.

The processes anterior to the formation of a healthy therapeutic alliance are especially difficult for these patients, for they possess little capacity to relate to others and are insufficiently self-critical. How to promote these capacities is the core of the treatment. There are a variety of descriptive theoretical models, and the decision which to use and apply should be congruent with the therapist's own philosophy and the nature of the patient's disorder. The relative roles of confrontation and empathy and their timing appear to be of central importance.

Battegay (1977) states that accelerating methods which intensify the emotional experience by more direct confrontation may be counterindicated in ego-weak patients. Stone and Whitman (1977) following Kohut's position, state that the therapist's "nonjudgmental acceptance of the patient's needs to idealize either the leader or the group, and to receive recognition and admiration also provides a theoretical basis for soothing and empathic intervention." Too early a confrontation or too vigorous an attempt to change a deviant personality pattern may result in rebellious denial and flight from the group. On the other hand, a continuance of unconditional empathy devoid of confrontation is likely to be equally futile.

Azima (1972) proposed the early alliance with the resistance, acting out, or the symptom. The therapist acknowledges, accepts empathically the need for the deviant pattern (at the present time), and does not make superego sanctions. In a way, the defense and underlying conflict are confronted; but this is a supportive, tolerant, and respectful way that does not threaten the individual or the group with the expected ridicule and chastisement. The stage is then set for collaborative working through, which, if successful, leads to the surrender of the entrenched defective personality traits.

COUNTERTRANSFERENCE

Acknowledgment of the therapist's evoked countertransference is the most direct and personal guide for the blocks and problems that occur in therapy. In group therapy, the complexity of response to a group of people is infinitely greater, and it takes considerable skill to decipher to what person or persons, to what group theme, and to what suggested dangers the therapist is being directed. Countertransference, reactions of despair, forgetting names or a session, feelings of rage, envy, and somatic reactions are hard to avoid, while overpositive feelings of grandiosity and erotic attraction are much more difficult to detect. The group members' critical response to the sporadic inappropriate therapist's behavior (verbal or nonverbal, slips of the tongue, blushing, stammering, etc.) must be accepted, without the usual rebuttal that they are the member's projection. The narcissistic, borderline, and histrionic personality disorders are much more confronting of the therapist than the guilt-ridden neurotic.

Specific Personality Disorders

PARANOID PERSONALITY

The major diagnostic characteristics of the paranoid are: (1) pervasive and unwarranted suspiciousness and mistrust of people, (2) hypersensitivity, and (3) restricted affectivity. Sadock states that, when the illness is not oversevere and there is no evidence of delusions, the paranoid patient may be more amenable to group than individual therapy. Suspicious projections are easily spotted by various members, and, when there is a group consensus, a group-as-a-whole interpretation has a forceful impact on the paranoid. However, Horwitz (1977), posited that paranoid features are a poor prognostic factor of good outcome.

The possible acceptance of a paranoid personality into a group will likely depend upon the composition of the group, the timing of the introduction into the group process, and the therapist's self-confidence and the match with his own personality. A paranoid patient may function well in a strong group whose members can tolerate dissonance, who do not enter into too vigorous confrontation or scapegoating, and where there are some members sympathetic to his feelings of mistrust. It is particularly difficult to introduce a cold, suspicious individual in an ongoing group that is in the midst of active confrontation. A new paranoid member remarked: "I'm getting out of here, you are all more suspicious than I."

In addition to the group's consensual validation, a forceful weapon for initiating change, a paranoid usually becomes less defensive when he is able to develop at least one friendship bond and does not have the feeling that "everyone is against him." Often it is the therapist who must ally with this patient in the early stages, to bring him under his umbrella of protection. A useful procedure is to bring two new members at a time into the group. In this way, there is the ready-made possibility of a positive dyad formation and less likelihood of group confrontation. Countertransference reactions in the therapist to the paranoid are likely to include feelings of irritability, anger, inattentiveness, hypervigilance, and many nonverbal behavioral signals to other group members of his helplessness and his need for protection. Oversilence by the therapist may provoke the membership to act out his unexpressed rage.

Cognizance of such countertransference reactions and group crescendos should signal the therapist that

he has now assumed that position of vulnerability that forces new understanding. These intense group crescendos cause a type of disequilibrium that breaks old homeostatic patterns and calls for new coping behaviors.

SCHIZOID PERSONALITY

The major DSM-III diagnostic criteria for the schizoid personality include: (1) emotional coldness and an absence of warm, tender feelings for others; (2) indifference to praise or criticism; and (3) lack of close friendships or family ties.

These individuals appear remote, detached, and uninterested in their social surroundings. They appear to live in an alienated dream world, seem unmotivated, dull, and passive. Precisely because of these asocial characteristics, they are prime candidates for a therapy group, provided they can be sufficiently motivated.

In interviewing the schizoid person, it is important to gain not only the relevant information but to judge the degree of affect and rapport. Subtle provocative statements may be used as a frustrating technique to assess the schizoid's capacity to verbalize and cope with stress. Knowledge of the patient's fantasies, dreams, sense of humor, personal diaries, art, etc., are important ways to learn about hidden conflictual material that the patient may not be capable of divulging.

The group matrix is precisely oriented to socialization and new parenting. Many of these patients profit from simply the exposure to other people on a consistent basis. They become more comfortable and less estranged. Attention to the decoding of facial and body language—such as blushing, lack of eye contact, rocking, and teeth gnashing—are ways that the schizoid soon learns from others how he communicates. Because of the schizoid's emptiness and lack of involvement, the therapist and group may similarly shut him out. By coincidence, the silent schizoid and passive personalities at times are seen as co-therapists because of their reflective manner. The silent member may also provoke the group and the therapist into efforts to get him to talk and self-disclose. "Ganging-up" may be fostered by the therapist over countertransference. A member is at times kept silent by the group when it is recognized that, each time he talks, he is enraged, bizarre, or inappropriate. A therapist with countertransference problems related to silence, activity, and passivity may alternatively become overaggressive or give no signals of communication to the shy, withdrawn member. It is also apparent that some inactive, silent members may be seen as welcome relief from the monopolistic, narcissistic, or histrionic personality type.

SCHIZOTYPAL PERSONALITY

The schizotype is a new classification intermediate between schizoid personality disorder and schizophrenia. The schizotype is more acutely disturbed than the schizoid and manifests oddities in thinking, perception, and verbal and social communication. The disturbances in cognition may include magical thinking, ideas of reference, or paranoid ideation. In the area of perception, there may be evidence of illusions, depersonalization, and derealization.

Speech may be vague and peculiar, words used inappropriately, and thoughts poorly articulated. Ability to relate to others is minimal, and there is evidence of social isolation. Contact with reality is preserved and, although there may be transitory psychotic or borderline intervals, the criteria for schizophrenia are not met.

Group therapy is indicated for the schizotype, as explicated for the schizoid, with counterindication when the disorder is very severe and when the peculiarities listed above verge on the bizarre and may be difficult for group members to tolerate. Depending on the strength of the group and the acceptance and guidance by the therapist, such patients often do well and become much more coherent.

An example of such a patient was a withdrawn, late adolescent who sat hunched over and rocked for most of the sessions. Joseph was largely silent, and his mutterings were impossible to comprehend and were mainly related to his rabbinical studies. The therapist's acceptance, support, and friendliness influenced other group members. When Joseph blushed one day, another group member spotted this and guessed his interest in a pretty girl. Through this provocative confrontation by a peer, Joseph gradually found some words and began to have eye contact. On one particular day, as he reached for his tiny Bible, another member quipped: "I bet you like to read and look at other books besides this one." The patient blushed crimson, and the group with good humor teased him into an explanation. He told them that he did read girly magazines and hid them under his mattress from his religious parents. During the following sessions, he revealed that he had been apprehended for voyeurism and that he could not prevent himself from sadistic sexual play with his dog.

Over a 2-year period, this 18-year-old made some dramatic changes. He was able to return to school, made an important friend, and was more readily accepted by his peers. At times, such a pathological member can function in a group when there is sufficient understanding, acceptance, and kindness prior to confrontation.

HISTRIONIC PERSONALITY

The essential diagnostic features of this category, formerly termed hysterical personality, are the presence of overly dramatic, volatile reactions and disturbance in the capacity to relate effectively to others. Initially, this personality appears charming, friendly, and sincere and is usually quickly chosen as a group candidate. Their behavior in group is apt to fluctuate dramatically, and they are prone to overexaggerate, complain, and show fits of temper. They are often fickle in their loyalties to group members, exchanging one ally for another simply to maintain a prominent image. They crave the limelight and enter into active rivalry with others, including the therapist.

The histrionic personality appears to be similar to the help-rejecting complainer (HRC) described by Berger and Rosenbaum (1967). These authors outline the frustration in dealing with these patients whose unconscious desires were to defeat the therapist and destroy the group. Yalom (1975) went as far as to say: "The help-rejecting complainer is an extraordinarily difficult and unrewarding task. If possible such patients should not be included in a therapy group."

More optimistically, Peters and Grunebaum (1977) present different techniques to cope with HRC's, and Bodganoff and Elbaum (1978) explicate the ways in which "role lock" develops in the group with character disorders and offer possible strategies that are helpful in disengaging these habitual reciprocal patterns. Stone and Whitman classify the HRC as a narcissistic disorder and apply the empathic, supportive model of Kohut to their treatment interventions. In all, the modification of techniques, an analysis of the defense, and an unmasking of the basic dynamics are essential to work through these problems.

It is interesting to note that nurses, medical students, and residents complain bitterly about the hysterical patient. They often cannot identify them as patients who are sick. They are easily seduced, then rejected, and thereafter commence a mutual competition and rejection pattern. Aside from these pitfalls, the dramatic, exploiting, monopolist and the victimized HRC are extremely useful group participants. They provide energy, activity, and a range of affects. They can be counted upon to re-enact and relieve past memories, and their seductive charms—although devious—act forcefully in the early stages to attract and bewitch the passive schizoid members.

Even though these patients are most problematic, a therapist should not encourage the group into silencing or rejecting these activists but, rather, should encourage them to perceive that their overtalkativeness, endless complaints, and inability to get satisfaction result in greater isolation and unhappiness because often people cannot relate meaningfully to them.

NARCISSISTIC PERSONALITY

The narcissistic and borderline personality disorders have received much attention in the last decade. DSM-III describes the narcissistic personality disorder as evidencing: (1) a grandiose sense of self-importance or uniqueness, (2) preoccupation with fantasies of unlimited success, (3) exhibitionism, and (4) disturbances in interpersonal relationships. The last may include a sense of overentitlement, interpersonal exploitativeness, alternating overidealization and devaluation, and a lack of empathy. There is some overlap with the histrionic personality, and the statements of the previous section apply in most instances here; however, the degree of disturbance and the outcome prognosis are much worse. Group treatment for the narcissistic and borderline presumably is difficult, at times hazardous, and often counterindicated unless specific precautions are made. In general, there is agreement that combined group and individual therapy may be the treatment of choice, although there is a difference of opinion as to whether the therapies should be concurrent or sequential.

Theoretical and treatment approaches include the more classical Freudian position (Spotnitz, 1957). Glatzer, although more traditionally using Freudian terminology, integrated some Kleinian concepts. Horwitz (1977) and Genzarain, among others, apply Kleinian object relationship concept, while the latter is an advocate of general systems application. In the last decade, group therapists working with the narcissistic and borderline type, have more or less become advocates of either the Kernberg or Kohut (1972) position. Some, including Wong (1979), have attempted an integration of these two approaches. Wong (1979) compares the theoretical positions of Kernberg and Kohut vis-à-vis the definition, development, and group treatment of narcissism. Roth (1979) has proposed a somewhat alternative model in the treatment of these identity-impaired individuals.

Kernberg maintains that the narcissist has an unusual degree of self-reference in his interaction with others and that his overneed to be loved and admired does not allow him to consider the therapist as a separate autonomous individual. Further, Kernberg maintains that the narcissistic personality has a specific pathological sort of infantile narcissism with no separate development of representations of the self and objects. Such personality disorders do not suffer from a deficit of structures in the ego and superego; rather, there is a maintenance and operation of pathological primitive structures. Kernberg emphasizes the need for analysis of positive and negative transference and focuses on the interpretation of the primitive idealization, omnipotent control, and devaluation of the therapist.

Application of Kernberg's theory to group therapy may be inferred as the need for the therapist to be cognizant of making transference interpretation relating to the narcissist's needs to devalue others, especially the authority figure, and to maintain omnipotent control. The therapist in this model must be willing to confront, interpret, and accept the patient's abusive, grandiose behavior in the here-and-now situation, which is then visible to the group.

Kohut, in contrast to Kernberg, postulates parallel separate developmental sequences for narcissism and object love and their corresponding libidinal states.

The course and outcome of these two developmental lines differ, one leading from autoerotism via narcissism to higher more complex transformations of narcissism and the other from autoerotism via narcissism to object love. Mature self-esteem is developed when the excessive exhibitionism is diminished and integrated into the adult personality. When, however, there has been severe narcissistic trauma, the grandiose self may retain its unaltered form and continue to strive for fulfillment of its archaic cravings.

Kohut's treatment pathway, congruent with his theoretical position, differs from the one proposed by Kernberg and stresses the recognition of the defense or resistance and the maintenance of correct understanding to avoid premature interpretation.

This model emphasizes the comprehension of and mastery of countertransference phenomena, and the role of the analyst is perceived and experienced as part of the patient's self. The consideration, therefore, is the need to foster the development of object love; consequently, the therapist adapts an empathic, caring, soothing, understanding attitude preceding the analysis of the resistance and transference.

Volkan (1980) stresses the dangers of inappropriate narcissistic leadership, whether it be in the personage of a group therapist or a political leader, for neither can relate in a meaningful way to others, as his own need gratifications are primary.

Depending on the deviancy of the narcissist, the group appears to be a potent therapeutic tool. Group members not only are seen as projective identifications but also as rivals who realistically demand and receive caring and attention from the therapist and force the narcissist to accept his lack of exclusivity. In this way the fantasy of omnipotence is interfered with. Additionally, the narcissist is often a needed stimulus to provoke the group members into an activation of their hidden feelings of intense deprivation, primitive envy, and greed.

BORDERLINE PERSONALITY

Borderline personalities are significantly ego impaired, relate minimally to others, and have erratic explosive behavior, sudden changes in mood, ambivalent feelings, and withdrawal into feeling states of emptiness and boredom. Diagnostically, they are positioned between the more intact neurosis and the psychosis. There may be transitory psychotic intervals, and this may occur in combination with the other personality disorders.

The DSM-III classification is made if five of the following criteria are evidenced: (1) impulsivity or unpredictability in at least two areas that are self-damaging, e.g., spending, sex, gambling, alcohol and drug use, shoplifting, overeating, physically self-damaging acts; (2) a pattern of unstable and intense interpersonal relationships; (3) inappropriate, intense anger or lack of control of anger; (4) identity disturbance related to uncertainties of self-image, gender identity, career goals; (5) affective instability; (6) intolerance of being alone; (7) physically self-destructive acts; and (8) chronic feelings of emptiness or boredom.

The controversy about the application of group therapy with the borderline and narcissistic character disorders has been related to many issues, including the theoretical one.

Horwitz (1977) states that group treatment can provide a helpful therapeutic preparation prior to entering individual therapy; because the group dilutes the intensity of the borderline patient's feelings for attachment and relationship with only one individual, he is better able to reduce the splitting of the self- and object representations to a point where he is eventually able to relate and form a transference in a dyadic relationship.

Kibel (1978) discusses the group treatment of borderline patients in a short-term inpatient unit where the goals are support, stabilization, norm setting, curtailment of acting out, and regression. For these reasons, the analysis is of here-and-now behavior, rather than the interpretation of unconscious motivation.

The difficulties encountered in dealing with borderline patients overlap with the explanations of treatment of the narcissistic character disorder but are likely more hazardous. The borderline member is usually seen by the group as offensive, angry, unpredictable, fear inducing, and disloyal. The constantly changing picture produces confusion, and the group cannot easily criticize the over-all personality portrait.

The constant attack, threat of suicide, substance abuse, and accident proneness are additional sources of difficulty for the therapist. The considerable stress on the countertransference indicates that only some therapists can work with this category successfully.

The following dream vignette and the group response to it illustrate the interactive nature of the group matrix and the emotional-cognitive feedback to a recovering borderline woman 40 years of age. Her previous treatment included 7 years of psycho-analysis, and at this point she was in her third year of group psychotherapy.

In my dreams last night my dark glasses were missing. I was going to go from one place to another ... it was part of a trip on a bus ... with a group of people.... I think they were talking to me.... I remember trying to get ready but everything was scattered all over, but I remember ending up collecting everything, but I couldn't find or see my dark glasses.... I could see my dark glasses on a park bench, and I wanted to go there right away before someone stole them.... It was an easy place to find, and I had to study the map, and I was afraid I would not get there on time."

Various members laughed and made these comments: "You saw well enough to get here on time tonight." "I love the word 'scattered,' do you remember how we used to call you 'flakey' and 'spinny' ... then you really were in pieces, spinning your wheels ... now I think you are still 'spinny' but in a fun way ... not boring but able to spin from one thing to another."

The patient laughed and said: "I see what you mean, and I do see that I am trying to put myself together and move ahead."

In the beginning, the patient was deaf and blind, in that she neither heard nor could see herself or others. She had been treated for deafness, but it was soon learned it was of psychological origin. She wore dark glasses for some time in the group and became aware of their protective hiding, as well as her disguised curiosity. The integration of the self may be inferred from her attempt to gather up and collect her own scattered pieces.

It is of interest to note the helpfulness of the specific naming of character traits by group members.

ANTISOCIAL PERSONALITY

Antisocial, rebellious, and acting-out behavior is seen in early childhood in the form of lying, stealing, and truancy, and in adolescence and young adulthood this is exhibited through increased delinquency, drinking, and drug abuse.

The DSM-III classification presents criteria for early onset of the disorder before the age of 15 and chronic antisocial behavior since age 18. In this latter category, four of the following nine manifestations are necessary for the diagnosis: (1) inability to sustain consistent work behavior; (2) lack of ability for responsible parenting; (3) failure to accept societal norms with respect to lawful behavior; (4) inability to maintain lasting attachments with one sexual partner; (5) irritability, aggressiveness, physical attack, and abuse; (6) failure to honor financial obligations; (7) failure to plan ahead and impulsive change of plans; (8) disregard for the truth; and (9) recklessness.

Julian and Kilman (1979) reviewed 32 group treatment studies of juvenile delinquents, and 9 positive outcome was found in only one-third of the cases. Overall, behavioral and modeling groups were the most successful, with the exception of demonstrated change on recidivism. Therapy groups were judged the most effective when achievement measures were used. Discussion groups were least effective. Across these three group approaches, closed milieu produced the best outcome.

In general, there is agreement that the antisocial personality is a high-risk patient who does not do well in either individual or group therapies because he lacks motivation and has little personal remorse or regard for group societal norms. Best results are most likely with the younger antisocial personality, for after the age of 20 this alloplastic structure is difficult to influence.

These patients, previously called psychopath or sociopath, are counterindicated for group psychotherapy except in certain well-structured closed therapeutic milieu settings.

AVOIDANT PERSONALITY

The diagnostic criteria include hypersensitivity to rejection, unwillingness to enter into relationships unless given unconditional guarantees of uncritical acceptance, social withdrawal, desire for affection and acceptance, and low self-esteem.

The avoidant personality makes a good group candidate, for, unlike the schizoid, he yearns for close social ties, even though he is shy and socially gauche. In the early stages of the group process, the therapist may have to be a positive, encouraging, protective ally not allowing undue early pressure from the group and permitting him to become comfortable in the participant observer role. Encouragement is often given to the avoidant by smiles, eye contact, and beckoning movements of the hands. This type of patient signals his growing intention for self-disclosure by moving closer to the therapist or an esteemed member, by improvement in his style of dressing, and by his degree of comfort in the group. These silent patients may encourage the group's avoidance and exclusion. The problem for the group therapist is to decide to what degree to encourage or delay the patient's inclusion and activity.

DEPENDENT PERSONALITY

This personality passively allows others to assume responsibility for the major areas of his life and subordinates his own needs in order to avoid any possibility of having to be self-reliant or independent.

Group therapy is the treatment of choice for such a patient, for his dependent cravings can be gratified by some members and his overclinging confronted by others. The danger of the group process is the fostering of a dependent attachment in the building of group cohesion and trust. In the early stage, the dependent personality may be overgratified, while in later stages he will be resentful of the risk taking demanded of him. The idealization of the therapist may induce grandiose and omnipotent countertransference reactions. It is well known that the termination phase is most difficult for the dependent patient, and therapists tend to overkeep them in treatment.

COMPULSIVE PERSONALITY

Four out of the following five criteria are needed to make this diagnosis: (1) restricted ability to express warm and tender emotions, (2) perfectionism and preoccupation with details, (3) stubborn insistence that others submit to his way of doing things, (4) excessive devotion to work and productivity, and (5) indecisiveness.

The compulsive patient often assumes the role of co-therapist, disguising his own competition for the leadership. Group members resent the compulsive's stubborness, arrogance, and workaholic attitudes. Usually, this patient becomes most vulnerable when his indecisiveness and underlying inferiority feelings are exposed. If this reaction formation is analyzed too prematurely, the patient may bolt from the group, rather than face his embarrassment, guilt, and shame.

Group therapists at times identify with the compulsive's needs of high attainment and perfectionism. His Achilles heel is also in the realm of decision making, which must be accurate and timely.

PASSIVE-AGGRESSIVE PERSONALITY

These individuals are characterized by their resistance to adequate performance in both occupational and social functioning. This resistance is expressed indirectly and covertly disguises aggression, or, conversely, the aggression hides the underlying passivity. In group therapy this character pattern can be effectively treated; the group can identify with both aspects of his passivity and aggressiveness. Alternatively, the group makes demands for an increase or a decrease in the desired or offensive activity pattern. Initially, the patient's passivity may be tolerated, but there is a gradual insistence for self-disclosure and self-assertion. What becomes problematic in their treatment is the sudden emergence of masochistic or sadistic needs (Glatzer, 1978).

Countertransference difficulties can be evoked by these hostile-withdrawn personalities, and Fried (1954) suggested the benefits of combined group and individual therapy. At times, the eruption of hidden rage may be catastrophic, and the therapist must be prepared to act as a protective shield which he gradually withdraws as the ambivalence within the patient is healed.

References

Azima, F. J. Transference-countertransference issues in group psychotherapy for adolescents. Int. J. Group Psychother., *1:* 51, 1972.

Battegay, R. Different kinds of group psychotherapy with patients with different diagnoses. Acta Psychiatr. Scand., *55:* 345, 1977.

Berger, M. M., and Rosenbaum, M. Notes on help-rejecting complainers. Int. J. Group Psychother., *17:* 357, 1967.

Bogdanoff, M., and Elbaum, P. L. Role lock: Dealing with monopolizers, mistrusters, isolates, helpful Hannahs, and other assorted characters in group psychotherapy. Int. J. Group Psychother., *28:* 247, 1978.

Buirski, P. Toward a theory of adaptation of analytic group psycotherapy. Int. J. Group Psychother., *30:* 477, 1980.

Carpenter, W. T., Gunderson, J. G., and Strauss, J. S. Considerations of the borderline syndrome: A longitudinal comparative study of borderline and shizophrenic patients. In *Borderline Personality Disorders,* P. Hartocollis, editor, p. 231. International Universities Press, New York, 1977.

Fried, E. Benefits of combined therapy for the hostile withdrawn and hostile dependent personality. Am. J. Orthopsychiatry, *24:* 529, 1954.

Glatzer, H. T. The working alliance in analytic group psychotherapy. Int. J. Group Psychother., *28:* 147, 1978.

Heckel, R., and Salzberg, H. *Group Psychotherapy: A Behavioral Approach.* University of South Carolina Press, Columbia, 1976.

Horwitz, L. Group psychotherapy of the borderline patient. In *Borderline Personality Disorders: The Concept, the synarome, the patient,* P. Hartocollis, editor, p. 399. International Universities Press, New York, 1977.

Julian, A., and Kilman, P. R. Group treatment of juvenile delinquents; a review of the outcome literature. Int. J. Group Psychother., *29:* 3, 1979.

Kibel, H. D. The rationale for the use of group psychotherapy for borderline patients on a short-term unit. Int. J. Group Psychother., *28:* 339, 1978.

Kohut, H. Thoughts on narcissism and narcissistic rage. Psychoanal. Study Child, *27:* 360, 1972.

Livingston, M. Working through in analytic group psychotherapy in relation to masochism as a refusal to mourn. Int. J. Group Psychother., *21:* 339, 1971.

Lothstein, L. M. Human territoriality in group psychotherapy. Int. J. Group Psychother., *28:* 55, 1978.

Ornstein, P. On narcissism: Beyond the introduction, highlights of Heinz Kohut's contributions to the psychoanalytic treatment of narcissistic personality disorders. Ann. Psychoanal., *2:* 17, 1974.

Peters, C., and Grunebaum, H. It could be worse: Effective group psychotherapy with help rejecting complainers. Int. J. Group Psychother., *7:* 471, 1977.

Rachman, A. Talking it out rather than fighting it out: Prevention of a delinquent gang war by group therapy intervention. Int. J. Group Psychother., *19:* 518, 1969.

Roth, B. Problems of early maintenance and entry into group psychotherapy with persons suffering from borderline and narcissistic states. Group, *3:* 1, 1979.

Spotnitz, H. The borderline schizophrenic in group psychotherapy. Int. J. Group Psychother., *7:* 155, 1957.

Stone, W. N., and Whitman, R. M. Contributions of the psychology of the self to group process and group therapy. Int. J. Group Psychother., *27:* 343, 1977.

Stubblefield, R. L. Antisocial personality in children and adolescents. In *Comprehensive Textbook of Psychiatry,* A. M. Freedman, H. I. Kaplan, and B. J. Sadock, editors, ed. 2, p. 2170. Williams & Wilkins, Baltimore, 1976.

Volkan, V. Narcissistic personality organization and "reparative" leadership. Int. J. Group Psychother., *30:* 131, 1980.

Wong, N. Clinical considerations in group treatment of narcissistic disorders. Int. J. Group Psychother., *29:* 325, 1979.

Yalom, I. D. *The Theory and Practice of Group Psychotherapy,* Ed. 2. Basic Books, New York, 1975.

C.8 Group Psychotherapy with the Old and Aged

JEFFREY R. FOSTER, M.D.
ROSEMARIE PÉREZ FOSTER, Ph.D.

Introduction

The approach of any topic concerning mental health aspects of older persons must be guided by several awarenesses. First, the convention of labeling "geriatric" all persons between the ages of about 60 and 100 years is, in fact, encompassing some 40 per cent of the entire human lifespan. There can be no simplistic generalizations about this magnitude and diversity of the human experience. Rather, clinical approaches must be guided and refined by specific studies that generate clinically meaningful data; such studies must take into account the enormous range of diagnostic heterogeneity, socioeconomic experiences, and resources, as well as adaptive capacities and physiological changes that characterize this broad sector of the population. Unfortunately, the available clinical literature is sparse, often unintegrated, frequently anecdotal, and often does not utilize adequate control or comparison groups. There is a pressing need for basic data to assess the applicability and effectiveness of group therapy with older persons.

Second, this is both the fastest growing age group in many countries and the group having the highest prevalence of mental disturbance of any age group in the population. This rapid growth of actual and potential patients requiring mental health services underscores the need for clinical data to guide the therapeutic effort.

Finally, the health needs of the broad age group being dealt with generate the highest per capita medical expenses in the population. The competition of health services within limited personal and national financial resources warrants close attention to the cost effectiveness of any treatment method. The availability of any cost-effective treatment, such as group therapy, must be systematically studied to demonstrate both its effectiveness and its limitations.

Review

Review of the relevant literature describes group therapy techniques which deal with the basic needs of the minimally verbal and inactive long-term geriatric inpatient, as well as the needs of the more congnitively intact and verbal older person. Group therapy as a treatment modality for the institutionalized geriatric patient has arisen in response to the repeatedly described phenomenon that the style of care offered in institutions for older patients often accelerates, rather than reduces, social isolation (Bolin, 1974; Weiner et al., 1978) and the general trend toward personality disintegration. The following specialized group treatments have been reported for use with the geriatric inpatient. These modalities commonly share the goal of enhancing concrete adaptation mechanisms to the environment.

Sensory retraining is a group therapy technique designed for severely regressed geriatric patients who have deficits in motoric and cognitive abilities and are thus compromised in discriminating basic sensory stimuli. Regardless of age or diagnostic category, patients who suffer multiple sensory losses cease to engage in normal interpersonal communications, and thus easily regress into isolated withdrawal (Folsom et al., 1978). Sensory retraining attempts to emerge the regressed older patient in an array of multisensory stimulation, so as to increase the sensitivity of his remaining senses and to increase his ability to respond appropriately to stimuli in his environment. The therapist typically works with a small group of five or six patients on a daily basis of 30 to 60 minutes, and in an orderly fashion stimulates the different sensory modalities. For example, differences in smell between two items are demonstrated, as are differences in color, shape, and texture. Hearing is stimulated by music or clanging instruments. Objects are verbally named. Sensory techniques are also applied to game activities. Huber reports on a sensory club for organic nursing home residents, and emphasizes the need for more than one sensory session per day to maintain continuity and sustain a high stimulatory level. She combined a sensory craft workshop with the regular sensory training, wherein interpersonal peer feedback and interaction reinforced strides made in the training group.

Reality orientation (RO) is a technique designed to return to the confused person the optimal use of his cognitive assets. The technique deals directly with the classic symptoms of confusion, disorientation, and memory deficits through intensive mental and memory stimulation. Reality orientation was designed by Folsom, who contends that no patient is totally confused; it is the job of the staff person to find the areas of wellness in the patient and try to expand its boundaries. Reality orientation was originally designed for institutionalized older patients, but the technique is also practiced in day care settings. In the RO process, every contact by the patient with the staff member is used to improve his patient's awareness of time, place, and person. All activities in which the person is engaged are continuously verbally labeled. Repetition of information and reinforcing the patient for correct responses is essential. Environmental aids—such as large clocks, calendars, and boards depicting date, year, and weather—are also used. Reality orientation group or classroom reality orientation is a supplementary, more intensive form of RO for more confused patients. Small groups, of optimally four patients, are usually seen daily. As with milieu reality orientation, patients are taught basic time, place, person, and object information. However, the group setting provides personal and interpersonal attention in which treatment objectives can be prescribed, attained, and practiced in a firm, supportive environment.

Anecdotal evidence in the form of case reports and staff observations indicates that RO is an effective therapeutic technique (Ireland, 1972; Letcher et al., 1974). In one of the few controlled experimental designs, Harris and Ivory (1976) report that 5 months of RO treatment significantly changed both the verbal orientation behaviors and the over-all clinical impression of female geriatric mental patients. No such changes were found in a control group who received traditional hospital care. Barnes (1974) found no significant changes in patients' overt behavior or informational ability after 6 weeks of classroom group RO treatment. This finding suggests that group RO treatment alone is not potent enough to produce cognitive-therapeutic changes, and that group RO must be used in conjunction with the sustained reinforcement effects of the environmental milieu RO approach.

Remotivation therapy is a structured group program used with institutionalized elderly individuals who can function on a verbal cognitive level. It aims to reach the intact interests of the patient in group discussions about everyday life (e.g., grooming, dining in public, current events, plant care, etc.). This group technique is an effort to resocialize the individual and arouse his interests in the environment by helping him learn or relearn a wide variety of informational knowledge. Remotivation was originally developed for administration by hospital aides. Groups range in number from eight to 15 and typically meet once or twice a week. Traditionally, this therapy follows a formalized plan of five steps, which evolves from establishing a climate of acceptance to introduction and discussion of a relevant topic of discussion geared to the group's interests, needs, and level of functioning. The group members are helped by the leader to explore the subject matter, to use their own available intellectual resources, and to apply the knowledge to their own immediate life circumstances. The results of Bovey's controlled experimental study show that remotivation therapy significantly enhances the self-concept of geriatric patients.

A remotivation group can be organized around the accomplishment of specific tasks. Patients with commonly poor personal appearance respond well to a grooming remotivation group. Previously, apathetic elderly female patients can be successfully motivated to plan and prepare ward social events. Lyon reports, however, that short-term task-oriented remotivation groups do not produce long-term motivation effects; instead, they generate islands of active participation which quickly disappear after task completion. Remotivation groups must be ongoing, Lyon notes, for higher level changes in behavior and attitudes to occur. Various offspring of the original remotivation therapy procedure are reported. Wallen (1970) describes a successful motivation therapy program for medically improved elderly veterans who were unmotivated to leave the hospital. The main goal was to develop more personal and social responsibility on the part of each patient, so that eventual courses of action could be taken for placement in the community. In an experimental design, Nevruz and Hrushka compared the effects of a motivation group specifically focused on leaving the hospital versus a nondirective verbal group on the discharge rate of geriatric psychiatric patients. Both groups were equally and significantly effective in producing an increase in the discharge rate. This finding suggests that the factors producing change in even the highly focused motivation and remotivation groups are based on certain emotional dynamics common to all types of group process.

Survey

The available clinical literature is helpful, but does not provide a practical or comprehensive overview for the reader to gain a picture of what it is like to be involved in verbal group therapy with the elderly. This was only compounded by a variety of different settings where group therapy is used that might effect the group process (e.g., senior citizen center, mental health clinic, skilled nursing facility). The treatment of similar diagnostic groups in these different settings raises other troublesome questions not clearly answered by the literature, e.g., is the group process of elderly depressives treated in an ambulatory setting different from that in a residential environment (nursing home, etc.)? Various other factors—such as dropout or turnover rate, attendance rate, time to reach cohesion, and patient selection variables—are often ignored in the literature. In short, if a new therapist starts a geriatric group, there is inadequate information about how to proceed and what to expect.

In an effort to help fill these gaps, Foster and Foster surveyed the available therapists, experienced in geriatric group therapy, in the metropolitan New York area. A total of 20 therapists were finally located by contacting all six medical schools in the city, as well as follow-up on all word-of-mouth referrals.

A questionnaire consisting of some 110 items was administered to all therapists, asking them to base their responses on the aggregate number of elderly group patients seen over their entire careers. A variety of settings were deliberately included: private office, senior citizen center, mental health clinics (free standing and hospital based), medical clinics, and nursing homes (health-related facility and skilled nursing facility components).

Any survey based on a small number of participants requires close attention to the therapists themselves, as well as to the collective clinical experience on which their answers are based. The 20 therapists treated an aggregate number of at least 3,065 elderly group patients. Their total years of group experience were 237 cumulatively (mean: 11.9 years; range: 2 to 30 years); and their total number of years working with elderly groups were 131 (mean: 6.6 years; range: 1 to 23 years). The average age of all therapists was 42.8 years (range: 26 to 62 years). Five, or 25 per cent, of the therapists had predominant experince treating residential patients (residential therapists), while the rest emphasized treatment of ambulatory patients (ambulatory therapists). A breakdown of the residential versus ambulatory therapists is given in Table C.8-1. These two therapist and patient categories are used to be consistent with the existing literature; also, residential patients—by virtue of 24-hour community contact—are exposed to many other factors impacting on group process that ambulatory patients do not encounter.

As can be seen in Table C.8-1, the residential and ambulatory therapists were of similar age and had comparable total years of group experience. Those with primarily residential experience have spent more years treating specifically older patients during their careers, and have each treated numerically more elderly patients than their ambulatory colleagues. The difference in number of elderly patients treated is substantially related to the greater number of years the residential therapists have devoted to elderly group therapy. For comparative purposes, the ambulatory therapist group has actually treated more elderly patients per average year than the residential therapists (253 patients per year versus 157 patients per year). Of the 3,065 elderly patients, 1,215 (40 per cent) were treated in ambulatory settings while 1,850 (60 per cent) were treated in residential environments.

The typical age of residential patients was approximately 1 decade greater (early 1980's versus early 1970's), although considerable overlap of the age ranges occurred. The sex composition was similar, with a clear preponderance of women in both ambulatory (82 per cent) and residential (89 per cent) patient groups.

As shown in Table C.8-2, the ambulatory and residential groups were quite similar diagnostically, in that 100 per cent of all therapists agreed that depression was their most frequently encountered problem. Both groups had a substantial frequency of mild dementia, but they differed in that the residential group had, as expected, a higher frequency of more severe dementia, while the ambulatory group had a higher frequency of personality and somatization disorders. The patient groups were also similar in the general frequency with which psychiatric treatment had been needed over the prior 20 years of the patient's life.

The socioeconomic matrix of this large group of patients is varied. The best generalizations again depict more similarities than differences. Both groups have a quite small upper-class component. The residential group was estimated to have a somewhat larger middle-class proportion, while the ambulatory sector had a larger lower-class constituency. Marital status again shows considerable commonality between groups. Most patients were married at some point in their lives. However, the residential patients have a higher percentage of widowed or separated spouses, while the ambulatory patients have a greater number of currently married spouses. Based on the above data characterizations, it seems that these are sufficiently comparable therapist and patient groups to permit meaningful comparisons of survey results. The results cut across theoretic orientations of the therapists by focusing on observable behaviors and other phenomena free of interpretations.

Foster and Foster used the responses from their survey to describe the following aspects of geriatric expressive group therapy:

(1) unique or distinctive features of techniques and process that typify work with elderly groups; (2) goals and effectiveness of group therapy; (3) patient selection factors, group composition, and group logistics guidelines; (4) initial patient rejection rates and reasons for not joining a group; (5) attendance, dropout, and turnover rates; (6) group cohesion; and (7) group process (behavior and themes).

DISTINCTIVE FEATURES

All therapists were asked if there was anything unique or distinctive about geriatric group therapy (using group treatment of persons under age 40 as a reference point). The responses were varied, and are best divided between those describing altered therapist techniques and those dealing with distinctive group process.

Modifications of therapist techniques

Two broad categories emerged regarding altered techniques: increased activity and heightened flexibility.

Table C.8-1
Therapist Demographics

	Ambulatory (N = 15)	Residential (N = 5)
Age	42.6 (26–62)*	43.4 (28–60)
Total group experience (years)	11.2 (2–30)	13.8 (8–23)
Elderly group experience (years)	4.8 (1–9)	11.8 (4–23)
Total elderly patients seen	1,215	1,850
Average number elderly patients/therapist	81 (15–200+)	370 (100–700+)
Average number elderly patients/therapist/year	253	157
Average age of elderly patients	early 70's (60–95)	early 80's (65–100)

* Numbers in parentheses are ranges.

Table C.8-2
Psychiatric Diagnostic Clusters (Rank Ordered)

	Frequent	Sometimes	Rare
A. Ambulatory	Depression Personality disorder		
		Mild dementia	
			Paranoia Somatization disorder (hypochondriasis) Psychotic Severe dementia
B. Residential	Depression Mild dementia		
		Severe dementia Paranoia	
			Personality disorder Psychotic

Increased activity. The term "activity" encompasses verbal and affective behavior in the group, as well as certain attitudes toward issues that often arise in elderly groups. When asked to rate themselves on a spectrum of active/directive versus passive/reflective, 85 per cent of all therapists unequivocally chose the former descriptor. Two therapists said they tended to be more active than with younger groups; and one felt her behavior oscillated between these poles.

When asked to rate their tendency to display or withhold emotionalism (warmth, energy, empathy, attempts to engage patients), 90 per cent of all therapists said they clearly actively displayed when appropriate to the group. One therapist felt she varied between displaying and withholding; one therapist felt her style was to be withholding. Regarding this display activity, a number of therapists mentioned their technique of using themselves more to give a personal concrete illustration, to become more a part of the group, to respond demonstrably to patients, and to encourage the continued engagement of their older patients. With some therapists this sometimes included physical touching, a hug, a song, or even a dance. One co-therapist would telephone a particular patient at home and sing an Irish lullaby to offset periods of depression and mobilize him to attend group that day. The same therapists did this to a far lesser or zero extent with their nongeriatric groups. This activity is consistent with reports that geriatric groups led by highly empathic leaders showed a significantly greater increase in their self-esteem than did patients whose groups were led by low-empathy leaders (Williams, 1979).

There emerged an often-reiterated activity that reflected a spontaneous attitude evolved by many therapists described as "advocacy." This included active encouragement of patients to take appropriate steps to seek proper medical attention, to deal actively with landlord problems, and to be aware of and utilize the political processes (e.g., elected officials) to correct certain problems. This technique was felt necessary to assure that correctable reality factors were not ignored and to help offset the erosive effects of needless passivity, excessive dependency, feelings of helplessness and lowered self-esteem, and the depressions so often seen in the elderly. This is consistent with the work of Forman, who encourages his group patients to use confrontation and active involvement in controversial social issues. As an aspect of advocacy, there was also the awareness in both groups of therapists that they were part of a team (often not well coordinated) that included other physicians, psychiatrists, nurses, social workers, other professionals, and concerned family members. Sometimes there was a need for a phone cell to express concerns or share information with other members of this team.

Heightened flexibility. The term "flexibility" refers to a willingness to rationally re-examine techniques from younger non-geriatric groups, and to sensibly retain or modify them in the light of special needs of the elderly. Seven examples were encountered with enough frequency to illustrate these modifications:

1. Food. Several ambulatory therapists have allowed the spontaneous interests of their patients in food to become integrated parts of group process to varying degrees. In one instance, the persisting interest in snacks became a full-fledged desire for an entire meal to be served as a 30-minute prelude to the more formal psychoanalytically oriented session that followed. These were more psychiatrically frail patients who were emotionally hungry in all respects; sometimes nonverbal behavior (e.g., stealing or hoarding of food) provided important clues to group process that were tactfully explored in the more formal session. In other settings, the

interest of patients in bringing in cakes and similar foods they had baked themselves to be shared with other members was encouraged. It was felt that this permitted the group to be viewed also as a positive social occasion where roles could be re-enacted (sometimes nonverbally) in ways acceptable and meaningful to both patient and group. In all these instances, it was the symbolic value of food that made it a potent therapeutic facilitator of group process. The use of food as a group process and group cohesion facilitator is described in the above literature review for both inpatient and outpatient group settings. Levine and Poston (1980), as well as Goldfarb and Turner, emphasized the narcissistic loss and deprivation of the senescent period which makes oral nurturing by the parent-leader or by group peers to be a positive and age-appropriate therapeutic tool.

2. Inclusion of ancillary nonpatient persons in the group. Several examples of this flexibility showed the helpfulness at times of including important caretakers (private nurses, attendants, close friend, spouse). The initial request for these persons to wait outside was modified to invite them in by the group, and the therapists noted positive results. Often these nonpatients directly participated in the group but did not always attend every time the patient was present.

3. Overstocking the group roster. This modification allowed the inclusion of a subgroup of patients whose attendance was irregular due mainly to emotional factors only. The emergence of predictable non-attendance cycles allowed the addition of new members and a swelling of the number of patients who technically could potentially attend any given session.

4. Outside session group member contact. A number of therapists report their support of the group's wish to visit a physically ill member who has been hospitalized. This has been extended by others to encourage social interaction between members that include visits to others' homes and invitations to dinner. Linden described in his report of inpatient groups that enhanced social interaction among geriatric group members outside of the group provided the first signs of therapeutic progress, despite the fact that group sessions were still marked by long silences and low patient activity.

5. Outside session therapist-patient contact. There is often increased communication between a therapist and patient or family. Typically, phone contact is used to ascertain why a patient did not attend a group meeting, to answer questions and provide guidance to concerned family members, to help solve transportation problems that may arise (often related to changing health status), and to follow medical progress during hospitalizations. The status of non-attending patients is usually shared discretely with the group, which often has an intense interest in such matters. If individual or family sessions are needed to supplement group attendance, they are promptly arranged until the crisis has resolved.

6. Use of goal-oriented focused techniques. Berman-Rossi, working with skilled nursing home facility patients, includes a task-oriented approach in helping her patients deal with the complex changes of frail aging and institutionalization. If, for example, complaints about food services and how to improve them are prevalent, she may invite an administrator to the next meeting to respond directly to the group. Rinehart, working with more chronic psychiatrically impaired ambulatory patients, uses goal-oriented tasks to focus topics of common concern or feeling. She feels these techniques are useful in prompting group process to achieve "a sense of agreement, of accomplishment, of closure and of self-affirmation."

7. Use of co-therapists. There are a variety of stresses that can deeply affect a single therapist working with an elderly group. An unusually large number of therapists have found a co-therapist to be of distinct help.

Distinctive group process

There is common agreement that powerful therapeutic processes are activated in many geriatric groups that are different from younger groups and fall into two main categories: ambivalence about engagement and style of engagement.

Ambivalence about engagement. This concept was best articulated by Berman-Rossi. The issues of time and losses complexly mix to leave many older persons hesitant to participate meaningfully in group therapy. Time includes a sense of one's longevity on one hand and an awareness of the growing imminence of death on the other. The dual themes that time is endless and time is short partly relate to these awarenesses. Clinical manifestations include a sense that things should be addressed quickly ("if not now, then when"); a sense that members might not meet again ("I'll see you next week, God willing"); and a feeling that, if one is not confident he will be alive, he will not invest in new group relationships. The issue of losses is quite broad, but includes a partial loss of role function due to decreased opportunities (e.g., widowhood, retirement) or decreased capacities (e.g., physical illness). This decrease in role function and opportunities to derive a sense of social supports seems to cause a positive pressure toward potentially utilizing group process to offset these losses. However, the prevalence of these and other losses also appears to engender a simultaneous fear of using the group. As Berman-Rossi paraphrases this concern: "I've lost so much, and I can't risk it again." Thus, ambivalence toward engagement is a powerful and sometimes chronic problem affecting the behavior of older persons in group therapy. It also contributes to problems of achieving and sustaining group cohesion.

Style of engagement. As engagement evolves and strengthens, there is often a stereotyped aspect of patient behavior commonly reported. Patients in both groups were typically described as being solicitous, deferential, polite, and appreciative in regard to the therapists. The patients were often uncomfortable with anger being expressed in the group. They were often reluctant to discuss or reveal personal problems to the group. The question arose during the survey whether these frequent behaviors related to the present age of the patients or were related to the cultural climate 60 to 100 years ago in which the patients were raised. All therapists that discussed this felt these behaviors were at least a partial cultural effect seen as a remnant from a time when cultural or social norms were different and mental health problems and services were not so publicly acceptable. Some felt it was entirely cultural. Others felt an aging-related influence was also showing itself. Charatan points out that, with age, one learns better control of negative behaviors and also that the drives are reduced, causing less pressure for many negative behaviors; he further noted the tendency for the elderly to conserve

psychic as well as physical energies to account for some of these group behaviors. Steinman feels that the tendency to keep problems to themselves was also age related by serving to enhance wishes to retain independence. It was the consensus that these phenomena were real and prevalent, and made geriatric group process distinctive from that with younger group patients.

GOALS AND EFFECTIVENESS

The therapists were asked to specify the tasks, functions, or goals they were trying to accomplish via group treatment. Five general goals emerged; they were highly consistent with those reported in the literature for both residential and outpatient groups:

(1) to decrease symptoms and deal with losses; symptoms of depression, exaggerated hypochondriacal-somatization complaints, and excessive feelings of passivity-dependency-helplessness were especially targeted; advocacy techniques were often used for the latter triad; (2) to encourage stable adjustments to the realities of environment, personal health, and stresses of aging at the highest functional level; there was particular emphasis among residential therapists on adjustment to chronic care hospital and nursing home environments; (3) to broaden the available social matrix and improve interpersonal relationships; included here are the goals of decreasing isolation, overcoming ambivalence to engagement, increasing social role opportunities, and increasing social supports (including the sharing of great commonalities of problems typifying this age group and the integrative stresses they create); (4) to provide a focus of hope for change; this was particularly emphasized by residential therapists where complaints were heard and active plans to correct problems (e.g., better food, disruptive patients) were encouraged; and (5) to help improve discharge rate from a skilled nursing facility; this was stressed by Charatan where group discussion of leaving the facility and adjustment problems to be anticipated were felt to be helpful.

Therapists were asked to rate the effectiveness of group therapy in realizing their goals (with group treatment of persons under age 40 as a reference point). Among the ambulatory group, 93 per cent felt group therapy was very effective, and 7 per cent felt it was moderately effective. Among the residential therapists, 80 per cent felt it was very effective, and 20 per cent felt it was moderately effective.

PATIENT SELECTION, GROUP COMPOSITON, AND GROUP LOGISTICS

All therapists tended to approach patient selection with an exclusionary emphasis. There were only minor differences between residential and ambulatory therapists and their results were combined. Table C.8-3A rank orders the frequency with which negative factors were specified. Table C.8-3B shows those positive selection variables that were noted.

It was generally felt that all potentially reversible disorders, especially those responsive to psychotropic drugs, should be adequately treated before considering group ther-

Table C.8-3
Patient Selection and Group Composition Guidelines
(Rank Ordered)

A. Negative factors:
    Substantial paranoia
    Active psychosis
    Severe dementia
    Narcissistic/angry borderline personality disorder
    Too physically ill
    Inclusion would create cultural rifts
    Intimacy problems and preference for anonymity
    Serious depression
    Marked voluntary social isolation
    Alcoholism
    Excessive chronic anxiety
    Uncorrectable hearing problems
    No rapport with therapists
    Passive-dependent personality disorder
B. Positive factors:
    Inclusion would enhance group homogeneity
    Good history of prior psychotherapy (group or individual)
    Good level of social skills
    Milder depression
    Somatization disorder (hypochondriasis)
    Nonvoluntary social isolation
    Reasonable command of English language
    History of losses/deprivations with group cohesion offering
      a potential second-chance family
    Some ability to recall the past

apy. Thus, serious depressions, substantial paranoid states, active psychoses, marked anxiety states, and potentially medically treatable severe organic brain syndromes should first be treated on an individual basis. These patients typically were not helped in a group setting, and their presence was often disruptive to group process by frightening other group members. It was often noted that strong hostility, especially when persistently directed toward the therapist, was poorly tolerated by the rest of the group. Often, the group members first ostracized and then eventually found ways to expel such hostile members.

Several therapists routinely saw potential group candidates in a series of two to five individual sessions to promote rapport before introduction to the actual group. The failure of the rapport to become manifest was felt to correlate with early group dropout.

The desirability of avoiding cultural rifts while promoting group homogeneity was often cited. Several examples of cultural rifts included disparate educational backgrounds that alienated group members, irreconcilable antagonisms that evolved when depressives with an Eastern European orthodox Jewish background joined a group of depressives with an American Jewish orthodox background, and one instance where black-white racial differences in an ongoing group suddenly became explosive, leading to group dropout and disruption. On the other hand, some therapists, especially Franklin and Kaufman, relate that deliberate promotion of homogeneity by cultural (e.g., all Hispanic) or common-problem (e.g., all obese) selection can enhance group process and speed cohesion. Groups homogeneous for dementia are often formed. Hegarty reports helpful group supports doing expressive group therapy with ambulatory Altzheimer patients suffering a moderate degree of organic brain syndrome. Folsom and Levine relate the spontaneous emergence of group dynamics and emotional themes among the more severely demented residential and ambulatory patients (from a variety of causes) who are being treated with a combination of reality orientation and attitude therapy.

Others have worked with groups dealing with problems of being widows. Mervis has worked extensively with groups having common problems of either themselves being cancer patients or a group consisting of spouses of cancer patients.

A final issue of group composition concerns group size. The typical size of an ambulatory group was eight members (range: six to 12), the average residential group was larger, having 12 members (range: six to 22, where the larger group involved an entire ward of a skilled nursing home facility). Several therapists, in both patient sectors, have experimented with overstocking their groups to accommodate a small patient subgroup whose attendance is regularly irregular for purely emotional reasons. Such patients may attend a group that is meeting weekly only every 3 weeks or every 3 months. They may come for one or two sessions and then not be seen for many weeks, only to repeat their cycle. The therapists felt the group was nonetheless helpful to such patients, and the group tolerated them as regular members.

A related aspect of group set-up concerns factors of session frequency, session length, and time of day of sessions. The typical group meets once each week, regardless of ambulatory or residential setting. The major exception concerns groups of the more severely demented (whether ambulatory or residential) where reality orientation is a major technique. These RO groups frequently meet several times weekly, sometimes almost daily, in sessions ranging from 60 minutes (residential) to 5 hours (ambulatory). Otherwise, the usual session length is about 60 minutes in residential groups (range: 35 to 90 minutes) and 90 minutes for outpatient ambulatory groups (range: 60 to 120 minutes). The time of day does not seem critical to ambulatory groups. However, a helpful comment from residential therapists was to avoid times immediately after meals where the postprandial effects of food often leave patients somewhat lethargic, sometimes dozing, soon restless from filling bladders, and generally not in optimal frames of mind for group therapy. A late morning time was often used.

INITIAL PATIENT REJECTION RATES AND REASONS FOR NOT JOINING A GROUP

Ambulatory therapists tended to recommend group treatment to more of their patients (69 per cent versus 56 per cent), to have a higher initial acceptance rate (84 per cent versus 72 per cent) and consequently to experience a lower initial rejection rate (16 per cent versus 28 per cent). The ranges for each figure are sufficiently broad and similar that the differences may not be significant.

To ascertain the reasons for refusal, the therapists were asked 10 potential factors associated with rejection and asked to identify any others they felt were important. First, it is of interest to note the following variables that were universally felt not to influence likelihood of initially rejecting group: (1) age (2) marital status, (3) socioeconomic status, and (4) prior exposure to group therapy.

Residential therapists cited two major rejection reasons: privacy concerns and general emotional resistance. "Privacy concerns" refers to a preference (unrelated to paranoia or other diagnosis) for not divulging any personal problems. This probably is a stronger example of a similar nondisclosure preference discussed regarding style of engagement.

Ambulatory therapists generated a lengthier nine-item list of refusal reasons that will be cited in order of the frequency with which they occurred:

(1) Diagnosis: patients with heightened narcissism, with severe dementia, and those who were actively psychotic regularly rejected group treatment; those with stable but severe chronic psychiatric disturbances were typical rejectors; patients who were stably recovered from a prior psychosis also often rejected groups; (2) privacy concerns; (3) independent/self-contained needs: this factor refers to strong preferences to view themselves as having no social needs they cannot take care of by themselves; these patients are not socially isolated or paranoid; this trait is separable from but probably closely related to privacy concerns; it relates to Steinman's view of the defensive aspects of non-disclosure tendencies in the elderly; (4) general emotional resistance; (5) claiming sufficient family or community supports to make group therapy unnecessary; (6) claims of excessive travel distance to attend the group (many regular patients in fact came from far distances); (7) voluntary social isolation of the patient; (8) fragile ego defenses leaving patients only interested in individual (not group) therapy; and (9) perception of cultural-educational rifts when group composition was described.

ATTENDANCE, DROPOUT, AND TURNOVER RATES

The typical attendance rates of all present members at each group session were 89 per cent for ambulatory patients (range: 65 per cent to 100 per cent) and 73 per cent for residential patients (range: 67 per cent to 85 per cent). The most frequent reason for absence in both groups related to illness (self or family). Other reasons for ambulatory patients concerned inclement weather, episodes of increased emotional resistance to treatment, and vacation traveling.

Once the group is started, there are an additional few patients who may drop out, mostly during the first 3 to 4 weeks. These patients are basically a continuum of those who outright reject the group initially, although they wait a few sessions before their emotional ambivalence mounts. As these early dropouts are replaced, new members will also have a similar small dropout potential due mainly to emotional factors. After the first month, group composition is relatively stable for ambulatory groups but not for residential groups.

The turnover rate was defined as the percentage of group patients (after the first month) that were not still group members after a 6-month time span since group start-up or any subsequent 6-month interval. The usual ambulatory turnover rate was 11 per cent (range: 5 per cent to 50 per cent), while the residential rate was 33 per cent (range: 17 per cent to 50 per cent). This extrapolates to annual turnover rates of 22 per cent and 66 per cent, respectively. The most typical reason for dropout after the first month was illness or death. It must be noted, however, that the residential patients are in more frail health and are on average 1 decade older; thus, a higher turnover rate, due to morbidity and mortality, is expected.

GROUP COHESION

Some 95 per cent of all therapists reported their groups became cohesive, although the time course was variable. Residential therapists reported that their groups took an average of 2.6 months (range: 1 to 5 months) to become cohesive. The ambulatory data were distinctly bimodal: one subgroup of four locations (seven therapists) had an average time of 1.9 months (range: 1 to 3 months), and the remaining subgroup reported an average of 10.1 months (range: 6 to 12 months). The non-overlapping disparity of some 8 months difference is dramatic. The short-cohesion time in the ambulatory subgroup is similar to that of residential groups. Residential groups have 24-hour daily contact between members, which probably facilitates group cohesion. Three of the four ambulatory short-cohesion time locations are characterized by frequent contact between patients of up to 5 to 8 hours daily, as often as 5 days a week.

The data thus suggest that total patient contact per week and, probably, homogeneity of groups are much

Table C.8-4
Behavior toward Therapist (Rank Ordered)

	Frequent*	Sometimes	Rare
A. Ambulatory	Solicitous Appreciative Deferential		
		Ignores/aloof Competitive Critical Angry/hostile	
			Suspicious
B. Residential	Solicitous Appreciative Deferential Angry/hostile		
		Critical	
			Suspicious Ignores/aloof Competitive

* Frequent, predominantly occurs every one to three sessions; sometimes, predominantly occurs every four to six sessions; rare, predominantly occurs only every seven or more sessions.

more important determinants of cohesiveness than are residential or ambulatory setting factors. It is striking that for residential groups the high turnover rate does not disrupt cohesiveness. This suggests the powerfulness of group member contact and homoge-

neity (all are in declining health and coping with institutionalization) in facilitating cohesion. At the other extreme, the data caution that, for ambulatory older patients where group sessions are their only contact, cohesion is typically delayed for sometimes

Table C.8-5
Patient-to-Patient Behavior (Rank Ordered)

	Frequent*	Sometimes	Rare
A. Ambulatory	Actively engaged Identifies with others' problems Reacts to absence, illness, death of member Shows clear affect		
		Competitive Deferential Aloof	
			Suspicious/angry/hostile
B. Residential	Actively engaged Shows clear affect Identifies with others' problems Reacts to absence, illness, death of member		
		Competitive Suspicious/angry/hostile	
			Deferential Aloof

* Frequent, predominantly occurs every one to three sessions; sometimes, predominantly occurs every four to six sessions; rare, predominantly occurs only every seven or more sessions.

Table C.8-6
Group Themes (Rank Ordered)

	Frequent*	Sometimes	Rare
A. Ambulatory	Losses (family/friends) Hope versus despair Loneliness Losses (health/function) Illness Reminiscing Dependency Family intactness Financial concerns Aging Quality of medical services Quality of nonmedical services Power versus weakness Passivity versus activity		
		Sexuality/romance Death/dying	
B. Residential	Losses (family/friends) Reminiscing Financial concerns Hope versus despair Dependency Aging		
		Loneliness Illness Quality of medical services Passivity versus activity Losses (health/function) Family intactness Power versus weakness Death/dying	
			Quality of nonmedical services Sexuality/romance

* Frequent, predominantly occurs every one to three sessions; sometimes, predominantly occurs every four to six sessions; rare, predominantly occurs only every seven or more sessions.

12 months, and the therapist should not be discouraged.

GROUP PROCESS

Table C.8-4 shows the rank order and frequency of eight behaviors shown by group members toward therapists. Solicitous, appreciative, and deferential behaviors were the most frequent ones in both groups; they occurred somewhat more frequently in residential groups. Also of note, is the tendency of residential patients to show more frequent evidence of angry, critical, and suspicious feelings than do ambulatory patients. Conversely, ambulatory patients more often ignore or appear sometimes aloof to the therapist than do their residential counterparts. It is possible the aloofness is a subtler display of angry feelings. Other behaviors reported included a variety of clear transference reactions that occurred with a low frequency in about one-half of all groups. Howell has noted mainly with ambulatory patients that transference reactions peak early in a group and decrease after approximately 6 months.

Table C.8-5 shows similar data for eight behaviors shown by group members toward each other. Both patient groups are much less deferential toward fellow members than they are toward their therapists. Again, the residential patients show more frequent evidence of suspicious, angry, and hostile feelings than do the ambulatory group. Charatan notes the frequent evidence of jealousy in and among residents in a teaching nursing home triggered by the perceived improvement in reality situations of other members (e.g., a move to a discharge home or to a different section or entirely different facility). Mervis discusses strong envy in ambulatory cancer patients when a group member no longer needs chemotherapy. Advice giving, sympathy, interest in the other's well-being, and general emotional supportiveness were behaviors noted by several therapists. Transference reactions between group members were rarely mentioned by therapists.

All therapists reported that group themes arose and evolved, although sometimes considerable therapist effort was needed to stimulate and encourage their continuation. Table C.8-6 shows the rank order and frequency of 16 themes in both groups. Of note is the higher density of frequent themes in the ambulatory group, an observation that means there are usually more themes per session than occur in residential sessions. Losses of family and friends were the highest ranking theme in both groups. This is consistent with Burnside, who crystallizes loss as a constant theme in group work with the elderly. The residential groups less often dealt with loss of personal health or functional status. Both groups were relatively disinclined to speak of death or dying; usually, discussion was stimulated by serious illness, death, or unexplained absence of a group member. When death was discussed by ambulatory patients, they often expressed fears of dying alone at home and not being found for a considerable time. An interesting theme in both groups concerned references to children and grandchildren; grandchildren were often used to deny tensions with children but to discuss those with the next generation; gratification

with the growth of the grandchildren was shared; and changes of life styles with their children was another variant theme. Residential patients elaborated on staff and roommate problems. Ambulatory patients spoke of fears of memory loss, of street crime, and of landlord problems. Both groups reacted quickly in seeking information about an absent group member.

Conclusion

Both the pertinent literature and survey data show geriatric group therapy to have distinct differences from younger groups concerning logistics and group process. Various effective group therapies are available to meet the differing needs of the healthier or more afflicted older patient. A number of modifications in therapist techniques are often required independent of the specific therapy being used. Various common behaviors and themes emerge in older groups, regardless of the specific therapy being used. It appears that group process has more similarities than differences, regardless of whether the patients are ambulatory or residing in inpatient facilities. These broader commonalities attest to the presence of strong developmental tasks and adaptive stresses that often characterize the senescent years.

The authors wish to dedicate this chapter to the memory of Dr. Alvin I. Goldfarb, who contributed the original chapter in the first edition. As teacher, mentor, colleague, and friend, his desire for quantitative clinical data has guided them throughout this project.

References

Barnes, J. Effects of reality orientation classroom on memory loss, confusion, and disorientation in geriatric patients. Gerontologist, 14: 138, 1974.

Berger, L. F. Activating a psychogeriatric group. Psychiatr. Q., 50: 63, 1978.

Berland, D. I., and Poggi, R. Expressive group psychotherapy with the aging. Int. J. Group Psychoth., 29: 87, 1979.

Bolin, R. Sensory deprivation: An overview. Nurs. Forum, 13: 240, 1974.

Deutsch, C. B., and Kramer, N. Outpatient group psychotherapy for the elderly: An alternative to institutionalization. Hosp. Community Psychiatry, 28: 440, 1977.

Folsom, J. C., Boies, B. L., and Pommerenck, K. Life adjustment techniques for use with the dynsfunctional elderly. Aged Care Serv. Rev., 1: 1, 1978.

Gugel, R. N. The effects of group psychotherapy on orientation, memory, reasoning ability, social involvement, and depression of brain damaged and non-brain damaged aged patients exhibiting senile behavior. Diss. Abst. Int., 40: 2365, 1979.

Harris, C. S., and Ivory, P. B. An outcome evaluation of reality orientation therapy with geriatric patients in a state mental hospital. Gerontologist, 16: 496, 1976.

Ingersoll, B., and Silverman, A. Comparative psychotherapy for the aged. Gerontologist, 8: 201, 1978.

Ireland, M. J. Starting reality orientation and remotivation. Nurs. Homes, 21: 19, 1977.

Lazarus, L. W. A program for the elderly at a private psychiatric hospital. Geronologist, 16: 125, 1976.

Letcher, P., Peterson, L., and Scarbrough, D. Reality orientation: A historical study of patient progress. J. Hosp. Community Psychiatry, 25: 801, 1974.

Levine, B. E., and Poston, M. A modified group treatment for elderly narcissistic patients. Int. J. Group Psychother., 30: 153, 1980.

Manaster, A. Therapy with the "senile" geriatric patient. Int. J. Group Psychother., 22: 250, 1971.

Saul, S. R., and Saul, S. Group psychotherapy in a proprietary nursing home. Gerontologist, 14: 446, 1974.

Turbow, S. R. Geriatric group day care and its effect on independent living. Gerontologist, *15:* 508, 1975.

Wallen, V. Motivation therapy with the aging geriatric veteran patient. Milit. Med., *135:* 1007, 1970.

Weiner, M. B., Brok, A. J., and Snadowsky, A. M. Working with the

Aged: Practical Approaches in the Institution and Community. Prentice-Hall, Englewood Cliffs, NJ, 1978.

Williams, C. L. Nurse therapist high empathy and nurse therapist low empathy during therapeutic group work as factors in changing the self-concept of the institutionalized aged. Diss. Abs. Int., *40:* 3095, 1979.

C.9 Group Psychotherapy with Couples

PETER A. MARTIN, M.D.

Introduction

Group therapy is defined by the thinking of the therapist in terms of the group, rather than by the number of persons in the room. In addition, therapists who work with groups have moved away from the relatively uninvolved attitude of psychoanalytic individual therapy. The therapist is much more active and is a member of the group. There is an awareness, not only that the therapist allows himself to get involved in the group process, but that it happens whether he is aware of it or not. In a group of married couples, the therapist becomes as vulnerable as the patients, because his own marriage and his parents' marriage are unknowingly called into play and become part of the group process. His own reactions become part of the psychotherapy process. Previously, such responses were interpreted in the negative, rather than being recognized as unavoidable.

Currently, when one speaks of marital therapy, what is meant is conjoint marital therapy. Husband and wife are seen together at the same time by the same therapist. However, there is great flexibility to this approach. Each mate is also seen individually. Parents or other members of the families of origin may be involved in therapeutic sessions. This flexibility can turn the usual triad into even larger groups. Thus, the marital therapist needs to be a group therapist whether he wishes it or not. Despite the acknowledgment of group aspects in all types of couples therapy, for the purpose of this chapter couples group therapy is defined in a strict sense as involving one or two therapists with two or more couples.

History

As the group therapy movement swept through the 1950's and 1960's, marital therapists participated in its growth. (Neubeck, 1954; Perelman, 1960; Blinder and Kirschenbaum, 1967). Many of the warnings and limitations declared by these pioneers have proven incorrect. With the passage

of time and accumulated experience, changing techniques were developed by innovative and creative therapists. Goller et al.'s (1956) conclusion that groups are considered useful only for the education of pairs of engaged couples or parents was soon bypassed. Treating each partner of a disturbed marriage in separate groups was soon outmoded, as was Hulse's warning against direct psychotherapeutic group approaches toward marital conflict. Later contributors to the literature described therapeutic successes with the group couples approach, thereby refuting the early conclusions (Flint and MacLennan, 1962; Leichter, 1962).

During the 1970's, there was a marked increase in published literature on group therapy with couples. Papanek concluded from the literature that the later authors seemed to agree that the therapist has to be an active participant to turn possible disadvantages into therapeutically useful interventions, and that an interaction between group members is dynamic and emotional, and, therefore, the therapist should not remain distant or neutral. Thus, workers moved away from psychoanalytic restrictions, and there was an emergence of general systems, behavioral, and several other theoretical approaches (Martin, 1976). This has led to the more eclectic approach of current therapists.

Technique

A couples group consists of two or more couples. There may be one or two therapists. If there are co-therapists, it is preferable that they be of different sexes. However, for purposes of training, same-sex co-therapists have been used. The couples may or may not be married. Cohabitation couples or premarital couples can be treated in separate groups or mixed with married couples. At times, only a single member of a couple may be a member of a couples group without the mate in attendance.

Many questions arise when using any of the different techniques of couples therapy, such as: Why this approach? What are its advantages, disadvantages, indications, and contraindications, and for which couples? In order to answer such questions with more than personal opinions, outcome studies are important. Unfortunately, there is a paucity of valid outcome studies in the literature. Gurman, in evaluating the outcomes of couples groups, first reviewed the goals of group marital therapy and indications and contraindications for group marital therapy. He concluded that psychoanalytic approaches fail to offer both a viable group treatment approach for couples and a foundation for clinically relevant research. He argued that the primary focus of change in couples groups should be on interactional dimensions.

Research and Training

Most of the material on which this chapter is based was obtained from two university training centers. The students have observed the author, through a one-way mirror, serving as a single therapist or a cotherapist treating a group of married couples (Martin, 1979). During the past 10 years, in addition to the educational function of this procedure and observing the effects of observers on the married couples group, an ongoing research project has been in effect. It consists of recording the dynamics and process of the observing group itself, and the effects of the couples therapy upon the personalities of the members of the observing group (Martin et al., 1977).

This research indicated that, during the observation of the therapy of married couples, education and personal change are interrelated. Changes occur spontaneously within the trainees and can be utilized constructively by the teacher. Process and reaction within the trainees' group allows them to learn meaningfully as future therapists and to mature as individuals. The powerful forces of marital and family relationships that unfold during the couples' therapeutic sessions forcefully awaken memories of similar forces within the immediate family or the childhood family of the trainee, and stimulate new, creative solutions, giving impetus to personal, marital, and family growth in trainees.

In an educational setting, the effect of the presence of the observing group is to split the responsibilities of the senior therapist, so that he is simultaneously a teacher to the observing group and a therapist to the couples group. However, an even-handed position is difficult to maintain. At times, he is aware of choosing an approach to the therapy group that fits the current educational need of the observing group. Frequently, however, as he is intensely involved in the therapeutic group process, he will disregard his role as a teacher.

It would seem that, when the group processes of the couples' group and the trainees' group are at the same point, the situation would be advantageous to the therapist from a teaching standpoint. Although this is usually true, it is not always true. Observers are not as broadly perceptive as they think they are or as has been reported in the literature.

Observers tend to over-identify with the patient group. The observing group experience helps them to learn this painful truth and to see that their own dynamics are involved in stressing the therapist's blind spots. As the trainees discover their own blind spots, they become more capable of working objectively with the technical problems being presented.

The wealth of process and reaction in the observing group can be tapped for training purposes. The professional training-personal growth dilemma encountered in training institutions is dealt with in an integrated fashion.

Indications and Contraindications

There is marked disagreement among practitioners about guidelines for selection of patients for a couples group. There is no empirical basis on which to evaluate the appropriateness of group therapy for couples. The following paragraphs include different ways of approaching the problems and include differing opinions.

This first classification follows Martin (1976):

INDICATIONS

1. Can be used routinely as a practical, efficacious form of marital therapy for all couples except when one of the contraindications listed below is present.
2. When other forms of marital therapy have reached an impasse and the advantages of the couples group can revitalize therapy.
3. When each mate is motivated to maintain the marriage and divorce is not to be considered.
4. When it is economically unfeasible for the couple to pay the fee required for the other forms of marital therapy.
5. When one or both mates suffer from social unease and can benefit from contact with other humans to effect socialization.
6. When the presence of a therapist of the same sex is essential for one member of the couples and the co-therapist approach of the couples group makes this available.

CONTRAINDICATIONS

1. When there is a family secret present which one or both mates do not want divulged.
2. When one mate is so narcissistically oriented that this mate cannot stand the attenuation of the patient-therapist relationship that occurs in a couples group.
3. When one mate is psychotic or verbally, unrestrainedly destructive.

A SECOND CLASSIFICATION

The second classification follows Gurman. He attempts clarification of the types of problems and types of people for whom group therapy is the treatment of choice.

Personality types

Outpatient couples group therapy is contraindicated when one spouse is psychotic. The stress of the group would be too great for a psychologically fragile mate.

It is also contraindicated when both members of the couple are immature and dependent, with feelings of inadequacy and confused sexual identities (Flint and MacLennan, 1962); Grunebaum takes the opposite view.

Some workers favor the group couples treatment of character-disordered couples despite the fact that others argue against including this most intractable patient subgroup.

Interactional styles

Here again there is wide disagreement, with Papanek finding an inability to communicate openly and an inability to relate to others, contraindicative for group therapy. Flint and MacLennan (1962) and Sherman feel that relatively withdrawn, noncommunicative couples with constricted social behavior are among the most likely to gain from such an experience.

Chronicity of Disharmony

Some writers state that only chronically experienced marital disharmony is appropriate for therapeutic intervention. There are no valid studies to prove or disprove either position.

Group Composition

Related to the question of selection of couples for group therapy is the question of the composition of the group. What couples should or should not be in a couples group together? Should the couples be about the same age, at similar developmental levels, and have the same sort of presenting problems? What sort of individual psychopathology is tolerable? Is it possible in group selection and compositions to select an ideal group? Is it possible to achieve therapeutic success with the worst combinations?

Grunebaum responds to this dilemma by commenting that these questions present the issues as though the decisions to be made were primarily diagnostic and were made by the therapist. He prefers approaching the issues by formulating the questions as follows: "Which sort of negotiations between the couple and the therapist are necessary and appropriate for the couple to agree to participate in group therapy (with the concurrence of the therapist) and to in fact follow through?"

He describes the individual attention given to one or both members of the couple before a referral to a group can be made. Grunebaum, Christ, and Neiberg state that many couples have to be shown that their problems are longstanding and require further intervention, and that a therapeutic alliance needs to be established in order to lower the attrition rate between the referral and true involvement in the group. Thus, negotiated aspects of referral to the group need attention.

Grunebaum responds to the question of the composition of the couples group by following the same principles that apply to individual group psychotherapy. First, a certain degree of homogeneity is desirable, since the individual who differs too greatly by virtue of degree of psychopathology, age, intellect, social class, work, or other characteristics is likely to leave or to be extruded. Groups offer opportunities for peer relationships, and they will not accept anyone who is too different. Couples groups can tolerate certain differences if they are not too extreme. Grunebaum correctly stresses that couples who are dealing with similar issues in the life cycle often do well together. For example, an older couple who are newlyweds could do well in a group of younger newlyweds if they are not too disparate in other ways.

Grunebaum's clinical experience indicates that (1) couples who have similar degrees of psychopathology do better than those with great differences in functioning; (2) the ability of couples to function socially is critical, probably more important than particular diagnoses; and (3) couples reasonably well matched in regard to mental issues tend to do well together in groups.

In summary, Grunebaum emphasized the negotiating process necessary for successful referral to couples group therapy. He suggested that the most useful criteria for the composition of well-functioning groups were similarity of developmental issues in the marriage and ability to relate to peers.

Dropouts

Many family service agencies, pressured by an overload of patients, have resorted to couples groups but found great difficulty in keeping such groups going. Couples tend to drop out in the first 3 or 4 sessions of group or will attend irregularly, leading to further dropouts and a demoralized group of one or two couples. Budman and Clifford (1979) have developed a pregroup preparation and screening approach which has reduced their couples group dropout rate to nearly zero. The Couples Communication Workshop is based on the fact that the best predictor of future behavior is present behavior. They have a workshop made up of 3 highly structured exercises. It serves as a preparation for the couples group and also as a screening process. Dropouts occur before the group ever begins, rather than hindering the process of the starting group. Budman states that a great deal more should go into starting a couples group then just setting a date and getting referrals. Good groundwork and preparation of agency personnel and patients enhance the likelihood of a successful program.

Each therapist develops his own style of forming and continuing couples groups. Framo (1973) has reported on his individual style. He structures a new group of three couples, who are all meeting for the first time, with a few simple ground rules. His aim is to develop a safe, trusting atmosphere which does not operate with the social facades and rules of ordinary social behavior. His rules include a premium on openness and expression of thoughts and feelings but no physical violence, a prohibition against talking about other couples in social situations, and a dictum that all criticisms of others in the group be made in a constructive fashion. Once his group is started, it becomes open ended.

Treatment

Having selected the couples for the group (whether by classic methods or by the pressures of service needs), the techniques of treatment come into focus. Every generalization on this subject found in the literature can be contradicted by specific examples. The exceptions to the rules are too numerous to catalogue. Each group is a new adventure to be explored with an open mind and a creative response by the therapist or co-therapists. Just as change is the goal for each member of the couple, so is change the goal in the therapists. The therapists are active participants in the process of change in each member of the group. An early clarification of this contract by the therapists is advocated. This is especially important in a couples group, because frequently the initial goal of each partner is to change the other person. Also, despite early clarification of the therapeutic contract, each member of the group will tend to establish his or her own contract with the therapists and with the group that is a duplicate of the type of contract the individual established with the partner (Martin, 1976). This will be observed through the individual's behavior. The work on contracts is helpful in the elucidation of this aspect of intimate relations.

For example, a common type of marriage relationship is where one spouse is completely controlling and dominates the passive spouse. As long as this contract is accepted by the passive partner, there is no marital disharmony. When such a couple comes into the group, the dominant one works feverishly to maintain control over the mate and initiate control over the therapists and other membes of the group. If, through the group process and support, the dependent spouse initiates changes toward separation, individuation, and independence, one of a number of different behaviors may be observed. In some instances, the dominant mate forces withdrawal from the group. The dependent mate is threatened by the loss of the spouse, accepts the old contract, and remains away from the group.

In some instances, the dependent spouse utilizes the support system of the group and the therapists, and returns to the therapy alone. This is a refusal to continue the old contract with the spouse. This may be a healthy change, with a breaking up of a fixed, rigid, psychopathological system, or it may in time turn out to be a maintenance of the same position and contract, but with a shift to the therapists or the group as the dominating, protective parent. Another recognizable course is where the dominant mate, recognizing the possible loss of the spouse, will return to the group and will accept a new contract with the spouse and the group. It may be merely a reversal, wherein the previously dominant mate gives up pseudoindependence and allows dependent needs to surface. However, with guidance of the therapists, it can become a developmental leap forward, with a gain of individuation for the self and an acceptance of individuation of the mate.

Papanek stated that the married couples group uses all the potentialities that the therapeutic group offers in an effort to help each spouse understand what he or she is missing in their relationship. This loosens the interlocking neurotic pattern and promotes healthier relationships by strengthening the sense of identity and self-worth, while also developing the ability for mutuality and cooperation. She describes communications and interactions in the married couples group as being at a high pitch, and asserts that group process develops by temporarily disrupting an unhealthy, conflict-ridden cohesiveness between the marriage partners. In her experience in the early sessions, the couples can hardly listen and relate to anybody else except each other. Thus, the other group members are perceived as audience or court of appeal, not as individuals. Then, when attention shifts and group members become individuals, the therapeutic process of insight—and correction of neurotic needs, expectations, and fears—can begin, and the unfinished maturation process can proceed. Papanek is

different from nonanalytic couples group leaders; she does not avoid dealing with unconscious material. Instead, she uses dreams as one method to help couples free themselves from their distorted images of one another and from neurotic binds that strangle their relationship. Group leaders who use unconscious material in this way can also use it to clarify distorted images which develop in both the nonspouse members of the group and in the therapists.

Leaders

A review of the leader concepts in the field of group therapy shows not only variations but contradictions in views. The claim of early leaders that group therapy ought to be limited to patients initially unknown to each other has been invalidated in practice. Wolf and Schwartz did concede, however, that it may be possible to treat married couples in groups when the leader plays some interpretive, supporting, guiding, and mediating role.

Kadis and Markowitz, as co-therapists, employed firm leadership roles even to the extent of limiting the number of sessions in couples groups. Grotjahn used his role to increase communication and to establish in-fighting. Everett and his co-therapists defuse hostile transference reactions by using some members of the group to serve as partisan lawyers and others to serve as objective and impartial judges and counselors.

Framo (1973), in his role as leader, confronts, challenges, and seeks to change. Strachstein uses both a directive and an analytic approach. The leader directs the mates to sit separately and assists emotional as well as physical separateness. She states: "Couples groups are 'chancey' but the results are often like turning on the lights in a dark room where each partner has been groping and stumbling against each other. Now he can see that the individual against whom he has been fighting for years is not his hated father, mother, or sibling, but a human being he could possibly love today."

Conclusion

Greater activity on the part of leaders of couples groups can be expended in different directions. The therapist can focus on interactions and become skilled and secure in confronting couples. At the same time, the therapist has available other members of the group to serve as co-therapists. The therapist can use flexible combinations of marriage dynamics and group dynamics to overcome resistance and to facilitate change. Papanek stated, "In the group, therapist and patients turn the searchlight of attention on the couple, on the individual and his past and present relationships, and also on his reactions in the group."

References

Blinder, G., and Kirschenbaum, M. The technique of married couple group therapy. Arch. Gen. Psychiatry, *17:* 44, 1967.
Budman, S. H., and Clifford, M. Short-term group therapy for couples in a health maintenance organization. Prof. Psychol., *10:* 49, 1979.

Cookerly, J. R. The outcome of the six major forms of marriage counseling compared: A pilot study. J. Marriage Fam., *41:* 608, 1973.

Flint, A. A., and MacLennan, B. W. Some dynamic factors in marital group psychotherapy. Int. J. Group Psychother. *12:* 355, 1962.

Framo, J. L. Marriage therapy in a couples group. Semin. Psychiatry, *5:* 207, 1973.

Goller, G., Sherman, S. N., and Hulse, W. C. Group approaches to the treatment of marital problems. In *Neurotic Interaction in Marriage*, V. W. Eisenstein, editor, p. 290. Basic Books, New York, 1956.

Leichter, E. Group psychotherapy with married couples. Int. J. Group Psychother., *12:* 154, 1962.

Martin, P. A. *A Marital Therapy Manual.* Brunner/Mazel, New York, 1976.

Martin, P. A. Training of psychiatric residents in marital therapy. J. Marital Fam. Ther., *41:* 43, 1979.

Martin, P. A., Tornga, M., McGlobin, J. F., and Boles, S. Observing groups as seen from both sides of the looking glass. Group, *1:* 147, 1977.

Neubeck, G. Factors affecting group therapy with married couples. Marriage Fam. Liv., *16:* 216, 1954.

Papanek, H. Group psychotherapy with married couples. Curr. Psychiatr. Ther., *5:* 158, 1965.

Perelman, J. L. Problems encountered in psychotherapy of married couples. Int. J. Group Psychother., *10:* 136, 1960.

C.10 Group Psychotherapy with Rape Victims and Battered Women

VIRGINIA A. SADOCK, M.D.

Introduction

Rape victims and battered persons are two different categories of victims. However, they have much in common. Both groups are predominantly—usually solely—female; both categories have suffered a combined physical and psychological trauma (inflicted by men); and both sets of victims have, until recently, been ignored by society in general. In addition, the two types of abuse can overlap. Battering husbands sometimes rape their wives, and 7 per cent of rapists are close relatives of their victims. Also, rapists usually inflict other forms of physical violence on their victims in addition to rape.

Feminist groups have been largely responsible for the recent attention focused on the problems of rape and spouse abuse. These groups are the most active anti-rape and anti-abuse factions in society in terms of consciousness raising, prevention, and immediate support for victims.

Rape

DEFINITION

In the third edition of the American Psychiatric Association's (1980) *Diagnostic and Statistical Manual of Mental Disorders* (DSM-III), rape is cautiously considered under the diagnosis of sexual sadism.

Rape or other sexual assault may be committed by individuals with this disorder. In such instances, the suffering inflicted on the victim increases the sexual excitement of the assailant. However, it should not be assumed that all or even most rapists are motivated by sexual sadism. Often, the rapist is not motivated by the prospect of inflicting suffering, and may even lose sexual desire as a consequence. These represent two poles of a spectrum; and for cases falling in the middle, it may be very difficult for the clinician to decide if the diagnosis of sexual sadism is warranted.

The legal definition of rape in the United States (Brownmiller, 1975) is:

The perpetration of an act of sexual intercourse with a female, not one's wife, against her will and consent, whether her will is overcome by force or fear resulting from the threat of force or by drugs or intoxicants; or when because of mental deficiency she is incapable of exercising rational judgment, or when she is below an artibrary age of consent.

The crime of rape requires slight penile penetration of the victim's outer vulva. Full erection and ejaculation are not necessary. Forced acts of fellatio and anal penetration, although they frequently accompany rape, are legally considered sodomy.

INCIDENCE

According to the Uniform Crime Reports for 1973 put out by the Federal Bureau of Investigation, rape is a highly underreported crime. The estimate is that only one out of four to one out of 10 rapes is reported. If the lowest estimated figure is taken, the reported incidence of 50,000 rapes a year increases to 200,000 rapes a year. The under-reporting is attributed to feelings of shame on the part of the victim.

Victims of rape can be any age. Cases have been

reported in which the victim was 15 months old and in which she was 82 years old. The greatest danger exists for women aged 10 to 29. Rape most commonly occurs in a woman's own neighborhood, frequently inside her own home. About 50 per cent of the rapes are committed by strangers and 50 per cent by men known, to varying degrees, by the victims.

Convicted rapists seem to be part of a general subculture of violence. Federal Bureau of Investigation records reveal that 70 per cent of arrested rapists have prior criminal histories, including records of assault, robbery, and homicide. Rape often occurs as an accompaniment to another crime. The rapist always threatens his victim with fists, gun, or knife and frequently harms her in nonsexual—as well as sexual—ways. The victim may be beaten, wounded, and sometimes killed.

Statistics show that 61 per cent of rapists are under 25, 51 per cent are white, 47 per cent are black, and the remaining 2 per cent come from all other races. A composite picture of a rapist drawn from police figures portrays a single, 19-year-old man from the lower socio-economic classes with a police record of acquisitive offenses. This composite picture of the rapist, however, is incomplete, due to the underreporting of the crime.

REACTIONS TO RAPE

It is sometimes difficult to separate previously existing pathology from reactions to the rape itself. Rape is sufficiently traumatic to do substantial damage to a psychologically healthy woman.

The woman being raped is frequently in a life-threatening situation. During the rape, she experiences shock and a fright approaching panic. Her prime motivation is to stay alive. There is a high incidence of submission, as can be expected, when the rapist uses a knife or a gun. In most cases, rapists choose victims slightly smaller than themselves. The rapist may urinate or defecate on his victim, ejaculate into her face and hair, force anal intercourse, and insert foreign objects into her vagina and rectum.

After the rape, the woman may experience shame, humiliation, confusion, fear, and rage. The type of reaction and the duration of the reaction are variable, but women report effects lasting for 1 year or longer. Many women experience the symptoms of a post-traumatic reaction. The rape overwhelms them with a sense of vulnerability, a fear of living in a dangerous world, and a loss of control over their own lives. They become preoccupied with the trauma, and it colors their future actions and day-to-day behavior. Some women feel defiled and unable to wash themselves clean. Many are afraid to walk through the neighborhood where the rape occurred, even if they lived there for years before the rape. Others cannot remain in their homes or apartments. They have a fear of being followed or a fear of being alone. They may be unable to sleep, afraid to shop in their usual stores, or unable to function at work. Some women are able to resume sexual relations with men, particularly if they have always felt sexually adequate. Others become phobic of sexual interaction, or develop such symp-toms as vaginismus or anorgasmia. Few women emerge from the assault completely unscathed. The manifestations and the degree of damage depend on the violence of the attack itself, the vulnerability of the woman, and the support systems available to her immediately after the attack.

GROUP THERAPY

Therapy is usually supportive in approach, unless there is a severe underlying disorder, and focuses on restoring the victim's sense of adequacy and control over her life and relieving the feelings of helplessness, dependency, and obsession with the assault that frequently follow rape. Group therapy with homogeneous groups composed of rape victims is a particularly helpful form of treatment.

The women, having shared similar traumas, quickly develop an empathic rapport. The group also effectively diminishes the shame that many victims feel; they know other group members will understand the answers to the disgraceful cultural accusations, "Why didn't you fight back?" or "Why did it happen to you?" The group provides a willing ear for the ventilation of feelings of rage and helplessness experienced by the victims. Also, group members are encouraged to provide a supportive network for each other between therapeutic sessions. For instance, if a rape victim is a single woman, living alone, she is encouraged to call group members when she feels panicky, particularly during the initial phase of recovery.

The homogeneity of the group comes from all members having been rape victims. In other respects, however, the group benefits from having members of different marital status, age, and socioeconomic background. For example, the trauma will have a significantly different effect on an adolescent girl with little sexual experience than on a 40-year-old woman who is married and has children. In a group with members of these two different backgrounds, the older woman can reassure the young girl about the possibility of having positive sexual experiences with men. She may be more effective in giving this reassurance than a therapist who has never been raped or the adolescent's family members, who may feel inhibited about discussing sex with her. By the same token, the presence of the adolescent in the group can help the older woman work through feelings of shame about facing her own children because she feels debased.

The group also provides an effective network with which to overcome phobias that rape victims may develop as a result of their experience.

Elaine, a 31-year-old divorced woman, worked as a junior executive for a large corporation. Her job occasionally required her to pick up material at a printer for presentation at work. The printing establishment was located near where she had been raped, and she experienced a sense of dread approaching a state of panic whenever she had to go there. Group members volunteered to accompany her until she overcame her fear. Although her anxiety diminished considerably over the course of a year, she never really felt comfortable with this chore, and eventually managed to assign it to someone else in the firm.

A number of behavioral techniques can be utilized within the group format to help members deal with the fears which have developd following the trauma. These techniques include using a buddy system to accomplish anxiety-provoking tasks, the full range of relaxation exercises, and the use of systematic desensitization. Modified sex therapy techniques also help women who develop sexual problems following rape.

Rape not only affects the victim herself but is frequently an emotional trauma for those close to her. The group provides an excellent forum for members to discuss and compare reactions of their family members. A group member's husband might even be invited to attend one of the group sessions. The group visit can be a therapeutic experience for the husband who feels that his wife should have fought off the rapist, or for the husband who fears his wife might have enjoyed the experience. This last fear is not uncommon in husbands whose wives develop sexual dysfunctions following rape.

The group visit offers the husband the opportunity to ventilate feelings about which he may be ashamed, and the couple, viewed as a traumatized unit, can receive support. However, such visits to the group must be approached with caution. They require vigilance on the part of the therapist, who must prevent scapegoating of the husband and also be alert to the reactivation of feelings of fear and low self-esteem in group members. An adjunctive technique is to form a separate group of rape victims' partners.

The therapist leading a group of rape victims deals with a variety of countertransference problems. The biggest danger is overidentification with the woman who has been brutalized. This can lead to infantalization of the victim, when what is necessary is the reestablishment of her sense of competence. Or angry feelings can be focused on to the exclusion of intrapsychic or interpersonal conflicts which the trauma has generated. The therapist has the difficult job of being supportive without being overprotective, of being empathic while maintaining objectivity.

The support systems a victim encounters following rape are critical to her ability to recover from the trauma. The sooner therapy is begun, the more likely it is to be successful.

Battered Women

Battered women are found, paradoxically, in the context of that structure designed to provide protection and security for its members: the family. Women are beaten by fathers or husbands or other male family members. Battering is often severe, involving broken limbs, broken ribs, internal bleeding, and brain damage. In this section, the focus is on battered wives.

This aspect of domestic violence has been recognized as a severe problem, largely as a result of recent cultural emphasis on civil rights and the work of feminist groups. The problem itself is one of long standing.

INCIDENCE

Spouse abuse is estimated to occur in from 3 million to 6 million families in the United States. Wife beating occurs in families of every racial and religious background and crosses all socio-economic lines. It is most frequent in families with problems of drug abuse, particularly where there is alcoholism.

CAUSES

Behavioral, cultural, intrapsychic, and interpersonal factors all contribute to the development of the problem. Abusive men are likely to have come from violent homes where they witnessed wife beating or were abused themselves as children. The act itself is reinforcing. Once a man has beaten his wife, he is likely to do so again. Although abusive husbands may not suffer from severe mental illness, they tend to be immature, dependent, and non-assertive, and to suffer from strong feelings of inadequacy.

Their aggression is bullying behavior, designed to humiliate their wives to build up their own low self-esteem. The abuse is most likely to occur when the man feels threatened or frustrated at home, at work, or with peers. Impatient and impulsive, abusive husbands literally and physically displace aggression provoked by others onto their wives. The dynamics include identification with an aggressor (father, boss), testing behavior (will she stay with me no matter how I treat her?), distorted desires to express manhood, and dehumanization of the woman.

An abusive husband considers his wife his belonging and may be particularly assaultive when she shows any sign of independence, talks about getting a job, leaves the house without telling him, or threatens to leave the marriage. By the same token, he is most destructive when she is most dependent—when she is pregnant or when she has small children—because the immature husband may feel he does not get enough attention or respect when his wife responds to the demands of their little children or has less time and energy for him.

The women who remain in such marriages do not necessarily come from violent homes. The trait most commonly found in abused wives who stay with their husbands is dependency. The woman perceives herself as unable to function alone in the world or without a man. Regardless of her occupation or talents, she sees marriage as an unequal partnership, with the man in the dominant position. She usually comes from a background that has supported traditional male-female (aggressive-passive) role models. On a deeper level, she defines herself by and takes her identity from her husband. That dynamic makes it extremely difficult for her to expose the problem. Revealing her husband as brutal and inadequate is tantamount to revealing herself as inadequate. Like the abused child, the dependent woman frequently blames herself for the abuse she receives.

Unfortunately, the culture has supported the distortion of the man who sees his wife as property and himself as manly when he is violent. It has also told the woman that she provokes the behavior and that she should maintain her marriage at all costs. That message has been given by mental health professionals, by pastoral counselors, and by police officers—all usually men—who are reluctant to interfere in domestic problems, and by society in general, which has largely ignored the problem.

GROUP TREATMENT

Group therapy for battered women is most effective when it is part of an over-all treatment program which provides medical assistance, emergency shelters, legal aid, access to child care facilities, and occupational counseling.

A homogeneous group of battered women provides an excellent support system for the abused woman who has decided to leave or restructure her violent home setting and must now navigate a complex legal system, withstand societal pressures to keep her marriage intact, and support herself and often her children, frequently without assistance.

Ideally, the group should be composed of members at different stages in resolving their problems. In that way, a woman who has been able to find a job and outgrow her feelings of helplessness and dependence on her husband stands as a role model for the woman in crisis who still bears the bruises from a recent battering.

Group members provide encouragement for each other. In addition, as in groups of rape victims, the members' sense of shame at being victimized diminishes as they share their experiences. Many feel able to ventilate feelings of humiliation, despair, or rage for the first time.

On a psychodynamic level, the group therapist focuses on issues of dependency and self-esteem. Group members support each other in taking what are often frightening steps for the women. For example, they may accompany each other to court, share child care, or help each other with resumes. Techniques such as role playing are used to help members prepare for job interviews or for meetings with their spouses.

Group members help each other withstand a husband's pleas to accept or return to the violent marriage. Some men feel remorse and guilt after an episode of violent behavior and become particularly loving. That behavior gives the wife hope, and she remains until the next cycle of violence, which inevitably occurs.

Other men become doubly intimidating when their wives try to alter the status quo and make threatening statements, such as, "I'll get you." The presence of another group member in a battered woman's first encounter with her husband after she has left the home—for instance, if he comes to see her at an emergency shelter—provides support for the wife and acts as a control on the husband.

Change in a husband's battering behavior is initiated only when the man is convinced that the woman will not tolerate the situation and when she begins to exert control over his behavior. The group is highly effective in helping a frightened, dependent woman confront that fact and recognize that she does have some means of controlling him. For example, she can do so by leaving for a prolonged period, with therapy for the man as a condition of return.

With relatively less impulsive and less brutal men, an external control, such as calling the police or a group member, may be sufficient to stop his assault. The group encourages the woman still living with her husband to call for help at the slightest indication of impending violence. She is reeducated to view a call for help as an act of strength. Before therapy, most battered women are too ashamed of their problem to ask for help and make the problem public: "How could I deal with my neighbors after they've seen a police car drive up to our house?"

As therapy progresses and the battered woman makes practical and emotional gains, she no longer conceptualizes her husband as all powerful. She begins to see his aggressiveness as the bullying of an emotionally immature, dependent, and frustrated person. This is a necessary step if she is to form a more satisfying relationship with another man or with her husband.

Concurrent groups for battering husbands are therapeutic for the men and essential if they want to change their behavior, or if the woman plans to stay in the marriage. Alternatives to this approach are concurrent family or marital therapy.

References

American Psychiatric Association. *Diagnostic and Statistical Manual of Mental Disorders,* ed 3. American Psychiatric Association, Washington, D.C., 1980.

Amin, A. *Patterns in Forcible Rape.* University of Chicago Press, Chicago, 1971.

Brownmiller, S. *Against Our Will: Men, Women, and Rape.* Simon & Schuster, New York, 1975.

Carmen, E., Russo, N., and Miller, J. Inequality and women's mental health: An overview. Am. J. Psychiatry, *138:* 1319, 1981.

Dobash, R. E., and Dobash, R. *Violence against Wives: A Case against the Patriarchy.* Free Press, New York, 1979.

Hilberman, E. *The Rape Victim.* Garamond/Pridemark Press, Baltimore, 1976.

Hilberman, E. Overview: The "wife-beater's wife" reconsidered. Am. J. Psychiatry, *137:* 1336, 1980.

Lowenstein, L. F. Who is the rapist? J. Crim. Law, *162:* 137, 1977.

Mulvihill, D. J. *Crimes of Violence: A Report to the National Commission on the Causes and Prevention of Violence.* United States Government Printing Office, Washington, D.C., 1969.

Murstein, B. I. *Love, Sex, and Marriage throughout the Ages.* Springer, New York, 1974.

Symonds, M. The rape victim: Psychological patterns of response. Am. J. Psychoanal., *36:* 27, 1976.

C.11 Group Psychotherapy of Psychosexual Dysfunctions

VIRGINIA A. SADOCK, M.D.

Introduction

In the past several decades, American society has experienced radical changes in its prevalent sexual attitudes. These changes in attitude are the result of many factors. The advent of effective birth control methods and the legalization of abortion have emphasized sexual activity as a pleasurable function separate from its procreative aspects. Studies such as those of the Kinsey Foundation and the Playboy Foundation published the degree, the type, and the frequency of sexual activity in this country, bringing sexual practices from the realm of inference and secrecy into accepted, if still private, reality. The Presidential Commission on Obscenity and Pornography (1970) advised against sexual repression, encouraging the candid discussion of sexuality in society and the acceptability of sexually stimulating material. The research and published reports of Masters and Johnson focused the attention of the medical profession and the general public on sexual physiology and on the distress caused by sexual dysfunctions. They also helped to create an optimistic climate for the treatment of sexual dysfunctions. In addition, cultural changes in the perception of women, stimulated by the work of feminist groups, and changes in the perception of the aged, accomplished by the efforts of geriatric groups, have affected the sexual expectations of women and of the aged.

Most medical schools now include lectures on sexual physiology and psychosexual disorders and the treatment of those disorders in their curriculums. Also, many medical centers have clinics specifically oriented to the treatment of sexual dysfunctions. The various sexual disorders amenable to treatment include the following: (1) inhibited sexual desire in a man and in a woman; (2) impotence or inhibited sexual excitement in a man; (3) inhibited female orgasm or anorgasmia; (4) inhibited male orgasm or retarded ejaculation; (5) premature ejaculation; (6) functional dyspareunia; and (7) functional vaginismus.

There are no reliable statistics on how often a particular sexual dysfunction has an organic cause, rather than a functional psychological cause, but a complete physical examination by a urologist, an internist or a gynecologist should be an integral part of the diagnostic work-up. And if an organic cause for the disorder is found, treatment should be directed toward ameliorating the physical cause of the disorder.

Theoretical Orientation of Groups

Group therapy is one of several modalities that have been successful in examining both intrapsychic and interpersonal problems in patients with sexual disorders. The therapy group provides a strong support system for a patient who feels ashamed, anxious, or guilty about a particular sexual problem. It is also a useful forum in which to counteract sexual myths and to educate patients regarding sexual anatomy, physiology, and varieties of behavior.

Groups may have different theoretical orientations. For example, groups may be psychodynamically oriented, behaviorally oriented, or primarily educational. And group composition can be organized in different ways. Members may all share the same problem (such as premature ejaculation), members may all be of the same sex with different sexual problems, or groups may be composed of men and women who are experiencing different sexual problems. Group membership may also be made up of couples or unattached persons.

The groups discussed in this chapter deal with sexual dysfunctions as they apply to heterosexual relationships.

Groups Oriented to Specific Psychosexual Dysfunctions

Groups organized to cure a specific psychosexual dysfunction are usually behavioral in approach (LoPiccolo and Lobitz, 1972; Barbach, 1975). Although those groups are usually homogeneous as to gender and sexual complaint, they can be heterogeneous regarding age, marital status, and sociocultural background. Reported ages of group members have varied from 19 years to 60 years of age. Members have been unskilled laborers, housewives, and professionals. Participants have had various religious, racial, and ethnic backgrounds. The majority of patients, however—as in traditional individual psychotherapy—have been white, middle-class people.

The sexual dysfunctions most frequently treated by behaviorally oriented groups are inhibited orgasm in women and premature ejaculation in men. The groups are usually composed of 5 to 10 members. The preorgasmic groups are generally led by a woman therapist or a female co-therapy team, and the groups for premature ejaculators usually have a male group leader.

The group leaders act as authorities, educators, and

role models for the program participants. As educators, they correct ignorance or misinformation regarding sexual physiology, anatomy, and behavior. Specific physiological information—sometimes with the aid of audiovisual materials—is presented to the group members. On a psychodynamic level, the group therapists represent parental figures who encourage the development of sexual expression that past experience has inhibited in the group members. And peer interaction provides support, confrontation, and validation of feelings that are a vital part of the therapeutic process.

PREORGASMIC GROUPS FOR WOMEN

Women suffering from anorgasmia participate with others suffering from the same problem in a short-term, intensive group experience. Group members share sexual histories, common feelings of low self-esteem, and concerns about body image. A woman's recognition that she is not alone in having this problem—that other women share her feelings of being incomplete or defective because they cannot have an orgasm—provides initial relief for many group members, and is a major source of group cohesion.

The review and sharing of histories helps some women become more conscious of those experiences and factors that contributed to their sexual dysfunction.

One patient, Anita, recalled that, as a child, she would gently rub her genital area with her hand over her clothing. She did not know she was masturbating; she just knew the sensations she felt were very pleasant. Each time her mother saw Anita masturbating, she would say, "Go to the bathroom, dear. You must have to go to the bathroom."
Anita quickly picked up the message that she should not masturbate in public. Unfortunately, she also learned to confuse the pleasant sensations she felt from masturbating with the functions of urinating and defecating. She had been taught that these were shameful acts. As a result, she began to inhibit her sexual responses.

In addition to group sessions—held 1 to 5 times weekly—members are given homework assignments to be performed in private. These assignments initially focus on helping the woman become comfortable with her body in general and later include exercises that involve stimulation of the genital area specifically. For instance, a patient may initially be told to take a long bath and caress her body with soap or lotions or to spend 15 to 20 minutes examining herself nude in front of a mirror, focusing on what she does and does not like about herself. Many women who are sexually inhibited ignore their bodies or magnify in their minds those aspects of themselves they consider physically unattractive. Those homework assignments and subsequent sessions can help diminish such distortions.

An early assignment usually includes suggestions that the women look at their genitalia with a hand mirror. Some women are squeamish about this exercise. Initial responses vary from disgust to surprise or pleasure. The group offers an arena for patients to talk about their reaction with their therapists and with other group members and to compare reactions. For example, some women who may not recall ever having looked at their genitals before become concerned about any asymmetry of the vaginal lips—a normal anatomical occurrence in many women. The group can provide reassurance and correct many misperceptions a member may have that she is physically abnormal.

Eventually, group members receive a homework assignment to masturbate. The therapists may describe a variety of techniques used in masturbation. The emphasis in discussing this exercise is on the uniqueness of each woman—the fact that each individual likes different areas caressed (although most women focus on sites on or around the clitoris), that different women respond to differing degrees of pressure during stimulation, and that some women—especially if they have never experienced orgasm—may require long periods of stimulation, sometimes up to several hours, before they are able to climax.

When this homework assignment is first given, the women are instructed not to have an orgasm—even if they feel they would be able to—in order to relieve performance pressure and avoid a repetition of experiences that have made them feel inadequate in the past. Instead, the group therapist will encourage the group members to focus on the slightest sensation that they feel. The use of fantasy is also explored.

Some women who have never allowed themselves to have conscious sexual fantasies are able to do so for the first time with the encouragement of the group. At first, some may borrow fantasies from group members and only later develop those that are more erotic for themselves.

A combination of group support and group pressure helps some of the women complete assignments they might otherwise avoid.

One woman, Betty, who had absorbed strong parental injunctions against masturbation, was nonetheless able to do the first masturbatory exercise and experienced intense, pleasurable sensations. Several sessions later, however, she angrily stated she was giving up because she no longer experienced any sensations when she attempted to masturbate. The group therapist reassured her that this was a frequent occurrence for many women, that old mechanisms of repression frequently take over after a first attempt at masturbation just because sexual sensations are experienced. Some of Betty's group members shared that they were having a similar problem and encouraged her to persevere. Equally important in getting her to continue was the challenge of one group member: "So give up. Just reconcile yourself to never having an orgasm."

Concurrent with exercises involving bodily stimulation, exercises are assigned which are designed to augment assertiveness and facilitate communication with partners. The group members are instructed to indulge in something they would ordinarily deny themselves; for one woman this might mean having a pedicure; for another it might mean spending an afternoon reading a book. Sometimes the homework assignment includes a discussion with one's mother—if she is available—regarding what the mother's sexual upbringing was like. Some women practice asserting themselves with their husbands. For example, they may ask that one weekend afternoon be devoted to brunch at a restaurant and a walk, instead of a scheduled television showing of a sports event.

With particularly resistant women, the use of vibrators or exercises such as sitting under water taps in the bath tub are sometimes suggested. These techniques provide unusual and intense stimulation and are then combined with exercises of manual stimulation.

As the group members become more comfortable with their sexuality, they are encouraged to talk about their experiences with their partners. The final exercises usually include members' partners if the woman is involved in a relationship.

GROUPS FOR PREMATURE EJACULATORS

These groups are organized similarly to the preorgasmic groups, with all the participants suffering from the same dysfunction. Sexual histories, feelings of inadequacy, and concerns about acceptance are shared. Many men with this problem find they share a history of initial sexual experiences in situations where discovery of themselves and their partners was a hazard. For example, they may have experienced sexual intercourse for the first time in the back seat of a car or in their girlfriend's home, where interruption by parents was a possibility. Experiences like those frequently condition participants to ejaculate quickly in order to avoid a potentially embarrassing situation. Other men are able to share more deep-seated feelings of inadequacy for the first time.

Robert, a 26-year-old man of average height, had reached puberty late. His early adolescence had been painful. He had not felt able to compete with other boys in sports because of his small size, and was not part of the popular social group when parties and dating began among his peers.

The group members were supportive of Robert and helped him to see that his adolescent feelings of inadequacy were coloring his current self-image and still affecting his life, including his sexual life. The group process enabled him to absorb this insight more rapidly than would have been possible in individual therapy.

Homework assignments for premature ejaculators focus on masturbating while using a stop-start technique. This technique is used to raise the threshold of penile excitability. In this exercise, the man stimulates the erect penis until the earliest sensations of impending orgasm and ejaculation are felt. Penile stimulation is then stopped abruptly. In one variation of this exercise, the penis is forcibly squeezed for several seconds when penile stimulation is stopped. This technique is repeated several times. Masturbation to the point of imminent orgasm raises the threshold of excitability to a more tolerant stimulation level (Semans, 1956).

If the men are involved in relationships, their partners are eventually included in the exercises. In this case, the woman stimulates the man, employing the squeeze technique. Communication between the partners is improved, since the man must let his partner know the degree of his sexual excitement, so that she can squeeze the penis before the ejaculatory process has started. Sex therapy, in general, has been most successful in the treatment of premature ejaculation.

OTHER DYSFUNCTION-ORIENTED GROUPS

Similar groups are also organized for the treatment of other sexual dysfunctions. The specific sexual exercises assigned as homework vary with the differing presenting complaints. In cases of vaginismus, for instance, the woman is advised to dilate her vaginal opening with her fingers or with size-graduated vaginal dilators as part of the therapy. In cases of impotence, the man—and later his wife—is instructed to tease the penis, to stimulate it for increasing periods of time, although not to organism. This same technique is used on men suffering from retarded ejaculation, sometimes including stimulation by a vibrator.

The over-all goal of treatment is always to initiate an educational process, to diminish fears of performance, and, when members are involved in relationships, to facilitate communication within the dyad in sexual and nonsexual areas.

Couples Groups

Groups have also been effective when composed of sexually dysfunctional married couples (Sadock and Spitz, 1976). The group provides the opportunity to gather accurate information, provides consensual validation of individual preferences, and enhances self-esteem and self-acceptance. Techniques such as role playing and psychodrama may be used in treatment. Couples groups are also effective as a form of follow-up treatment for couples who have been through individual sex therapy. Such groups are not indicated when one partner is uncooperative, when a patient is suffering from a severe depression or psychosis, when there is a strong repugnance to explicit sexual audio-visual material, or when there is a strong fear of groups.

Psychodynamically Oriented Group Therapy

Intensive group psychotherapy explores the psychodynamic personality make-up of the members involved. Denial and projective mechanisms are frequently used by patients with sexual anxieties. Member-to-member and member-to-therapist transferences and interactions allow for the rapid emergence of sexual conflicts related to past experiences with siblings, parents, and other significant persons. Single people who have not had much experience in close, sexual relationships have a unique opportunity to correct misperceptions about attitudes or behavior of the opposite sex. Psychodynamically oriented groups require a greater time commitment from patients and are less focused on a specific sexual dysfunction than are behaviorally oriented groups.

Results

The reported effectiveness of various treatment methods for a problem of sexual dysfunction varies from study to study. Barbach (1975) reports on statistics compiled by the Human Sexuality Program at the University of California Medical Center, indicating that 93 per cent of anorgasmic women who entered the program were able to experience orgasms through self-stimulation after 5 weeks of therapy.

Some workers have studied empirical criteria which they feel are predictive of outcome when behavioral approaches are used. According to these criteria, persons who regularly practice assigned exercises have a much greater likelihood of successful outcome than do more resistant patients or patients whose interactions involve mechanisms of blame or projection. Flexibility of attitude is also a favorable prognostic factor.

In general, the more severe the psychopathology associated with a problem of long duration, the more adverse the outcome. In cases of successful therapy, the gains are reinforced by a continuation of the therapy exercises, even after treatment has stopped, and by scheduled follow-up sessions with group leaders or group members.

References

Barbach, L. G. *For Yourself: The Fulfillment of Female Sexuality.* Doubleday, New York, 1975.
Commission on Obscenity and Pornography. *The Report on the Commission on Obscenity and Pornography.* United States Government Printing Office, Washington, D.C., 1970.
Ersner-Hirschfield, R., and Kopel, S. Group treatment of pre-orgasmic women. J. Consult. Clin. Psychol., *47:* 750, 1979.
Lobitz, W. C., and Baker E. C. Group therapy of single males with erectile dysfunction. Arch. Sex. Behav., *8:* 127, 1979.
LoPiccolo, J., and Lobitz, W. The role of masturbation in the treatment of sexual dysfunction. Arch. Sex. Behav., *2:* 163, 1972.
Meyer, J. K., Schmidt, C. W., Lucas, M. J., and Smith, E. Short-term treatment of sexual problems: Interim report. Am. J. Psychiatry, *132:* 172, 1975.
Sadock, B. J., and Spitz, H. I. Group psychotherapy of sexual disorders. In *The Sexual Experience,* B. J. Sadock, H. I. Kaplan, and A. M. Freedman, editors, ed. 2, p. 1569. Williams & Wilkins, Baltimore, 1976.
Sadock, V. A. Treatment of psychosexual dysfunctions. In *Comprehensive Textbook of Psychiatry,* H. I. Kaplan, A. M. Freedman, and B. J. Sadock, editors, ed. 3, p. 1799. Williams & Wilkins, Baltimore, 1980.
Semans, J. H. Premature ejaculation: A new approach. South. Med. J., *49:* 353, 1956.
Smith, E. P., and Meyer, J. K. Attitudes and temperaments of non-orgastic women. Med. Asp. Hum. Sexual., *12:* 66, 1978.

C.12 Group Methods in the General Hospital Setting

ALLEN H. COLLINS, M.D., M.P.H.
JERALD GROBMAN, M.D.

Introduction

Two historical trends have led to the use of small groups on the medical-surgical units of general hospitals. One trend has been the increasing use of a group approach in the psychiatric consultation-liaison process. Shulman (1975) notes that, since the 1950's, consultation-liaison psychiatrists have recognized that the most effective consultations involve both patients and the medical, nursing, and other ward support staff. To improve their consultations, many consultation-liaison psychiatrists began to use weekly meetings with members of the health care delivery team to augment their patient-oriented consultations. These regularly scheduled meetings between the consultation psychiatrist and the medical team are now well recognized as an important component of the consultation-liaison service process.

Another trend has been the use of small groups to help the medical staff cope with many sources of emotional stress that are a real part of their work environment, to reduce frequent staff turnover, and to improve patient care (Eisendrath et al., 1970; Craig, 1973; Abram, 1974, Kilgour, 1975; Weeks, 1978; Berarducci et al., 1979; Eisendrath and Dunkel, 1979; Gardner et al., 1980). These groups are usually established on the most acute medical-surgical units which treat the sickest patients.

In the literature, these groups are referred to as "consultation conferences" (Simon and Whiteley, 1977), "nurse support groups" (Caldwell and Weiner, 1981), "liaison teaching conferences" (Strain, 1975), and "ombudsman (medical-psychiatric) rounds" (Strain and Hamerman, 1978). They are led by liaison psychiatrists, psychiatric residents, psychologists, and psychiatric liaison nurse clinicians. Group meetings vary in frequency, from once a week to once a month, and are approximately 1 hour in duration. They may exist for several sessions or may go on for several years. Membership is open to all interested medical and nursing staff who work on the inpatient unit. In this chapter, these groups are referred to as psychiatric liaison groups.

Many authors have written about both the need for and usefulness of psychiatric liaison groups (Bibring, 1956; Issacharoff et al., 1972; Lipowski, 1974; Rosini et al., 1974; Strain, 1975; Simon and Whiteley, 1977; Strain and Hamerman, 1978). Several authors have described the psychodynamic and group process aspects of these groups in general terms. However, little has been written about the unique developmental stages and phase-specific leadership tasks in these specialized groups. Mohl (1980) leads these groups by relying heavily on the use of group process interpretations. He feels that such group process interpretations can be used to alter the "values, norms, and behavior of a unit system." In addition, he discusses the dynamics of alliance formation, handling resistances, and the grounds for success and failure in these groups.

Purposes of the Psychiatric Liaison Group

There are two purposes of psychiatric liaison groups: to educate medical, nursing and support staff in the psychodynamic and psychosocial factors involved in patient care and to help staff deal more effectively with work-related stresses so as to improve unit morale and cohesiveness, enhance individual staff members' functioning, decrease staff turnover, and ultimately effect better patient care.

Why a group setting? There are several reasons: The small group setting is the most efficient one for involving staff providing patient care. The group setting promotes communication and information sharing between members; this sharing allows for more integrated patient care, reduces individuals' anxiety and isolation, and facilitates collaboration. Finally, the group setting helps the liaison psychiatrist more effectively gather different levels of information about patients' problems. In addition, individual staff members' dynamics and the unit's group dynamics evolve in the here and now of the group setting; consequently, the liaison psychiatrist can intervene in ways that enhance the positive and diminish the negative aspects of these dynamics.

Group Composition and Size

The optimal group size is between five and 12 members. Five members are sufficient to provide meaningful member-to-member dynamic interaction. More than 12 members dilutes such interaction. All members of the medical-nursing team are encouraged to attend. The core group usually consists of nursing staff and social workers, although occasionally physicians attend.

Developmental Stages

First stage

There are a variety of contexts within which psychiatric liaison groups develop. The most frequent one is that in which the liaison psychiatrist has been performing patient consultations on the unit at the request of the medical staff for at least several months. As the psychiatrist begins to demonstrate his diagnostic competence, his knowledge of medicine as it interfaces with psychiatry, his comfort in the medical setting, and especially his unique ability to provide workable alternatives for improved patient care, the medical-nursing staff come to trust and respect him. This trust

and respect provide the basic framework within which a liaison group can develop.

During the initial stage of the psychiatric liaison group, the leader provides direction and structure. He may suggest different topics for discussion or specific types of problem patients for presentation. At this point it is important for the leader and group to arrive at a mutually agreed-upon working contract. Frequency of group meetings, length of each meeting, over-all goals of the group, membership of the group, and suitable topics for future discussion should be discussed.

Liaison groups may meet anywhere from once a week to once a month and may last from 50 to 60 minutes. Membership varies from meeting to meeting, although the group is most effective when a core group of unit staff provide membership continuity. Once the initial working alliance between the leader and the group members has been established, the leader's main goal is to help members become comfortable with him and each other, so that the group can continue to function.

To achieve this level of comfort, the leader must address the sources of anxiety which arise in this first stage of the group's development. The two principal sources of anxiety for members at this point are fear of having their professional work criticized and fear of being personally analyzed by the psychiatrist-leader. By focusing the discussion on how to approach patients' clinical data, the leader discourages the exploration of staff's personal responses to patients and difficulties staff have with each other. By doing so, the psychiatrist allays fears that his hidden agenda is to analyze each of them and the unit as a whole. Mohl (1980) gives several examples of how the use of group process interventions at this stage can lead to a serious regression and disruption in the group's development. Rather than use group process interpretations, the leader's task is to keep the discussions quite structured and act as a teacher. He encourages members to share their views of the patient being discussed. Most of the interactions in the group involve the leader. However, he carefully encourages members to share information and opinions with each other. He allays members' fears about their professional competence by speaking to the constructive aspects of the staff's efforts to manage difficult clinical situations. His criticisms are gentle and muted. He is especially interested in synthesizing clinical material so that he can provide the staff with workable practical approaches to their patients. As members' anxieties are alleviated by the leader, members become more comfortable with him and each other.

Second stage

In this stage, group members begin to take more responsibility for providing structure in the group. As anxiety diminishes, they more readily volunteer case material, and resistances to full participation decrease. Member-to-member interactions occur more frequently. Members ask each other questions and add to each other's observations and descriptions of clinical situations. A major task of the leader is to facilitate these member-to-member interactions. He acknowledges but limits exploration of the interpersonal conflicts which inevitably arise when a team approach is used in patient care. At this stage, exploration of interstaff conflict may increase the group's anxiety to the point where serious regression occurs. Examples of such regression include members' withdrawal from participation, irregular attendance, unavailability of suitable case material for presentation, and even cancellation of meetings.

As stage two unfolds, group cohesiveness begins to solidify, member-to-member trust increases, and anxiety further declines. Members are more willing to share their professional uncertainties in difficult clinical management situations, and some personal responses to patients are verbalized. Members begin to more frequently volunteer how they reacted to specific problematic patients and share personal resonses which proved disappointing or distressing to them. It is important for the leader to respectfully and empathically acknowledge these experiences as ones to be expected in providing care to sick patients. He may facilitate this process by sharing a similarly distressing clinical experience. Even though the group has matured considerably, psychodynamic exploration or interpretation of these personal responses can still result in significant regression in the group process and can threaten the viability of the group itself. However, it is constructive for the leader to encourage all members to share their personal responses to patients. By doing so, group members become more accepting of their emotional responses and understand them as a manifestation of the patient's psychodynamics. The leader introduces the concepts of acting out of these personal feelings and facilitates group members' recognition that these are not always helpful to the patient. It is important for the leader at this point to enable the group to formulate alternative practical approaches in the interpersonal management of the patient.

Suggested practical management alternatives can be tested by members in the clinical setting of the unit. As these alternatives prove useful to the clinician, she experiences a sense of gratification and mastery. This experience is shared with the group members and provides a source of accomplishment and gratification for all members. This increasing sense of mastery and cohesiveness in the group becomes a source of improving morale for the unit as a whole. These steps are outlined in Table C.12-1.

Third stage

With solidification of group cohesiveness, more member-to-member interactions take place. Group members have established a firmer foundation of trust by revealing and accepting their uncomfortable personal responses to patients. By formulating alternative interactive approaches to avoid the acting out of these responses, a new sense of mastery has been achieved. Up to this point, the leader has been careful to avoid any psychodynamic exploration of the meaning of these responses. In this manner, the group's anxiety has been contained.

In the third stage, the leader introduces the concepts of transference and countertransference. The issue of transference was introduced in the preceding stage, when the leader helped the group understand patients' inappropriate attitudes and behavior toward staff. Now the leader more formally outlines the concept of transference as the process of feeling and behaving toward people in the present as if they were important people from the past.

The leader may ask group members for examples of patients who may have reacted to staff members in transferential ways. These cases are discussed in detail by making use of the patient's developmental and family history. The leader may also amplify the discussion by sharing with the group examples of transference from his own clinical experience. Applying the concept of transference to specific case material goes a long way in making the theoretical concept real for group members. However, when members raise transference material in the here and now of the group's interactions, the leader acknowledges it but is careful not to further explore or interpret it.

Up to this point, group discussions have revolved around patient-centered material. The introduction of the concept of countertransference is the next step in the evolution of

Table C.12-1
Steps in Establishing Group Cohesion

Member presents clinical problem to group
↓
Group discusses and formulates alternative approaches
↓
Member tests out alternative approach in clinical setting
↓
More workable clinical situation results
↓
Member experiences new sense of gratification and mastery
↓
Member shares experience with group
↓
Group experiences new sense of mastery and gratification
↓
Increased group cohesion results

stage three. This changes the group's focus from patients' experiences to the psychological experiences of the group members themselves. It is a particularly sensitive transition, and, if not handled properly, it can lead to severe regressions in the group process.

Balint's concept of countertransference, cited by Sandler et al. (1973) as "the totality of the analyst's attitude and behavior toward his patient," is useful in the psychiatric liaison group. The introduction of the concept of countertransference raises the level of the group's anxiety by rekindling members' fears of being analyzed by the leader and of being exposed to other group members. However, the leader makes clear that the purpose of discussing countertransference responses to patients is to help members identify, accept, and separate the sources of these responses. He explains how this process will enable group members to decide when their responses are appropriate or inappropriate and when they are or are not interfering with patient care.

As he did with the earlier case examples of transference, the leader asks members for examples of countertransference. However, he must carefully maintain the boundaries of these inquiries by limiting members' tendencies to bring up sensitive material from their own pasts. To set appropriate limits, the leader uses his clinical judgment to determine the capacity of members to use this personal material within the educational and didactic framework of the group. He makes clear that one's personal material will not be explored. To do so would violate the working contract and turn the group into a therapy group. When anxiety about this material gets too high, the group may want to return to more case-oriented material. This should not be seen as a regression but merely as an expected aspect of the group's dynamics in this stage.

The final evolution of the third stage of group development may come when the principal focus of the group changes from patient-staff problems to staff-staff problems. At this point, the group becomes what many authors have called a "nurse support group." Having gained a new sense of mastery in the interpersonal management of patients, the staff members now want to address problems in their work relationships with each other. The desire may not be explicitly verbalized but may simply become the focus of the group process. Up to this time, the leader has contained extended discussion of interstaff problems because of the fragile state of group cohesiveness; now, however, he may elect to proceed with this new undertaking.

Certain special circumstances must exist in order for the nurse support group phase to be a constructive outgrowth of the third state: (1) The group members must have adequate ego strength and psychological sophistication. (2) The group members should be well motivated. (3) An adequate level of group cohesiveness and functioning must be established. (4) The leader, members, and unit administration must feel that the nurse support group will be useful to the individual members and the unit as a whole.

If these four conditions are present, then the group can operate within the following guidelines: members must commit themselves to regular attendance; the nurse support group cannot be run as an open-ended group with variable membership. Members must maintain a code of strict confidentiality of all material discussed in the group. The group must be time limited, but this limit can be renegotiated. The nurse support group is not a therapy group; current personal problems with family and friends outside the work setting are not appropriate material for the group.

The primary goal of this type of group is to help its members deal more effectively with the work-related stresses of the hospital environment. By doing so, the group helps individual member functioning, unit cohesiveness, and staff morale and may reduce staff turnover. Group discussions focus on personal, emotional, and interactional responses of the members to patients and each other; when appropriate, members' own past developmental experiences may be discussed.

In the nurse support group, the leader may explore and interpret psychodynamic aspects of the group interactions. He may use group process interpretations to point out the many levels of these interactions. At all times, however, he must maintain the group's anxiety at a manageable and workable level. The group's main focus is on the here and now of the interactions within the group and in the work setting. The leader discourages members from externalizing and projecting their problems onto the unit as a whole. He makes members aware of their desires to find scapegoats outside the group. In these ways, the nurse support group resembles training groups that are conducted in other settings (Horwitz, 1967).

It is useful for the nurse support group to reserve its last few sessions for a review and self-critique. In these concluding sessions, the leader and members share their over-all experiences of the group. The important events of the group history are highlighted.

Conclusion

The natural evolution of psychiatric liaison groups has been divided into three stages so that leaders of these groups can more easily understand the dynamic issues and leadership tasks appropriate to each stage. In the first two stages, the leader must be quite active in providing structure and direction for both content and group interactions. This is done so that individual members can become comfortable with him, with each other, and with the group as a whole. This setting allows the group process to develop, mature, and unfold without undue resistance.

The leader makes use of his knowledge of group dynamics to formulate the level of the group's development but does not interpret this process. Instead, he uses these formulations to directly structure and guide the process to ensure the group's natural evolution. The use of interpretations in the first and second stages of the group's development, despite their accuracy, usually raises, rather than lowers, the group members' anxieties and generally leads to severe regressions that may threaten the group's existence. It is not until the third stage—and especially in the nurse support group phase—that the leader can profitably use interpretive interventions without risking severe regressions.

In reality, there are no pure stages in the development of psychiatric liaison groups. Each stage contains some elements of the others. Moreover, each medical-surgical unit has its own distinct character. The realities of the physical environment and of the administrative and clinical structure (especially the relationships within the nursing hierarchy and between nurses and physicians) greatly influence the developmental process of each psychiatric liaison group. Under certain circumstances, such as a unit in crisis (Issacharoff et al., 1972) or a unit with a psychologically mature and cohesive staff, psychiatric liaison groups may begin in the third or even nurse support stage.

Finally, one must keep in mind that the purposes of psychiatric liaison groups are to teach nursing and medical staff about the psychodynamic aspects of all levels of patient care, and to enhance the interpersonal functioning of the health care delivery team. They are not and should not become therapy groups.

References

Abram, H. S. Psychological aspects of intensive care units. Med. Ann. D.C., *227:* 860, 1974.

Berarducci, M., Blandford, K., and Garant, C. A. The psychiatric liaison nurse in the general hospital: Three models of practice. Gen. Hosp. Psychiatry, *1:* 66, 1979.

Bibring, G. L. Psychiatry and medical practice in the general hospital. N. Engl. J. Med., *254:* 366, 1956.

Caldwell, T. A. and Weiner, M. F. Stresses and coping in ICU nursing; I. General. Hosp Psychiatry, *3:* 119, 1981.

Craig, T. J. Psychiatric consultation to the nonphysician staff on an outpatient oncology clinic. Int. J. Psychiatry Med., *4:* 291, 1973.

Eisendrath, R. M., Tapor, M., Misfeldt, C., and Jessiman, A. G. Service meetings in a renal transplant unit: An unused adjunct to total patient care. Psychol. Med., *1:* 53, 1970.

Eisendrath, S. J., and Dunkel, J. Psychological issues in intensive care unit staff. Heart Lung., *8:* 751, 1979.

Gardner, D., Parzen, Z. D., and Stewart, N. The nurse's dilemma: Mediating stress in critical care units. Heart Lung, *9:* 103, 1980.

Horwitz, L. Training groups for psychiatric residents. Int. J. Group Psychother., *17:* 421, 1967.

Issacharoff, A., Redinger, R., and Schneider, D. The psychiatric consultation as an experience in group process. Contemp. Psychoanal., *8:* 260, 1972.

Kilgour, D. Y. Nursing in intensive therapy units: Personnel problems. In *Intensive Care*, W. F. Walker and D. E. M. Taylor, editors, p. 228. Churchill Livingstone, London, 1975.

Lipowski, Z. J. Consultation-liaison psychiatry: An overview. Am. J. Psychiatry, *131:* 623, 1974.

Mohl, P. C. Group process interpretations in liaison psychiatry nurse groups. Gen. Hosp. Psychiatry, *2:* 104, 1980.

Rosini, L. A., Howell, M. C., Todres, I. D., and Dorman, J. Group meetings in a pediatric intensive care unit. Pediatrics, *53:* 371, 1974.

Sandler, J., Dare, C., and Holder, A. *The Patient and the Analyst: The Basis of the Psychoanalytic Process.* International Universities Press, New York, 1973.

Shulman, B. N. Group process: An adjunct in liaison consultation psychiatry. Int. J. Psychiatry Med., *6:* 489, 1975.

Simon, N. M., and Whiteley, S. Psychiatric consultation with MICU nurses: The consultation conference as a working group. Heart Lung, *6:* 497, 1977.

Strain, J. J. Building the alliance. In *Psychological Care of the Medically Ill: A Primer in Liaison Psychiatry.* J. J. Strain and S. Grossman, editors, p. 185. Appleton-Century-Crofts, New York, 1975.

Strain, J. J., and Hamerman, D. The application of psychological concepts in the hospital-inpatient setting. In *Psychological Interventions in Medical Practice*, J. J. Strain, editor, p. 179. Appleton-Century-Crofts, New York, 1978.

Tuckman, B. W. Developmental sequence in small groups. Psychol. Bull., *63:* 384, 1965.

Turquot, P. M. Leadership: The individual and the group. In *Analysis of Groups*, G. S. Gibbard, J. J. Hartman, and R. D. Mann, editors, p. 354. Jossey-Bass, San Francisco, 1974.

Weeks, H. Dealing with the stress. Matern. Child Nurs. J., *3:* 151, 1978.

AREA D

TRAINING, RESEARCH, AND SPECIAL AREAS

D.1 The Qualities of the Group Psychotherapist

MARTIN GROTJAHN, M.D.

Introduction

The study of the group therapist as a person is of central importance because group psychotherapy, more than almost any individual therapy, is based on the dynamics of interaction: the therapist is the central and decisive influence in the group process.

Qualities of a Psychotherapist

A psychotherapist must be reliable; only then will he invite trust and confidence. He must have trust and confidence in himself and in other people. He must be an expert in the mastery of communication, whether it be the therapist's communication with himself or with the people he tries to understand.

The therapist ought to be a person who has experienced life to the fullest. He may be young, or he may be old, but he must have the courage to experience life in all its shades, and he must know how it feels to be alive. He must have known fear and anxiety, mastery and dependency. Most of all, he must not be afraid to love, and he does not need to be a stranger to hate.

The therapist ought to be well-read, since the experience of having lived with the great figures of literature is a part of his knowledge. The images he must learn to understand can be found among friends, lovers, patients, colleagues, and enemies; but the models of true integration are still the characters documented in the great literature of mankind.

In the end, an analyst should look back on his life as a proud expression of a lifelong creative effort. He should consider himself as his own favorite patient, one who has to learn as long as he lives. He should learn how to treat himself as his best patient, and how to treat his patient as he would himself.

In his honesty, the therapist must have the courage for what Carl Jaspers describes as "unlimited communication," both consciously and unconsciously. He must be a master in what Franz Alexander (1946) calls "dynamic reasoning." He must learn how to see people not only in the here-and-now and in their relationship to him (but also in their long-term psychological development). His understanding may start with the understanding of a particular person here-and-now, but it must extend to understanding how people became what they are. In this sense, the psychologist is a historian.

In order to safeguard his own mental health and the health of his patients and his own family, he must be aware of himself. This awareness must include parts of his unconscious. It is this awareness that is a tool of his trade, and that Theodor Reik called the "third ear."

The true psychologist must be driven by the wish to understand, and in that way he is a scientist. At the same time, he must be able to stand the tension of not understanding. As Reik says, it is better not to understand than to misunderstand.

The therapist must offer himself as a more or less blank screen in order to invite the development of transference. And, as Zetzel and Greenson note, he must simultaneously be human and real enough to establish a working alliance. If he only tries to remain a blank screen, he will lose his patient, since nobody wants to be analyzed by a blank screen. If he offers himself too loudly as a helper or teammate in the working alliance, the patient may feel dominated; he may become fearful and withdrawn. It is this bipolarity that makes the work of the therapist difficult.

Qualifications of the Group Psychotherapist

SPONTANEITY

The group therapist should be a person of spontaneity or responsiveness. As the word implies, responsiveness is connected to responsibility. The response must be spontaneous, natural, and direct, but it must be combined with an always ready sense of responsibility not to hurt the psychological atmosphere that engulfs both the therapist and group simultaneously.

Perhaps there are advantages for a group therapist in being schizoid—that is, in being able and willing by nature to split himself and endure contradictions. It is easier for the schizoid therapist to perform this rather deep splitting of his person with ease and with grace. He always has to remain firmly grounded in his identity; at the same time, he ought to be able to split off parts of his personality, which he then projects onto different members of his group in order to understand them by partial projective identification. He has to perform this splitting process at all times in order to remain simultaneously both a participant and an observer, both an active member of the group and the central figure—perceiving, interpreting, and integrating.

The experienced psychoanalyst who starts working in a group has to learn something that can be learned best by years of experience: the use of spontaneity as a technical device. Many therapists have the impression that they are getting better in their relationship to the people they are trying to understand when they develop a certain trust in their spontaneous responses. An analyst in a one-to-one relationship may take time to wait, to think, to speculate, like a slow-moving chess player. The group response to such a slow-moving therapist is to slow down. The efficiency of a group therapist is much more dependent on the quick and correct use of his spontaneous responses, growing out of his intuition, empathy, trust, and feeling for the situation. He learns to trust his group and his hunches more and more, and he will begin to act like the conductor of an orchestra.

The group therapist is nothing if he is not spontaneous. He depends on his immediate, intuitive, emotional, and honest responses. As a rule, he cannot wait, think, and consult with himself, as in analysis. To do so would interfere with the group process and slow it down to a standstill. He cannot test and probe, correct, and finally integrate and interpret, as in psychoanalysis. He shoots from the hip, and experience will show that he frequently hits the target with the right interpretation or interaction, and does so at the right moment.

TRUST

The free use of spontaneity is possible only in a therapist who trusts himself, as he also must have trust and confidence in the group. This trust demands courage and the ability to withstand bad experiences without despair.

The question of basic trust leads directly to the central problem of group therapy. A trusting therapist invites trust. Just as a trusting mother gains the confidence of her children, so does she give to her children the basis for their self-confidence. Only the well-mothered child, as Winnicott (1965) has shown, develops the kind of basic trust that is necessary for mental health in later life. And, as Erikson (1950) notes, nobody can develop this basic trust by himself. A person can develop everything else in the process of individuation, but the basic trust, says Fairbairn (1963), has to be started with the experience of the mother-infant symbiosis. If this relationship is traumatized or even destroyed,

it cannot be restored in analysis. In the specifically different mother transference of the group, such basic trust and self-reliance may possibly be invited and developed. At least, it can be better developed from tender beginnings in the group than in one-to-one relationship. The analyst may be astounded to find that members of a group begin to trust the group more than they trust the therapist alone. It is this trust that the therapist must be able to invite, handle, and, finally, deserve. The group therapist must know how to develop and protect the trust of the group—primarily to the group and secondarily to himself, as the parental and central figure.

The therapist's spontaneity, his responsiveness, his ability to trust and to identify—these are the tools of the therapist's trade, and determine the efficiency of the therapeutic group process—more so than in individual therapy. In the group, the therapist is like the conductor of an orchestra. In analysis, a therapist is like a critic who sits in the audience and occasionally gets up, stops the concert, makes a remark, and sits down again to listen. He does not conduct. He limits himself more or less to interpretations. But the group therapist reacts first and interprets later; this is why only a therapist who has learned to trust the different aspects of his countertransference is fit to work well in groups.

The basic faith or basic assumption of a therapist should be his belief in the quintessential goodness of people or, at least, in their wish to be good. In this sense, the therapist has to also believe in himself. If he cannot do so—and he may have good reason to doubt his good intention—he should not work with people. His assignment is to try to restore his patients' belief in their fellow men and in themselves.

PERFORMANCE

There is a clear difference between an actor and a performer: A good performer is not somebody who acts as if he were somebody else. A performer performs a task that has to be done, and he does it carefully, with skill and elegance. He chooses to do it in a way that can be observed and understood by others. He not only does something, but shows what is done and how it is done. A conductor communicates with the language of his body what he hopes and wants the orchestra to do. He shows what he does, but what he does is real and not pretended. He performs his duty. But an actor behaves as if he were conducting. The trust of the group is partly based on seeing the therapist in his performance.

A group of psychiatrists met one day after some of them had viewed together—unrelated to the group—four movies from a research institution on sexual information for physicians. They told the men who had not seen the movies what they were all about. One member of the group came 20 minutes late, listened to the talk for a while, and said with indignation: "I have an emergency on my ward—that's why I was late—and I have lots to do. I did not come down here to listen to this locker-room nonsense."

With slightly overemphasized and pointedly polite superiority, the group therapist turned to him and said:

"I am well aware that this conversation is not quite up to the high standards of our group. It was my intention to prepare the field in this way to loosen up the resistance against discussing questions of sexuality in this group of men, who all know each other outside of the group and whose wives are also known to everybody. From there I planned to open the way into the secrecy of everybody's marriage and sexual behavior."

The therapist used his responsive annoyance about the criticism to demonstrate what he was doing. At the same time, he performed the difficult task of showing his annoyance to a group of psychiatrists who tended to behave like a board of experts. Almost immediately, somebody looked at the therapist and said, "All right, what do you want to know?" The group leader continued the performance by addressing each member of the group with a pointed question about something that he guessed was a sore point for him and was carefully kept taboo and so far excluded from the group discussion. After a fruitful and rather deep-going session, the therapist turned once more to the young man and asked him whether the progress of the group justified the introduction of the "locker-room" atmosphere. He and the group agreed that the procedure was right—and so was his challenging it.

FIRM IDENTITY

The central firmness of the group therapist allows him to be recognized for who he is—namely, as a real person and not only as an imagination of the transference. This is of importance for the growth and maturation of the group, its cohesion, its trust, and its relation to reality. The therapist is the central figure, symbolizing the parent in all the shades of various transferences. His peripheral openness toward the different members of the group will allow him to perform his duties by being father to one, mother to all, affectionate friend to somebody who may need one, disciplinarian to somebody who may at that time be working on problems of authority. He must not get lost in the pitiful spectacle of a multiple personality. His central firmness or ego identity will protect him against that. He must remain what he is—he is himself and nobody else.

Naturally, this firmness does not exclude his constant readiness to learn, to change, to develop, and to grow and mature. The therapist is not a patient in his group, but, just as a good parent allows the members of his family to recognize him in strength and in weakness, so the good therapist—more than the analyst—shows himself as a real person. Doing so invites the members of the group-family to become independent and to avoid the danger of regressive infantilization, which is so prominent in standard analysis. The therapist as a real person also counteracts the patient's suspicion that he is being manipulated when he sees what the conductor does. This—the real person that is the therapist—is the basis for the group's working alliance.

HUMOR

Another character trait which may help the group therapist to keep his group from infantilization is the group therapist's sense of humor. It is needed in group therapy to a higher degree than in individual therapy, because it helps the group to see the therapist as a real person. It counteracts the transference that idealizes the therapist as an omniscient parental figure. A therapist with a sense of humor invites the group to look at him realistically and to correct transference distortions. It also shows everyone that the therapist himself knows his limitations, and can smile about them.

Humor leaves the situation open for changes as the transference demands. The therapist's sense of humor reassures the group that he can stand multifaceted transference trends without being destroyed. Only then can the group, unlike the patient in individual therapy, use the therapist as a transference figure and simultaneously as a teammate in the group team effort. No therapist can remain a blank screen within the group forever. This makes it difficult for therapists who have been trained or who have worked in traditional, individual therapy to make the transition to group work.

The therapist has to be somewhat on guard with his always ready wit and his fondness for the sharply pointed and often painfully penetrating remark. Such remarks show his incompletely resolved ambivalence and perhaps some sadistic traits, which have no place among the tools of a therapist. He may employ his wit occasionally to counteract the trend to infantilization or hero worship, which is such a convenient way to hide hostility.

A therapist under observation behind a one-way screen was once confronted by one member of an unruly and rebellious group with a mistake a group member was convinced the therapist had made. The therapist answered with a haughty-sounding and, in my mind, humorous remark: "I always considered the possibility of making a mistake. It would be the first time."

Such ironic remarks are not meant to be taken seriously. They are, therefore, dangerous in a therapeutic group setting because they imply a certain indirectness. Kidding alerts the therapist for danger, since it does not lead to free communication, which he tries to develop. He also does not join in meaningless social laughter, which covers embarrassment or anxiety. If the therapist resists the temptation to join such laughter, then his group will probably laugh less than the groups of other therapists. He joins in the laughter only when he truly feels like it and when something funny has happened. It is a good sign in the development of group cohesion when all members and the therapist join in laughter once in a while. Laughter and the telling of jokes and funny stories may become a resistance, and must be interpreted as that.

A humorous attitude shows the therapist not as a sadistic, cutting wit but as an understanding and kind mother.

COUNTERTRANSFERENCE

With his central identity, the therapist offers himself as a screen for different transference-projections. He is aware that in every group three transference relatioinships must be differentiated: transference to him as a central figure, similar to the situation in analysis; transference to the peers in the group, as among siblings in a family; and transference to the group as a whole and as a mother symbol.

In the analytic situation, the analyst can slowly and deliberately interpret the transference, but the group therapist must react spontaneously; otherwise he is lost. To react spontaneously, he must feel the meaning of his position in the group at all times.

The group situation does not facilitate the transference relationship to regress to the degree of a transference neurosis, as in standard analysis. This makes the assignment of the group therapist different from that of an analyst conducting a standard analysis. There the analyst has to focus on the interpretation of the transference neurosis.

The group therapist should not fight with the members of the group for dominance by narcissistically displaying his brilliance or by showing his superiority in other ways. His only and almost silent superiority should be his honesty, courage, and frankness to understand the unconscious. The group therapist should use the peer relationship as an effective way to exercise therapeutic pressure. He should be able to handle this relationship not with envy and not with interference, but rather by guarding it. A jealous parent is not a good parent. The analyst in the analytic situation almost invites resistance; the patient feels he must defend his sickness against the father who wants to destroy it. The peer relationship in the group situation invites cooperative effort, and is one of the most effective therapeutic potentials in group work.

The group is the symbol of the mother, and a great part of the group therapeutic efficacy is based on a preoedipal maternal transference. The symbolic meaning of the group as a mother helps to steady the course of the group's progress.

The therapist's maternal attitude facilitates his acceptance of the group and his trust. The final dissolution of the mother-infant symbiosis may amount to an experience of rebirth in the group. In his maternal identification, the group therapist can be passive, indulgent, waiting, or silent. It is a time of rest and saturation for him, awaiting the group's delivery. The therapist is helped in his motherliness by the group as a symbolic mother. The group's benevolent indifference, expressed in its tolerance, supports the therapist's attitude.

A good mother has to learn that a child is a going concern, in Winnicott's (1965) words, and the good therapist, as mother, must learn how to trust the group, just as he would trust a child who is developing his own drive for mastery. Trust in the well-mothered child is rewarded by the child's self-confidence—a good model for the therapist to understand the progress of individuation in a well-conducted group.

In the strictest sense of the word, the countertransference of the therapist is his response to the transference feelings of the patient or patients. However, it has become customary to summarize all feelings of the therapist toward his patients under the term "countertransference."

It is important that the group therapist has the inner freedom to use his feelings toward his patient to further the therapeutic process in the group. When the therapist is open, honest, and frank in his self-expression, the group will honor this confidence and follow his example. It should be evident that such self-revelations are allowed only so far as the group process benefits from them. Anything more would have the character of acting out, and the therapist would become a burden and finally destructive to the group.

FALLIBILITY

The group therapist may make mistakes; he is expected and allowed to do so. His honesty makes it possible for him to accept the correction of his mistake by the group, the way the head of a family listens to others in the family council. The therapist does not lose his position by admitting to a mistake. On the contrary, his central position may be confirmed. The only unforgivable mistake he can make is to pull rank, which a group of growing-up people will not tolerate.

The most frequently committed mistakes one sees when watching group therapy being conducted behind a one-way screen is the passive, waiting, analytically neutral attitude of the therapist. No individual patient is more dependent upon the activity of the therapist than the group. It seems especially difficult for therapists who have gone through analytic training and work to change from watching and waiting and interpreting the transference neurosis to interpreting the interaction of the group. The activity of the group therapist is justified, since the group does not allow the development of a full-blown transference neurosis. If it is not the therapist, then the peers in the group will constantly correct the transference phenomena without bothering to interpret anything.

Another mistake, limited mostly to beginners, is berating the group as lazy or sleepy. It is advisable that the therapist at first consider his own, possibly unconscious resistance, which may affect the behavior of the group. It is the therapist's duty to realize resistance, then not to bemoan it but try to understand its motivation. If he is able to do that, then he is ready to give an interpretaion.

SPLITTING MECHANISM

Unlike an individual analyst, the group therapist must not consider himself always in the focus of all the multiple transference trends. It would be a mistake if he concentrated on the one transference trend in the group that relates to him, as in analysis. The therapist must be aware that approximately two-thirds of the interaction leaves him in the role of the observing bystander. Besides the transference to him as the central figure, the group re-enacts interfamily attitudes toward the family of peers and toward the group as a mother symbol. Therefore, the analytic group therapist has great freedom to work as an observer and participant, instead of an interpreter. He may interpret by his participation.

Ross and Kapp suggested that the therapist use inner visualization to catch his own unconscious reaction to the free associative material of the patient or of the group process. This inner visualization while listening, this view with the third eye, helps the therapist to find understanding first in visual form and then in verbal formulation.

The Group Therapist As a Patient

A good physician learns how to use the experience of having been sick. As a rule, the medical man is a poor patient. The situation is the same in the development of a good group psychotherapist. Psychoanalysis teaches insight and understanding, but group psychotherapy offers therapy to the therapist.

When a physician goes to another physician because he is sick, he inevitably says to his colleague, "I want you to treat me like any other patient of yours." To which the consulted colleague is honor bound to answer, "That was my intention anyhow." Then they both promptly relate to each other like two colleagues discussing a most interesting third person. In the case of serious illness, fateful disaster may result.

The problem for the physician is how to become a patient. The physician actually is different from the average patient, who knows little about his body and nothing about the function of his inner organs. He is also different from the neurotic patient, even if he has read something about his unconscious.

The physician in medical treatment and the therapist in training each have to learn how to split themselves into two parts: One part remains a therapist and joins his colleague as co-therapist; another part becomes a patient in therapy. This splitting makes the working alliance in the training and therapeutic situation different from other treatment situations. If not handled correctly, it seriously limits the therapeutic efficacy of training analysis. The therapist in training or therapy has to be aware of it. If the teacher accepts his therapist-students only as students, they will never become patients, since they want to become what the training analyst is—an accepted member of the analytic community. To be effective, training must combine the therapeutic alliance with a learning alliance.

THE ANALYTIC GROUP EXPERIENCE

It has been said that a psychiatrist passes through three stages: Young psychiatrists talk about their cases, established psychiatrists talk about money, and senior therapists talk about themselves.

One analyst does not seem to be enough in the terminal stage of an analysis for an analyst. Repeated analysis of different analysts has been recommended and tried by Kubie (1968), among others. But analysts learn how to deal with their analysts and how to disarm them, so another analyst is not the solution to this phenomenon. Equally unsatisfactory is an always-longer training analysis. Neither is a friend able to continue the analysis of an analyst where his training left off. In such a friendship, there is too much mutual affection, too much relaxation, too little freely expressed hostility, and not enough working through of the transference phenomena.

A new transference situation is needed and could be provided by the one-of-us relationship in the group. The transference of peers to each other and to the group as a mother image is needed in order to analyze the analyst within the family transference. Most analysts growing older in their profession lose the trust, confidence, and faith in their colleagues that they had when they started as young men and accepted an analytic working alliance to older training analysts. As they grow older, a certain therapeutic skepticism takes hold. In the one-to-one relationship, this skepticism becomes even stronger. It is easier to reactivate confidence and trust in a group relationship than in an individual setting.

CONFLICT-FREE PERSONALITY TRENDS

Many areas that do not cause special conflict in the analyst may never appear in the associations of a therapist in training analysis; they will show up in his relationship to his patients. They also may not become visible under supervision, though they will certainly become obvious in the relationship to the peers in the group. These areas involve such things as the distribution and combination of activity and passivity, maleness and femaleness, other-directedness and inner-directedness, enthusiasm and sobriety, masochistic and sadistic trends, sensitive and insensitive social consciousness, tolerance and intolerance, loving and hostile trends, spontaneity and intellectualization, patience and impatience, and many variations of prejudice.

NEGATIVE TRANSFERENCE

The transference to the training analyst is by implication of transference to a parental figure in a position of authority. Since the student therapist wants to become like his analyst, he submits to him and seems to do so willingly. But secretly and out of reach, he harbors a trend to rebellion; he postpones this negative part of his attitude, which is typical in the analytic training situation. Often, this rebellion is expressed only later in the life of an analyst, and rarely is it accessible to analysis. But in the group situation, where the peer relationship prevails, it comes to the surface of consciousness and can be analyzed.

An ever-deepening criticism of analytic training is becoming apparent. Analysts have failed in the therapy that is a part of training. Clinical evidence is given by the majority of analysts and the pathology of analytic group behavior. Analytic training, which serves here as a model for the training of therapists, tends to be infantilizing and, therefore, stimulating to hostile, rebellious trends in the student. Due to his dependency, these negative trends are postponed until after the training analysis, meaning they are postponed for an indefinite future. The analytic group experience offers an opportunity to correct this defect.

The problem of the analysis of negative transference is also a countertransference problem: Fathers want to be loved by their student-sons, who, after all, represent the future. Therefore, analysts tend to relate differently to their training candidates in action, behavior, and interpretation than to most of their other patients.

Kubie (1968) has discussed these problems and confessed that the transference neurosis is never really dissolved in a training analysis. As a remedy, he asks for a real relationship in the form of a controlled, disciplined, low-intensity friendship after the formal analysis. He also suggests a change of analyst during the terminal stage of training. The new analyst is supposed to take a better look at the residual transference to the first analyst.

THE FAMILY ROMANCE

Analytic training liberates the individual analyst in training from the tyranny of his unconscious, but his family romance remains largely unanalyzed. The transference of the infantile past into the psychoanalytic training situation is accomplished in the setting of individual analysis. The family romance, however, is neglected in standard training. As a rule, the family romance is projected onto the family of analysts, symbolized by the institute, the society, or the educational training committee. The analytic group experience offers the possibility of a belated analysis. This opportunity should not be missed by any student of therapy.

Freud may have known this; the minutes of the early meetings of the Viennese Psychoanalytic Society show that these seminars were originally organized for the purpose of teaching and learning psychoanalysis, but they soon assumed the character of modified therapeutic group sessions. Another example of an early analytic group experience was the intimate daily discussions of Freud, Jung, and Ferenczi on their ocean crossing to America.

DIDACTIC GROUPS

Psychotherapists in training frequently use intellectualization as a form of resistance. An often-heard phrase in a didactic group is: "We all talk like a bunch of smart professionals."

The avoidance of intellectualization, after it has been repeatedly called by that term, may lead to a new form of resistance: Insights are resolutely rejected because they may sound too intellectual to a board of experts. There are sometimes episodes of resistance in a group of therapists where every interpretation is labeled a rationalization, and only emotions are considered therapeutically valid.

In a group, colleagues have to learn how to place questions to each other by associative responses. In the first stage of group formation, professional members try to confirm their impressions and planned interpretations by fishing for more clinical evidence. They soon realize that their spontaneous response is more important and usually contains the proper interpretation. They then develop the courage for human response, overcoming the handicap of the medical person who is suspicious of spontaneity and who has been trained to filter his response carefully.

Work in groups of psychiatrists or psychoanalysts is difficult for the central figure. Whether experienced or inexperienced, a group of colleagues will recognize the therapist's weak spots. They use their therapeutic skill to put their finger where it hurts most, and the narcissistic therapist in charge may feel in need of a hiding place. If he is open, responsive, and ready to learn, he will succeed—like a father who does not pull rank but who accepts democracy and freedom in his family. Only then can the group become a learning and therapeutic experience.

The conduct of a training group for therapists is excellent postgraduate training for the central figure, as well as for the members of the group. The therapist has to perform in the presence of 6 or 8 alert and specially trained critics. At times, the experience almost amounts to a board examination. Anyone who passes such a test has received a baptism under analytic fire. Only total honesty and sincerity save the therapist. The analyst who has difficulty in allowing himself to feel his hostility or his need for tenderness benefits the most. He can learn how to be more free, spontaneous, trusting, and responsive. The same group that exposes him also protects him until he finds his way to an attitude appropriate for him. A therapist may satisfy his need for intimacy in the one-to-one relationship, but in the group he satisfies his need for participation in the growth and maturation of a family.

When working in groups, the analyst's narcissism takes a severe blow. When he steps out of his professional isolation, he sees that he is not the only good therapist. But he also realizes that he is not making many more mistakes than his colleagues. He may find that people he has not especially respected are quite different in the intimate interaction of a group, and this is a worthwhile human experience. After the group experience, a new, somewhat humble, and realistic attitude replaces his narcissism, and makes him a better therapist.

THE THERAPIST'S SPOUSE

Group therapy seems especially suited to satisfy the specific needs of therapists and their spouses because it offers them an extended family. The therapist's spouse has to learn that nobody can be a therapist in his own family, even if he is considered an expert and "The Professor" by his spouse and his community. In the extended family of the group, a learning experience is offered to him—how to be helpful and understanding without using the tools of his trade. To learn this is important for the happiness of his family, as it will benefit his therapeutic attitude later.

Furthermore, analytic group work with therapists and their spouses brings relief from the burden of secrecy. The partner in the analyst's marriage often feels left out. His work may be shrouded in confidentiality and may appear mysterious to the outsider. Frequently, the children pay the price for their parents' competitiveness.

The identification with the mother is probably the

basis of creative work, as it can be studied so strikingly in the life and work of Sigmund Freud. Nevertheless, the therapist must be aware of how destructive competition with his spouse at home may become if not analyzed and changed. Besides endangering his relationship, the competition may have the most destructive influence on the growth of the children and their sexual identification. A mother or father needs support, not competition.

A therapist at home can be dangerous when he treats his spouse by a method that is often called "gaslighting." Gaslighting is driving somebody slowly, consistently, deliberately, and occasionally successfully into madness by skillfully undermining his or her self-confidence and identity.

A therapist works, as a rule, in utter isolation and, therefore, may lose the benefits of feedback from his colleagues. This line of communication can be re-established in group work. With increased freedom, the therapist's dialogue in his group, in his family, and, finally, with his patients becomes less defensive, freer, deeper, and more spontaneous and fulfilling. He may even learn how to overcome his isolation and how to be more trusting, open, and ultimately more loving.

THE THERAPIST'S MENTAL HEALTH

The therapist does not need to be a paragon of mental health. He can proceed in the face of his own anxiety, just as he can proceed efficiently with all kinds of psychosomatic symptoms, such as high blood pressure, migraine, and even a gastric ulcer. It is preferable for a therapist to overcome his symptoms, and he sometimes does. The analysis and correction of conflict-free areas takes time, and the therapist may work well before his own therapy is completed. As a matter of fact, the therapist should remain his own favorite patient for the rest of his life.

A slight and perhaps even chronic depressive position may actually be a qualification for a therapist. In the face of so much often unnecessary suffering, a sensitive person is almost bound to become slightly depressed. It is a kind of existential despair, a way of being human, an acknowledgment of our impossible profession. It does not interfere with the therapist's functioning. It may give him that kind of maturity a child expects from his parents.

The group therapist may be a person who knows anxiety and fear, as well as depression and despair. In the therapeutic alliance with his patients, he must not fear his fears. He may forever feel guilty that he is inadequate in his ability to understand people in their complexity.

Growth and Maturation

Many therapists develop the belief that they are superior to all others. Some become bitter and cynical about therapy, or they become exhibitionistic and narcissistic and may think that everything is allowed to them. Others may become depressed or resigned. Their reputation by then may be affirmed, and an encounter with these great men of therapy may still be worthwhile for the patient.

A therapist is mature when he has learned how to deal with the inner and outer reality of himself and his patients. He also must learn how to deal with his ever-present guilt at not being "good enough." One has to accept—albeit reluctantly—one's limitations.

There is a similarity between a friendship and a therapeutic alliance. When one has a good friend, one does not need an enemy, because fighting is a special kind of friendship. The main difference is that a friendship is two-sided, but a therapeutic alliance is for the benefit of the patient mostly. Therapists are not lovers, not even friends, to their patients. Neither are they enemies. A working relationship is a fighting relationship, the way a friendship is. The healthy ego of the patient fights in alliance with the therapist against the sick. In group therapy, this attitude is a necessity.

It is easier to grow old gracefully as a group therapist than in the isolation of the one-to-one relationship. The therapist must not abuse his groups as tools of treatment for himself, but he must accept the help of the group in the continuation of his never-ending self-analysis.

Beethoven is supposed to have said, "If you understand my music, you are saved." Applied to the therapeutic situation, this means that, when the therapist is understood by the group, both have benefited. This is the promise group therapy holds for both the group and the therapist.

References

Anthony, J. Reflections on twenty-five years of group psychotherapy. Int. J. Group Psychother., *18:* 277, 1968.

Alexander, F. The principle of flexibility. In *Psychoanalytic Therapy,* F. Alexander and T. French, editors, p. 25. Ronald Press, New York, 1946.

De Maré, P. *Perspectives in Group Psychotherapy.* Jason Aronson, New York, 1972.

Durkin, H. E. *Therapeutic Group Analysis.* International Universities Press, New York, 1964.

Erikson, E. H. *Childhood and Society.* W. W. Norton, New York, 1950.

Fairbairn, W. R. D. Synopsis of an object relation theory of the personality. Int. J. Psychoanal., *44:* 224, 1963.

Foulkes, S. H. *Therapeutic Group Analysis.* International Universities Press, New York, 1974.

Garetz, C. Group rounds versus individual medical rounds on a psychiatric inpatient service. Am. J. Psychiatry, *128:* 119, 1971.

Greenson, R. R. The selection of candidates for psychoanalytic training: A panel report. J. Am. Psychoanal. Assoc., *9:* 135, 1961.

Greenson, R. R. The working alliance and the transference neurosis. Psychoanal. Q. *34:* 134, 1965.

Grotjahn, M. The process of maturation in group psychotherapy and in the group therapist. Psychiatry, *13:* 63, 1950.

Grotijahn, M. Mistakes in analytic group therapy. Int. J. Group. Psychother., *29:* 317, 1979.

Grotjahn, M. The best and the worst in analytic group therapy: Clinical observations about suitability. In *Group and Family Therapy,* L. R. Wolberg and M. Aronson, editors, p. 58. Brunner/Mazel, New York, 1980a.

Grotjahn, M. The dream in analytic group therapy. *The Dream in Clinical Practice,* J. M. Natterson, editor, p. 427. Jason Aronson, New York, 1980b.

Kohut, H. The evaluation of applicants for psychoanalytic training. Int. J. Psychoanal., *49:* 54, 1968.

Kreeger, M. *The Large Group.* Constable, London, 1975.
Kubie, L. Unsolved problems in the resolution of the transference. Psychoanal. Q., *37:* 331, 1968.
Pines, M. Overview. In *The Large Group,* L. Kreeger, p. 291. Constable, London, 1975.

Winnicott. D *The Maturational Processes and the Facilitating Environment: Studies in the Theory of Emotional Development.* International Universities Press, New York, 1965.
Yalom, I. *The Theory and Practice of Group Psychotherapy.* Basic Books, New York, 1970.

D.2 Ethical and Legal Issues in Group Psychotherapy

EDWARD L. PINNEY, JR., M.D.

Introduction

With group psychotherapy now an established practice, issues of ethics and legal aspects have become increasingly important. While the American Group Psychotherapy Association is in the process of formulating a code of ethics, group psychotherapists must rely on the ethical codes promulgated by their specific professional organizations. Psychiatrists and psychologists already have explicit ethical codes. Other professionals in the field of group psychotherapy follow codes of ethics of their particular oganizations; however, codes for psychiatrists and psychologists provide principles significant for all. In this chapter, the principles of ethics for psychiatrists will be followed, since they are applicable to the many categories of behavioral scientists who work in the group psychotherapy mode.

Issues

At the beginning of the series of new group psychotherapy sessions, the therapist and the group members work out a contract. This agreement specifies the time and place of the group meetings, the duration and frequency of the sessions, arrangements as to fees and missed appointments, how tardiness is to be handled, the confidential content of the discussions, and prohibition of physical assault or sexual contact between group members. Principles of ethics demand that the therapist keep his part of the contract as perfectly as possible; he is supposed to be in control.

AGGRESSION

Rarely should a therapist have to physically restrain a group member. It seems faintly possible that a severely ill group member with almost nonexistent self-control may become assaultive. Physical restraint or assault in self-defense could conceivably be required by the therapist. Assaults between group members are known to have happened.

Technically, the group psychotherapist must scrutinize his behavior in relation to assaults between patients. Assaults cannot always be averted or predicted. If they happened repeatedly in a group, the therapist would be ethically bound to examine himself and his therapeutic techniques.

SEX

Sexual activity is a more complex issue than aggression. A group psychotherapist should not have sexual relations with a member of his group. Group patients can be vulnerable to suggestions both overt and unwitting from the therapist, and sexual activity can often be provoked by the therapist. Again, training can help a therapist know how to avoid provocative behavior.

Certain clients and patients by their nature can be seductive, sexually and otherwise. They not only can excite the therapist to join their protest against whatever perceived wrongdoer they find, but can suggest a closer personal relationship. These approaches are antitherapeutic and can lead to unethical and illegal behavior.

Of course, group psychotherapists have the potential to be provocative and seductive themselves. Training and a sense of ethical behavior serve to attenuate these trends.

As to sexual relations between group members, this cannot always be avoided. The therapist is responsible for this behavior, due to his position as the leader of the group. He is like the captain of a ship, ethically—and sometimes legally—responsible for all that goes on.

The therapist must try to avoid this kind of activity. Patients come to group psychotherapy for help with the cognitive and emotional disturbances they have in interacting with other people in their everyday lives. Group psychotherapy cannot provide an adequate substitute for worthwhile social relationships; to make the relationships in the therapy group a substitute for the real thing is to jeopardize the goals of a healthy therapy.

CONDUCT

Ethics refers to the moral relationship of each individual to his social group. Acceptable conduct is determined by ethical and moral standards. Legally, behavior is regulated by common law (judicial precedent) and statutes. Unethical conduct has no specific penalty, nor is it enforced by government agencies, such as the police. What is unethical is frequently not illegal, and at times what is legal appears grossly unfair, immoral, and unethical.

In group psychotherapy, the ethical and legal issues generally concern the group psychotherapist. Patients in group psychotherapy are assumed to be ethical suffering people who can be relieved by group treatment. The contract between the group members and the group leader is similar to legal issues involving the group therapist in that the contract is specified and made definite, usually at the beginning of the therapy group. Confidentiality is legally required of the therapist, and ethically required of the patients in a group.

LICENSURE

Legal requirements for a group psychotherapist vary according to the location of the practice of group psychotherapy. For example, in Texas, psychotherapists are licensed as a special occupation. In New York, anyone can call himself a psychotherapist without restriction. Group psychotherapists are included in both areas, either regulated or unregulated. Group psychotherapists must be aware of the local requirements or run the risk of legal action.

Ethical qualifications to practice group psychotherapy are in effect everywhere. They have to do do with the ideals for group therapists; the ethical requirement that the group psychotherapist should be adequately qualified is an example of this.

Obviously, the ethical requirements concern preparation to do group psychotherapy. Specific training in psychotherapy and group psychotherapy is required. To put one's self forward as a group psychotherapist when one is not trained and has but his own very private approach not only deprives the patients of adequate treatment, but prevents their getting adequate treatment elsewhere and can leave the patients disillusioned with group psychotherapy.

Syllabi are generally related to the standard textbooks of group psychotherapy. The training usually emphasizes supervision, observation of groups in progress, sometimes co-therapy experience, a personal group experience, and didactic material imparted by lectures, reading, discussions, and workshop seminars.

Qualifying organizations for group psychotherapists exist. They are sufficiently flexible to permit individual variation in style, and are accessible to new developments yet emphasize the known and reliable techniques. In the United States, the American Group Psychotherapy Association standards for membership emphasize the training requirements for membership, while leaving the content to the training institutions.

Basic training is not sufficient to meet ethical standards for continuing practice. "A lifetime of learning" is the expression of the principles of ethics of the American Psychiatric Association.

Technical expertise and ethics are inseparable. In psychotherapy, integrative insight-oriented psychotherapy requires that patients and clients be helped to understand the outer reality of the external world better, as well as to understand better the inner reality of the psyche. Supportive psychotherapy in groups requires that clients and patients be assisted in better using their perceptions of reality in a practical way.

In both great areas of group psychotherapy—integrative or insight-oriented therapy and didactic, inspirational, or supportive therapy—the reality orientation is ethically required. Therefore, ethical treatment is reality oriented. Truth demands statements that correspond to objective reality. Philosophically, the truths of psychotherapy and mental activity are so overdetermined as to allow much flexibility in the supportive therapy of unrealistic patients.

Generally, honesty and fair dealing are required of the group psychotherapist. The group psychotherapist must be an ethical person for his patients to benefit from the example he shows.

The group psychotherapist is also ethically obligated to observe proper behavior as to fees, time obligations, and the formal requirements of all therapists. If appointments cannot be kept, or time commitments for the duration of sessions have to be curtailed, arrangements should be made for remission of all or part of a fee.

EXPLOITATION

The therapist is also required to avoid exploiting his group to further his political or other special interests. Unusual forms of dress or behavior on the part of a group psychotherapist also serve to inject into the lives of patients an unnecessary complication.

Personal problems of the psychotherapist that interfere with his ability to give his full attention to his patients should be dealt with elsewhere. At times, the group psychotherapist should avoid seeing patients when a personal problem distracts him from using his full capabilities. He should not see patients when he is only half-alert or half-competent.

Patients frequently are troubled by their fears of others and by their difficulty in being able to trust. Ideally, they succeed in group psychotherapy when they are basically honest and able to trust the group psychotherapist. The group psychotherapist must be above reproach to meet his part of the therapeutic contract. Mutual trust and respect can lead to meaningful handling of intimate personal data by the patients in the group. This effort at trusting the several strangers within the group is a basic tenet to group psychotherapy. (This differs from individual psychotherapy, in which the therapist alone has to be trusted.)

A tentative kind of trust between group members occurs at the beginning if a group is to develop. Group members try out one another and the therapist. Ideally, trust develops as the group proceeds. Untrustworthy members of a group reveal themselves as unreliable. They may work with whatever makes them untrustworthy, drop out, or be asked to leave.

CONFIDENTIALITY

Confidentiality, based on trust, is considered essential to successful treatment. In two cases of individual treatment, Lifshutz and Caesar illustrate some of the problems.

In early December 1969, Lifschutz had been sent to jail for contempt of court for refusing to disclose the content of his therapeutic communications with a person alleged to be a former patient. The patient had entered his emotional condition into a lawsuit for damages. Lifschutz was ordered to produce his records. He refused on the basis that to release the information would seriously damage other current and future patients by causing them to fear that what is told to the therapist may be revealed on the witness stand. He argued also that the patient cannot possibly know the full content of the information he is releasing and, therefore, cannot give informed consent.

By May 1970, Lifschutz's situation had been clarified by several court appeals, so that extraneous or potentially embarrassing information would be excluded. Lifschutz testified that he had treated the patient and gave the dates of treatment but no further details. This satisfied Judge Melvin Cohn, and contempt of court charges were dismissed.

George Caesar's experience was described as a one-man test of the law on privileged communications. In December 1969, Caesar saw a patient for psychiatric examination and treatment following an automobile accident. He saw her 20 times for psychotherapy. The following July and August 1970, she filed personal injury actions to recover damages in the Supreme Court of California. In April 1972, her attorneys questioned Caesar. He refused to answer information which would be harmful and detrimental to the patient, since no consent had been obtained from the patient, and answers might not be relevant.

He was ordered by the court to answer the questions. In the meantime, the patient saw another psychiatrist and based her claims on his findings.

Later, Caesar answered some questions for the defendant's attorneys but refused to answer others he thought would be unethical to answer, and he was held in contempt of court. He appealed the decision through the courts to the United States Supreme Court, where in April 1977 his petition was denied.

Caesar then spent 3 days in jail, after which he still refused to testify in the case. His legal fees were reported to total $28,000.

The therapist is ethically and legally bound to keep confidential the material of what transpires in group sessions. If he reveals confidential information about his treatment, he likewise exposes his unreliability.

TRAINING

Group experiences for training purposes illustrate the importance of confidentiality. Members of experiential groups for training become very much aware of their concern about exposure of weaknesses they fear might impair their potential capability as therapists. These vulnerabilities can be exposed in the training group, though they are not carried out to such an extent as in a therapeutic group. It is undesirable and potentially unethical for the therapist in a training group to allow development of an intensity of emotional reactions that will interfere with the functioning or interpersonal relations of those in the group. In training institutions, serious damage to the careers of beginning therapists has resulted from improvident occurrences in experiential groups for training.

Legal Aspects

Confidentiality as an issue leads from the ethical to the legal aspects of group psychotherapy. Confidentiality is both an ideal and a technical requirement; and the legal aspects of group psychotherapy stem from this aspect.

There are two sources for our laws: (1) laws enacted by various law-making bodies or governmental administrative regulations based on delegated legal mandates and (2) law based on judicial decision and precedent.

It is instructive to remember that our system of courts and trials is an adversary system, stemming from the ancient trial by combat. Intrinsically, there is no relation between what is legal and what is ethical. It is the ideal in a representative government that the lawmaker will be just and fair. The combat in the courts and of the elective process continues to be our safeguard in this area.

The group psychotherapist who does not keep the content of group sessions confidential is legally and ethically liable. He can be sued for his breach of confidence if he betrays his patients, though this kind of suit is not common.

Legal cases, based on the involvement of a member of a psychotherapy group in a case in which other members of the group are to be called as witnesses, raise issues of privilege and confidentiality. Privileged communications legally occur in English and American common law only between an attorney and his client. This means that a court cannot force an attorney to tell anyone what his client has told him about what has already happened. This privilege has been extended to include information given by a patient to his doctor, but this is not absolute. A third person present when a communication occurs that would ordinarily be privileged can take away the privilege and make the communication available to a court. Various aspects of this dilemma in group psychotherapy are apparent.

Confidentiality was voided in a case of joint therapy of husband and wife. In early 1979, a Virginia circuit court judge ruled: "When a husband and wife are in counseling session with a psychiatrist which is between the husband and wife, there is no confidentiality because the statements were not made in private to a doctor but in the presence of the spouse."

Although this decision does not directly involve group psychotherapy, it has a potentially inhibiting influence on clients and patients who need to speak freely to gain the benefit of their group psychotherapy.

An attorney who is told by his client that the client intends to commit a crime is ethically obligated to take action to prevent the commission of such crime. From this legal practice came the recent decision that psychiatrists were similarly obligated.

In a pre-1970 decision (Tarasoff), the California Supreme Court held that "when a therapist knows that his patient is likely to injure another and the therapist can ascertain the identity of the intended victim, he must use reasonable care from causing the intended injury."

In 1978, Daniel Greenson was said to have the duty, based on the Tarasoff decision, to warn the parents of a patient that she was potentially suicidal. The California Apellate Court dismissed the case against Greenson, commenting that "the court did not hold that such disclosure was required where the danger presented was that of self-inflicted harm or suicide or where the danger consisted of a likelihood of property damage." Instead, the court recognized the importance of the confidential relationship which ordinarily obtains between a therapist and his patient, holding that "the therapist's obligations to his patient require that he not disclose a confidence unless such disclosure is necessary to avert danger to others . . .." It continued that "Tarasoff requires that a therapist not disclose information unless the strong interest in confidentiality is counterbalanced by an even stronger public interest, namely safety from violent assault."

Conclusion

In group psychotherapy, there are practical consequences of legal and ethical realities that can interfere with treatment. Though these issues seldom arise, the group psychotherapist must be taught and know these ethical and legal mandates for both himself and his patients. Since good treatment is ethical, then ethical behavior is a requirement for competent group psychotherapists.

References

American Psychiatric Association. The principles of medical ethics with annotations especially applicable to psychiatry. American Psychiatric Association, Washington, D.C. 1981.
Group for the Advancement of Psychiatry. *Report No. 45: Confidentiality and Privileged Communication in the Practice of Psychiatry.* Group for the Advancement of Psychiatry, New York, 1960.
Meyer, R. G., and Smith, S. R. A crisis in group therapy. Am. Psychol., *32:* 638, 1977.

D.3 Research in Group Psychotherapy

DONALD B. COLSON, Ph.D.
LEONARD HORWITZ, Ph.D.

Introduction

Researchers on the various modalities of psychotherapy are confronted with the fact that their studies seldom become influential in clinical practice. Training institutions teach the accumulated clinical wisdom of their faculties, who in turn rely mainly on clincal literature for keeping abreast of new ideas.

In fact, some research findings have recently appeared which indicate the relatively small impact of formal research upon clinical practice. Wolfgang and Pierson surveyed group practitioners in a metropolitan area about their use of group therapy research, and discovered that 75 per cent of the respondents regarded the research literature as irrelevant to their clinical practice. Additional evidence comes from Dies (1980), who surveyed group therapists for their opinions about various training methods. He found that the overwhelming number of clinicians surveyed failed to include research references in their recommended readings for beginning group therapists. In addition, the respondents seldom mentioned the use of research tools (inventories, rating scales, leader or group assessment techniques) in their training and supervisory practices.

How may we understand the relatively weak impact of a fairly extensive research literature? In part, the problem stems from the fact that a large portion of the group literature derives from sociological and social psychological sources where clinical relevance is minimal. The efforts to build connecting links between basic and applied research in our field have not been notably successful. But even avowedly clinical research has frequently failed to address itself to the most pressing and significant issues in our field. Certainly the question of outcome or treatment effectiveness looms as a central problem, but, as will be shown, few researchers have taken seriously the need to formulate sufficiently specific questions with regard to the appropriateness of special techniques with particular patient problems. For example, despite the growing interest in the group treatment of borderline patients, there is a dearth of research studies regarding the most appropriate methods for this population or, even more narrowly, for subtypes of these patients. On another issue which continually confronts the clinicians—the use of group versus individual intervention—with the exception of the important Malan study, there is little hard data (although much clinical material) available.

There is a great complexity of tasks confronting the researcher seriously interested in investigating clinically relevant issues. Compared with individual therapy, the problems for the group researcher are far more complex insofar as each therapy group is unique by virtue of the interactions of seven or eight idiosyncratic individuals.

The state of the art and science of research, whether in individual or group or family therapy, is still relatively undeveloped. Two basic needs in the research field have remained largely unfulfilled. First, there is no agreement on standardized instruments for measuring change, nor is there any agreement on even more complex instruments of evaluating the treatment process. Dies and MacKenzie may have taken an important step in this direction with their CORE Battery, an instrument for evaluating change in group patients, a development which is sponsored by the American Group Psychotherapy Association. A comparable effort was made several years ago by the National Institute of Mental Health (NIMH) group headed by Waskow and Parloff, in which a battery of initial and outcome instruments was adopted by a group of researchers in individual psychotherapy. Second, the need for replication of studies by individual investigators remains a major problem. The repetition of studies using similar methods and comparable populations by researchers in diverse settings is well recognized as essential for research progress. Some steps in this direction have been taken by the NIMH Collaborative Study on the treatment of depression and may be the start of comparable work by other investigators. Until these problems have been surmounted, research may remain relegated to a peripheral position in the clinical field.

It is commonplace for clinicians and researchers to judge the research on group psychotherapy on the basis of its success or failure to cumulatively provide clear answers, a goal which seems to be unrealistic and guarantees disappointment. It is more reasonable to expect the research to provide hints, confirm or disconfirm clinical hunches, and add to the conceptual background for clinical work.

Outcome

THERAPEUTIC BENEFITS

Early in the 1970's, Bednar and Lawlis reviewed the research on group therapy and concluded that there was clear evidence that therapy in general and group therapy in particular were effective, leading to behavioral and personality changes in a variety of patients treated by therapists of different persuasions working in diverse settings. Subsequently, Lewis and McCants argued that researchers should stop evaluating the effect of globally defined group therapy on broad classifications of patients (inpatients, outpatients, schizophrenics). They also maintained that the use of different outcome criteria across studies made it nearly impossible to compare results. They recommended an individualized approach to the study of change, resting on a diagnosis of each individual's maladaptive pattern of interpersonal behavior and an assessment of change in that behavior in the group.

In 1974, Black examined reviews, research articles, and case studies related to outcome. In contrast to Bednar and Lawlis, he concluded that it was premature to answer the question of whether group therapy was an effective method of treatment. He described patient variables, therapy variables, instrumentation, behavior change, and follow-up evidence, and made three recommendations which have been echoed in nearly every review since: (1) Specify patient variables in more detail; (2) use multiple measures of therapeutic effectiveness and change; and (3) use control techniques and follow-up data collection. In the same year, Fielding emphasized that the variety of theoretical orientations and differences among group approaches contribute to difficulty in defining group therapy. Also, he advocated assessing individualized outcome appropriate to each patient. So far, his recommendation has not been pursued, except by some studies which include multiple measures of outcome to allow for assessment of more than one kind of therapeutic benefit.

Grunebaum summarized the research on group therapy to facilitate its use by clinicians. He addressed the question of whether the use of group therapy is warranted by its effectiveness and answered affirmatively, citing studies which show that certain patient and therapist characteristics facilitate or obstruct successful outcome. More specifically, he reviewed the research relating to the client, the therapist, the quality of the group experience, and the outcome measures. Among his conclusions were the following: Clients have better outcomes if they are from a higher social class, have fairly realistic expectations, are not susceptible to scapegoating, experience some degree of distress but are not impulsive, and receive some preparation for group therapy. The clients will also tend to do better if their therapists have a positive, empathic orientation, help the clients to think about themselves in new ways, and foster a supportive group atmosphere including attention to group rules and boundaries. Frank notes that, despite some gain in methodological rigor, there has been little improvement in the relevance of research to clinical problems, in part because of having to contend with so many variables and types of treatment. However, he stated that with the increased sophistication in research methods, more clinically relevant research was beginning to appear, and he referred in particular to Lieberman's work.

On the negative side of the ledger, Parloff and Dies surveyed group therapy outcome studies from 1966 to 1975 and concluded that in a variety of patient groups (neurotic, schizophrenic, juvenile or adult offenders, and addicts) there is no cumulative and compelling evidence for the effectiveness of group therapy. They conclude that researchers should abandon efforts to demonstrate that all group therapies are equally effective with all classifications of patients. Like Black, they advocate clear statements of what characterizes various group treatments. Subsequently, in a much-quoted passage, they write that the basic research questions should be: "what kinds of changes are produced by what kinds of interventions provided by what kinds of therapists with what kinds of patients/problems under what kinds of conditions?" Lieberman makes a similar point—that no one therapeutic technique, type of group, or orientation succeeds for the majority of group participants.

Bednar and Kaul (1978), in a review which focuses on relatively well-designed studies, strike a cautiously optimistic note. They conclude that a large number of studies indicate that group treatments work. They add that these studies do not allow confident conclusions about the curative forces, group contexts, and other circumstances leading to positive changes in the members of these groups.

It may be concluded from these reviews that the general issue—of whether positive changes result for group therapy patients—is too vague, because of the diversity in types of groups and research efforts. The variability of responses to the question of the usefulness of groups comes in part from the particular interests and perspectives of the reviewers and variations in the stringency of their criteria for defining evidence of positive outcomes. But it seems that all reviewers agree that more clinically sophisticated and ultimately more useful questions and answers lie in greater refinement and specificity, particularly in regard to treatment techniques and patient types.

HARMFUL EFFECTS

An issue central to studies of outcome—and one of crucial interest to the clinician—is that of negative effects. Every group therapist has had experiences with patients which provide compelling reasons for attention to negative effects. Bergin and Garfield determined that, in studies of a variety of types of groups with diverse populations, there was clear evidence of psychological deterioration in a significant number of patients (about 10 per cent). The Lieberman, Yalom, and Miles study of encounter groups found that casualties were related to the leader and his technique. Casualties often resulted when the participants evoked a scapegoating process, in which they were attacked or rejected by the leader and the group. Often the leader was oblivious to a group member's deterioration, although the group members often tended to be aware of it. An important contribution to casualties, then, may lie in the therapist's failure to recognize a patient's psychological vulnerability, which in turn leads the therapist to proceed in an insensitive manner without providing adequate support or protection for the patient. One clinical observation is that groups may frequently scapegoat one or more members, often the most disturbed members, and that the therapist may unwittingly collude with this process, primarily because of countertransference reactions. Hadley and Strupp conclude that negative effects may stem from the failure to conduct adequate diagnostic assessment and screening prior to referring a patient to group therapy. This view is well supported by a cluster of studies of negative effects in individual psychotherapy.

A relevant but seldom-mentioned study conducted by Malan and his colleagues created considerable controversy in the community of psychoanalytic group therapists. The investigators conducted a follow-up study of 55 outpatients who had obtained insight-oriented group therapy at the Tavistock Clinic in London. They found no evidence that these groups were helpful, unless the patients had prior individual psychotherapy. Moreover, the majority of patients experienced the group as depriving, harsh, and frustrating. It is important to recognize that the technique employed was a rather literal adaptation of psychoanalysis to the group, in which the therapists confined interventions primarily to interpretations and emphasized group-as-a-whole phenomena with relative neglect of individuals. The therapists avoided entering discussions, asking or answering questions, providing support, or giving advice. The researchers concluded that the therapists should offer greater warmth, encouragement, individual attention, and participation in group interactions. This study may have limited generalizability, because the Tavistock approach differs in important ways from the type of psychoanalytically oriented group therapy usually practiced in this country, which is more balanced in attention to the group as a whole and to individuals. Nonetheless, the findings have considerable import for group therapists, and the points made by Malan relating to technique derive support from several other studies.

PREMATURE TERMINATION

Those who leave treatment prematurely are frequently viewed as failures, sometimes even as casualties. While it is crucial to assess qualities in the patient, the group, or in the therapist's personality and technique which may be associated with premature termination, the research should also assess whether the terminators are better or worse off at the time of termination. The bulk of the research in this area can be faulted for disregarding the patient's psychological state or reasons for leaving the group.

Bednar and Kaul (1978), in a section on premature termination and casualties, discuss relevant research, including five studies on patient characteristics associated with premature termination from group therapy. These studies yield an array of findings which collectively suggest that these patients may have been fearful and excessively different from others in the group or may have had expectations which could not be fulfilled. The assumption is supported that patient behaviors and outcomes require consideration of the group context.

An additional study of interest reported that patients who perceive their therapists as open, responsive, and confident are less likely to drop out, while therapists viewed as less accepting and maintaining rigid professional role behavior had more dropouts. One might note the parallel between this study and the findings of diverse studies like the Malan research, Lieberman's findings about the group leader's role in casualties, and Truax and Mitchell's work on therapist interpersonal skills in relation to process and outcome. It seems likely that for therapists, regardless of specific orientation, a proper balance between professionally prescribed distance and responsive, judiciously measured involvement is important for favorable outcomes.

The research literature also suggests that prevention of premature termination and casualties may lie in greater attention to criteria for referring patients to group therapy and adequate screening. Countertransference dispositions and institutional priorities may also affect referral to group therapy. Green et al. (1980), in the most recent report of a series of studies of such matters, find that the process of referring patients to group therapy is influenced by myths and assumptions about the efficacy of the modality, and infer that, particularly in clinical contexts where groups are not understood, the referral process may be infused with irrational ideas. For example, such referrals may be influenced by an assumption that group therapy is a second-rate treatment. This cluster of research is reminiscent of Yalom's well-known earlier study, showing that therapists with a high percentage of dropouts had less training, did little or no screening of group members, communicated less with their co-therapists, and had less supervision.

One final issue of relevance to premature termination and casualties is the research evidence that pregroup preparation of patients for group therapy is important. Curran studied videotape presentations to assist in preparing patients and concluded that the number of premature terminations would be reduced by the preparatory experience. Strupp and Bloxom demonstrated that two role-induction procedures facilitated a more favorable therapy experience for lower class patients than for those in a control condition. Nichols (1976) provides a summary of research evidence supporting the benefit of pregroup preparation. It has been observed that a patient's integration into group therapy is aided by several preparatory meetings with the therapist, which serve a diagnostic purpose and facilitate exploration of fantasies and reservations about the group. However, there are no studies of this kind of pregroup diagnostic process, screening, and preparation, which in clinical settings typically accompanies referral to group therapy.

Treatment Variables

Other variables may be categorized as therapeutic factors, the therapists, the patients, the groups, and the process.

THERAPEUTIC FACTORS

This section deals with research on factors which may lead to either a favorable group process or to good outcomes. Much of this work has recently been reviewed and summarized for a period from 1955 to 1979, including research on self-disclosure, interaction, cohesiveness, insight, catharsis, guidance, altruism, vicarious learning, and instillation of hope. Among the factors most frequently subjected to empirical study are self-disclosure (by patients and therapists) and group cohesiveness.

Studies of self-disclosure by patients, although not uniform in their results, tend to show that there is a relationship between self-disclosure in patients and the development of group cohesiveness and that therapist behavior seems to affect self-disclosure. However, various studies suggest that therapist transparency and self-disclosure are far more complex than many theoreticians and researchers imply. Dies writes "without specification of the 'when,' 'where,' 'why,' 'by whom' and 'to whom' facets, the more general question (does self-disclosure make a difference?) seems

anachronistic." In an earlier article he remarks that the impact of therapist self-disclosure will depend on a variety of considerations, including length of time in the group; level of therapist competence and experience; type, purpose, and composition of the group; and the content of the self-disclosure. In the same study, Dies noted that while self-revealing therapists were viewed as more friendly, trusting and intimate—they also were viewed as less relaxed, less strong, and less stable, these findings lead to questions about the fit of therapist self-disclosure with patients' psychological needs and expectations.

Yalom's review of the literature emphasizes the importance of cohesiveness (positive feelings of the group members about the group). Cohesiveness is likely to be fostered by therapists who intentionally reinforce cohesiveness, attempt to increase compatibility among group members, and promote interaction and member self-disclosure. However, Bloch et al. conclude that, while the therapist's influence on cohesiveness is obviously important, the link between group cohesiveness and outcome remains largely unexplored. Clinical experience suggests that group cohesiveness is indeed related to therapeutic effectiveness, but should not be equated with the expression of positive feelings. Tolerance and support for a certain amount of group conflict and anger are a necessary part of therapy groups, particularly those which have as a goal the resolution of internal conflicts of the group members.

In order to increase the clinical relevance of issues of cohesiveness and self-disclosure by patients and therapists, these issues might be conceptually reframed as contributions of the therapist's personality, technique, transference, and countertransference phenomena to the therapeutic alliance. In group therapy, in contrast to individual therapy, the alliance consists not only of collaborative attitudes toward the therapist and the work of therapy but also the patient's positive working attitudes toward other group members. Marziali et al. (1981) present research findings from individual therapy, showing that the alliance is related to therapeutic gains, suggestive of the use of such an approach for group therapy research.

Of special interest to psychodynamically oriented clinicians, and the subject of numerous investigations, is the extent to which a group is oriented toward developing insight. Roback reviewed the research literature to compare the influence of insight and non-insight psychotherapies on outcome, and he concluded, on a tentative note, that an orientation toward a combination of insight and member-to-member interaction produced most positive change. More recently, Bloch provides an excellent discussion of the complexity of the subject of insight and research in the area. One of several studies in this area focuses on the relationship between psychological mindedness and benefit from insight-oriented group therapy. This study reveals that more psychologically minded group members gained more from insight-oriented therapy than from a group oriented primarily toward learning from interpersonal interaction without therapist emphasis on insight. However, the participants in the groups were college student volunteers, somewhat diminishing confidence in generalizing the findings to clinical groups. Nonetheless, the findings do support the role of insight specifically in those groups which are conducted with the goal of acquisition of insight, and which are composed of carefully selected patients. This type of research finding, emphasizing the fit of therapeutic factors with specific patient attributes, may well be the most fruitful yield of future research in the area. From the point of view of clinical practice, such findings support not only the necessity for the matching of patients and groups, but also that therapists be judiciously flexible in the use of specific therapeutic techniques depending on the needs of their patients.

Bloch describes a potentially useful process approach for studying therapeutic factors: At regular intervals, patients and therapists prepare descriptions of events in treatment they regard as particularly important. These reports are then assigned by independent judges to a classification of therapeutic factors. The feasibility, validity, and reliability of the method are discussed, but the application to group therapy research awaits further study. Much can be learned about technique and specific interventions by assessing aspects of the group process at important choice points, when actions by the patients or therapist may have significant and lasting consequences. Several related studies use a group incident questionnaire, in part to assess skill in group facilitation (Stokes and Tait, 1979), to analzye choice points which require the therapist to take action (Tauber, 1978), and to examine nodal points in group therapy. None of these process measures has yet been applied in studies of outcome.

THE THERAPISTS

Lieberman's review of change induction in small groups concludes that there is little clear evidence of the effect of specific leader behavior on outcome. Bednar and Kaul (1978) note the paucity of work in the area and refer the reader to Lieberman's article. However, it seems that on the basis of the aforementioned articles reviewed, there is good evidence that leaders who are accepting, who are relatively active, who are selectively supportive, and who facilitate greater cohesiveness and self-disclosure set the stage for a better working alliance with some tentative suggestions of better outcomes as well. Lieberman's study of encounter groups showed some relationships between types of leader behavior and normative qualities of the groups, although this could not be shown to be a cause-and-effect relationship. Specifically, while leader theoretical orientation was unrelated to the leaders' behavior and member outcome, leaders who scored high on measures on caring and attribution of meaning had groups from which members derived greater benefit. It may be concluded that effective group leaders facilitate supportive group interactions and are accepting and non-intrusive, in part because they appreciate the self-preserving function of defenses and the necessity for the working through which is essential for positive changes. The

study also suggests that the most successful leaders helped members make their own decisions about what work and how much work they wished to do, a finding which may be viewed as suggesting the crucial importance of the leaders' respect for individual autonomy. Casualties occurred with greater frequency in groups where the leaders were insensitive to the members' needs, tended to approach resistances head-on in a critical way, and tended to minimize their responsibility for the course of the group. Such leaders seem to display an investment in having a successful group at all costs determined by their unresolved narcissistic needs and vulnerabilities. Although such findings should be applied to group therapy with caution, they are supported by other studies and fit closely with Malan's prescription of corrective measures for group therapies which may be too depriving and frustrating.

Studies of the effects of therapist and patient matching are relevant to the study of therapist variables. Two recent studies in the area offer promising findings, one by McLachlan on matching conceptual level ratings and the previously cited study on insight orientation. A study by Peake (1979) of aspects of therapist-patient agreement yields more ambiguous findings. McLachlan's work focused on groups of 92 alcoholic inpatients. The conceptual levels of the therapists and patients were assessed by means of a paragraph completion test and were scored according to a bipolar variable with conceptual dependence and independence as the extremes, a dimension weighted heavily on degree of cognitive complexity. Patients who were matched with therapists on conceptual level improved more in social functioning and perceived their therapists as more socially competent. The better group process of patients and therapists matched on cognitive style may stem in part from the importance of interventions and therapist styles being tailored to the patient's level of psychological functioning and specific treatment needs.

Finally, while a review of this literature reveals little conclusive research, evidence of the kinds of training, professional experience, or personality factors which combine to create the most effective therapists, it may be tentatively inferred from a cluster of findings from diverse sources that therapists might best be patient, flexible, sensitive to group conditions which facilitate work by the members, adept at management and structure setting, and not distant or narcissistically aloof. Although there is no consistent evidence that training or experience make a difference, these issues have yet to be adequately tested, particularly in longer term psychodynamically oriented group therapies where such variables may emerge as more compelling and influential than in briefer processes.

THE PATIENTS

Within recent years, specialized reviews of research on groups for particular types of patients have begun to appear. Among these are reviews which focus on group therapy with children, a variety of rehabilitation clients, amputees, homosexuals, juvenile delinquents, patients with cardiovascular disease, and patients diagnosed as schizophrenic. There is a growing literature on group treatment of adolescents and the elderly. With the current use of groups in psychosocial treatment of physically or terminally ill patients, particularly those suffering from cancer, we may expect to see a rapid growth of research in that area. Also, given the heightened attention to the psychology of women, there will be an increase in the number of studies of groups specifically for women.

Parloff and Dies, in a discussion of outcome research, conclude that studies with neurotics, schizophrenics, delinquents, adult offenders, and addicts have not demonstrated the efficacy of group psychotherapy. In spite of the lack of cumulative and unambiguous evidence, much research on group treatments with various patient and client populations is relevant to clinical practice. Two examples of useful work from studies of group therapy with cancer patients and with patients diagnosed as schizophrenic will be elaborated.

Spiegel studied the effects of weekly supportive group meetings for women with metastatic carcinoma of the breast. The design consisted of a 1-year, randomized, prospective-outcome assessment. Patients in these groups, which focused on the shared profound problems of a potentially terminal illness, became less confused, anxious, fatigued, and fearful as compared with a control group. There were no suggestions that such treatment groups were demoralizing or otherwise destructive. Such findings should support the application of group treatment in psychosocial programs for people with serious physical illnesses, and one wonders what information might come from such research to enrich group therapy with other populations. More could be learned, for example, about how social, group, and psychological factors interface with biological functioning and physical illness.

Reviews of research on the effectiveness of group therapy with psychotic patients have not been encouraging. However, it seems that it is not reasonable to assume, as many do, that a study with positive findings is necessarily canceled by one with negative findings. Rather, discrepant findings should be judged in the context of the kinds of results which are realistically expectable given particular types of groups and patients. For example, it is far more reasonable, in the case of group therapy with schizophrenics, to expect demonstrations of improvement in social functioning than in hospital readmission rates. The need for rehospitalization is a complex matter heavily influenced by the severity of initial levels of psychological disturbance. In a study of group treatment for psychotic patients, O'Brien compared group and individual therapy with schizophrenic patients discharged from a state psychiatric hospital. He discovered that the group patients were rated as more socially skilled than those treated in individual therapy. Neither treatment made a difference in readmission rates. On the basis of further clinical experience and research, O'Brien concluded that therapists and patients in groups composed of schizophrenics became enthusiastic about group therapy, with consequent improvement in communication and socialization.

THE GROUPS

The research on group characteristics, rather than therapist or patient variables, focuses primarily on group size and composition. Generally, the research literature suggests that therapy groups function best with 5 to 10 group members and with some degree of heterogeneity in types of people. Homogeneity of certain specific patient variables may facilitate the work of the group, depending on the treatment goals—for example, in groups designed for people who abuse alcohol or drugs.

An area of research most useful in conceptualizing the type of group which might be best for particular types of patients includes investigations of the interaction between specific patient attributes and treatment characteristics. One such cluster of studies deals with groups which vary in the provision of structure (instructions, rules, guidelines) to group participants. A number of these studies show that the type and extent of structure interacts with patient characteristics and group variables. For example, Lee and Bednar show that, in the early development of groups of college students, a high degree of structure is most helpful for low risk-taking members. Then, in a study which may be viewed as an elaboration of these findings, DeJulio suggests that high structure (audiotaped instructions) facilitated a higher level of group interaction in early group sessions but a less productive interaction over time. Conversely, the groups without the structured preparation began more slowly but progressed to better group functioning over time. Although once again the subjects were college students, the findings are consistent with the clinical observation that some optimally functioning groups, of the expressive variety, work through an initial phase of dependent behavior, which may eventually lead to greater peer interaction and autonomy in subsequent stages.

A limitation in the study of influential group attributes is that the overwhelming majority of studies involve short-term groups or assess change early in the group process. Consequently, many questions relating to the efficacy of long-term versus short-term groups have not been addressed, although there are some studies relevant to longer term therapy.

Studies comparing group therapy with other treatment modalities are described in the excellent recent reviews by Bednar and Kaul (1978), Lieberman, and Parloff and Dies.

THE PROCESS

Process studies of events and perceptions linked to different stages of group development are of particular interest to the many therapists who work with relatively long-term groups. One study employed a factor analytic approach to identify process issues typical of early and late stages of group development, and showed that quite different factors emerged during the two stages. Such work underscores the importance of therapist flexibility in shifting interventions, depending on specific stages of group development.

Increasing attention is being devoted in the research literature to a cluster of influential process variables referred to as group norms, group atmosphere, or group climate. This area of interest seems to have derived its impetus in part from the Lieberman, Yalom, and Miles study, which suggested the significance of leader behaviors in shaping such norms. Their factor analysis of a device for assessing norms resulted in five factors: (1) intense emotional expression; (2) open boundaries; (3) hostile, judgmental confrontation; (4) counterdependence/dependence; and (5) peer control. They found that groups with norms supporting flexible group boundaries (discussion of issues outside the group and of personal material) and peer control yielded more positive group results. Leaders who provided coherence in understanding individual feelings and behavior (conceptual explanations) had groups which favored open boundaries. Caring leaders seemed to have groups characterized by greater emotional expression. More recently, MacKenzie (1979, 1981) and Silbergeld also suggest that qualities of group climate or of the implicit rules of group conduct, are effective predictors of individual behavior. An assessment device developed by Silbergeld, the Group Atmosphere Scale, has recently attracted attention. MacKenzie stresses the use of the instrument to measure the impact of leader styles on group climate and ways in which the climate mediates the leaders' influence on the members. This work is particularly important because it is directed at understanding aspects of group life, in contrast to dyadic interaction, which facilitate positive change in members. Although MacKenzie focuses on that which is distinct to group process, it is possible to view the functioning of group atmosphere in ways comparable to the effects of the therapeutic alliance in individual therapy. With increasing awareness of changes in group norms, qualities of group atmosphere at different phases of group life may be identified, and the progression versus impasses in group development related to outcome.

A potentially rich approach to the study of process seems to be clearly underrepresented in present research; this is the kind of systematic clinical conceptualization first demonstrated in the early work of Powdermaker and Frank. Certain crucial events and patterns of change involving patients, the group, and the therapist are noted in sequence, and subsequent events are carefully traced, a procedure which Powdermaker and Frank refer to as situation analysis. Such disciplined and selective running accounts of events can be made as rigorous in method and instrumentation as more traditional research design, analogous in some ways to the single-case design in research on individual psychotherapy.

Methodology and Instrumentation

Bednar and Kaul (1978), like other reviewers, conclude that meaningful investigation of group work requires "precise, comprehensive, relevant descriptions that preserve the essentials of the very phenomena we hope to investigate." Lewis and McCants argue that we should develop process and change measures unique to group therapy and emphasize that change measures should be individualized.

In response to such recommendations, the research does show increased sophistication, indicated, for example, by the numerous useful guides available which attend to methodological issues and problems. Hare includes an encyclopedic list of references to methods, variables, and assessment techniques. Lieberman lists instruments frequently used to study change in groups. Weigel and Corazzini (1978) present suggestions for solving common methodological problems and include sections on instrumentation and assessment procedures. Parloff and Dies (1978) provide a useful set of guidelines for assessing the adequacy of research on group therapy outcome. They include checklists, rating scales, and worksheets relevant to many aspects of group research. Lieberman also provides numerous examples of issues to consider in the design of research on groups, particularly in the area of instrumentation. Finally, Dies suggests techniques to foster a working alliance between the researcher and subjects over the course of a project. He offers specific recommendations for the recruitment, pretesting, group assignment, post-testing, and debriefing stages of research.

Several methodological issues are underscored by our clinical perspective. First, studies which are based on psychodynamic concepts are relatively scarce. Few researchers include assessment of such patient variables as ego strength, quality of interpersonal relations, superego functioning, motivation to change, impulse control, preferred defensive styles, and prominence of narcissistic or borderline features. It is as though study of the group has made the goal of clarifying interpersonal processes so compelling that attention to individual characteristics and psychopathology pales in comparison. Bellak (1980) has suggested the use of his Ego Function Assessment Scales to compare dyadic and group treatments.

A second problem is the infrequency of follow-up assessments to determine the persistence or absence of treatment effects over time. Outcome measures at the time treatment ends are vulnerable to complex influences associated with the termination process itself. Some studies suggest that a certain percentage of group therapy patients continue to improve after treatment. Of six follow-up studies reviewed by Bednar and Kaul (1978), three indicated that early treatment effects persisted into a follow-up period. Malan's study might be interpreted as showing that negative reactions can be more confidently assessed at follow-up.

Finally, there is an issue which has been mentioned by several reviewers of group therapy research: namely, a lack of theoretical and conceptual richness which might serve as a base for more coherence in the research (Bednar and Kaul, 1978). While group therapy does not have as extensive a heritage of theoretical scholarship as that on individual psychotherapy, there is a body of theory about groups which often is ignored. It is rare to see articles which take as their starting point premises deriving from classic works like those by Bion, Ezriel, Foulkes, Bennis and Shepard, and Whitaker and Liberman.

Conclusion

The research in group therapy provides few conclusive answers about the efficacy of various types of therapists and groups in the treatment of different kinds of patients. However, given the relatively early stage in the history of this research, the enormous diversity of variables, and the lack of major programmatic efforts, this comes as no surprise. This is not to say that the existing body of research is of little use; rather, it lays a groundwork for increasingly sophisticated research and provides much information of use to the clinician who is willing to attend to the empirical work. Where the research fails to provide indisputable evidence for a particular treatment approach, it does furnish many suggestions bearing on clinical practice—for example, about negative effects, the utility of pregroup preparation, and therapist behaviors which facilitate a productive group atmosphere or therapeutic alliance. Evaluating existing research against the criterion of providing conclusive evidence is not justified in the realm of psychological research, at least not in its current formative stage. Indeed, it might be better to examine how the present contributions enrich the therapists's conceptual field and thereby improve clinical work.

A brief sketch of some clinical implications of the group therapy research is as follows. A large number of studies indicate that group treatments are useful to the participants. While a properly conducted group therapy can be beneficial, groups, like any form of treatment, may have adverse effects. Negative effects are most likely when therapists—because of a lack of training, insufficient diagnostic data, or countertransference reactions—are insensitive to the patient's psychological needs. In this regard, adequate patient screening and preparation is often useful. Frequently, casualties result from a patient occupying a deviant position in the group, thereby becoming the object of scapegoating. Therapists and groups fostering patient self-disclosure and cohesiveness contribute to a high degree of collaboration, which in turn fosters other beneficial group processes. Self-disclosure or transparency in the therapist is a more complex and ubiquitous matter. Therapists would do well to have a caring, non-intrusive, and supportive attitude toward the group and its members and should be attentive to the patient's needs for new or alternative explanations for their maladaptive behavior. The extent to which the therapist is directive versus nondirective, imposes structure, or emphasizes interpretation of unconscious material should be closely tied to specific patient qualities and treatment needs—admittedly a difficult task when working with groups of idiosyncratic individuals. Numerous studies may be interpreted as supporting the tailoring of interventions to the patient's level of psychological functioning. The group atmosphere or climate is likely an influential factor in a group's effectiveness, and thus the therapist should assess those interventions which will foster a productive climate—for example, through occasional attention to group norms. When evaluating gains in one's group members, it is best to think in terms of those changes which are expectable, given the type of group and types of patients involved. For schizophrenic patients, it is more reasonable to assess changes in social skills than to expect a direct influence of the group on readmission rates.

Advances in methodology and measurement of the last decade have made the field ripe for major programs of research. Working in the same direction as the improved methodology, there are increased social, professional, financial, and legal pressures to demonstrate formally the efficacy of various forms of psychotherapy. There is a particularly notable deficit of research on long-term psychodynamically oriented groups characteristic of outpatient treatment centers and the private practice realm. Finally, it would be useful to heighten our awareness of the increasing division in theory and research between attention to individual psychological processes and group processes. The current burgeoning literature in systems and family dynamic perspectives may provide opportunities for greater conceptual integration of individual and group dynamics.

References

Barbach, L., and Flaherty, M. Group treatment of situationally organsmic women. Sex Marital Ther., 6: 19, 1980.

Beck, A. P., and Peters, L. The research evidence for distributed leadership in therapy groups. Int. J. Group Psychother., 31: 43, 1981.

Bednar, R. L., and Kaul, T. J. Experimental group research: Current perspectives. In Handbook of Psychotherapy and Behavior Change, S. L. Garfield and A. E. Bergin, editors, ed. 2. John Wiley & Sons, New York, 1978.

Bellak, L. On some limitations of dyadic psychotherapy and the role of group modalities. Int. J. Group Psychother., 30: 7, 1980.

Corder, B. F., Haizlip, T. M., and Walker, P. A. Critical areas of therapists' functioning in adolescent group psychotherapy: A comparison with self-perception of functioning in adult groups by experienced and inexperienced therapists. Adolescence, 15: 435, 1980.

Dies, R. R. Group psychotherapy: Reflections on three decades of research. J. Appl. Behav. Sci., 15: 361, 1979.

Dies, R. R. Current practice in the training of group therapists. Int. J. Group. Psychother., 30: 169, 1980.

Fisher, B. A., and Werbel, W. S. T-group and therapy group communication. Small Group Behav., 10: 475, 1979.

Goldberg, S., editor. The Psychology of Self: A Case Book. International Universities Press, New York, 1978.

Greene, L. R., Abramowitz, S. I., Davidson, C. V., and Edwards, D. W. Gender, race and referral to group psychotherapy: Further empirical evidence of countertransference. Int. J. Group Psychother., 30: 357, 1980.

Hecht, M. A cooperative approach toward children from alcoholic families. Elem. School Guid. Counsel., 11: 197, 1977.

Horwitz, L. A group-centered approach to group psychotherapy. Int. J. Group Psychother., 27: 423, 1977.

Ingersoll, B., and Silverman, A. Comparative group psychotherapy for the aged. Gerontologist, 18: 201, 1978.

Julian, A., and Kilmann, P. R. Group treatment of juvenile delinquents: A review of the outcome literature. Int. J. Group Psychother., 29: 3, 1979.

Kellerman, H. Group Psychotherapy and Personality: Intersecting Structures. Grune & Stratton, New York, 1978.

Lieberman, M. A., and Gourash, H. Evaluating the effects of change on the elderly in groups. Int. J. Group Psychother., 29: 283, 1979.

Mackenzie, R. Group norms: Importance and measurement. Int. J. Group Psychother., 29: 471, 1979.

Mackenzie, R. Measurement of group climate. Int. J. Group Psychother., 31: 287, 1981.

Marziali, E., Marmar, C., and Krupnick, J. Therapeutic alliance scales: Development and relationship to psychotherapeutic outcome. Am. J. Psychiatry, 138: 361, 1981.

Mosher, L. R., and Keith, S. J. Research on the psychosocial treatment of schizophrenia: A summary report. Am. J. Psychiatry, 136: 623, 1979.

Parloff, M. B., and Dies, R. R. Group therapy outcome instrument: Guidelines for conducting research. Small Group Behav., 9: 243, 1978.

Peake, T. H. Therapist-patient agreement and outcome in group therapy. J. Clin. Psychol., 35: 637, 1979.

Stokes, J. P., and Tait, R. C. The group incident's questionnaire: A measure of skill in group facilitation. J. Counsel. Psychol., 26: 250, 1979.

Tauber, L. E. Choice point analysis: Formulation, strategy, intervention, and result in group process therapy and supervision. Int. J. Group Psychother., 28: 163, 1978.

Weigel, R. G., and Corazzini, J. G. Small group research: Suggestions for solving common methodologic and design problems. Small Group Behav., 9: 193, 1978.

AREA E

INTERNATIONAL GROUP PSYCHOTHERAPY

E.1 Group Psychotherapy in Argentina

GUILLERMO FERSCHTUT, M.D.

History

There are two Argentine histories, which sometimes parallel each other and sometimes run in opposition. The first Argentine history is a story of independence and national consolidation, and was the task of both the Spanish people and the *criollos*, the Americans born of Spanish parents. They conquered and liberated the country and established its frontiers. The second history begins with the appearance of immigration. The first wave of immigrants were the conquerors of the agricultural soil; the second were poor and unwanted, linked to the first only by religious beliefs. The last wave of immigration resulted from the Spanish Civil War. Argentina's new arrivals were made up of intellectuals and traders impoverished by the misery of war and destruction but enriched by their ancestral cultures.

Health Care

Argentina is characterized by a multiplicity of health care systems. These public and private resources exert an influence on all levels of the society. The state, through its public health administration policies and according to modern health precepts, is trying to change the traditional concept of medicine.

The ultimate goal of these changes is healing—and the prevention and avoidance of—illness. Since the end of the last century, Argentine medicine has been considered one of the most advanced in Latin America. Because of the economic postwar welfare and massive European immigration, important centers of social and cultural evolution have emerged in Argentina.

Psychiatry

Psychiatric hospitals are centers devoted to the healing and recovery of patients suffering from psychological problems, but these institutions have little or no social community penetration. They do not follow the modern tendency of preventing psychiatric illness and establishing early treatment plans for psychiatric ailments. These factors contribute to the high hospital occupancy rate, the high incidence of mental illness, and the high percentage of chronically ill patients.

In 1957, several groups of psychiatrists organized the Instituto Nacional de Salud Mental (National Institute of Mental Health), thus initiating a period of renewal; unfortunately, this revival became stagnant due to the lack of economic resources and the presence of political agitation. At present, the most renewing impulse comes from the general hospitals, where psychiatry is being infiltrated with a more dynamic sense of community. The creation of psychology schools in the different universities has increased the interest in medical psychology. Although psychologists collaborate in many institutions and wards, their number is still small.

At present, only the psychiatrist can practice psychotherapy. Psychologists can participate in the treating team only under the direction of the doctors who are responsible for the patients.

Group Therapy

Group therapy was born in Argentina under the aegis of psychoanalysts who started to implement the different ways for learning this science. Psychoanalytic theory is still the major theoretical basis of the various groups in the Argentine Association of Psychology and Group Psychotherapy; other theoretical bases include Freud, Melanie Klein, Bion, Ezriel, Foulkes, and Slavson.

In the 1960's, a great variety of different techniques began to appear, including sensitivity groups, marathon groups, LSD groups, and gestalt groups. Simultaneously, social psychiatry applied group techniques in the prevention of mental illness within the community, schools, factories, and neighborhood associations. Besides the use of therapeutic groups with neurotic or psychotic patients, groups are used with adults, children, teenagers, families, couples, multi-family groups of psychotic patients, and children with learning difficulties.

Group techniques

The main approach is an interpretative technique based on psychoanalysis, with one or two 90-minute weekly sessions that may continue for an unspecified period of time. No dramatization or role playing is used. There is only one therapist, who generally acts as a nonparticipating observer.

The fundamental role of the therapist is the interpretation of the here and now of the unconscious aspects of the group behavior, taking into account both the group structure and the group dynamics. The interpretations are related to transference situations.

The objective or group task is the healing of the members of the group. This can occur through the projection into the group situation of the inner world of each one of the participants, and the relation of this inner world to the momentary situation.

Family therapy

In Argentina, Enrique Pichon Riviere and Jorge Garcia Badaracco can be considered the two pioneers in family group therapy. The former started working by the end of the 1950's, the latter by the mid-1960's. Riviere developed his theories from concepts of social therapy; Badaracco developed his from his experience in the psychoanalytic therapeutic community with psychotic patients.

The goal of family group therapy is to increase the discrimination of the patients through the interpretation of intrapsychic events and psychopathological interactions with other members of the group.

Psychodrama

Two trends exist in psychodrama—the psychodrama of Moreno and psychoanalytic psychodrama, which utilizes psychoanalytic concepts in its interpretation.

Along the lines of Moreno's theory, the group is defined as a sociometric structure offering a psychotherapeutical matrix where the roles that have been structured with difficulty in the successive matrixes of social and family identity can be modified or developed; and in this new matrix they will find those elements that were lost or absent in the previous ones. The finding of nuclear conflicting scenes is the touchstone in the psychodramatic process.

Conclusion

Group therapy is now widely used in many hospitals and with all kinds of patients in Argentina. Its influence has also been felt in the heightened interest in the fields of sociology and psychology. The growing popularity of group therapy is attested to by the various professional associations existing today in the country, and by Argentina's active and ongoing participation at international congresses.

References

Berman, G. *Problemas Psiquiatricos*. Paidos, Buenos Aires, 1966.
Dellarossa, A., and Ferschtut, G. *Estructuracion de una Institucion para la Formacion de Coordinadores de Groupo*. Breviarios, Asociacion Argentina der Psicol. y Psicot. de Groupo, Buenos Aires, 1979.
Ferschtut, G. *Formacion de Terapeutas de Grupo*. Acta Psiquat. y. Psicol. de Americalatina, Buenos Aires, 1973.
Grinberg, L., Langer, M., and Rodrigue, E. *Psicoterapia de Grupo: Se Enfoque Psicoanalitico*. Paidos, Buenos Aires, 1957.

E.2 Group Therapy in Australia

FRANCIS WALTER GRAHAM, M.B., B.S., D.P.M., F.R.C. Psych.

History

Australia, sometimes called the smallest continent and the biggest island in the world, is almost the size of the continental United States. It has a population of almost 15 million.

When Captain Cook arrived in Botany Bay in 1788, he found there a very ancient and primitive race, later called Australian Aborigines. About that time, they were estimated to number approximately 300,000. In the 1970's, there were between 40,000 and 50,000 full bloods, and 100,000 mixed bloods. In the early days of colonization, they lived a very uneasy coexistence with the whites, marked by occasional violent clashes, and even sporadic warfare from time to time, as pastoralists pushed further outward from the original settlements. In the 1830's Protectors of Aborigines were appointed in most colonies and on outlying settlements, and Aborigines started to be tapped as a work force.

In 1897, control of Aboriginal Reserves passed from mission stations to government. In the 1960's, increasing public concern turned Aboriginal rights into a political issue with the eventual granting of citizen rights, wage equality, and access to social services and public schools. In 1973, the federal government established the National Aboriginal Consultative Committee (NACC), which acts in an advisory capacity to the Minister for Aboriginal affairs.

Health Care

The first organized health service to be established was in 1788, for the penal settlement off the coast of New South Wales. From that point, development was along lines, 19th-century British, with increasing but limited government involvement and considerable reliance on charity. From the late 1940's, ideas influencing health care tended to come from North America.

The years 1972 to 1975 saw the establishment by a Labor government of Medibank, a federal agency that was part of a universal health insurance scheme, which included a number of private, government-registered health insurance organizations. The insured are covered for practically all hospital, medical, surgical, and dental expenses. The cost has proved enormous, and has led to desperate attempts to cut down and cut back. Government funding of hospitals has been markedly reduced. Psychoanalysis and other long-term, frequent-sessions-a-week psychological methods of treatment have come under strong criticism as doubtful allowable items for health insurance purposes.

In Australia, the most widely used services are provided by private practitioners. Medical practitioners and specialists are remunerated on a fee-for-service basis, and at least 85 per cent of a government-set scheduled fee is recoverable. Doctors may charge a fee higher than this on their own judgment or according to a schedule recommended by the Australian Medical Association, but, in this case, the patient accepts responsibility for the difference.

Group psychotherapy in Australia comes within the above insurance scheme as long as it is carried out by a registered medical practitioner, which includes medical psychotherapists, medical psychoanalysts, and psychiatrists. No insurance funds are available for the payment of fees of lay psychotherapists. The psychotherapy groups must contain no more than nine patients; there is no limit on the number of sessions per week and no limit on length of time of treatment.

Public health services are concerned with environmental control and a limited range of personal health care. They are primarily the responsibility of state health authorities, assisted by local government bodies. Their activities extend to regulation and surveillance of water and air quality, waste disposal, housing and occupational hygiene, radiation, food and drug standards, immunization programs, school medical and dental services, maternal and child health clinics,

and health education campaigns. A federal initiative supported by state and local government and non-government bodies, known as the Community Health Program, aims at providing health services to disadvantaged groups—such as the aged and the Aborigines—and at developing preventive and rehabilitation services. Quarantine services are the responsibility of the federal government.

An ambulance service by road and air covers most of the population. For a small annual fee, a patient earns the right to travel to a hospital or doctor for treatment without further charge if ambulance travel is necessary. Additionally, Australia's unique aerial medical service, the Royal Flying Doctor Service, covers more than two-thirds of the Australia continent.

Another important service in Australia, but one that seldom even rates an honorable mention, is the Commonwealth Rehabilitation Service. This has its headquarters in Canberra, the Australian Capital Territory, and has branches in all states, staffed by doctors trained in rehabilitation with a paramedical staff of occupational therapists, physiotherapists, speech therapists, nurses, and recreational personnel. They have both outpatient and inpatient services, and the latter are usually run along the lines of therapeutic communities. They are staffed also by part-time rehabilitation medical consultants from private practice, who do sessional work at the various institutions. Patients from 16 to 65 years of age are eligible. They are usually referred by doctors in general practice, have a preliminary assessment, and, if accepted, can be taken into training for anything up to 3 years, all expenses paid.

Overview of Psychiatry

The Royal Australian and New Zealand College of Psychiatrists (R.A.N.Z.C.P.) has a membership of about 850. Most of the states have branches of the college, holding regular scientific meetings and conducting training courses in general psychiatry for psychiatric registrars. The membership of the college consists mainly of state mental health-trained consultants, but includes also most of the psychiatrists in private practice, who, for the most part, have migrated into private from state-run psychiatric clinics. These psychiatrists have their own independent association.

Some of the universities still give a Diploma of Psychological Medicine (D.P.M.), but this is widely being replaced by the longer, more thorough 5-year course of the college. The professorial departments are all linked with college activities, and some have a close working relationship with state mental health institutions.

Some of the small number of professors of psychiatry are locally trained, having had overseas experience also; but most have come from the United Kingdom, with the background of a strong London Maudsley Hospital tradition, which has had a dominant influence over the younger generation of·psychiatrists.

Role of Psychiatric Hospitals

Most of the psychiatric hospitals are state-run, with a full-time salaried staff of psychiatrists and paramedical personnel. Private psychiatric hospitals are few. These state hospitals cope with the greater bulk of psychiatric illness, particularly severe psychoses. Apart from the large mental hospitals in every city, there are an ever-increasing number of state-run clinics treating ambulatory psychotic, neurotic, and drug-dependent patients. Among the inpatient population, there is an ever-increasing interest on the part of the staff in establishing therapeutic communities, particularly in convalescent wards, and in trying out group methods of therapy not only with neurotic but with even severely psychotic patients.

Private psychiatric hospitals fulfill a limited but useful role, making available all standard forms of physical treatment and making use of group methods with inpatients and with former patients who return on an outpatient basis.

Group Therapy

Paul Dane, the well-known Melbourne psychiatrist and a director of the Melbourne Institute for Psychoanalysis, introduced group psychotherapy to Australia. He was most impressed by the analytical approach to group psychotherapy in the United States.

Later, the author started group psychotherapy with psychiatric outpatients at the Royal Melbourne Hospital. This was the first time such therapy had been introduced at a university teaching hospital in Australia. During this period, the author was joined in this work by another psychoanalyst, Ian Martin, who later became chief psychiatrist at the hospital. Doctors and clinical psychologists would occasionally sit in on their groups to study the method and get some introductory training. Both have maintained from the beginning that a sound personal analysis or analytical group experience is essential for this work.

Interstate conferences are a regular feature of the life of this association. Clinical and theoretical themes receive about equal consideration, including some of the following: (1) suitability of patients for an analytical group experience—the possibility of trauma to patient or group; (2) frequency of sessions; (3) tensions arising in patients and therapists; (4) group therapy sessions combined with individual sessions; (5) adjunct drug therapy—e.g., antidepressants in endogenous depression, lithium in manic-depressive conditions; (6) stance and emotional expression of the therapist—e.g., a poker face or a natural play of facial expression, eye-to-eye contact or Rodin's "Le Pen-seur" pose; and (7) interpretations to individuals versus those to the group as a whole and optimal conditions for mutative interpretations.

All universities in Australia have professorial departments of psychology, most of which make a close study of group phenomena. They do little in the field of group therapy proper, but they organize workshops in group dynamics, and this can form a sound basis for those relatively few psychologists who wish to move into the field of group therapy. Most academics who have a bent toward treating patients seem to prefer to practice behavior therapy.

State mental health authorities run comprehensive courses of training in psychiatry for their own personnel. These courses focus only on basic theory and skills. They are designed to be useful for running the usual kinds of group meetings formed in mental health clinics and to prepare those who may want additional training in group psychotherapy.

The encounter group experience is very popular and is widely practiced, proving of considerable benefit to the average person. T-groups are most sought after and widely used, particularly in industry and in many situations where there are problems of organization and administration.

Alcoholics Anonymous (AA) is also widely active (together with its associated Al-Anon and Alateen groups) in all cities, suburbs, and large towns throughout the country. AA works closely with the staffs of general hospitals, psychiatric clinics, mental hospitals, and prisons, and is deeply involved in trying to combat the ravages of alcoholism, not only in the general community but also among the Australian Aborigines.

As in other countries, many groups are being formed and encouraged along the lines of the original AA to help in other problems of adjustment, e.g., Gamblers Anonymous and Parents Anonymous. A much greater proliferation of these sorts of groups can be expected, and this growth points to a need for a greater understanding of the processes involved in their undoubtedly therapeutic effects.

References

Blansfield, O. H. D. Group: The more primitive psychology—a theory of some paradigms on group dynamics. Aust. N. Z. J. Psychiatry, 6: 238, 1972.

Christie, G. Group psychotherapy in private practice. Aust. N. Z. J. Psychiatry, 4: 43, 1970.

Graham, F. W. Observations on analytical group psychotherapy. Int. J. Group Psychother., 9: 50, 1959.

Graham, F. W. A case treated by psychoanalysis and analytic group psychotherapy. Int. J. Group Psychother., 13: 25, 1964.

Rampling, D. R., and Williams, R. A. Evaluation of group process using visual analogue scales. Aust. N. Z. J. Psychiatry, 11: 189, 1977.

E.3 Group Psychotherapy in China

WU CHEN-I, M.D.

Introduction

Ancient Chinese medical literature contains several valuable records that describe the concept and practice of psychotherapy. The doctor, according to traditional Chinese medical philosophy, should consider the patient's mind and body as one; any physical change will affect the psyche.

In "Lin Shu," a famous ancient medical essay, it is said that the patient must be told where his trouble lies, what the parameters of his illness are, and how to take care of it. He must also be instructed not to feel distressed by his trouble. Moreover, the doctor should explain in detail to the patient the proper attitude toward the disease and help the patient eliminate or alleviate his own pain. The purposes of the dialogue between the patient and the doctor are to enable the patient to understand those factors which will be beneficial in treating his case, to encourage the patient to take an active role in combating his illness, and to restore his self-confidence. Traditionally, Chinese medicine is predicated on a patient-centered approach to the treatment of both mental and physiological disorders; it is precisely because of this psychotherapeutic approach that traditional Chinese medical practice has been so widely accepted and has had so much success among the Chinese people.

Prior to 1949, the use of psychotherapy was restricted chiefly to individual therapy; group psychotherapy was used only in the treatment of special cases. During this period of time, the theory and practice of psychotherapy were primarily influenced by foreign schools of psychoanalysis and psychobiology.

Since the People's Republic of China was established in 1949, psychiatric services and research have developed tremendously. Because of the extensive use of psychotropic drugs, however, psychotherapy is still relegated to a subordinate role in the treatment of mental illness. In 1958, during the state of economic readjustment and consolidation, China's psychiatric workers decided to give priority to the study of those mental illnesses which had comparatively high incidence and prevalence. Consequently, a great deal of research concentrated on schizophrenia and neurosis. Moreover, during this period, several institutes combined resources and experimented with combined psychotherapy in a group mode to treat neurosis and psychosomatic disorders. The ensuing years of practice, experience, and success laid the foundation for the contemporary form of group psychotherapy used in the treatment of chronic and paranoid schizophrenia.

Theoretical Considerations

Two precepts are accepted today as the fundamental principles on which Chinese therapists base their practice. If the patient understands that mental disorders may be a manifestation of pathophysiological functions and that the use of correct methodology is the key to understanding problems, he will learn how to recognize his own illness and how to adopt a proper attitude toward it. The function of the medical workers—including psychologists, doctors, nurses, and occupational therapists—is, therefore, to help patients develop a correct understanding of their disease, and to encourage patients to utilize their initiative in an effort to eliminate the illness. The key to successful treatment lies in the relationship between the doctor and the patient, and this interaction is especially important in psychotherapy.

Selection of Patients

Group psychotherapy is today the principal form of treatment used in China. Each patient's educational, social, cultural, and family background, combined with individual personality traits, causes him to react differently to various stimuli. In selecting the appropriate form of treatment, one should consider all these factors. Therefore, although group psychotherapy is the principal form used in China, it has become a psychiatric truism that better results can be achieved through the use of a combination of different treatment modalities.

Through group psychotherapy, the patient becomes fully aware of all the manifestations and ramifications of his illness. With the assistance of the doctor, the patient is encouraged to recover his insight; this allows him to understand the source of his disease and permits him to willfully struggle against it.

Generally, groups composed of neurotic patients or patients with a physical ailment consist of 10 to 20 individuals. However, groups of schizophrenic patients are smaller, containing only about 10 people. The group discussion usually takes place once or twice a week, with the group leader being selected by the patients. This is crucial to group morale, since patients believe that having control over both the selection of a group leader and the discussion proves that they are trusted and respected.

Group therapy may not be appropriate for all patients. Some patients require individual care. For these patients, individual consultations with their doctors are necessary but may not be sufficient. Indeed, therapy is adapted to the individual's specific needs. Individual sessions are usually held once or twice a week and are alternated with group sessions.

Results

Clinical practice has shown that many etiological factors are concerned with the patient's family or his work unit. Family therapy aids in recognizing and clarifying the patient's symptoms. Positive results may be obtained if the patient's relatives and colleagues participate in group discussion. After this participation in the group discussion, they may become aware of their own prejudices and may gradually acquire a sympathetic attitude toward the mentally ill. They consequently learn to observe and to care for the patient, to detect the early signs of illness in order to avoid a relapse, and to help him cope with his life. Most importantly, they learn to create a healthy and harmonious environment that is conducive to successful recovery.

Contradictions exist everywhere in daily life, which may create pathological factors, in turn precipitating mental troubles. Social therapy includes the follow-up care of the patient. This kind of therapy is basically a mental checkup, which can take place either in a doctor's office or in an outpatient clinic. The purpose of this form of treatment is to help the patients to reconcile themselves with the contradictions in their environment and to thus prevent relapse.

Accumulated experience shows that group therapy is the core of psychotherapy. However, under special circumstances, in order to increase the curative effect and to prevent relapse, better results are achieved if this group therapy is combined with other forms of therapy, such as individual psychotherapy, family therapy, social therapy, and pharmacotherapy.

Conclusion

Group psychotherapy has demonstrated a clear and definite effect in the treatment of neurosis and psychosis. Group therapy seems helpful in accelerating the eradication of symptoms, in recovering insight, in increasing the effect of treatment, in shortening the course of treatment, in maximizing the curative effect, and in preventing relapse.

References

Slavson, S. R. *Analytic Group Psychotherapy.* Columbia University Press, New York, 1950.
Slavson, S. R. *A Textbook in Analytic Group Psychotherapy.* International Universities Press, New York, 1964.

E.4 Group Psychotherapy in Egypt

MOHAMMED SHAALAN, M.B., B.Ch., D.P.M.

History

Egypt has been an integrated social entity for many centuries. It is truly a gift of its own geography or, as Herodotus put it, a "gift of the Nile." A constant source of water, irrigating a black fertile valley, contrasts with vast expanses of flat desert.

This insulation both preserved Egypt's unity and permitted periodic incursions from beyond. While the continuity of its pharaonic heritage persisted, it was not immune from fertilization by other cultures.

Egypt has grown into a senior member among a larger group in expanding spheres of identification: the Arabic, the Islamic, and, more recently, the Afro-Asian, the Third World, and, indeed, the international community at large.

Health Care System

To the extent that Egypt is socialistic, health care, like education, is the responsibility of the state, through the Ministries of Health and Education. Such service is available freely and randomly; understandably, this affects its quality.

Recent interest in improving public service is paralleled by an increased interest in prevention and primary care, with an attempt to evolve medical education accordingly. Thus, well-equipped, large hospitals and private offices are complemented by numerous and dispersed health units and outpatient clinics. Individuals who can afford it are thus able to obtain top-quality care, which is not completely barred from those who cannot. Physicians, while allowed to profit from tertiary and secondary care for such individuals, are under obligation to contribute to the larger group's health in the form of primary care, prevention, and education.

Psychiatry, as a recent import attendant to modern medicine, has been geared even more to the tertiary and secondary care model. Its precursor was the old British model, with a heavy leaning toward the organic, as opposed to the psychological and social orientations.

This shift is attributable partly to the demands of society for help at the primary level, and partly as a reflection of the medical profession's growing awareness of the importance of caring for the individual as a whole.

Psychotherapy

Psychotherapy in Egypt, as a specialized profession, has been associated with nonpsychiatric therapists, such as psychologists and social workers. Physicians, in an effort to assert their modern identity, tended to neglect psychotherapy.

This trend is changing as a result of psychoanalysis and associated schools, such as existential psychotherapy and, more recently, learning theory-based behavior modification.

Psychotherapy remains restricted to a class of people who are privileged both in education and economics. Those who are economically able tend to be newly rich, often uneducated, and migratory, especially to neighboring oil-rich countries; this makes for generally poor candidates for psychotherapy.

On the other hand, the increasing alienation of educated people, as well as the expanding youth sector of the population, is creating a demand for psychotherapy. There are limits beyond which drugs can no longer help people reorganize their attitudes to themselves, to others, and to life. This creates a real need in a rapidly changing society, a need which group psychotherapy may help fill.

The original appeal of group therapy was that it appealed to those who needed psychotherapy but could not afford it privately and individually. In addition, the rapid social changes in Egypt uprooted the rural population—a milieu that was group oriented—to the cities, where physical crowding, paradoxically, created a shift toward individualism. The young educated individual was yearning for a recapitulation of the group context. The group, as a therapeutic medium, filled this need. This was not the case with the semicultured newly rich, who were eager to display the power of their newly acquired wealth by emphasizing their capacity for individualism, privacy, and appropriation of services.

On the training level, group psychotherapy provided a feasible format where experiential, technical, and didactic approaches could be combined as a way of introducing psychodynamics and psychotherapy. Heretofore, psychotherapy was considered a highly developed specialty which could only be acquired abroad in special institutions. It was, moreover, very costly, requiring individual analysis of the candidate, as well as supervision for individual therapy.

On the research level, the medical practitioner, particularly the psychiatrist, was becoming aware of the role of psychosocial factors in the dynamics of illness. The psychiatrist who had familiarized himself with the groups had already equipped himself with a tool for psychosocioanthropological research as a clinician by diagnosing and seeking to solve a problem and, as a participant-observer, by being involved in the problem and its solution. In response to a large group need, society sought the assistance of psychiatrists in an effort to understand and solve the many problems of living that a rapidly changing society was facing.

Group Ambition beyond Therapy

The group psychotherapeutic approach in psychiatry was itself an expression of rapid change within psychiatry; this in turn reflected the rapid social-historical process. The polarization without would, understandably, be reflected in a polarization within.

The group psychotherapy movement gradually gave rise to two distinct trends—one addressing the medical model, the other the psychosocial, educational, and growth model.

If group psychotherapy could appeal to the psychiatrist as another tool in his therapeutic armamentarium, then it must keep its connection with the medical school. And, in time, group therapy was essentially for patients who sought treatment through a basic cause-and-effect method of healing illness and reducing suffering. Personal growth, expanded awareness, and other such positive directions were secondary byproducts, resulting from the negation of the negative, or treatment of the illness.

This was the point of view represented by Rakhawy and his associates, and was complemented by a system of thinking termed evolutionary psychiatry. The group was one aspect of the whole, albeit a prominent one; and group therapy occupied an important position in both inpatient and outpatient treatment settings, mostly private.

The pull in the other direction, which was more radical and socially oriented, was based on the philosophy that the medical model was often in danger of serving the medical profession at the expense of society. Although it was not necessary that the whole profession must abolish itself and cease to become an institution, it was imperative that socially oriented viewpoints be voiced by at least some members of the profession.

Group psychotherapy, closely mirroring social processes, could serve this end. Proceeding in this direction, toward society and away from the hospital and clinic, the appeal was to seek the positive as such and not merely as a negation of the negative—for well people to be better, for grown individuals to grow further and evolve, and for normal consciousness to expand.

This trend in group psychotherapy expressed itself in various directions. These could be defined as, first, growth and enhancement of sensitivity to others as provided in groups attended by nonpatients; second, a similar process but one geared toward facilitating human relations among managers and workers, with a view to facilitating organizational development;

and, third, education as a way of acquiring self-knowledge or insights and affective skills. The last was further expanded to allow students and young physicians to carry over their skills in group processes to the public.

Conclusion

With the vicissitudes of a rapidly changing society and the natural laboratory that such a society is, group psychotherapy in Egypt may perhaps have a role in resolving social conflicts at varying levels of magnitude.

References

Rakhawy, Y. T. *Group Therapy: An Introduction.* Dar-El-Ghad, Cairo, 1978.
Shaalan, M. Egypt. In *World Studies in Psychiatry*, G. L. Usdin, editor. Warner/Chilcot, 1979.
Shaalan, M. *Psychiatry and Group Therapy.* El-Arabi, Cairo, 1981.

E.5 Group Psychotherapy in France

CLAUDE PIGOTT, M.D.

History

France, generally considered a land of individualism, is actually a country of tight centralization and administrative uniformity; and historically, it is a country that is the consequence of a complex and, in many ways, paradoxical process.

The story of France is the story of an idea, of a symbol—the King. This kingship culminated in the 18th century, during the reign of Louis XIV, when the kingdom fell under the authority of one sovereign, the Roi Soleil, and when the restless princes were put into the golden cage of Versailles. It was during this period that France achieved a great empire with the power in the sole hands of one man, the King. Surprisingly, neither the Revolution nor the Republic changed anything about this basic structure; subjects still submit to the same laws, to the same government, and to the same central power.

Health Care System

The French health care system is in constant evolution. In 1945, a health project was put into effect; it is still working but has been modified several times, owing to the evolution of medical science and social needs. This project has instituted a medical national insurance system; the attribution of family allowances related to the number of children; the implementation of a system of compulsory medical examinations for various circumstances and at various levels of life; pregnancy testing and a series of medical tests and examinations during pregnancy and after childbirth; examinations for newborn children every month during the first year of life at a decreasing rate until the age of 6; and annual examinations of every person living in France over the age of 6.

France is divided into 20 regions, each of them comprising 4 or 5 traditional departments, which are themselves partitioned into towns, wards, and villages. This system is designed to recognize needs at different levels and to design the application of the decisions that have been faced.

The departmental level is the most important. It must cope with a wide variety of problems, from the building of a hospital to the verification of the bookkeeping of a mental health institution. It must also coordinate activity between other ministries connected with social and medical problems.

Psychiatry

In 1949, breaking with the traditional training based solely on the experience gathered in mental hospitals, a special qualification certificate of neuropsychiatry was instituted. In 1968, neurology and psychiatry were separated into two different specialties, and in 1972, a special diploma in child psychiatry was created. At the end of 1980, there were 2,246 neuropsychiatrists and 2,906 psychiatrists in France.

In the practical and organizational fields, psychiatrists operate in all the institutions where mental health is concerned as directors, consultants, or psychotherapists, provided they can prove a convenient training and that the institutions are prepared to accept it. They may also be in private practice.

Psychiatric hospitals

There are 104 state psychiatric hospitals in France—a little more than one per department. In addition, private clinics offer various financial contracts with the social security system.

Admission to psychiatric hospitals is regulated by strict rules which preserve the patient's rights. The hospital is still the center of administration, and psychiatric dispensaries, which were the first outer agencies created, remain bound to it. It also has the leading role as far as teaching is concerned, and psychiatric hospital directors are also professors in their specialty.

Various forms of psychotherapy can be found in France, ranging from the somewhat solemn individual psychanalytic setting to the nude marathon group. The predominant trend, however, is toward psychoanalysis, which itself is divided into different theories and practices, such as post-Kleinian concepts and the linguistic concepts of Jacques Lacan.

Another current is related to the traditional trend of French psychiatry, based on empathy and rational elaboration. Experimental psychology has also developed, and behavior therapy is further extending its range of action.

Group therapies

Group psychotherapy has had two illustrious predecessors in France. One is the famous Mesmer, who came from Vienna and who attracted the fancy of grand ladies and fine gentlemen of Parisian high society at the end of the 18th century by magnetizing (hypnotizing) them in group settings; the second is the Marquis de Sade, who was authorized by the director of the Charenton psychiatric hospital to organize theater plays in which mentally ill persons could act. The director very much appreciated the Marquis's initiative, and he commented in a letter that this gentleman wanted to bring "to the stage the mentally ill" and contemplated "to cure them by this type of remedy."

Indeed, this forms a surprising if not questionable inheritance. Fortunately, a century and a half has passed since these extraordinary times, and after World War II the interest in group therapy developed among more stable personalities who were eager to know what had been elaborated in the free nations of the world during the years of oppression. The inheritance was by then more substantial and came along several lines, originating in the United States and Great Britain.

French group therapists looked eagerly in the direction of British authors, such as Foulkes and Bion, in regard to the subject of early mental stages of the child. Anzieu, with his concept of group illusion, attempted to define organizers of the group unconscious. Winnicott's transitional object was translated into René Kaës's transitional analysis.

Concepts of individual therapy were recognized in group therapy as well; and the therapeutic conclusion in this direction was that the group setting is particularly efficient in dealing with the elaboration of archaic processes, such as projective identification.

Recently, the contributions of Bateson and the systemic school to the treatment of schizophrenic patients were reexamined, with notable results. It has been known for a long time that their curable liability included the care of the entire family. The illuminating of the paradoxical communication is considered here as a major contribution to family therapy, but, although many therapists apply Palo Alto's or Maria Selvini's methods, others—especially the psychoanalysts—reject the premise of the black box, preferring, instead, to explore the unconscious roots of the paradox and its appearance in the transference. This has led to the formulation of a group paradox transference by André Ruffiot.

Since 1960, the new American humanism movement has found increased expression in the use of nonverbal techniques, bioenergy, transactional analysis, and primal scream therapy, to cite a few methods.

This wide and diversified interest explains the numerous applications of group therapy in France; however, it is almost impossible to evaluate its extent. Its status is even less defined than for individual therapy, and its introduction into a therapeutic institution is dependent on such factors as whether it is accepted as a therapeutic means, the existence in the institution of trained personnel, and agreement from the paying agency, generally the social security system.

The various group therapy methods have been created in the framework of the various institutional settings. The psychiatric hospitals, for example, provide ventilation, occupation, and recreational groups. Parents of these severely ill people are grouped with the aim of disentangling complex family situations and quickly releasing the patients. Outpatients can participate in more elaborate methods, such as group analysis and psychodrama.

Regular meetings of the staff often have a therapeutic value, and, in a case of deep paralyzing tensions, a therapist from the outside may be asked to come and solve the crisis. The psychiatric dispensaries and the day and night hospitals, which are extensions of the hospital, offer the same possibilities as the outpatient services. Their particular importance is in the treatment of groups of alcoholics in cooperation with antialcoholic associations. These associations were the first in France to consider groups as having a therapeutic role, and have existed since the beginning of the century.

Another example of group therapy functioning within the framework of an institution is in prisons and institutions for delinquents, where sociodrama enables the participants to act out their problems concerning the authority figures of the prison or the institution. These groups generally concern patients with severe pathology, and require strong motivation from the therapists to continue to work.

Less burdensome, more efficient, and perhaps more interesting are groups which deal with children and adolescents. They are scattered throughout the different health regions where child guidance and medicopsychopedagogic centers have been created. Group therapy is not performed in each of them, and it is difficult to evaluate its extent, but the positive aspect is due to the fact that the children are taken care of and generally live with their families.

Psychodrama is the main therapeutic method practiced. Others have appeared lately, such as the aforementioned family therapy and child evolution groups. These groups do not use conventional role playing.

They have as their aim the analysis of what spontaneously occurs in a group of six or eight children and
the gradual elaboration of their various symptoms
and problems. This method gathers the advantages of
different methods, such as interaction and modeling,
around an understanding of psychoanalytic inspiration. It can be applied to very young children, and is
particularly beneficial for those suffering from autistic
tendencies, from predominant nonverbal communication, and from a lack of capacity to symbolize.

Adolescents may have the same treatment opportunities, but the evolution groups cannot take place
in the same setting as for children. The appropriate
treatment setting is closer to group analysis intended
for adults. Speech is the natural way to elaborate
things at these ages, whatever its level and whatever
the communication may be.

Another way of handling groups is through non-state-
sponsored practices. These generally concern adult patients.
If a therapist wants to start a group on his own, he may do
so in his consulting room or any other convenient place. He
can lead it alone or choose a colleague as co-therapist.
Several therapists can gather and create a private association
and promote various techniques. An association which is
officially registered as providing group therapy must necessarily be sponsored by a medical authority; others, which
are not therapeutic, do not need such sponsorship.

Conclusion

Group practice has a great variety of forms. Some
are stable and long-living societies; they have been
working along clear lines with recognized techniques
and have gathered consistent experience. They usually propose regular weekly sessions throughout the
year or are spaced out over weekends or entire weeks
of intensive group work. Often, techniques are combined, and group analysis, psychodrama, and relaxation therapy can alternate with an estimated optimum frequency. In various cities of the country,
workshops and seminars are organized periodically
by the local societies to make them known and to
promote group therapy.

References

Anzieu, D. *Le Psychodrame analytique chez l'enfant.* Editions Presses
    Universitarie de France, Paris, 1956.
Anzieu, D. *Le Groupe L'Inconscient.* Editions Dunod, Paris, 1975.
Decherf, G. *Oedipe en Groupe: Psychoanalyse et groupes d'enfants.*
    Editions Claneire-Guenaud, Paris, 1981.
Kaes, R. *Etude Bibliagraphique et Documentaire sur les Groupes
    Huamains (1946–1975): Evolution des recherches dans l'aire fran-
    cophone.* Universite de Provence, Provence, 1976.
Kaes, R. Introduction a l'analyse transitionnelle. In *Crise, Rupture et
    Depassement.* Editons Dunod, Paris, 1979.
Ruffiot, A. Le groupe-famille en analyse: l'apparail physicque fami-
    lia. In *La Therapie Familiale Psychanalytique.* Editions Dunod,
    Paris, 1981.

E.6   Group Psychotherapy in Germany

KARL KONIG, M.D.
REGINE TISCHTAU-SCHROTER, M.A.

History

Germany is divided into two parts: the western Federal
Republic of Germany and the eastern German Democratic
Republic. While some group psychotherapy is being done
in the eastern part of Germany, chiefly along behavioristic
lines, this chapter concentrates on the western part.

Health Services

Government insurance pays for analytically oriented group psychotherapy for most persons. Usually,
120 to 150 sessions of 100 minutes each are covered.
Group psychotherapists who want to take patients on
government insurance basis must be certified for psychotherapy or psychoanalysis.

There are numerous psychiatric state hospitals and
university clinics; universities are all run by the states

which constitute the Federal Republic of Germany.
A majority of psychoanalytically oriented hospitals
for the treatment of neurotic and psychosomatic disorders are privately owned.

University psychiatry is largely organic or descriptive. A psychodynamic orientation of psychiatry is
prevalent in a minority of university psychiatric hospitals; some university hospitals specialize in social
psychiatry, rehabilitation, and community health
care. Most state psychiatric hospitals are biologically
oriented; they also do social psychiatry, rehabilitation,
and community psychiatry in their outpatient departments.

Most psychiatrists in private practice are phenomenologically oriented; but there are also a considerable number of psychiatrists who are certified in

analytically oriented psychotherapy or in psycho-analysis.

Development of Group Psychotherapy

Persecution by the National Socialist Party brought great hardship upon psychoanalysts and their families, and prevented Freud's ideas from becoming known to the younger generation of physicians and psychologists. Thus, psychiatry was for a long time quite separate from psychoanalysis.

Apart from the Jungians—who, for a long time, remained in esoteric confinement—and the Adlerians—who, up to now, have not gained much importance—there are two large psychoanalytic societies in Germany. Germans who became interested in group psychotherapy after the war were faced with a choice; this choice was influenced by professional affiliations more than by anything else. German students of psychoanalysis, who went to Britain for didactic analysis, were very much influenced by the teaching analysts they happened to have found in London.

Theories of Group Therapy

The German analyst Argelander, himself a Freudian, acknowledged the importance of Bion's and Ezriel's concepts, but developed a theoretical model of his own which has gained considerable currency. He viewed the group as a single person with a psychic apparatus consisting of id, ego, and superego—a single person talking to the therapist. In this concept, transferences among group members which cannot be connected with the therapist are of little account. Argelander sees no difference in indications between individual and group analysis; besides being an interesting field of study to him, the group is important because it can reach more patients during a given period of the therapist's time.

Annelise Heigl-Evers' model of group psychotherapy is divided into three parts: one stresses ego functions, using an interactional approach, and addresses itself to conscious processes; one concerns subconscious and preconscious processes reflected in multiple transference; and the third is based on an analytic method encompassing unconscious fantasy directed onto the therapist or the whole group.

Konig, trained in the Gottingen school of Annelise Heigl-Evers, developed a concept of working relationships applying Greenson's idea of a working alliance to groups. This can serve as a technical guide to timing and dosage of interventions; strong working relationships may coexist with deep regression, whereas in Bion's concept of basic assumption and working groups, both appear to be mutually exclusive.

Konig has described the beginning of the group process in terms of a low level of information the group members have about each other, which makes each member see the rest of the group as a global, undifferentiated large object. Later, a higher level of information about individual members enhances the perception of them as individuals, and the perception of the group as a global object recedes into the background.

On the whole, Kleinian influence, which was once strong, has diminished during the last 10 years in Germany. Therapists are no longer exclusively concerned with the here-and-now; they pay increasing attention to how life in the therapeutic group and life outside the group interact.

On the other hand, object relations theory in concert with ego psychology as described by Kernberg is beginning to make itself felt in analytic group psychotherapy.

Ammon, an analyst and group therapist trained at the Menninger Clinic, has been active in group psychotherapy since his return from the United States; his theories pay particular attention to the group supplementing and developing ego functions for the individual patient. Although he has many followers and students in the various institutes he founded in Germany, his ideas are not discussed as much among the larger body of group psychotherapists as they would perhaps deserve from a theoretical point of view.

Other types of groups used include: behavioral group therapy, which has largely remained a domain of psychologists; Rogerian group therapy, which is also mostly done by psychologists; and encounter groups, in which there have been casualties reported. In addition, transactional analysis has been increasing during the last few years both in individual therapy and in group psychotherapy. Existential psychotherapy was very prominent after the war, when Heidegger and Jaspers were the chief figures on the philosophical scene, but has been declining in use. Psychodrama is also practiced in Germany and is derived directly from Moreno.

Conclusion

Group psychotherapy in its various forms is used in various settings—inpatient therapy, outpatient therapy, and combinations of the two. Various patient populations (heterogeneous and homogeneous groups of people with various neurotic and psychosomatic disorders) are treated. Future trends will probably be directed toward an empirical validation of theory, and toward further differentiation of therapeutic methods in order to reach patients having more severe forms of pathology.

References

Ammon, G. Ich-Entwicklung in der Gruppe. In *Analytische Gruppendynamik*, p. 53. G. Ammon, editor, Hoffmann und Campe, Hamburg, 1976.

Argelander, H. Gruppenanalyse unter Anwendung des Strukturmodells. Psyche, *22:* 1968.

Brocher, T. *Gruppendynamik und Erwachsenenbildung.* Westermann, Braunschweig, 1967.

Cohn, R. *Von der Psychoanalyse zur themenzentrierten Interaktion. Von der Behandlung einzelner zu einer Padagogik fur alle.* Klett, Stuttgart, 1975.

Ermann, M. Die themenzentrierte Interaktion (TZI) in Gruppenarbeit und Gruppenpsychotherapie. Gruppenpsychother. Gruppendynamik, *12:* 266, 1977.

Foulkes, S. H. *Introduction to Group-Analytic Psychotherapy.* William Heinemann, London, 1948.

Heigl-Evers, A. *Konzepte der analytischen Gruppenpsychotherapie,* ed. 2. Verlag für Medizinische Psychologie im Verlag Vandenhoeck und Ruprecht, Göttingen, 1978.

Heigl-Evers, A., and Heigl, F. Gruppentherapie: interaktionell-tiefenpsychologisch fundiert (analytisch orientiert)-psychoanalytisch. Gruppenpsychother. Gruppendynamik, *7:* 132, 1973.

Kernberg, O. *Object Relations Theory and Clinical Psychoanalysis.* Jason Aronson, New York, 1976.

Konig, K. Ubertragungsausloser—Ubertragung—Regressionin der analytischen Gruppe. Gruppenpsychother. Gruppendynamik, *10:* 220, 1976.

Konig, K. Le travail thérapeutique dans l'analyse de groups. Connexions, *31:* 25, 1980.

Leutz, G. A. *Psychodrama: Theorie und Praxis.* Springer, Berlin, 1974.

Kutter, P., and Roth, J. K. *Psychoanalyse in der Universitat. Psychoanalytische Selbsterfahrungs—und Supervisionsgruppen mit Studenten in Theorie und Praxis.* Kindler, Munchen, 1981.

Mahler, E. Interdependez von Klein- und Gronzgruppenprozessen aus psychoanalytischer Sicht—Am Beispiel einer Gruppenarbeit in der Lehrerausbildung. Gruppenpsychother. Gruppendynamik, *10:* 25, 1976.

Ruger, U. Indikationsmoglichkeiten fur eine stationar-ambulante Gruppenpsychotherapie. Gruppenpsychother. Gruppendynamik, *16:* 335, 1981.

Sandner, D. Theoriebildung in der Gruppenanalyse: Gegenwartiger Stand und Perspektiven. Gruppenpsychother. Gruppendynamik, *17:* 234, 1981.

E.7　Group Psychotherapy in Hungary

GABOR SZONYI, M.D.
TEODORA TOMCSANYI, Ph.D.

History

The Magyars, or Hungarians, arrived in several streams in the Carpathian Basin during the period of the Great Migration of the Peoples, and occupied their present homeland in the central part of the Basin by 896. Eventually, they gave up their nomadic style of life, adopted Christianity, and came to consolidate their rule in the Carpathian Basin.

In medieval times Hungary was a great regional power of Central and Eastern Europe, but lost her independence under the onslaught of the Turks in 1526. The country broke into three parts and remained divided for 150 years, with part conquered by the Turks and the rest dependent on the Hapsburg empire. Several wars of liberation followed, spanning several centuries.

In an environment of Indo-European peoples, largely Slavic and Germanic, the Magyars have no kin and are isolated in their language. The resulting antagonisms were often fanned by the well-known great-power policy of divide and rule.

After World War II, a close alliance was established with the Soviet Union. A radical social transformation took place. For a while, an economic and intellectual isolation restricted development in a number of fields, but since the 1960's there has been a growing openness in every area. Hungary belongs to the alliance system of the socialist countries.

Health Care System

The basic principles of Hungary's socialist health service are worked out by the Council of Ministers on the basis of the party program. With only a few exceptions, most of the health and medical institutions in the country are under the shared jurisdiction of the councils and the Ministry of Health.

In the Hungary of today, every citizen has the right to free medical and health service, including free hospitalization.

The system is organized according to regional principles. A physician or a panel of medical doctors is responsible for the care of the local population in any given area. Although this practice ensures adequate care, it limits the free choice of physicians. With 24.6 physicians for each 10,000 of the population, the physician-resident ratio is good in Hungary by international comparison.

Psychiatry

Psychiatry has always occupied a marginal position within the health facilities as a whole, and its development has always been much slower in comparison with other medical specialties. The first private mental institution was established by Jozef Polya in 1841 and was then followed by a succession of similar institutions. Later on, however, the organizational pattern favored government psychiatric departments, rather than independent institutions. These were ill-equipped, however—the general attitude was that funds would be more usefully spent on the other departments in a given hospital.

An organic neurological approach has dominated psychiatric practice in diagnostics and in choice of treatment, in the organization and operation of hospital departments, and in the development of outpatient services. A psychiatric care system did take shape eventually, but it has not yet gone further than offering traditional types of psychiatric treatment for mental patients.

Provisions for neurotic cases are still virtually nonexistent, and an effective psychotherapy network functions only for children. There are about 1,180 psychiatrists for the 10,688,000 people of Hungary. In the outpatient services, one psychiatrist is in charge of a district of about 90,000 people.

The rapidly changing needs in psychiatry and the growing access to models of foreign development in the field have led to the accelerated development of interdisciplinary psychotherapy. This has modified psychiatric approaches and created a number of new treatment forms, such as therapeutic communities. Greater professional and organizational independence of psychiatry has resulted, and the formation of the independent Hungarian Psychiatric Society in 1980 was a milestone in this direction.

Psychotherapy

In the first decades of the century, psychoanalysis had a striking impact. The Association of Hungarian Psychoanalysis was formed in 1913. Sandor Ferenczi was appointed in 1919 as professor to head the world's first university department of psychoanalysis. In addition to Freudian orientation, the influence of Alfred Adler was also significant.

Under the influence of developmental psychology, an increasing number of psychologists became active in educational institutions, where they also did therapeutic work. The development of psychology in the 1930's contributed to the development of psychotherapy. However, by the end of the 1940's, the Hungarian Psychological Society and the training of psychologists were discontinued. The training of psychologists was resumed at the University of Budapest in 1962. The interval had been too long; psychotherapy in Hungary had a long way to go to catch up with international developments in the field.

There is still no institutional training of psychotherapists, and no special examination in the field. Training, which took place earlier only through informal channels according to the standards of the International Psychoanalytical Association, has been gradually assumed by the Psychotherapy Section of the Society of Hungarian Psychiatrists. Additionally, there are work groups specializing in psychoanalytic therapy, behavior therapy, family therapy, group therapy, individual psychotherapy, child psychotherapy, hypnosis, and relaxation approaches.

Group therapy

Starting in the late 1950's, group psychotherapy developed along several pathways in Hungary. The first trend relied on the traditions of individual therapy and the influence of psychoanalysis. The second line of approach was based on experimentation with new approaches, such as group therapy, that might hold some promise of therapeutic results. The third orientation resulted from occupational and work therapy to humanize the treatment of mental patients. The fourth pathway was that of social psychology.

At the start, psychotherapy was ideologically unaccepted, a discipline regarded with suspicion and subject to attacks. Group psychotherapy also had to pass through a phase in which it had to demonstrate the reason for its existence and its validity.

Beginning in 1970, the practice of group psychotherapy underwent extensive development, and became an accepted practice in hospitals. Physicians leading departments of psychiatry were no longer averse to group psychotherapy. In addition, training groups were started for psychologists and psychiatrists. Between 1975 and 1981, more publications appeared on group psychotherapy than in the prior 20 years.

In recent years, group psychotherapy has clearly been more accepted. The method has also gained ground in other branches of medicine.

Various group methods are used, including analytic, psychodrama, autogenic training, group hypnosis, transactional therapy, behavioral therapy, and movement therapy. Other groups are composed of special groups of patients, such as managers retired early because of disability, parents of mentally handicapped children, alcoholics, and postsuicidal patients.

The most urgent problem for group psychotherapy is the lack of channels for the training of psychotherapists. The group plays an important role in methodological and theoretical training of therapists. It provides many students part of their essential personal experience, which includes participation in a group and theoretical studies and supervision. Participation in a group also provides a chance for direct observation as a participant, and for functioning as a co-therapist. The Hungarian Psychiatric Society also organizes seminars for therapists.

Some private training has always been available, chiefly in Freudian psychoanalysis but also in Jungian analysis and in hypnosis. These models were also followed by the training groups started in the 1960's, in which both physicians and psychologists participated.

Further, a unique educational experience is gained from psychotherapeutic weekends, an experimental program started in 1975, which consists of two or three weekends a year, each of them in a different town, attended by groups of physicians, nurses, psychologists, and university students from all parts of the country. During the weekends small and large groups meet and can be seen in action almost nonstop for 48 hours. At the end there is an evaluative discussion.

Despite some similarities and shared problems in neighboring socialist countries, the development of group psychotherapy has taken different paths. To increase professional contact between the different countries, the Psychotherapeutic Work-Group of the Socialist Countries was formed in 1973 to exchange experiences.

References

Boszorményi, Z., editor. *Az Orszagos Ideg- és Elmegyógyintézet (100 Years of the National Neurological Clinic and Psychiatric Hospital).* Budapest, 1968.

Fulop, T. *Social Medicine (Egeszsegugyi Szervezestan)*. Medicina, Budapest, 1973.

Hock, K., editor. *Psychotherapie and Gesellschaft*. Seidel, Berlin, 1976.

Ministry of Health. *Guidelines on the Development of the Mental Health Service*. Ministry of Health, Budapest, 1969.

Paal, J. Psychoanalyse in Osteuropa. In *Die Psychologie des 20 Jahrhunderts*, A. Heigl Evers, editor. Kindler, Zurich, 1979.

Pataki, F. Some timely lessons from the history of Hungarian psychology. In *Institute of Psychology of the Hungarian Academy of Sciences 75 Years Old (75 eves az MTA Pszichologiai Intezete)*, I. Dance, editor. Budapest, 1978.

E.8 Group Psychotherapy in India

A. VENKOBA RAO, M.D., Ph.D., D.P.M., F.R.C. Psych.

History

India—comprising 31 states with 684 million people (1981 census), speaking 15 major languages and hundreds of dialects—is a land of paradox in which opposites exist side by side. The average Indian simultaneously practices the doctrines of modernism and primitivism, reflecting both the strength and the weakness of the country.

Psychiatry

Mental illness in India is estimated to affect some two to seven persons per 1,000 population. There are 38 mental hospitals in the country, two of which (National Institute of Mental Health and Neuro-Sciences at Bangalore and the Central Institute of Psychiatry at Ranchi) are managed by the government of India. Four others are managed by private agencies, and the remainder by the individual state governments. Psychiatric services are poor in the country. Many of the hospitals continue to be understaffed and are primarily custodial, although a few have begun to modernize their services. There are about 20,000 total beds in these hospitals.

Although voluntary entry for treatment is encouraged, admission into state mental hospitals is regulated by the Indian Lunacy Act of 1912, which is fashioned after the British Lunacy Act of 1890. A new mental health bill, incorporating progressive measures, is now before the Indian Parliament for enactment.

In the late 1950's, general hospital psychiatry emerged as a growing force in India. Today, Indian psychiatrists are being trained in ever-increasing numbers. There are more than a score of centers for training postgraduates in psychiatry. Many contemporary psychiatrists have trained either in the Western nations or in Indian centers under Western-trained Indian teachers. The advent of new training centers will allow psychiatric care to be offered that conforms to the needs of the country.

The traditional extended-family system is being replaced by the nuclear family as the prevailing way of life. India is thus presently in a period of transition, with the attendant loss of the benefits of extended-family living and the inability to manage living as a nuclear family. However, the dynamics of extended-family life continue to work in the nuclear-family system. Family participation in the care of the sick, both physically and mentally ill, is still possible to some extent. This is a great asset and carries potential for fostering community services. Family involvement in the care of patients in mental institutions was pioneered by the late Vidyasagar, and is now practiced in many other centers. Most of the mental hospitals and the psychiatry departments in general hospitals have adopted a revolving-door policy; patients stay for only a brief period during acute stages of their illness, but are readmitted when they relapse, and this relieves the family's burden.

Therapeutic outcome is believed to depend in large part on social care and drug dosage, the two being inversely related. For example, it has been observed that family care contributes to a favorable prognosis in schizophrenia, and this may also be the reason for the lower dose requirements that have been noted for psychotropic drugs, such as the phenothiazines and lithium.

It is a strange but accepted fact that certain ancient methods and modern therapeutic ways exist side by side when it comes to the care of the mentally ill. Many patients visit well-known shrines, and some practice rigorous austerities in the temples for specified periods. Divine command in dreams is awaited. Shamans have a large clientele. Offerings are made to the deities, and talismans and amulets are worn by the sick even today. Certain barbaric treatments, such as branding and the use of bodily restraints, are still practiced in the villages. Many patients resort to these measures before seeking psychiatric consultation.

Syphilitic infection of the central nervous system continues to be encountered, although in less magnitude than 25 years ago. Addiction to various drugs and alcohol is common, according to individual reports; however, according to a recent report from the National Committee on Drug Addiction, dependency on drugs is not currently a major issue, although it has the potential to become one. The government of India has adopted a policy of total prohibition of the use of drugs, and this has been implemented in many states. The cultivation of cannabis is forbidden, and during the next 2 decades the indigenous cannabis will not be available for use.

India is the home of yoga, but little scientific work has been published on application of the Patanjali's yogic principle to the prevention and treatment of disease. Several centers in India have recently initiated research programs into this ancient technique for health and personality development. Advocates of yoga believe that, for meditation to be effective, it must be repeated regularly because its benefits are short lived. Emphasis is on the spiritual and ethical aspects of the practice. It is to be viewed as a total way of life, rather than an intermittent and whimsical exercise.

There has been a tremendous increase in the use of psychotropic drugs in India by psychiatrists, as well as by other specialists and by general practitioners. This has contributed in no small measure to the success of general hospital psychiatry.

Psychotherapy

During the last 3 decades, Indian psychiatrists have expressed concern over the suitability of Western psychotherapy for Indian patients. This has inevitably led to publications on the ingredients of a psychotherapeutic system which would be appropriate for the Indian culture.

Surya and Jayaram drew attention to the basic considerations for the practice of psychotherapy in an Indian setting. They emphasized language, expectations of the average Indian patient, and conceptual references which are based on India's culture and philosophy. These authors stress the need to understand the religion and faith of patients. They feel that the Western concept of ideal mental health involves a search for intrapsychic integration, which is at variance with Indian concepts, because it fails to take into account faith and religion. Without sufficient attention to these areas, psychotherapy, according to these authors, is not likely to be effective.

India offers a rich field for the development of a relevant and culturally congruous psychotherapeutic system from its own philosophies, folklore, and systems of medicine. There are many psychiatrists who have made serious attempts to use this valuable material for psychotherapeutic purposes. There are others who have commented extensively on the psychotherapeutic principles enunciated in the Bhagavad Gita. Venkoba Rao and Parvathi Devi (1974) have drawn attention to the concepts of total surrender, eagerness of the pupil for enlightenment, liberty to interrogate intelligently, desire for knowledge, and, finally, absence of coercion on the part of the counselor. These concepts from Gita are taken as a paradigm for the psychotherapeutic system practiced by Venkoba Rao and Vidyasagar, as well as others. Gita exemplifies the Guru-chela relationship or the traditional relationship between the teacher and disciple.

Group psychotherapy

The practice of group psychotherapy is not very much in evidence in India, as the paucity of publications on the subject indicates. Nevertheless, group organizations and group discussions are arranged in mental hospitals, psychiatric departments of general hospitals, educational institutions, industries, and prisons. The same is true among the religious groups and in the monasteries. There appears to be a fundamental conflict between the principles of conventional group therapy and the principles of the primary unit of living in India—namely, the family. The family in India is arranged anatomically and functionally in a hierarchy, with the head of the family at the top. From him are derived the support, the authority, and the decision making. Many of the members in the family unit turn to him for guidance and for their educational, marital, and occupational choices. The head is the repository of the total family responsibility. It is evident from this that the constituents of the family owe their allegiance to one individual and await guidance from him, without too much of a mutual exchange of ideas between themselves or assuming of individual responsibility.

Adherence to tradition is strong. The crust of custom resists easy cracking. Such a system is at variance with classical group setting, where the group leader enables the members to learn to take responsibility and allows them to develop individuality, while minimally exercising his own authoritarian role.

Although groups exist in India in different walks of life, the relation between group leader and the members is one of Guru-chela type. Members prefer to be led en masse, rather than deciding between themselves and relying little on the leader. The father figure (or God figure) dominates in all the group settings. This pattern of Guru-chela relationship is the cornerstone of individual psychotherapy, which continues to operate in the context of the group. The classical model of individual psychotherapy, enunciating the concept of total surrender on the part of individual to the teacher, is exemplified in Gita. Similarly, in the ancient Indian philosophical treatises, like Vedas and Upanishads, dyadic relationship between the teacher and the pupil stands out, although several disciples assemble around him. For example, the word "Upanishad" means sitting near the master for transmission of secret knowledge.

In the Indian psychophilosophical system, emphasis is laid on the understanding of the self by techniques of introspection and meditation. This discovery of self needs a teacher. The need for group is rarely stressed. It is natural that this dyadic relationship persists in the group also. Members of the group are collectively attached to the leader, but, between themselves, the cohesion may not be strong and durable. There is a superficial gregariousness, but at deeper levels there is social isolation. This is the significant feature of both the group organization and group therapy in the Indian context, where the leader is looked upon as a source of inspiration, endowed with authority and omnipotence. This type of functioning runs through a spectrum of groups—through the family, through educational areas and psychiatric hospitals, and to the political organizations. This feature considerably hampers the development of a therapeutic community in psychiatric settings. In mental hospitals, groups are organized for schizophrenic and neurotic patients, for the aged, and for drug dependents; recreational, occupational, or industrial therapy units are available in many centers. Day hospitals function in several places. In Indian settings, female patients usually do not mix freely with male patients, and hence groups are arranged for them separately. There are also Alcoholics Anonymous organizations in major cities like Delhi, Bombay, and Madras.

The features of joint or extended-family living modify rehabilitation programs for the mentally handicapped. Hence, the ideal of rendering a patient self-reliant, responsible, and gainfully employed is never realized, but is replaced by attempting reintegration of the individual into the family.

References

Bose, G. The concept of repression. Doctoral dissertation, Calcutta University, 1921.

Hoch, E. M. Psychotherapy in India. In *Indo-Asian Culture 12.* Indian Council for Cultural Relations, New Delhi, 1963.

Neki, J. S. *Psychotherapy in India.* Presidential address, Calcutta, 1977.

Saytanand, D. *Dynamic Psychology of the Gita of Hinduism.* I.B.H., New Delhi, 1972.

Venkoba Rao, A., and Parvathi Devi, S. Body and mind in the Bhagavad Gita. In *The Science of Medicine and Physiological Concepts in Ancient and Medieval India,* N. H. Keswani, editor, p. 2. 1974.

Vidyasagar. Challenge of our times. Ind. J. Psychiatry, *15:* 95, 1973.

E.9 Group Psychotherapy in Israel

ATARA KAPLAN DE-NOUR, M.D.
J. P. BROWN, M.B., M.R.C. Psych.

History

Israel is one of the most ancient and yet most modern countries in the world. Its history is divided into three periods: ancient statehood, the diaspora, and modern Israel.

Ancient Israel, commencing in the 14th century B.C. with the conquest of Canaan by the 12 tribes and continuing up to 70 A.D. with the destruction of the second temple, was characterized by many internal struggles, with only a brief united kingdom around 1000 B.C. (population 2 million), and by repeated invasions. These invasions led to the destruction of the first temple by the Babylonians (586 B.C.) and subsequent exile, with only a minority remaining in the Holy Land to represent the spiritual, cultural, and material center of the Jewish people. At the time of the conquest by the Romans, it is estimated that 2.5 million of the more than 8 million Jews lived in Israel without statehood. This disproportion of Jews in the diaspora continued from 70 A.D. until the 19th and 20th centuries. Initially, the Jews of the dispersion were located in the Mediterranean region, and, by the time of the Crusaders, the majority lived in countries under Moslem rule. Subsequently, Jewish communities extended to central and Eastern Europe and beyond. Throughout these many centuries of exile, there were repeated movements to return to Israel or, more precisely, to Zion (Jeru-

salem). Toward the end of the 19th century, what had largely been an emotional and traditional national trend merged with a rational and intellectual one to give birth to Zionism, a movement committed to the cultural Hebraic renaissance and to the gradual building up of Jewish settlements in Palestine, while continuing to work toward the establishment of a Jewish state.

A century ago the Jewish nation was about 7.7 million, and the Jewish population of Palestine was 25,000. At the outbreak of World War II, the respective numbers were 16.6 million and 400,000. The state of Israel was established in 1948 with a Jewish population of about 600,000. At that time, the total world Jewish population was about 11.5 million. Thirty years later the Jewish population of Israel was more than 3 million, about half of them born outside Israel. The impact of massive immigration has been even more pronounced on the adult population, i.e., only 5 per cent of the adult population are second generation or more Israeli born, and 30 per cent are Israeli-born first generation, half of them of Asian-African origin and the other half of European-American origin. The rest, about 65 per cent of the adult population, are immigrants, many of them refugees of persecution, i.e., survivors of the Holocaust in Europe and refugees from the Moslem countries. Thus, the recent history of Israel is characterized by newly gained independence, mass migration, clash of cultures, and repeated wars.

Health Care System

The local medical association had already been established in 1912, but, up to the establishment of the state, practically all physicians were immigrants who had grown up and received their medical education in the many different countries of the diaspora. Even today, with the four state medical schools, the local graduates comprise less than a third of the total of about 7,500 practicing physicians.

In the prestatehood period, the following two organizations supplied most of the medical services to the Jewish population: The Sick Fund of the Labor Federation (to which the members paid nominal membership fees) and the American Hadassah Women's Zionist Organization. These two organizations built clinics and hospitals and provided outpatient treatment and hospitalization, child health care, and school health services.

The establishment of the state, with its ensuing huge wave of immigration, demanded a fast expansion of the health care services. Several hospitals and outpatient clinics were founded by the newly established Ministry of Health, while the Hadassah Medical Organization gradually withdrew from the national services and concentrated on founding, together with the Hebrew University of Jerusalem, the country's first university hospital and medical school.

At the present, almost every citizen has medical insurance with one of the sick funds (that of the Labor Federation having remained by far the biggest, and the only one to have its own hospitals). Thus, most of the population has ready access to medical care in outpatient clinics and in hospitals.

Group Therapy

The development of group psychotherapy in Israel must be considered in its social and cultural context. Fundamental to the Israeli way of life has been the difficulty in integrating occidental with oriental mentalities and behaviors. Cross-cultural themes show in the form and intensity of mental illness, the degree of tolerance toward frustration and trauma, and the differing abilities for patients to understand explanations and interpretations. In addition to immigration, economic stress, political insecurity, and the ever-present military alert complicate treatment and rehabilitation. Despite the fact that most Israelis grow up in groups (the Kibbutz is the prototype), action and rational thought have prevailed over emotional expression and motivation, and the strong pressure to conform, particularly to aggressive and authoritarian norms, has had particularly restrictive consequences for coping with the ubiquitous stresses of trauma and loss. Furthermore, Israeli attitudes regarding mental illness have been ambivalent, and the authority of the rabbinate, state, and military have reinforced values often incompatible with group psychotherapeutic attempts to foster both initiative and cooperation.

Additionally, restrictions from within the mental health field itself have come from traditional adherence to individ-

ual case study approaches, within the context of a vertical hierarchy of professional activity. Lack of training opportunities has left group therapy in the hands of a well-educated, generally occidental professional elite. Nevertheless, all methods of group psychotherapy have been used. The principal areas of both clinical and nonclinical application of group work have been in acute adaptational problems, and in crisis intervention with soldiers, parents, teachers, and mental patients and in facilitating social contact and aiding in rehabilitation with adolescents, soldiers, and patients with heart disease. Thus, group psychotherapy has been applied to survival and to maintaining active social functioning in the face of many national problems.

Resocialization of withdrawn psychiatric inpatients has been attempted, using a combination of music, art, and subsequent group discussion. Weekly group meetings for schizophrenic patients and their families were instigated. The therapeutic aim was to shift conflict out of the intrapsychic world of the patient and back into the interpersonal domain. A therapeutic community ward for adolescents was run where milieu activity, particularly large groups, was able to meet both transference and reality-based needs. Over a period of time, adolescents were reabsorbed into society. In a day hospital in Ramat Chen, intensive existential individual and group psychotherapy was used to provide a halfway-in psychiatric service for schizophrenics and the chronic mentally ill. The treatment goal was patient self-realization, achieved by accepting anxiety and suffering as universal and by integrating illness into their lives. Working with difficult psychiatric outpatients in traditional group psychotherapy stressed the importance of overcoming resistance to behavior change, as well as the better-known resistance to insight. Group analytic psychotherapy has been developed for specific categories of psychiatric patients.

Summit, a charity-based organization, runs several therapeutic community units for adolescents and young adults suffering from mental illness and minimal brain damage. Their milieu and rehabilitation programs use small and large group methods extensively, with a predominantly psychoanalytic orientation. Clinics for drug and alcohol abuse similarly use group methods (in up to 30 per cent of patients), although the individualized approach is primary.

Within military psychiatry, a traditional neuropsychiatric approach (hypnosis plus psychopharmacology) with a psychosocial treatment basis (group psychotherapy) is used for the assessment and treatment of soldiers with combat reactions. Group treatment of the soldier in his combat unit demonstrated more rapid and complete rehabilitation.

Group psychotherapy has also found diverse application in the medical world, particularly in education, prevention, and rehabilitation. Health education was supplemented by small group discussion meetings with mothers and their newborn babies. By focusing on new parental roles and relationships, these mothers were spared the need for routine medical consultations during the puerperium, when compared with nongroup attenders. Group psychotherapy and graded exercises for patients suffering acute myocardial infarct trauma led to fewer emergency room consultations and inpatient admissions, as the quality of life improved for both patients and their spouses. Large group meetings in a chronic-stay hospital (mostly patients suffering from strokes and over 70 years) helped with patient assessment, stimulation, socialization, and rehabilitation.

Training in group psychotherapy has been a haphazard affair. In 1958, at a time of rapid development of psychiatric services, an in-service training program in group psychotherapy in a psychiatric hospital was successfully established. Over a period of 2 years, participants formed analytic small groups and attended weekly supervision and theoretical seminars. Core members of the program also attended their own weekly psychotherapy group.

Another effort to introduce some order in the chaos of group psychotherapy was the establishment of the Israel Association for the Advancement of Group Psychotherapy in the late 1950's. This association, which opened its doors to all professionals in the behavioral sciences, required a certain number of hours of participation in group psychotherapy. The association was quite active, organized a few workshops a year, and had a membership of a few hundred.

The Association for Analytic Group Psychotherapy was also established, but this group has greatly restricted its membership (presently under 30) and requires previous group analysis. During the late 1970's, a fruitful training connection was established in Shalvata Hospital with visiting group analysts from the United Kingdom.

More recent developments have taken place in the universities, where training in group psychotherapy is now on the curriculum. A training program in child psychotherapy for clinical psychology students has been established in Tel-Aviv University. This extended traditional lecture, seminar, and small-group methods for instruction, employs a body awareness and movement group to facilitate the integration of traditional skills and knowledge into the primarily nonverbal therapeutic encounter with the child.

For several years at the Hebrew University of Jerusalem, experiential (particularly gestalt) groups have been a part of clinical psychology training. In Beersheva University, the Department of Behavioral Science has been involved in applying psychodrama to teaching and research into mass group activity, and in developing the field of family therapy. Recently, an official 2-year program for group psychotherapy was opened at the School of Social Work at Tel-Aviv University. The prerequisites for this course include an academic degree (in social work, psychology, or psychiatry), previous exposure to group dynamics, and at least 2 years experience in social treatment. This course includes didactic teaching, participation in group dynamics, and moderating groups under supervision.

The Association of Clinical Psychologists, in conjunction with the Ministry of Health, recently ran training workshops in group psychotherapy, including existential, dynamic-analytic, Rogerain, and gestalt orientations. Several private institutions, such as the Adler Institute, provide training in group psychotherapy. A group of psychodramatists regularly meets for mutual supervision, research, and occasional training workshops. In-service group therapy training for psychiatric residents has been provided recently in most areas. Programs included experiential (T-group), supervision with role playing, and semididactic approaches.

The major part of group psychotherapy is done in private practice, either organized in private institutes—such as the Adler Institute—or by private practitioners. Most of the group work is done by social workers and psychologists, and only a small part is done by psychiatrists. This also holds true for public clinics.

References

Chazan, R. A group family therapy approach to schizophrenia. Isr. Ann. Psychiatry, *12:* 177, 1974.

Davidson, S., and Behr, H. Group analysis: An Israeli experience. Group Anal., *13:* 121, 1980.

Erlich, H. S. Growth opportunities in the hospital: Intensive inpatient psychotherapy of adolescents. Isr. Ann. Psychiatry, *14:* 173, 1976.

Kugelmass, S., and Schossberger, J. Problems in initial training for group psychology in Israel. Int. J. Group Psychother., *8:* 179, 1958.

Neumann, M., and Gaoni, B. Types of patients especially suitable for analytically oriented group psychotherapy: Some clinical examples. Isr. Ann. Psychiatry, *12:* 203, 1974.

Springmann, R. R. Psychotherapy in the large group. In *The Large Group Dynamics and Theory*, L. Kreeger, editor, p. 216. Constable: London, 1975.

E.10 Group Psychotherapy in Norway

JARL JORSTAD, M.D.
SIGMUND KARTERUD, M.D.

History

Norway comprises the fifth largest land area in Europe, but the population density is the lowest except for that of Iceland. Of the 4 million inhabitants, half a million live in the capital, Oslo, and another 1 million in the Oslo region. The population and the society are unusually homogeneous; indeed, except for the Laps in the North of Norway, the minority ethnic groups (due to recent immigration) are small.

Since World War II, Norway has oriented itself strongly toward the West, specifically toward the United States. It occupies a stable position within the North Atlantic Treaty Organization. Economic conditions were favorable even before the large oil reservoirs in the North Sea were discovered in the 1960's, and today Norway is one of the richest countries in the world.

The social-political field is characterized by strong values of egalitarianism and unity. The conditions of life with respect to housing, the health care system, educational facilities, available food and goods, and leisure opportunities should be the same everywhere and for everybody, regardless of geographic position and social class. In order to realize these values, a strong state administration is necessary to cope with the task of transferring resources from productive agricultural, industrial, and cultural areas to the poorer regions.

In Norway, almost everything is modified into one main stream: There is one labor union organization, one state church, one broadcasting organization, one medical organization, one psychoanalytic organization, and one academic professional organization. The income tax policy, which limits high income benefits, causes most foreigners to experience Norway as one of the most socialistic or most welfare democratic societies in the world. This implies a well-developed capacity for overcoming individualistic strivings and for resolving social contradictions in groups and between groups.

Health Care System

Membership in the National Health Insurance System is compulsory for all residents of Norway. Members and their families receive free medical care in all hospitals, compensation for most doctors' fees, and almost free medication for certain chronic illnesses. Furthermore, wage earners are included in a system giving cash benefits during illness and pregnancy. Insurance premiums are paid by the insured persons; in addition, contributions are made by employers, the municipalities, and the state. The national insurance system also covers allowances for old-age pensioners, children under 16 years of age, single parents, surviving spouses, and disabled and unemployed people.

The government health services are administrated by the Health Directorate, a division of the Ministry of Health and Social Affairs, presided over by the Director of Health. The Health Directorate has numerous subsections and also acts as supervising authority for medical personnel, dentists, and pharmacists and for the building of new hospitals and other health institutions. This central health administration has local representatives: the County Health Officer (Fylkeslege) and the County Mental Health Officer (Fylkespsykiater). Every municipality or city has a local Health Officer or District Medical Officer (Distrikslege, Stadslege) who also engages in private practice. Each of these District Medical Officers is chairman in the local municipal Board of Health. Norway has about 8,400 licensed physicians, or one doctor per 476 inhabitants. Further, the number of general practitioners is declining, and the number of specialists is increasing.

Almost all Norwegian physicians are members of the Norwegian Medical Association, and within this organization every specialty has its own subdivision. The Norwegian Psychiatric Association refers to one of the largest of these specialty groups, with 450 members and with several subcommittees, the most important being the sections for psychotherapy and for postgraduate training programs. The Norwegian Psychiatric Association has been very advanced and has done pioneer work in Scandinavia.

Psychiatry

Until World War II, Norwegian psychiatry was mostly German dominated and Kraepelinian, engaged in descriptive elaborations and diagnostic work. The influence of psychoanalysis was more evident in the public debate and literature of the 1930's than in psychiatry. Nearly all the psychiatrists were working in mental hospitals or inpatient clinics; very few worked in private practice.

After the war, the picture changed rapidly. The German trend in psychiatry decreased, and influences from the United States and England had greater impact on theory and practice. From the late 1950's, this development was characterized by an increased integration of psychodynamic and social psychiatric teaching. Three trends emerged: (1) More individual psychodynamic psychotherapy was introduced and was practiced mostly within institutions by doctors and psychologists. This was mostly a consequence of the geography of the country and the lack of specialists in private practice; (2) Milieu therapy and the therapeutic community model were introduced and established all over the country; this changed most psychiatric institutions. The larger psychiatric hospitals were decentralized, and the wards became more independent; and (3) Community psychiatry promoted a transfer of interest and resources from institutional to outpatient work. Consequently, aftercare homes, rehabilitation programs for long-term patients, day centers, and sheltered workshops were enlarged, particularly in Oslo.

The contemporary psychiatry health care system in Norway is now sectorized in catchment areas. In Oslo, 10 outpatient clinics are set up.

Over the last 10 years, the psychiatric hospitals have used a decreasing number of beds, and the length of stay has been markedly shortened. However, this process has been hallmarked by serious problems, such as a lack of enthusiasm and a declining recruitment of nurses and doctors.

The sectorization has caused dramatic changes, such as increasing number of emergency admittances, and shortened the length of the average hospital stay. This development represents a challenge to psychiatric hospital treatment, particularly to the adaptation and further development of the therapeutic community model.

After World War II, the psychoanalytic group in Oslo was not very advanced. The consequent slow pace of development was due to trained analysts. The first analysts were trained at the Berlin Institute. An increasing number of psychiatrists and psychologists desired training in psychoanalysis, and in 1967 the Norwegian Psychoanalytic Institute was founded. Today, there are 40 fully trained psychoanalysts and the same number of candidates-in-training. A holistic Norwegian Institute for psychotherapy was founded in 1963, and since 1968, it has also offered more advanced training in psychotherapy.

Within the Norwegian Psychiatric Association, a keen interest among young psychiatric residents and psychiatrists succeeded in integrating more psychodynamic psychotherapy and supervision in general psychiatry. The formal curriculum for the contemporary Norwegian psychiatry resident has a basic psychodynamic orientation; every psychiatric teaching institution must have one accepted supervisor on the staff or a part-time consultant and must offer at least one weekly supervisory hour individually for every psychiatric resident.

For psychologists, psychodynamic psychotherapy has had to compete with behavior therapy and other theoretical orientations, and the scene seems more complex. Some of the specialists in clinical psychology have been licensed by the health authorities, which guarantees (with certain limitations) that the psychotherapy fees are paid for by the general insurance system. Therefore, an increasing number of psychologists have started private practice.

Group Psychotherapy

In patient group therapy was introduced to Norwegian psychiatric institutions in 1954, when several influential psychiatrists returned from studies in England, Germany, and the United States. As a result, there evolved two different modes of working with groups in institutions.

The British-oriented psychiatrists (Dahl, Froshaug, and Thomstad) were eager to integrate group treatment into the over-all organization of the therapeutic community. The group became a fundamental organizational principle for the community and represented the primary place of belonging and identity for the patients. In this context, group therapy was not a special treatment modality with its own indications and contraindications; rather, every patient became a member of the group from the very day he or she entered the community.

The German-influenced psychiatrists (Astrup, Retterstol, Ugelstad, and Alnaes) hesitated to abolish the medical model as an organizational principle of psychiatric hospital treatment and introduced, according to this basic view, group therapy as an addition to the total therapeutic armamentarium. Patients presumed suitable for this mode of therapy were selected for specially designed closed or slow-open groups. These different organizational principles converged in the early 1970's, when the therapeutic community model was at the height of its vitality. The milieu therapy groups then dominated the field. In addition to the different tasks and activities of the groups—such as group planning, group occupational work, and food preparation—the groups met three to five times a week for an unstructured group session lasting 1 hour. Usually, there was no selection of patients in the groups. People in acute psychotic states were sheltered but usually became full participants within a week after admission to the ward. The groups were open ended, with a turnover of approximately one member a week. The size was larger than the classical small group, varying from 10 to 15 members. The leadership was most often shared among the two to five staff members, the one resident, and the two to four milieu therapists. Indeed, the primary task of these groups was poorly defined; they were said to be an integral part of the over-all milieu therapy. This implies that the ideal focus would be the here-and-now events on the ward. In spite of the widespread use of groups like these, however, the principles governing the aim, structure, management, and therapeutic technique were scarcely stated in the literature.

These groups contributed to a rapid country-wide acceptance of the importance of interpersonal relations in psychiatry, and counteracted the authoritarian and custodial medical model. Under favorable circumstances, the groups could develop a culture which represented a warm and tolerant place for new patients, which secured possibilities for social and interpersonal learning and which stimulated the capacities in each patient for mutual support and care. Several follow-up studies show that patients themselves emphasize this last point very strongly in their recovery process.

In spite of the enormous popularity of the milieu therapeutic way of thinking, some institutions continued with closed small groups, where patients were selected according to vulnerability, capacity for insight, and interpersonal learning. These institutions experimented with the length of the therapeutic contract, the firmness of the group boundaries, and the composition according to symptoms, age, and common focal conflicts. A cross-sectional therapist system was adopted: the group therapist should not have individual therapeutic responsibility for any patient in the group.

One serious drawback concerning the development of group therapy in Norway is the lack of formal training and education. No institute or organization for group therapy is in existence; indeed, only a handful of Norwegian psychotherapists have completed formal group therapy training abroad. This means that training and supervision must rely on local initiatives at the different institutions. A few places have organized in-service training programs, but most of the institutions ignore this basic need. On the other hand, there is a well-organized supervisory system for individual psychotherapy. The result is inevitably a tendency toward psychotherapy in the group, rather than psychotherapy through the group.

The use of additional expressive group therapies within institutions—such as psychodrama, gestalt, encounter, dance, and music groups—varies widely in place and time. As in other countries, the treatment units for young people and drug addicts have developed confrontational and expressive group therapies.

Outpatient group therapy

Outpatient group therapy plays a significant but nevertheless limited role in the over-all treatment system. Social workers, milieu therapists, and psychologists dominate this field. After care units and outpatient clinics run supportive and activity-based groups for less resourceful and isolated patients. Within the health care system for alcoholics, which is organized separately from the psychiatric health care system, there are a variety of groups—confrontational and social learning groups influenced by behavioral therapy, self-help groups, and alcoholics anonymous groups, to name a few.

Outpatient psychotherapeutic groups are quite rare, however. A few established psychiatrists and psychologists in family therapy agencies, child guidance clinics, and outpatient clinics run marital and parental groups, child groups, and occasionally some gestalt-oriented groups. This limited group psychotherapy activity is due in part to a lack of experienced and confident group therapists, and to the absence of a formal training and educational institute.

Self-experience groups

Self-experience groups, which focus on both personal growth and professional training, represent a field of group therapy which is diffuse and difficult to define. A one-half-year self-experience training course for students of psychology exists only in one of the four universities of Norway. The most widely used group modality for persons in human relations occupations is probably gestalt-oriented groups; no training institute exists in this domain either. Visiting foreigners, mostly American gestalt therapists, have provided inspiration and guidance. There are, however, local training groups, mostly consisting of psychologists, in some areas of the country.

Since Wilhelm Reich lived in Norway for some years, an established individual characterological vegetotherapy tradition exists. In recent years, this has mingled with bioener-getics, gestalt, and rebirthing, resulting in a highly expressive group modality. Like the other new group therapies, this mode is difficult to evaluate, since it is not presented in the literature. The lack of scientific investigations holds true, however, for almost all group therapy in Norway.

T-groups

T-group activity in the industrial and administrational sphere resulted in the organization of a center in the late 1950's which offered a 9-week residential workshop, with emphasis on sensitivity training and on learning about group and organizational dynamics and group-related topics of management. The organization was quite influential in the 1960's, but seems to have lost some of its vitality in recent years.

Conclusion

Group therapy in Norway is mainly confined to psychiatric institutions—inpatient and outpatient clinics and mental hospitals. The private practice of group therapy is almost nonexistent. The reasons for this are not entirely clear; one reason may be the difficulty in finding less severely disturbed patients able to deal with the emotional turbulence connected with group therapy.

There should be a distinction made between group work and group therapy. Group work includes task and activity groups, which are properly led by psychiatric nurses and occupational therapists. Group therapy lies more within the domain of the psychiatrist, and adequate training is necessary. There appears to be some difficulty defining rules—who should lead which groups.

The increasing impact from Scandinavian Tavistock conferences—with their strong emphasis on role, authority, and boundary issues—may be helpful in overcoming the obstacles connected with the smooth operation of selected and differentiated groups within the psychiatric institutions.

References

Albretsen, C. S. Couples and multifamily groups: Therapeutic and administrative viewpoints. J. Oslo City Hosp., *31:* 27, 1981.

Astrup, C. Group therapy in mental hospital with special regard to schizophrenics. Acta Psychiatr. Neurol. Scand., *33:* 1, 1958.

Borchgrevink, M. Description and evaluation of group psychotherapy with 10 long-term patients: Follow-up after 10 years. J. Oslo City Hosp., *31:* 21, 1981.

Brown, G. J., Yeomans, T., and Grizzard, L., editors. *The Live Classroom: Innovation through Confluent Education and Gestalt.* Viking Press, New York, 1975.

Jorstad, J. Psychotherapy in a psychiatric institution: Attitude and process. Psychother. Psychosom., *24:* 281, 1974.

Karterud, S. The primary task of open heterogeneous groups in a therapeutic community. J. Oslo City Hosp., *31:* 71, 1981.

Ugelstad, E. Some experiences in group psychotherapy with psychotic patients. Acta Psychiatr. Scand. Suppl., *40:* 239, 1965.

Vaglum, P., and Boe, L. What was helpful and what was harmful? Patients evaluate the process of recovery in a therapeutic community. J. Oslo City Hosp., *31,* 55, 1981.

E.11 Group Psychotherapy in Poland

JERZY W. ALEKSANDROWICZ, M.D.

History

After World War II, Poland became a socialist state, all but ethnically homogeneous; and, as in past centuries, the cultural influences of the West (this time largely the English-speaking world) were integrated with those of the East. The country concentrated its efforts on a crash program of industrialization. Changes within its socioeconomic system, as well as an explosive birth rate (20,000,000 in 1945 to about 36,000,000 today), have resulted in a rapid and frequently frenzied sociocultural growth.

Health Care System

The health care system developed within the last 35 years consists of medical services provided free of charge. At the same time, private practice has been largely curtailed. The basic health care framework is divided into a system of regions which, in principle, correspond to administrative territorial units. A single general practitioner, for example, takes care of between 3,000 and 5,000 inhabitants. The regional structure of the health care system also covers hospitals which generally contain four basic departments: medicine, surgery, obstetrics and gynecology, and pediatrics. Additionally, there is a network of specialty clinics, including psychiatric clinics. Employees of major industrial plants, students, and soldiers have their own medical care systems.

Psychiatry

Presently, the specialized psychiatric health care system has at its disposal 41 psychiatric hospitals and departments within about 70 general hospitals (including wards for drug addiction and for child psychiatry), in addition to separate long-term centers for chronic mental illnesses. In major population centers, there are specialized psychiatric units integrating the work of local hospitals and outpatient clinics. The over-all supervision and leadership in the development of psychiatry is carried out by the Psychoneurological Institute in Warsaw, which consists of more than 20 clinics and units, cooperating with 11 psychiatric faculties and clinics at medical academies.

Throughout Poland, there are about 70,000 doctors. 2,500 work within the psychiatric sector and 1,700 of those are specialists. Specialization in psychiatry is achieved in two stages, lasting a total of about 6 years. In addition, the psychiatric medical service employs an increasing number of clinical psychologists, who are trained at eight universities.

The psychiatric medical service is mainly oriented toward treatment of psychotics, while neurotics and other groups are still relatively neglected. A particular problem is the lack of adequate inpatient services for the large number of patients. Therapy is generally dominated by pharmacological methods, even though other therapeutic modalities—especially psychotherapy—may be more appropriate.

One of the most serious social problems in Poland is a dependence on alcohol. Addiction to other drugs has not been, at least for the last several years, a major problem. Compounding the problem is the fact that the network of medical services for treating alcoholics is still very poorly developed, and its methods are far from satisfactory.

Large psychiatric hospitals, generally handling more than 1,000 patients at a time, are usually situated far away from major urban centers, and their role is still chiefly custodial. Many of these hospitals have introduced the principles of the therapeutic community, and occupational or work therapy is utilized, with an aim toward social rehabilitation. However, these are limited by the large number of patients, insufficient personnel, and economic difficulties.

In an effort to avoid isolation of patients and staff of those hospitals within the regional community, the tendency has been to establish only small wards within large regional hospitals providing multispecialized services, and to organize so-called intermediary forms of medical care, such as day hospitals and workshops for the handicapped. In such settings, psychotherapy is introduced much more frequently and with greater ease than in larger hospitals, particularly in treating neuroses, personality disorders, and various types of dependencies.

Psychotherapy

After World War II, psychotherapy hardly existed in Poland. Most psychiatrists (and in particular those with a psychoanalytic background) had either died or emigrated. Indeed, most psychiatrists gained their knowledge of psychotherapy through self-education.

In this early period, the mainstream of psychotherapy developed in the academic environment of psychiatrists. For example, in the Psychiatric Clinic in

Cracow, Kepinski initiated its development in a holistic direction, integrating biological, existential, and sociocultural approaches, including psychotherapy. Until the late 1950's, psychotherapy was dealt with and promoted by very few; a handful of doctors in other specialties introduced elements of psychotherapy—such as autogenic training, relaxation, and hypnosis—to the treatment of psychosomatic illnesses.

Starting in 1960, the Polish Psychiatric Association (PPA) launched its Psychotherapy Scientific Section. It became the hub of exchange of experience, training, and research. Paralleling this was the Section of Psychotherapy of Children and Adolescents of the Polish Society of Psychic Hygiene.

During this initial period, a considerable influence on the growth of psychotherapy in Poland was exerted by psychotherapists from Czechoslovakia and the Leningrad School of Psychiatry. The Czechoslovaks assisted largely in the training of Polish psychotherapists. Of importance also were contacts with psychotherapists from other countries. Within the last decade, an important role in the development of psychotherapy was played through participation in world congresses of psychotherapy and through scholarships abroad (England, France, and the United States). Cooperation with psychotherapists of socialist countries, meeting every 3 years at their congresses (Prague, 1973; Warsaw, 1976; Leningrad, 1979) organized by the Permanent Working Group, also influenced its development. Since 1974, the Psychotherapy Section of the PPA has organized national symposia of Polish psychoanalysis therapists scheduled to meet every 4 years, and since 1970 the Section has published articles relevant to psychotherapy. All these factors affected the evolution of views concerning psychotherapy and the practice of psychotherapy itself. Until the 1960's, the practice of individual psychotherapy based on the dynamic and so-called rational-realistic approaches was dominant.

In the 1960's and the 1970's, group therapy began to acquire a greater following, and this applied also to other forms of group activities, particularly the therapeutic community. Besides psychoanalysis, concepts based on learning theory and existential and phenomenological approaches were also gaining ground. The therapeutic systems taking into account specific Polish cultural and sociological aspects were also developed.

The mid-1970's witnessed the spread of views related to the antipsychiatric trend. Numerous disputes were caused by the tendency to pay more attention to the development of patients' personalities while bypassing the significance of their troubles. Arguments were fueled further by a spreading belief that in the psychotherapist's activity, his personality—and not his clinical knowledge—was of primary importance. This approach resulted in an increased interest in psychotherapy among psychologists.

The dissemination of such nonprofessional views was also affected by the relatively limited possibility of acquiring training in psychotherapy. In 1972, the Psychotherapy Section of the PPA started a training course of weekly classes based on the activity of T-

groups. The participants were exposed to psychotherapeutic techniques such as psychodrama, music therapy, pantomime, choreotherapy (dance therapy), art therapy, hypnosis and activity therapy.

Group therapy

Group psychotherapy in Poland began between 1956 and 1958, when it was introduced by Kepinski at the Psychiatric Clinic of the Medical Academy in Cracow. It was used mainly for psychotic patients or for groups that combined neurotic and psychotic patients. Since 1959, group psychotherapy has been the leading form of therapy in the Neurosis Clinic of the Psychoneurological Institute, which evolved into the center for the development of this form of psychotherapy. In the early 1970's, group psychotherapy became the form of psychotherapy most frequently applied in treating neuroses and personality disturbances.

Various methods are used in group psychotherapy. At the present time, groups are usually heterogeneous regarding sex and homogeneous as to the type of disturbance. Quite frequently, separate groups are formed for adolescent and aged patients.

Group psychotherapy of neuroses sometimes uses the closed-group method, but, because of organizational reasons, most centers utilize the open-group method. Treatment is conducted in groups of eight patients and usually lasts for about 3 months, ranging from one meeting per week to 3 hours of psychotherapy daily; this is free of charge to the participants.

Generally, however, group therapy becomes one element of a complex treatment program. Such a therapeutic system is made up of individual psychotherapy, pharmacotherapy, movement and occupational therapies, behavioral training, and other therapeutic activities.

Techniques. Methods of group therapy use various techniques. Most frequently used is the verbal technique, or talk therapy. Psychodrama is also frequently used.

Among nonverbal techniques, pantomime is quite popular, as is music therapy, both active and passive. Art therapy—including individual and collective drawing and clay modeling—is simultaneously treated as a projection technique permitting a better understanding of each patient's problems by the group, and as a technique facilitating working through. An original technique called choreotherapy consists of a combination of dance and rhythm routines which makes possible treatment of mobility disturbances of neurotic patients.

Relaxation techniques and group hypnotherapy are also used by some therapists.

Interpersonal training, introduced in the early 1970's to educate psychotherapists, gained popularity rather quickly as an autonomous form of group therapy. However, its frequent incompetent application provoked relatively rapid disenchantment, and its use as a therapeutic modality became limited. Currently, some therapists use some elements of interpersonal training in their work with groups of patients. Most often, however, interpersonal training is used with various professional groups (sensitivity training) or as a means of integrating different groups, i.e., students.

Next to group psychotherapy, the most frequent form of group activity is the therapeutic community as it applies to inpatient services. Concepts of the therapeutic community were introduced in the early 1960's at the Psychiatric Clinics in Cracow, Warsaw, and Poznan. Its development is coordinated by the Scientific Section of Social Psychiatry of the Polish Psychiatric Association. In the 1970's, many large psychiatric hospitals introduced the principles of the therapeutic community. Currently, however, a kind of retreat from operating wards according to these principles is occurring.

Other forms of group therapy are used only with specific patient populations. Ex-patients' clubs, for example, serve psychotic patients. Often they function as posthospitalization rehabilitation centers, enabling the ex-patient to find understanding for his experiences and difficulties. At the same time, however, they may create problems for less disturbed patients in terms of returning to the community by reducing their motivation to make adaptive efforts, and also by creating the opportunity to live exclusively within the therapeutic environment.

Alcoholics Anonymous groups exist in many cities, and form supportive units for those who try to stop drinking. They do not, however, play as important a role as they do in some other countries; this is perhaps due to poor national motivation for treatment of alcoholism. As in other countries, however, such groups largely derive their strength from the cohesion of the group. In the treatment of alcoholics, there is also a special form of group therapy, utilizing the method of large-group meetings combined with behavioral techniques and social pressure.

Conclusion

All forms of group therapy, particularly group psychotherapy, are currently among the main trends in Polish psychiatry. Their introduction into general practice is one of the principal aims of the Psychotherapy Section of the Polish Psychiatric Association.

References

Aleksandrowicz, J. W. Some remarks on the development of hypnotherapy and autogenic training in Poland. Hypnos, *3:* 4, 1978.

Aleksandrowicz, J. W., Bierzynski, K., Kolbik, I., Kowalczyk, E., Martyniak, J., Miczynska, A., Meus, J., Mis, L., Niwicki, J., Paluchowski, J., Pytko, A., Trzcieniecka, A., Wojnar, M., Romeyko, A., Romanik, O., and Zgud, J. Minimum of information about neurosis patients and treating them. Psychoterapia, *1:* 371, 1981.

Bomba, J., Badura, W., Mamrot, E., and Orwid, M. Results of psychotherapy in adolescent schizophrenia. Psychother. der Schizophrenie, Munchen, 1980.

Godwood-Sikorska, C., Pawlik, J., and Tworska, A. Psychotherapy of girls with neurotic emotional disturbances. IX International Congress of Psychotherapy, Oslo, 1973.

Kepinski, A., Orwid, M., and Gatarski, J. Group psychotherapy as an approach to a psychotherapeutic community. Group Psychother., *3:* 4, 1960.

Orwid, M., Badura, W., Bomba, J., Mamrot, E., and Jaworska-Franczak, E. The main psychotherapeutic trends in Poland with special attention to the Department of Child and Adolescent Psychiatry in Cracow. J. Adolesc., *1:* 4, 1981.

Pohorecka, A. Characteristics of the image of significant persons and of the self in neurotics. Psychoterapia, *3:* 2, 1980.

E.12 Group Psychotherapy in Portugal

EDUARDO LUIS CORTESÃO, M.D.

Introduction

The development and gradual acceptance of group analytic psychotherapy methods and practice have had a strong influence in various aspects of medicine, mental health, and psychiatry in Portugal. The impact of group methods has resulted in alterations in hospital and institutional psychiatric structures. Team work, group discussion, day hospitals, assessment of diagnosis, and therapeutic evaluation by multidisciplinary and multiprofessional approaches have been some of the more conspicuous changes.

Other developments include: (1) group methods introduced in both undergraduate and postgraduate medical education; (2) group counseling and group psychotherapy taught and practiced by social workers; (3) group analytic approaches and group methods introduced in the field of occupational therapy; (4) permanent education curriculums for nurses which take into account the teaching and practice of group work; and (5) since 1956, group analytic psychotherapy and group analysis which provide treatment of neurotic, psychosomatic, and borderline patients.

Group Analysis

The nature, structure, and technique of group analysis as developed by Cortesão take into account the initial coining of the term "group analysis" by Burrow and the influence of Foulkes's group analytic framework.

Cortesão emphasized the analyzability of transference neurosis, early object relations, developmental processes, and their working through in a specific group setting. By so doing, he offered to group analysis a challenging perspective both for therapy and research.

In this framework, some theoretical and technical constructs were devised as, for instance, the concept of group analytic pattern and the mutable levels of experience and interpretation. The level or levels on which the psychotherapist is going to operate will define what sort of group psychotherapy he is doing. This, in turn, will demarcate a psychotherapeutic variation.

Transference interpretation

Transferences are a latent and changing phenomenon in an analytic group or in any psychotherapeutic group. The analyst has to induce the recollection of past experience embedded in object relations, the fixations in pregenital phases of development, the quality of oedipal regression, and, by therapeutic elaboration (working through), the evolution of the self in different phases and situations of life.

The group analyst may be aware that what is verbalized here and now is not especially relevant in its manifest content. Rather, what it reveals is a displacement of affect (even in the simple form of diffuse anxiety) invested (cathected) in fantasies, screen memories, or actual specific conflicts to this new object relation as it is furthered by the group matrix and pattern. To bind or not to bind these transference phenomena may be done by the work of transference interpretation. Transference interpretation is a means for rearrangement and reshaping of unconscious motivation, object relations, and self-organization of inner and past conflicts. The procedures are carried out in three sessions per week, usually for not less than 4 to 5 years. The working through and transference neurosis are the core of this group analytic technique, and interpretations are the important contribution of the group analyst.

An instance of a specific transference development is given by the splitting of the mother unconscious object representation (imago). By the nature of the transference neurosis roots in the group analytic matrix, there is a splitting of the mother imago into two unconscious object representations, projected onto the group and onto the analyst. The first object representation, its structure and functioning, belongs to the realm of the ego. The second object representation is anchored in the deep grounds of the id, superego, and ego ideal.

Narcissistic conditions

Patients with predominant narcissistic disturbance tend to carry on with long-term group analysis. The narcissistic structure is not always easy to detect even by the experienced analyst, before group analysis is indicated. In many cases, intellectual functioning and pragmatic development of ego functions in external reality are unimpaired. Once in group analysis, they may reveal those narcissistic structures and modes of functioning. Yet these structures offer a unique possibility both for the investigation of their nature, structure, and functioning in the particular narcissistic patient, and for the assessment of the narcissistic nuclei and roots in self-development in every member of the group.

Termination of analysis of these patients is always particularly painful, both for the patient and for the group. It is likely to embarrass even the experienced analyst, who may find himself in serious doubt about how to terminate such an analysis. The patient seems to have settled inside a new narcissistic network, where he has woven himself into the group analytic matrix. Nevertheless, the outcome of analysis and its mourning process are described positively, with these persons coping reasonably well with the demands of life and external reality once the actual analytic tie has finally been broken.

References

Abse, W. D. Trigant Burrow and the inauguration of group analysis in the USA. Group Anal., *12*: 218, 1979.

Burrow, T. *Neurosis of Man.* Routledge & Kegan Paul, London, 1949.

Cortesão, E. L. Transference neurosis and the group analytic process. Group Anal., 7, Appendix, 1974.

Cortesão, E. L. Group psychotherapy, group analysis and the vicissitudes of transference. Acta Psiquiatr. Port., *27*: 31, 1981.

Ferreira, A. G. Survey of group psychotherapy in Portugal. Group Anal., *3*: 126, 1970.

Foulkes, S. H. *Therapeutic Group Analysis.* George Allen and Unwin, London, 1964.

Foulkes, S. H., and Anthony, E. J. *Group Psychotherapy: The Psychoanalytic Approach,* ed. 2. Penguin Books, London, 1965.

Leal, M. R. A selection of good questions and some suggestions. Group Anal., *4*: 54, 1971.

E.13 Group Psychotherapy in Sweden

BO SIGRELL, Ph.D.

History

Sweden is the largest of the Scandinavian countries, and the fourth largest country in area in Europe. The population of Sweden is slightly over 8 million people. The country has a low birth rate and a slow rate of population growth. A considerable proportion of the country's population growth since World War II has been the result of immigration.

Sweden has a Lutheran state church, of which all Swedes are members, provided they have not formally withdrawn. Five per cent of the population are nonmembers of the church. Sweden is a constitutional monarchy with a parliamentary form of government. After general elections or the resignation of the cabinet, the leadership of the government is awarded to the party leader capable of forming a cabinet with the greatest possible support in Parliament.

Health Care System

All residents of Sweden are covered by a compulsory health insurance system. A sick person is guaranteed a daily allowance during illness, with an aim toward providing about 90 per cent of income lost from illness.

Health insurance also covers hospitalization, which in principle is free of charge. Visits to doctors at outpatient clinics cost a set fee for the first 15 visits, after which they are free of charge. During the 1960's, large parts of the public health system were transferred from the jurisdiction of the national government to the county councils.

Health care is provided on three levels. The first is primary care, comprised of all the public health and medical care which can be provided outside of hospitals and central nursing homes. All home care and most long-term care also fall under this heading. The second is county-level medical care, which is responsible for almost all general medical care and inpatient psychiatric care. The county general hospital or county hospital receives inpatients and has access to facilities unavailable in primary care. County general hospitals are normally able to provide care in every medical specialty. The third level is called regional medical care, which comprises about 1 per cent of short-term inpatient care and a fraction of 1 per cent of outpatient care. Facilities for remote consultations are provided, and patients with unclear symptoms or with complicated medical conditions are admitted to regional hospitals, which also serve as teaching hospitals.

Psychiatry

Swedish psychiatry is presently undergoing change. The resources of psychiatry are the result of past times and are very much conditioned by outdated forms of care. The goal, however, is more open forms of care where the patients, as much as possible, will be able to maintain links with their normal setting. A census made in March 1979 showed that the number of persons admitted to inpatient care has decreased by approximately 8,000 compared with 10 to 12 years previously. One of the reasons for this is that elderly patients with organic brain syndromes are now, to a greater extent, being treated in the long-term care program. However, long-term schizophrenic patients account mainly for the reduced need for inpatient care. At the separate mental hospitals, the number of beds has been reduced during the last few years by up to 4,000; this trend is continuing. Integration into the rest of the health care system is an important aim for psychiatry. In November 1979, the National Board of Health and Welfare adopted guidelines for psychiatric care in the 1980's, in which the principles for such development were established. Psychiatry is to be organized according to the sectorized model. A psychiatric clinic would, in this way, have total responsibility for specialized psychiatric care within each county.

Psychiatric short-term care, including emergency service, will work in cooperation with general inpatient services. It is important that the clinics be organized in such a way as to give systematic assistance to primary health care and social services. In order to classify and to treat mental patients, a holistic view is required, along with a consideration of medical, psychological, and social factors. This implies that a psychiatric team should consist of doctors and other medical staff, as well as psychologists and social workers.

Psychotherapy

Until 1960, psychotherapy had little impact on psychiatric treatment. There was also little academic training for psychiatrists, psychologists, and social workers in Sweden. The Swedish Psychoanalytic Association was established in 1934, but it had only a few members for many years. However, from 1960 to the present, development has been extremely rapid.

The increased interest in psychotherapy started with group psychotherapy. A group of psychoanalysts had studied group psychotherapy in Boston and London and started to work with analytic group psychotherapy in Stockholm. At the same time, a number of psychotherapy groups were set up in prisons, also as a result of experiences in other countries, especially in the United States.

The most common theoretical frame of reference in Swedish psychotherapy is a psychodynamic-psychoanalytic one. Other forms also exist, such as nondirective, gestalt, psychodrama, and behavioral therapy. During the last 10 years, a growing interest in behavioral therapy has developed, especially at psychological institutions at some of the universities.

The Swedish Association of Group Psychotherapy was formed in 1960. When group psychotherapy first came to Sweden, there were a number of trained psychotherapists interested in participating in the theories and practice of this alternative to individual psychotherapy. In 1968, the association started an educational program in group psychotherapy, together with the Department of Education at the University of Stockholm. The course was offered on the graduate level. In 1978, the first federal training program started in Sweden. Today, this program is at two universities, Stockholm and Umea. Plans are to have similar group therapy training programs at each of the five universities in Sweden and, later on, at a number of university affiliates.

Now that the federal training program in psychotherapy has been established, the program of basic education for group psychotherapists is no longer of primary concern. The discussion now is focused on how to plan a program for specialists in analytic group psychotherapy, a program aimed at psychotherapists who already have basic training in individual psychotherapy.

From the beginning, the Swedish Association of Group Psychotherapy had members from all over the country. They started training programs and weekend seminars. In 1969, an association was formed in Lund; in 1971, another in Gothenburg; and in 1972, a third one in Uppsala. In 1975, a cooperative organization called the Swedish Union for Group Psychotherapy was formed, which at present has 11 different member associations and about 700 members.

Today, group psychotherapy is one of several different types of psychotherapy methods, but it is widely used in different areas of psychiatry throughout Sweden.

References

Backa-Tellefsen, K., and Sigrell, B. An evaluation of an educational program in group psychotherapy. Presented at the Fourth European Symposium of Group Analysis, Stockholm, 1979.
National Swedsh Board of Health and Welfare. *The Swedish Health Services in 1980's.* National Swedish Board of Health and Welfare, Stockholm, 1976.
Sigrell, B. *Group Psychotherapy: Studies of Processes in Therapeutic Groups.* Almqvist & Wiksell, Stockholm, 1968.

E.14 Group Psychotherapy in Switzerland

RAYMOND BATTEGAY, M.D.

Introduction

Psychiatrists in Switzerland recognized as early as the 1920's the importance of the group milieu for the resocialization of psychiatric patients. They correctly evaluated the importance of collective psychotherapy in psychiatric hospitals and in attached houses outside the hospital for helping the patients to remain in or to learn social contact. Many psychiatrists stressed the necessity of social training in the psychiatric wards or in free colonies outside the hospital. Since the beginning of the 20th century, the psychiatric hospitals had also organized a family care system in the countryside for chronic schizophrenic patients.

A sign that the medical profession, as well as other professional disciplines, began to discover the possibilities which the group offered as a milieu for therapy and for training was the publication of books concerning group psychotherapy since the early 1950's, and the founding, in 1973, of the Swiss Society for Group Psychology and Group Dynamics, in which all professions and all directions of group approaches were represented.

Influences

In the beginning of group psychotherapy in Switzerland, only physicians were engaged in group approaches. Therefore, people participating in group psychotherapy were then recruited only from a population of hospitalized or ambulatory psychiatric patients. It was intended to help neurotics and psychotics gain insight into their psychopathological mechanisms and to develop social skills.

The initial period was mainly influenced by the psychoanalytic school. The early group psychotherapists tried to transmit their own experiences with individual psychoanalysis or psychotherapy into the field of group psychotherapy.

In addition, many nonpsychoanalytic methods came into use, especially the theme-centered interactional method, group approaches derived from Gestalt therapy, transactional analysis, and sensitivity training and psychodrama. By these methods, which tend to accelerate the emotional involvement of the participants, group members are supposed to undergo behavioral training in an effort to more openly express their emotions and to better cope by developing a deeper sensitivity toward others. Therefore, many interested people aside from patients became involved in different types of groups.

Training

In almost all psychiatry outpatient and inpatient institutions, in the universities, and in many training institutes, group psychotherapy or group training methods are offered. Group psychotherapy is practiced in Swiss psychiatry with all the different diagnostic groups.

Mostly, there are small groups of seven to nine patients. In almost all psychiatric hospitals and outpatient clinics, doctors-in-training run mostly analytically oriented groups under supervision. This is a requirement in each psychiatric institution for the purpose of specialization. In most of the psychiatric hospitals, therapeutic communities have developed. In the last few years, formerly hospitalized patients, especially those who had been drug dependent, have been aided in creating living communities, which help them to overcome their dependency needs and their loneliness.

Research

The literature published in Switzerland shows that some therapists were interested in studying spontaneous group formation. Others were concerned with technical problems, such as how to motivate and prepare patients for group psychotherapy and how to preserve the balance between analysis of deep psychological conflicts and reconditioning of behavior. Still others concentrated on group psychotherapy with hospitalized patients, where the aim is to reestablish social contact.

Other areas of study include the so-called group dream, in which the dreams of an individual are linked to the group. In addition, theoretical problems of group psychotherapy, couples and family therapy, and group work with antisocial members of society have also been described.

Results

Little has been done to evaluate the results of group psychotherapy on a quantitative basis. However, such studies are being undertaken currently, especially with schizophrenics.

The trend toward doing therapy in a social system—the group—reached Switzerland from surrounding countries. Switzerland followed the general trend in a way adapted to the character of the Swiss population, where groups play an enormous role in political and social life. In the future, research and evaluation of group methods and solid training of group psychotherapists will be emphasized.

References

Balint, M., and Balint, E. *The Doctor, His Patient, and the Illness.* Pitman, London, 1957.

Battegay, R. The group dream. In *Group Therapy*, L. R. Wolberg, M. L. Aronson, and A. R. Wolberg, editors, p. 27. Stratton Intercontinental, New York, 1977.

Foulkes, S. H., and Anthony, E. J. *Group Psychotherapy.* Penguin Books, London, 1957.

Friedemann, A. Gruppentherapie und Gruppendiagnostik an Kindern (Group therapy and group diagnostics of children). Z. Diagnost. Psychol. Pers. Forsch., *5:* 295, 1957.

Guggenbühl-Craig, A. *Experiences with Group Psychotherapy.* S. Karger, New York, 1956.

Jones, M. *Beyond the Therapeutic Community.* Yale University Press, New Haven, CT, 1968.

Lebovici, S. L'utilisation du psychodrame dans le diagnostic en psychiatrie (The use of the psychodrama as a means of diagnostics in psychiatry). Z. Diagnost. Psychol. Pers. Forsch., *5:* 197, 1957.

Lieberman, M. A., Yalom, I. D., and Miles, M. B. *Encounter Groups: First Facts.* Basic Books, New York, 1973.

Moreno, J. L. *Psychodrama.* Beacon House, New York, 1946.

Schindler, W. Transference and counter-transference in "family-pattern" group psychotherapy. Ref. Int. Psychotherapie-Kongress, Zurich, 1954. Acta Psychother. *3*(suppl.)*:* 345, 1955.

Slavson, S. R. *The Practice of Group Psychotherapy.* Pushkin Press, London, 1947.

E.15 Group Psychotherapy in the United Kingdom

MALCOLM PINES, M.D., F.R.C.P., F.R.C., Psych., D.P.M.

Introduction

The United Kingdom is a politically and socially stable society whose institutions have allowed for constant development in the past century without major social and political upheaval. A powerful and prosperous middle-class, based on the Industrial Revolution and the wealth of empire, endowed the schools and universities for the education of their descendants.

The great achievements of 19th-century medicine in the United Kingdom have included advances in neurology and psychiatry made by such outstanding figures as Hughlings Jackson and Henry Maudsley. As the specialty of psychiatry developed, the physician, then termed the alienist, largely practiced within the confines of the mental hospitals. These hospitals were often isolated, large institutions built on cheap land on the outskirts of the large cities whose function was more custodial than therapeutic. The very existence of these hospitals represented a retrograde step from the advances of the humane period of moral psychiatry of the 18th century as exemplified by the retreat at York, where individual care and attention was given to patients and great emphasis was placed on the creation and maintenance of an optimistic and caring atmosphere.

In the early years of this century, psychoanalytic views were enthusiastically accepted by a small group of psychiatrists in London, headed for very many years by Ernest Jones, one of Freud's close disciples and supporters.

The small British Psychoanaytic Society received a large influx of continental pschoanalysts in the 1930's. This produced many tensions and controversies, as the British Society had, in the 1920's, already begun to develop along lines that diverged from those of Vienna. Ernest Jones had supported Melanie Klein, and an English school began to develop that the Viennese analysts could not accept. The intensities of these controversies detracted from the development of group psychotherapy through the decade that followed World War II.

Health Services

Prior to the establishment of the National Health Service in 1948, there was a large network of local medical services. The majority of the population received low-cost medical treatment from their general practitioners, and, if they needed hospital care, it was provided by the local municipal hospital, where treatment was free. The medical schools, situated in London and the large provincial cities, were called voluntary hospitals, where patients were expected to make a contribution to the cost of treatment based upon their capacity to pay; however, the bulk of the cost of these hospitals was provided by public voluntary support.

The psychiatric hospitals were almost all large municipal institutions until the Maudsely Hospital opened its doors in 1917, becoming the United Kingdom's first metropolitan, centrally located hospital that admitted only voluntary patients. The Maudsley became a center of research and teaching affiliated with the University of London and the Institute of Psychiatry.

Before the National Health Service (NHS) came into being in 1948, there were numerous small private psychiatric hospitals of varying standards, a few of which have survived. The most important of these, The Bethlem Royal Hospital, originally Bedlam, combined with the Maudsley to form The Royal Bethlem and Maudsley Hospitals.

A great majority of the population receive free care under the NHS, although all adults contribute to the cost of the service through compulsory insurance contributions. The cost of individual and group psychotherapy for outpatients above a small yearly amount is not covered by insurance, and, therefore, the patient must pay the bulk of the cost himself. This fact partly accounts for the relatively small demand for psychotherapy outside the NHS; among other deterrents is the cultural factor, the notion that seeking psychotherapeutic help for emotional problems is still not yet widely accepted as a sensible and practical procedure. The number of trained therapists is still small—slightly over 600 for the whole country (population 50 million)—and the great majority are in or near London.

Psychiatry

Psychiatric services are fairly well distributed throughout the United Kingdom by a network of psychiatric hospitals and clinics. All these hospitals are inspected by the Royal College of Psychiatrists, and have to meet College standards if they seek approval as training situations for junior psychiatrists. The official policy for the past 20 years has been to reduce the size of the old mental hospital, and to develop small psychiatric units within the new large modern district general hospitals. These psychiatric units are intended as early treatment centers serving the local community, and are integrated with the local community social and welfare services. Patients can much more easily attend as outpatients at these clinics, and the stigma of mental illness is, to some extent, reduced by the fact that the psychiatric clinic is situated within the same building as the general hospital. The disadvantages are that these small units often have a high turnover and the emphasis is usually on pharmacotherapy. The United Kingdom also has a well-established tradition of child guidance clinics, where children up to the age of 16 can be seen, and where the tradition is for the treatment team approach to be used.

The general orientation of British psychiatry is far less dynamically oriented than in North America. Medical schools and psychiatric hospitals teach and practice diagnostic and treatment skills that emphasize the organic aspects of mental illness, and the psychotherapy provided is more supportive than insight directed. The dynamic approach has, however, made a considerable advance in the past 20 years, and the Royal College of Psychiatrists, which advises the government, has proposed a psychotherapeutic service based upon one consultant psychotherapist to a population of 60,000 persons. Training for consultant posts in the NHS is through the position of a senior registrar (equivalent to a senior resident). The 4-year period of training in psychotherapy is open to persons who have already completed their basic training in medicine and postgraduate psychiatry. These training posts can be established only when the training scheme has been inspected and approved by a special committee appointed jointly by the Royal College of Psychiatrists and the Association of University Teachers of Psychiatry. This committee has produced guidelines for psychotherapy training, designed to equip the future consultant with skills relevant to the role of a consultant psychotherapist in the NHS. Thus, apart from basic skills in psychodynamics and individual psychotherapy, the trainee should have experience in group psychotherapy with small analytic groups, with large groups (ward groups milieu therapy), and with marital and family work. The provision of personal therapy, individual or group, for the trainee is often difficult away from London and Edinburgh. There is an informal system of collaboration between the NHS and the private psychotherapeutic training establishment, such as the Institute of Psychoanalysis, the Society of Analytical Psychologists (Jungian), the Institute of Group Analysis (all of which are in London), and the Scottish Institute of Human Relations in Edinburgh. The trainees may train at these establishments while holding their NHS posts and will be partly reimbursed by the NHS for the expense of training, although not for the cost of the personal therapy component.

Psychotherapy

The predominant psychotherapeutic tradition is psychoanalysis. The Institute of Psychoanalysis in London is the main training center outside the NHS, and many of its graduates are part-time employees of the National Health Service.

Formal training in group analytic psychotherapy has been possible in London for the last 8 years. It is provided by the Institute of Group Analysis, founded by S. H. Foulkes and his colleagues, and is based upon Foulkes's work, which represents a synthesis of psychoanalysis and social psychology. Full training, leading to membership in the Institute of Group Analysis, consists of: (1) personal group psychotherapy for a minimum of 3 years as a member of an ordinary psychotherapeutic group conducted by a senior analyst; the trainee is never a member of a therapy group constituted solely of other trainees; (2) a theoretical program consisting of seminars lasting 2½ years; and (3) careful supervision of the trainee's own work.

The trainee can enter this program after completing a 1-year general group work course. In recent years, this introductory general course can be taken in one of several provincial centers, such as Oxford, Cambridge, Northampton, and Manchester.

Group psychotherapy

Developments in the United Kingdom have been of outstanding importance to group psychotherapy as a whole. The work of Bion, Ezriel, and Foulkes in psychoanalytic group psychotherapy; of Maxwell Jones and T. F. Main in therapeutic community; of Bierer in day hospitals; of Clark in administrative psychiatry; and of Taylor in research collectively represents a considerable contribution to psychodynamic psychiatry. These developments can be traced through the work of these individuals and the institutions with which they have been connected.

Tavistock Clinic

The Tavistock Clinic, an outpatient clinic for the treatment of the psychoneuroses, and the Cassel Hospital, originally an inpatient hospital for the treatment of the psychoneuroses, were both founded after World War I when the medical profession first recognized that shell shock and the traumatic neuroses of war could best be understood and treated psychodynamically. Both these institutions were at first centers for individual psychodynamic psychotherapy, but both adopted group models after World War II and for the same reason: the massive impact of the experience of military psychiatry in the British Army from 1939 to 1945.

Many of these military psychiatrists had been on the staff of the prewar Tavistock Clinic, and, on their return, the orientation of this clinic turned decisively toward group dynamics. The outstanding influence was undoubtedly that of W. R. Bion. Ambitious plans were made for a psychiatric clinic that would be a center for research and therapy in this new field of social psychiatry, using the new understanding of group dynamics. Psychological illness was now seen as the symptom of disturbances in social groups, such as the family, the work group, and other social institutions. Treatment in a group and of a group was given prominence. The study of interpersonal relationships, the relationship of the individual to society, and the use of the tools of psychoanalysis and of social psychology were central to the planning of the postwar Tavistock Clinic.

A separate facility, the Tavistock Institute of Human Relations, was created to further research the application of group dynamic concepts to industry and to other institutions. It was partly created to maintain the independence of this work from the National Health Service when the Tavistock Clinic became part of it in 1948. The journal *Human Relations* began as the house journal of the Tavistock Clinic.

What has become known as the Tavistock model is based upon the work of Bion, Ezriel, and Sutherland. They shared a psychoanalytic approach which is strongly influenced by object relations theory (Melanie Klein and Ronald Fairbairn). The amount of group psychotherapy carried out at the Tavistock Clinic is now less than before, when enthusiasm for the theories of these pioneers was high; new models are being sought. A rapprochement between the Tavistock approach and the group analytic (Foulksian) approach may emerge. Bion's and Ezriel's theories, however, continue to stimulate thought and research.

The Tavistock Clinic has been a center of innovation in other fields. John Bowlby pioneered family therapy in the Department of Children and Parents, and the work of Michael Balint in sensitizing general practitioners to the psychodynamic aspects of their work was carried out in groups and has had a great influence in this country and in Europe.

Therapeutic community

The concept of the therapeutic community itself and its practice originated in Great Britain, again in response to the demands and opportunities of military psychiatry. There were two separate sources, and the distinction between them has continued to influence the development of therapeutic communities until today. One group of workers—Foulkes, Bridger, Main, Bion—was psychoanalytic in origin and orientation; the other group, led by Maxwell Jones, was innocent of psychoanalysis and reached their practice empirically.

Northfield Military Hospital was the setting where Bion and Rickman—followed by Foulkes, Bridger, and Main—were able to reform and to redesign the practice of hospital psychiatry. The notion that the institution itself, the hospital, can be either therapeutic or antitherapeutic, according to the ways the roles of patient and staff are defined, originated there.

Maxwell Jones's pioneering work at Henderson Hospital was the subject of the most important single piece of research into therapeutic communities, Rappaport's *Community as Doctor.* Henderson Hospital gradually developed into a treatment center for psychopathic personalities and for other character disturbances, and has survived as a significant center of treatment and research in the face of what at times has been considerable opposition.

Therapeutic communities in the United Kingdom have combined to form an Association of Therapeutic Communities (ATC), which now sponsors a journal, *The International Journal of Therapeutic Communities.* The ATC cooperates closely with Dutch therapeutic communities and holds regular international meetings. The therapeutic community movement has also had its failures, and some units have closed, either because of local opposition or because of mismanagement and maladministration.

Forensic psychiatry

An outstanding example of group psychotherapy within an institution is Grendon Underwood, a prison to which prisoners are sent who are thought likely to benefit from intensive psychotherapy. Group psychotherapy has an important place with the patients of Broadmoor Hospital, a special hospital to which persons are sent when they are convicted of crimes committed in abnormal states of mind. The Portman Clinic specifically treats psychopathic personalities and sexual deviants, and has an extensive program of group psychotherapy.

Group analytic psychotherapy

S. H. Foulkes, the originator of psychoanalytic group psychotherapy, founded the Group Analytic Society, the Institute of Group Analysis, and the journal *Group Analysis.* For many years, he taught at the Maudsley Hospital, where he influenced many generations of psychiatrists. The Institute of Group Analysis is now the major center of training in group psychotherapy in the United Kingdom, and it graduates therapists after a 3-year training program which involves personal group analytic psychotherapy, theoretical training, and supervised work. The Institute of Group Analysis has sponsored the International Library of Group Psychotherapy and Group Process.

Foulkes was trained as a psychoanalyst in Vienna in the mid-1920's, and he came to the United Kingdom as a refugee in 1933, after having worked in Frankfurt as Director of the Psychoanalytic Clinic. He began group analytic psychotherapy in 1938, in Exeter, putting into practice ideas that had been developing for several years. He was significantly influenced by Gestalt psychology through his work with Kurt Goldstein, whose work with brain-injured patients after World War I had shown the importance of Gestalt concepts in evaluating impaired central nervous system function. Foulkes extended Goldstein's neuropsychological theories of the individual to the group situation. He was also a sophisticated student of modern sociology and was able to make a personal synthesis of sociology and psychoanalysis through which he placed the group as the prime unit of study, rather than the isolated individual who was the object of study of psychoanalysis.

Foulkes also played an important role in military psychiatry between 1939 and 1945. At Northfield Military Hospital, where he followed Bion and Rickman, he was more successful in gaining support and acceptance than his predecessors had been. The work of Foulkes, Main, Bridger, and their colleagues led to the concept of the therapeutic community, which has had world-wide effects on hospital psychiatry.

Foulkes's concepts can be summarized as follows: (1) The essence of the individual is social, as he develops only in a social context and is defined as a person by this context. The individual is a nodal point in the social network; (2) Neuroses and psychological disturbances in general have their origin in disturbed social relationships; (3) These disturbed relationships develop from the unconscious forces of love and of hate that affect the relationships of the individual and of his social network; he now becomes a nodal point of disturbance. The neurotic position in its very nature is highly individualistic; it is group disruptive in essence, for it is genetically the result of an incompatibility between the individual and his original group. It is at the same time an expression of destructive and aggressive tendencies; (4) The resolution of the individual's conflict is possible in a social network, either that of the group in which the disturbance arises, e.g., the family, or in a therapeutic (proxy, stranger) group; (5) The symptom or disturbance will be reactivated in the group. It will be located in the communicative processes and relationship patterns and appear as a characteristic disturbance of these. The symptom will be translatable into communicational processes, since the person's inner world is actualized in the group context; (6) The healing properties of the group situation lie in the uncovering of the interpersonal disturbances and their resolutions in the relationships context of the group. New modes of relating are available once the old patterns have been recognized, analyzed, and transcended; (7) As each member of the group represents a deviation from the norm of the community to which all members belong, collectively they are the norm from which each one is a deviant; and (8) The therapist's role is predominantly to be of service to the group as a whole. He is able to identify processes which obstruct free communication and fuller understanding between its members. With his help, the group as a whole and, consequently, its individual members, will develop and mature.

Conclusion

Group analytic psychotherapy is well established and of growing significance in the United Kingdom. The therapeutic community movement developed in England has weathered setbacks and continued to be of significance, although limited to a few centers. Training in group psychotherapy has been recognized as an important component of the training of all psychiatrists. However, academic interest and involvement in group psychotherapy have been limited, and there are few signs as yet of a change in this attitude. Although few important advances in small-group psychotherapy have been made since the influential work of Bion, Foulkes, and Ezriel, some headway has been made with medium and large groups.

References

Barnes, E., editor. *Psycho-Social Nursing (Studies from the Cassel Hospital)*. Tavistock Publications, London, 1968.

Clark, D. H. *Administrative Therapy: The Role of the Doctor in a Therapeutic Community*. Tavistock Publications, London, 1964.

De Mare, P. B. *Perspectives in Group Psychotherapy*. George Allen and Unwin, London, 1962.

Dicks, H. V. *Fifty Years of the Tavistock Clinic*. Routledge and Kegan Paul, London, 1970.

Hinshlewood, R. D., and Manning, N., editors. *Therapeutic Communitis: Reflections and Progress*. Routledge and Kegan Paul, London, 1979.

Kreeger, L., editor. *The Large Group: Dynamics and Therapy*. Constable, London, 1975.

Taylor, F. K. A history of group and administrative therapy in Great Britain. Br. J. Med. Psychol., *31:* 153, 1958.

Whitely, F. J. The Henderson Hospital. Int. J. Ter. Commun., *1:* 38, 1980.

Glossary

ROBERT JEAN CAMPBELL, M.D.

Abreaction. The re-entry of repressed material into consciousness; the material that is recalled is accompanied by appropriate affect, whose discharge or expression gives the emotional relief characteristics of abreaction.

Abstinence. Denial or avoidance of gratification, sometimes encouraged in psychotherapy as a way to maintain an optimal level of anxiety for the treatment process. When applied to persons who are dependent upon alcohol or other substances, abstinence means complete cessation of intake of the substance.

Abstinence syndrome. Withdrawal syndrome; the various symptoms that develop in a person who has been physiologically dependent upon any substance when intake of that substance is stopped.

Abstract thinking. Higher-level thinking, such as the ability to categorize, generalize, or extrapolate from a single immediate experience to the likelihood that future experiences may follow the same pattern; to grasp the essentials of a whole, even while recognizing the distinctions between the parts that make up the whole; to plan ahead and consider various alternatives to action; to think or perform symbolically. Abstract thinking is often impaired early in the course of a degenerative brain disorder, as well as in schizophrenic disorders.

Abuse. Improper treatment or handling; mismanagement or misuse, often with the implication that some injury is likely to ensue. Alcohol abuse refers to abnormal, excessive, intemperate intake of alcohol that has not yet reached a degree where physiological dependence or addiction has been established. Substance abuse refers to similar abnormal use of other drugs. Child abuse refers to behavior of parents or parent substitutes that results in physical injury or even death of the child; the abuse may; consist of intentional acts of omission or of repeated, excessive beatings.

Accelerated interaction. An alternate term for marathon group session that emphasizes one result of the intensity of the marathon approach.

Accountability. A participant's responsibility for his behavior within the therapy group and for reporting the reasons for that behavior.

Acting out. Behavior that is determined unconsciously by a situation other than the one to which the subject appears to be responding in the present; the behavior often represents a displacement of affect onto the current situation from an earlier experience and typically produces relief from tension. Transference reactions are examples of acting out that occur in the treatment situation.

Action group (A-group). A group organized around a specific problem that it faces as a community, an industry, an agency, etc. Emphasis is on problem solving and formulation of a plan of action, rather than an understanding of self or group process.

Actional-deep approach. The use of nonverbal behavior as a communications vehicle in group therapy, either in addition to or as a substitute for language. Psychodrama employs this technique extensively.

Actional-superficial approach. The use of specific nonverbal activities in addition to language to achieve limited goals in group therapy. Groups using such an approach tend to be large and place minimal emphasis on participants' awareness of psychodynamics.

Active. As applied to psychotherapy or therapist, referring to the use of a directive and focused approach, such as clearly defining leadership role, providing a model and encouraging its imitation, setting specific goals and establishing a time frame for their accomplishment, and shifting techniques to conform to the shifting needs of the patients.

Activity group therapy. Developed by S. R. Slavson for use with children, an approach that emphasizes emotional interaction in guided, permissive activities as a way of developing socialization skills and promoting personality development. The therapist uses action interpretation, nonverbal reactions to the child's statements or behavior, to encourage reality testing and ego strengthening.

Activity, immobilizing. In activity group psychotherapy, an environment designed to bind energy and libido, rather than to release or activate them, typically by emphasis on specific, concrete activities.

Activity-interview method. Screening and diagnosis of a child based on observational analysis of his group behavior and interactions in a group setting and on his reactions to the interviewer.

Actualization. Fulfillment or realization of one's potential, the major thrust of many self-help groups.

Adapted child. In transactional analysis, the dependent, inhibited, constrained, compliant, procrastinating, withdrawing part of the Child ego state that is subservient to parental influence.

Adult ego state. In transactional analysis, the part of the ego that analyzes and makes decisions; like a computer, it has no feelings and emphasizes the objective and the rational. While the Child ego state creates the wanting part of the person, the Adult ego state decides whether the want can be fulfilled and determines how fulfillment can be achieved.

Affective interaction. Emotionally charged interpersonal experience and exchange.

Affectualizing. In transactional therapy, pseudoemotionally or the expression of feelings as part of a pastime or game, it is contrasted with the expression of authentic feelings that are characteristic of intimacy.

After session. A meeting of the participants in a therapy group without the therapist, usually held immediately after a regular session with the therapist.

Aggression. Aggressivity, aggressiveness; forceful, dominant, controlling, provocative, or hostile behavior. In psychoanalytic psychology, the energy of the death instinct, as contrasted with libido, the energy of the erotic instinct or drive.

Akathisia. Inability to sit down or sit still; it may occur as a side effect of treatment with neuroleptics.

Alanon. A self-help fellowship, modeled after Alcoholics

Anonymous, whose focus is on meeting the psychosocial needs of adult members of the families of alcoholics.

Alcoholics Anonymous (AA). A self-help group founded in 1935 by two former alcoholics, a New York broker and an Akron physician, for the purpose of rehabilitating alcoholics. Abstinence is the cornerstone of the AA approach, which uses inspirational-supportive and other group techniques. Since its inception, AA has expanded into an international movement and is an essential or, at least, significant part of many alcohol rehabilitation programs.

Alienation. A feeling of being estranged, separated from, or out of touch with oneself and consequent uncertainty about one's appropriate role, identity, or ability to influence the outside world.

Allport's group relations theory. A holistic psychology of human behavior, developed by Gordon Willard Allport (1897–1967), that emphasized the influence not only of the subject's personality but also of the social demands to which he must conform. Allport doubted that the therapeutic discovery of infantile motivations would always be effective, and he favored the idea of challenging the relevance of those earlier forces to current behavior in group therapy experiences.

Alternate session. A regularly scheduled meeting of a therapy group held without the therapist. The technique was introduced by Alexander Wolf.

Alternating role. Inconsistency of social behavior or switching from one type of behavior to another, as from giving to taking, leading to following. Alternation of role can often be observed among participants in a therapy group, where such changes can be used to promote insight and initiate modification of self-limiting behavior patterns.

Alternatives, illusion of. A type of strategic intervention in which the patient is presented with two alternatives, either one of which is likely to initiate change in his behavior, such as asking him, "When will you tell your superintendent about your feelings, this week or next?"

Ambivalence. Coexistence of antithetic feelings (ambivalence of affect, the most common form), ideas (ambivalence of intellect), or impulses (ambivalence or the will). Everyone has ambivalence to some degree, at least in some areas, but it is seen clearly to be abnormal when both sides of an ambivalent attitude coexist in consciousness and the subject seems aware of the incongruity or when the ambivalent subject tries in a single action to give vent to both sides of an ambivalent impulse.

Analytic psychodrama. A technique that employs the therapeutic stage to bring a patient's underlying psychic process and conflicts to expression. The analyst observes the action as a member of the audience and later comments on it with the purpose of clarifying, promoting insight, and interpreting the material that has been produced.

Ancillary group. A form of group therapy that is used as an adjunctive or accessory part of a comprehenisve treatment program, usually with a defined task to accomplish (such as discussion of the anxieties the group members feel about discharge plans).

Antiexpectation technique. A type of paradoxical or strategic intervention in which the therapist expresses an attitude about the patient's symptom(s) that appears to encourage and reinforce them, rather than the more usual approach of urging the patient to join forces with the therapist in resisting or ignoring them. Some authors refer to this technique as paradoxical positioning.

Attitude. A predisposition to act, think, judge, or believe in a specific direction. One of the early functions of group

therapy is to help each participant recognize his attitudes, to explore how they have affected his relationships in the past, and to experiment with different attitudes in his intragroup exchanges.

Attitude therapy. Originally, an indirect method of child therapy in which disturbed parental attitudes were the main focus of therapy sessions. Currently, a type of reeducative therapy, often utilized in groups, that focuses on the patient's distorted attitudes and finding more harmonious or less abrasive substitutes for them.

Authority figure. A person, group, or idea that exerts power or command over others; such a person's power may be illusory more than real because, more than anything else, it is a projection onto him of the authority the subservient one's parent (especially the father) exerted during the childhood years. Such irrational authority may be the source of a cult's blind obedience to their leader, who may himself need and crave such power, whether or not he warrants it by reason of his competence or skill.

Authority principle. The theory that in an organization each member complies with what he assumes or fantasizes are the wishes of his superior and, in turn, exerts the same kind of irrational authority on those below him in the hierarchical scale. One goal of sensitivity training or T-groups in organizations was to open channels of communication between all participants and thereby reduce the irrationality of decision making and the automaton quality of workers' performances.

Autoplasty. Adaptation achieved through alteration of the self, rather than alteration of the external world.

Auxiliary ego. In psychodrama, a person (usually a trained member of the staff) who consciously identifies with the subject's needs and expressions to promote more adequate presentation of the subject's situation. The auxiliary ego is an extension or prolongation of the subject's own ego, lending strength when that is necessary and assisting, sometimes in a concrete way and at other times in a symbolic way, in bringing the subject to a more complete presentation of his world. The auxiliary ego may emphasize the subject's unconscious wishes, his unrecognized assets, his disguised inadequacies, and even his hallucinations or delusions if that will help to portray more accurately and more concretely the subject's psychodramatic world.

Aversion therapy. Negative conditioning, a form of behavior therapy in which painful or unpleasant situations are consistently paired with the undesirable behavior (e.g., smoking, alcohol overindulgence, overeating) until the latter is suppressed or eliminated. Many styles of aversion therapy use group techniques as ancillary aids in their attack on the behavior they aim to eliminate.

Basic anxiety. According to Karen Horney, a feeling of loneliness and helplessness toward a potentially hostile world and the origin of the intensity and pervasiveness of neurotic trends.

Basic mistakes. According to Alfred Adler, the childhood concepts and attitudes that have molded one's lifestyle that therapy must correct if it is to be successful.

Basic skills training. Education in leadership functions, communication, relatedness, openness to new ideas, experimentation with new approaches, and other interpersonal methods and group techniques. In the T-group or sensitivity group, such training aims to replace automaton conformity with a willingness to take risks and thereby promote effective decision making within the organization to which the participants belong.

Behavior therapy. An empirical approach to treatment that emphasizes overt behavior, rather than understanding of unconscious conflicts, and directs itself to the inhibition or extinction of neurotic symptoms through a variety of techniques based on behavior and learning theory. Among those specific techniques are reciprocal innervation and systematic desensitization, aversion therapy, assertiveness training, flooding, implosion, exposure in vivo, contingency contracting, anxiety management training, social skills training, covert sensitization, overcorrection, biofeedback, shaping, and symptom substitution.

Behavioral group psychotherapy. Any form of treatment that focuses on external behavior, rather than internal feelings, in an attempt to achieve symptom alleviation through alteration of maladaptive habits. If a stereotypic repetition of "tsk, tsk, tsk," for example, causes others to avoid a person who complains that he cannot get along with people, the therapeutic task is to stop the "tsk, tsk, tsk" and not worry about how it got started or what it may mean unconsciously. Behavioral group psychotherapy combines conditioning and anxiety-eliminating techniques with didactic discussions, based on learning (behavior) theory.

Bibliotherapy. The use of books or other reading material as a significant portion of the total treatment program. The reading matter is suggested by the therapist on the basis of the particular needs of the patient.

Bioenergetic group psychotherapy. The use of various body exercises to promote coordination of physical with mental functioning and to facilitate verbal interchange and the expression of feeling. The method was developed by Alexander Lowen.

Blank screen. The neutral backdrop presented by the classical psychoanalytic treatment setting that invites maximal projection of the patient's transference attitudes onto the relationship with the analyst, and minimizes the likelihood that the patient's feelings will be reactions to the real aspects of the therapist's personality. The passivity of the analyst and his apparent lack of reactivity to the patient's productions encourage the development of the transference neurosis.

Blind self. The aspects of a person that he is unaware of, even though they are known and recognized by those around him. The blind self is one quadrant of the Johari Window, a diagrammatic conceptualization of human behavior.

Boundary. A defined border of line of demarcation between one element or system and another; in group therapy, any physical or psychological factor that separates the group from the surrounding environment (an external boundary) or one that separates members of a group from one another. A major internal boundary is one that in some way separates the group leader from the rest of the group; a minor internal boundary separates members of the group from other members of subgroups.

Brief psychotherapy. Any form of individual or group therapy that is time limited, usually to a maximum of 20 sessions. Short-term therapy, as it is also called, is usually active, directive, circumscribed in its goals, and focused on immediate crises and the here and now, rather than on the genetic-developmental antecedents of attitude and personality traits.

Casualty. In group therapy, a subject whose group experience had a psychologically destructive effect on him.

Category method. A technique of structured interactional group psychotherapy in which members are asked to rate each other verbally on appearance, intelligence, relatedness, and any number of other qualities.

Catharsis. Release or discharge of unconscious material in actions and behavior accompanied by appropriate affective or emotional response. Such a breakthrough may occur in group or individual therapy and is generally perceived as a lifting of oppressive tension by the patient.

Cathexis. Investment or concentration of psychic energy onto an idea, an object, or its intrapsychic representation.

Chain-reaction phenomenon. Passing of information from one therapy group to another, with resultant loss of confidentiality. It occurs when members of different groups have the opportunity to socialize with one another.

Choreography, family. A technique adapted from psychodrama for use in family therapy to help in clarification of nonverbal manifestations of family relationships. Closely related is a techniqe called family sculpting.

Clarification. In transactional analysis, the attainment of control by the Adult ego state so that the patient understands what he is doing, is able to monitor the effect of his hidden Parent and Child ego states on what he is doing, and can decide whether or not to continue his games.

Class method. An instructional type of group therapy in which the leader, teacher, or lecturer provides information to patients and encourages them to adhere to their prescribed treatment regimen. The method was first used by Joseph Pratt in Boston, with his tuberculous patients.

Client-centered psychotherapy. A type of counseling, devised by Carl Rogers, predicated on the belief that the client's inherent potential for growth needs only to be released by the counselor for improvement to occur. It is also known as nondirective therapy.

Closed group. A treatment group that forbids the introduction of new members once treatment has begun.

Clouding of consciousness. Defective awareness or disturbed ability to maintain level of attention. Differing degrees of clouding include inattentiveness, preoccupation, and semistuporous or semicomatose states, any of which is suggestive of underlying organic disorder.

Coercive expectations. A reaction of some group therapy members who become therapeutic casualties; they feel unable to meet what they interpret as the demands of the leader or other members to display emotions and come to feel that they are shallow, artificial, emotionally void, or lacking in some other basic way.

Coexistent culture. Any system of values, perceptions, or behavior patterns that is different from one's own. The group therapy experience promotes acceptance of such different systems as acceptable alternatives to a member's own system.

Cognitive behavior therapy. Derived from the work of Ellis, Wolpe, Eysenck, Beck, and Lazarus, an approach based on the assumption that the person's faulty ways of thinking and perceiving reality determine his disorder and not his behavior *per se.*

Cognitive responses. In cognitive therapy, the evaluative labels a person attaches to self-perceptions or perceptions of reality. Such labels are powerful antecedents in that they make it probable that the person will react to a situation according to the way he has labeled it, rather than as it exists. Thus, a person who has labeled himself "a loser" tends to see only the negative, self-defeating side of situations, and that in turn perpetuates self-defeating behavior.

Collaborative therapy. Marital therapy conducted by two therapists, each of whom sees one of the spouses. Usually, the therapists confer frequently with one another and thereby gain a double view of each spouse—that given by the husband, for example, to his therapist and that given by the wife's therapist on the basis of what she has reported about her husband.

Collective experience. The emotions and reactions shared by participants in a group, including the identifications, mutual support, reduction of ego defenses, sibling transferences, and empathy that promote the therapeutic process by helping the individual to become integrated within the group. One function of the group leader is to prevent the collective experience from submerging individuality or from being used by a member as a means of escape from his own autonomy and responsibility.

Collective family transference neurosis. Projection of irrational feelings and thoughts onto other members of the group by a participant who transfers family psychopathology from his early childhood into the therapeutic group situation. Psychoanalytic group therapy focuses on the interpretation and analysis of such transference phenomena.

Combined therapy. The use of more than one form of treatment for a patient, such as the simultaneous use of group therapy and individual therapy with either the same or different therapists. In marriage therapy, for example, married couples group therapy is often combined with individual sessions with one spouse or with conjoint sessions with the marital pair.

Coming on. The appearance or the assumed reasons or motives for acting in a certain way. In transactional analysis, for example, the person who points his finger and says "should" is often labeled as coming on Parent; that is, the particular way in which he presents himself is assumed to reflect the Parent ego state.

Common group tension. The anxiety level of the group as a whole, to which each participant contributes by projecting his unconscious fantasies onto the other members of the group and trying to manipulate them accordingly. The group therapist effects change by interpreting the projections and the attempts at manipulation.

Communion. The act of joining with one or more others, as in participating in an organization or group and becoming integrated with it. In group therapy, both leader and member must experience communion if the experience is to be successful.

Communion-oriented group psychotherapy. A type of group therapy that emphasizes the development of a spirit of unity and cohesiveness among members, rather than performance of a task.

Complementarity of interaction. Harmony or balance in relationships between people. No person is only a responder to what goes on around him; he is also an instigator and a stimulator. In consequence, the void created by the passivity of one person is likely to be filled by the activity of another, and the balance thereby achieved is termed complementarity of interaction.

Compliance, strategic. In paradoxical therapy, change that is a result of the patient's acceptance of or obedience to the therapist's request or directive.

Composition. Make-up of a group, often defined in terms of sex, age, cultural or ethnic background, or type of psychopathology.

Concretization of living. In psychodrama, the actualization of life in the therapeutic setting, with integration of time, space, reality, and cosmos.

Concurrent therapy. A type of family therapy in which the therapist is the same for two or more of the family's members, although each of them is seen separately in therapy sessions.

Confidentiality. In a treatment situation, the secrecy accorded a patient's productions and the steps taken to ensure that his privacy will be protected. Confidentiality is both a tradition of medical ethics and a matter of legal definition, which varies from one jurisdiction or state to another. In general, the ethic of confidentiality is assumed to apply to the members of a group to the same degree to which it applies to the therapist or group leader, subject to the laws of the land and the decisions of the appropriate court.

Confirmation. In transactional analysis, the repetition of confrontation that may be initiated by the patient himself.

Conflict. Battle or struggle between opposing forces. In a group, the conflict may be between members or between one or more members and the leader. The latter is particularly likely to reflect the significant intrapsychic conflicts of the group member.

Conflict-free area. Any portion of the personality or ego that is well integrated and smoothly functioning, in contrast to those portions where clashes between opposing forces give rise to displeasure or symptoms. The conflict-free areas are a source of strength to the person and are more likely to be exposed, and thus subject to analysis, in group therapy than in individual therapy.

Confrontation. Forceful presentation of facts, observations, evidence, conclusions, etc., with an insistence or demand that the patient give his attention to what is being presented. Used in group and individual therapy, the technique is often a potent force in effecting behavioral and attitudinal changes. The material presented typically involves letting the patient know how others see him and how he affects them and, thus, himself. Although a threatening or hostile attack on the patient, such potentially negative elements are tempered by the spirit of deep involvement and meliorative intervention that motivate the therapist or other members of the group to utilize the maneuver.

Conjoint therapy. A form of marriage therapy in which the therapist sees the two partners simultaneously, in the same session. Because there are three people involved, conjoint therapy is sometimes called triadic or triangular therapy.

Consensual validation. Confirmation of the reality of a thought, perception, or interpretation by comparing one's own conceptualization with others'. In group therapy, group members tend continually to compare their feelings and reactions, and the consensual validation thereby achieved may modify and correct interpersonal distortions. The term was introduced by Harry Stack Sullivan; Trigant Burrow had used the phrase "consensual observation" to refer to the same phenomenon.

Consequence. In behavior therapy, the result or after effect of action that itself becomes a modifier of that action or affects the likelihood of its repetition. When the consequence of behavior increases the likelihood that the same behavior will be repeated, it is termed a reinforcer or reward; when the consequence decreases the likelihood that the same behavior will be repeated, it is an extinguisher, and the process of punishment or extinction is in operation.

Contamination. In transactional analysis, acceptance by the Adult ego state the attitudes, prejudices, and standards that originated in a Parent or Child ego state as facts. Instead of recognizing them for what they are, the Adult ego state incorporates them uncritically as part of its own information base.

Conversational catharsis. Emotional release through verbal interchange, such as occurs in both individual and group psychotherapy.

Corrective emotional experience.   A type of brief psychotherapy, introduced by Franz Alexander, in which the therapist encourages the patient to relive an emotional experience that was traumatic in the past, on the assumption that the guidance, support, and reality testing afforded by the therapist will foster more effective coping and mastery of the situation than was possible when it was originally experienced.

Co-therapy.   A form of psychotherapy with more than one therapist treating the individual or group. It is also known as combined therapy, cooperative therapy, dual leadership, multiple therapy, and three-cornered therapy.

Countertransference.   The therapist's reactions to a patient that are based on the therapist's unconscious needs and conflicts, rather than on the patient's needs. An example of countertransference occurs when an analyst unearths in every patient the impulses and conflicts that he cannot recognize in himself.

Co-worker.   A professional or paraprofessional who works in the same clinical service setting.

Crisis intervention group psychotherapy.   Group therapy with a focus on transitional-developmental and accidental-situational demands for novel adaptational responses, such as helping the survivors of a disaster cope with their reactions to the traumatic events.

Crystallization.   In transactional analysis, a definition or summarization by the Adult or the therapist of the patient's position to the latter's Adult ego state.

Cultural conserve.   Social heritage; the repository of a group's creative achievements that serves as a guide to conduct in the present, as well as a sculptor of accomplishments in the future.

Dance therapy.   The use of rhythmical body movement in rehabilitation of people with emotional or physical disorders. Dance therapy was introduced by Marian Chase in 1940, and has been used in both individual and group therapy.

Day hospital.   A clinical setting that provides a full range of hospital-related services for use by the patient during the day. The patient returns home at night.

Decision.   In transactional analysis, a childhood commitment to a life style based on the verbal and nonverbal messages received from parenting figures about how to behave. Such decisions are incorporated into thinking and feeling and become the entire life pattern of the person.

Decontamination.   In transactional analysis, freeing a person from the interferences with optimal functioning by the Parent or Child ego state.

Defense mechanism.   An unconscious process that develops in the ego as a way of protecting against anxiety or conflict that might otherwise overwhelm it.

Defiance-based strategy.   A form of paradoxical therapy whose use is based on the expectation that the patient will rebel against a directive or resist the therapist's influence. One of the pioneers in the development of such an approach was Jay Haley.

Derivative insight.   Spontaneous insight that the patient achieves on his own, without interpretation by the therapist. Derivative insight is characteristic of activity therapy groups.

Deviance.   Deviation; variance; abnormality. In group therapy, deviance is sometimes used to refer specifically to the group's perception or evaluation of one member as being different or unacceptable, often because that member demonstrates behavior in opposition to the norms of the group. The group tries at first to influence the deviant member to conform; if he does not conform, he may be ejected from the group or isolated psychologically from it, even though allowed to remain.

Devil's pact.   A compliance-induction procedure of paradoxical therapy employed by the Palo Alto group in which the patient is induced to promise that he will carry out a plan before he is told what the plan is.

Diagnostic and Statistical Manual of Mental Disorders.   The classification and nomenclature system authorized by the American Psychiatric Association. The World Health Association publishes the International Classification of Diseases (ICD) that is in general use throughout the world. The ninth edition (ICD-9) is the most recent and became effective in 1979. ICD-9-CM is a Clinical Modification developed for use in the United States. The most recent (1980) edition of the *Diagnostic and Statistical Manual* (DSM-III) is generally compatible with the mental disorders section of ICD-9-CM. In some areas, however, DSM-III is more detailed and reflects more recent clinical data; in addition, it provides a multiaxial coding system that ICD-9-CMK does not use.

Didactic technique.   Emphasis on tutorial methods in group therapy, as advocated by J. M. Klapman. Textbooks, outlines, and audiovisual aids are used to teach participants about themselves and their functioning.

Differential reinforcement.   A technique of behavior therapy that, in addition to reward or reinforcement of desired behavior, utilizes extinction of punishment for problem behavior.

Dilution of transference.   Reduced concentration of transference projections onto the therapist that some believe occurs routinely in group therapy because some or many of those projections are directed instead to other members of the group.

Direct analysis.   A technique advocated by John Rosen in which the patient was encouraged to re-enact aspects of his acutely psychotic phase.

Directive-didactic approach.   In group therapy, emphasis on guided discussions and other educational methods, as well as active involvement of the therapist in making suggestions and planning for the patient. Such an approach is often used with regressed, hospitalized patients.

Discussion model.   In group therapy, a technique that emphasizes rational understanding of problems, attained through deliberations over problems, their probable explanations, and their possible solutions.

Dissociation.   An unconscious defense mechanism consisting of separation of an idea from its accompanying affect or of splitting off a group of mental processes from the rest of the person's thinking. The split-off portion may then operate with relative autonomy, as in the case of double or multiple personality.

Distortion.   Disguising or modifying unconscious material that would otherwise be denied entrance to consciousness; misinterpretation or misrepresentation of reality, as is typical in presenting the history of one's development, childhood incidents, and memories.

Distractibility.   Rapid, uncontrolled shifting of ideas and attention, seen commonly in mania and also in organic mental disorders.

Divorce therapy.   The principles and methods of treating couples contemplating divorce or coping with its consequences.

Dominant member.   The person in a group who tends to monopolize certain group sessions or situations.

Double bind.   A dilemma produced when contradictory, incongruent, and mutually exclusive messages emanate from the same source. Originally described by Gregory Bateson, the double-bind occurs frequently, although not exclusively, in familes of schizophrenic patients. Example: A mother gives her son two ties for his birthday, and, when he appears wearing one of them the next morning, she asks, in an aggrieved tone, "What was wrong with the other tie I gave you?"

Double-bind, therapeutic. Application of the double-bind type of communication to the therapeutic situation by enjoining the patient to change by remaining unchanged; if he complies and remains unchanged, he demonstrates that he can, in fact, control the situation, whereas, if he defies by changing, he has accomplished the purpose of therapy.

Double-blind. Referring to a type of drug research in which neither the person receiving the medication nor the clinician rating its effect knows whether the medication administered is the drug under study or a placebo.

Drug therapy. Treatment with pharmacological agents or chemical substances; chemotherapy.

Dual-sex therapy. A form of psychotherapy developed by William Masters and Virginia Johnson for the treatment of sexual disorders. A core feature of the method is the round-table session including a male therapist, a female therapist, and the couple in treatment.

Dyad. A pair of interacting persons, such as husband and wife or therapist and patient.

Dyadic session. Individual therapy involving only two persons, therapist and patient.

East Coast-style T-group. A group that follows the traditional National Training Laboratories model, with focus on awareness of group process. The first T-groups were held in Bethel, Maine.

Ego. In the structural hypothesis of psychoanalytic psychology, one of the three subdivisions of the psyche, the other two being id and superego. The major tasks of the ego include reality testing, replacement of the primary process of the id by the secondary process, and cognitive functions, including perception, memory, and thinking. Among the mechanisms the ego develops to accomplish its various tasks are the defense mechanisms that assist it in controlling drive energy in the ego's mediation between the person and reality.

Ego model. A person after whom another person patterns himself. In group therapy, a member with a weak ego often takes the therapist or a healthier group member as a model. In psychodrama, the auxiliary ego may act as the ego model.

Emotional support. Encouragement, hope, exhortation, and inspiration given by one or more people to another. Members of a therapy group often give such support to another member who needs encouragment in trying a new mode of behavior or in facing some truth about himself.

Empathy. Capacity to put oneself into the psychological frame of reference of another person and thereby understand his thinking, feelings, and behavior. Empathy is believed to be a major element in success as a therapist, facilitator, or helpful group member.

Enactment. Under the direction of the therapist, the carrying out of behavioral tasks that have direct bearing on the patient's or family's problems. The family of a patient with anorexia nervosa, for example, may be asked to have lunch together while the therapist observes their interactions.

Encounter group. An outgrowth of sensitivity training that emphasizes how individual relationships are experienced within the group, in the here and now, rather than concentrating on the past or the outside problems of its members. J. L. Moreno introduced and developed the idea of the encounter group in 1914 and recognized it as a complex psychosocial system.

Encounter tapes. Tape recordings to provide leaderless, self-directed groups with guidelines for progressive interaction that will engender a nonthreatening and cohesive climate. The taped program may include structured exercises in interrelating among the group as a whole, between pairs, or among other subsets within the group.

Esalen encounter group. An eclectic form of encounter group developed at the Esalen Institute, a growth center at Big Sur, California. It emphasizes limiting somatic restrictions that ordinarily inhibit the development and deepening of interpersonal relationships.

Existential group psychotherapy. A technique that emphasizes here-and-now interaction and confrontation and feeling experiences, rather than rational thinking.

Expanded group. The social network to which the patient relates outside a formal therapy group. It includes immediate family, friends, and interested relatives.

Extended family therapy. A type of family therapy that involves family members beyond the nuclear family because of their association with and influence on the family itself.

Facilitator. A group leader, who may be the therapist or a patient, who emerges during the course of an encounter and channels group interaction. The facilitator is also called the session leader.

Family diagnosis. Assessment and evaluation of the family unit and of its members, not only in terms of specific mental disorders that may exist but also in terms of how the family functions.

Family homeostasis. Maintenance of the family as a functioning unit, reflective of a systems approach which maintains that change in any individual member of the family is not possible without change in the rest of the family. A derivative of that concept is the belief that change in a family will alter the balance between its members and will effect changes in the pathology of individual members of the family.

Family neurosis. Emotional disorder or psychopathology of one member of a family that reflects the interrelationships within the family as a whole.

Family therapy. Treatment of a family with conflicts as a unit, rather than individual treatment of one or more members of the family. The therapist meets with the whole family to explore its relationships and style of functioning. Focus is on resolution of current reactions to one another, rather than individual symptoms.

Father surrogate. Substitute for the father or the internalized representation of the father. In psychoanalysis, the patient may project his father image onto the analyst and respond to the latter unconsciously in an inappropriate and unrealistic manner, with feelings and attitudes held for the real father.

Feedback. Information given to a person about the nature and effects of his behavior; communication to the sender of the effect his original message had on those to whom it was relayed.

Feeling-driven group. A group in which little attention is given to rational processes, thinking, or cognition and in which the expression of any kind of emotion is rewarded.

Field theory. Kurt Lewin's hypothesis that a person is a complex energy field in which all behavior can be viewed as a change in some state of the field during a given unit of time. Lewin also postulated the existence of psychological tension within the field, expressed in states of readiness or preparation for action. The field theory is primarily concerned with the present field, the here and now, and it has been used as a point of departure for many theorists in group psychotherapy.

Fixed membership. A closed group in which no new patients are added in the course of treatment or after treatment has proceeded for a set period.

Flashback. Hallucinosis consisting of the spontaneous recurrence, after a drug-free period, of hallucinations similar to those experienced during an acute toxic episode. It is often associated with repeated LSD use. The hallucinations are predominantly visual and may last for months after the last use of the drug.

Focal psychotherapy. Short-term, brief psychotherapy that is limited to the exploration and resolution of a specific area of intrapsychic conflict.

Focused exercise. Encounter group technique used to break through participants' defensive behavior and help them to express their feelings of anger, affection, joy, etc. In similar fashion, psychodrama may focus on a specific problem that a participant has with his wife. In playing out both his part and her part, he becomes aware of the emotion he has been blocking.

Forced interaction. Behavior that occurs within a group setting because the therapist or other members demand that the particular patient respond, react, and be active.

Free association. The fundamental technique of psychoanalysis devised by Freud, in which the patient is urged to tell the analyst everything that comes to his mind, to leave out nothing, regardless of whether he thinks it relevant or not. The conflicts that emerge while attempting to fulfill this mandate consitute resistances that are the basis of the analytic interpretations.

Freud, Sigmund (1856-1939). Austrian psychiatrist and found of psychoanalysis. With Josef Breuer, he explored the potentialities of catharsis as therapy and then developed psychoanalysis as a technique of investigating the mind, as a method of treatment for psychological disorders, and as a system of psychology. He introduced such fundamental concepts as unconscious, infantile sexuality, repression, sublimation, id, ego, superego, Oedipus complex, and transference.

Fulfillment. Satisfaction of needs, whether real or illusory.

Future projection. Psychodrama technique in which the patient demonstrates what he believes his life will be like in the future. He chooses, sometimes with the help of the director, the point in time, the place, and the people with whom he expects to be involved.

Gallows transaction. A transaction in which a person with a self-destructive script smiles while narrating or performing a self-destructive act. His smile evokes a smile in the listener, which in turn encourages his self-destructive behavior.

Game analysis. In transactional analysis, exploring and exposing the ulterior messages that go on between people. People actively seek stimulation, but often that stimulation is not socially condoned and must be attained in deviant ways. The sought-after stimulation or payoff is often not clearly understood by the Adult of the acting person, a game analysis attempts to reveal the games that go on between the subject and other people.

Gestalt therapy. A type of psychotherapy that emphasizes heightened emotionality, understanding the autonomic and musculoskeletal messages transmitted by the body, and helping the patient get in touch with the primitive wisdom of the body. It was developed by Fritz Perls and is used in both individual and group therapy. Change is viewed as a subintellectual process, and the here-and-now

as all important. Gestalt therapy employs role playing and other techniques to promote the patient's growth process and to develop his full potential.

Go-around. A group therapy technique in which the therapist directs each member of the group to respond in turn to another member, a theme, a statement, etc., as a way of encouraging participation by all members in the group session.

God complex. A belief that one can accomplish more than is humanly possible or that one's word should not be doubted. The God complex of the aging psychoanalyst was first discussed by Ernest Jones, Freud's biographer.

Group action technique. Use of the group to help participants achieve skills in interpersonal relations and improve their capacity to perform certain tasks better on the job or at home. Physical interaction is often employed to enhance involvement or communion within a new group.

Group analysand. A person in treatment in a psychoanalytically oriented group.

Group analytic psychotherapy. S. H. Foulkes's term for his method of therapeutic group analysis in which the group is used as the principal therapeutic agent and all communications and relationships are viewed as part of a total field of interaction. Interventions deal primarily with group forces, rather than individual forces.

Group apparatus. Guardian(s) of a group, those who preserve order and ensure the group's survival. The internal apparatus focuses on intragroup cohesiveness; the external apparatus focuses on the environment to minimize the threat of external pressure. In a small therapy group, the therapist usually serves as his own apparatus, just as a teacher keeps order in the schoolroom. The therapist usually acts as his own external apparatus also by setting the time and place for meetings and making certain that outsiders do not interfere.

Group balance. The result of grouping patients in accordance with clinical and personal criteria, in order to prevent intensification of a specific problem.

Group bibliotherapy. Use of selected readings as stimulus material for group participants. Outside readings and presentations by the therapist or patients of written material encourage verbal interchange in the sessions and hold the attention of severely regressed patients. This technique is particularly useful in treating large groups of institutionalized patients.

Group-centered psychotherapy. A short-term, nonclinical form of group therapy developed by followers of Carl Rogers and based on his client-centered method of individual treatment. The therapist maintains a nonjudgmental attitude, clarifies the feelings expressed in the sessions, and communicates empathic understanding and respect. The participants' disorders are not diagnosed, and uncovering techniques are not employed.

Group climate. Emotional tone and general atmosphere or feel of a group therapy session.

Group cohesion. Effect of the mutual bonds between members of a group resulting from their concerted effort toward a common goal. Until cohesiveness is achieved, the group cannot concentrate its full energy on a common task.

Group dynamics. The sum total of all the interactions between members of the group—termed by some, group process—plus the structure that evolves from such ongoing interaction. The group equilibrium is constantly changing because of the tensions aroused by interrelations between different members and the therapist. Various phases of group development have been identified: orientation of members to the group; learning to trust the therapist; trying to manipulate the therapist to satisfy dependency needs; rebellious anger toward the therapist when those needs are not met and a turning to other members of the group; gaining independence from the therapist and, finally, independence and separation from the group. Each of those phases is highly influenced by individual participants' psychological make-up, unconscious drives, motives, and fantasies. The understanding and effective use of group dynamics is essential in group treatment.

Group grope. Belittling reference to some of the body manipulation procedures advocated by certain encounter groups. The procedures are aimed at providing emotional release through physical contact.

Group growth. Development of trust and cohesiveness in a group, leading to increased awareness of self and of group inter-relationships and to more effective coping with conflict and intimacy problems.

Group history. Chronology of the experiences of a group, including the rituals, traditions, and themes that have developed during its existence.

Group marathon. Group meeting that typically lasts between 8 and 72 hours and is interrupted only for eating and sleeping. The leader encourages the development of intimacy and open expression of feelings, and the time-extended group experience tends to heighten and intensify feelings of excitement and elation. The participant often describes a peak experience that he views as a turning point in his life when the experience is successful. Encounter group leaders tend to support such a view and believe that the intense togetherness induced by the method can effect more far-reaching changes than can be produced by years of less intensive treatment.

Group marital therapy. A type of marriage therapy that uses the group for implementation of its two basic techniques: (1) The marital partner of a group member is invited to a group session, thus affording the participants new insights and awareness as they observe the neurotic interactions of the marital partners. (2) A husband and wife are placed together in a traditional group as a way of encouraging more meaningful intimacy by reassuring them that they will not lose their individual identities within the marriage any more than they have within the group.

Group mind. The dynamic structure of the group emanating from the group process, consisting of an autonomous and unified mental life in an assemblage of people bound together by mutual interests. It is a concept used by group therapists who focus on the group as a unit, rather than on its individual members.

Group mobility. Spontaneity, modifiability, adaptability, and emotional growth within the group brought about by changes in the functions and roles of individual members, relative to their progress.

Group-on-group technique. A T-group technique in which one group observes a second group in action and then gives it feedback on what has been observed. The technique is often applied within the group by breaking it into two sections, each taking turns watching the other in action. The device is used to sharpen participants' awareness of individual behavior and group process.

Group pressure. Influence exerted by group members as a whole on individual members. Acting as a unified force, the group is able to wield considerable power in demanding that a member conform to its standards and values.

Group psychotherapy. A form of treatment for problems assumed to be emotional in nature in which a specially trained practitioner deliberately establishes a professional relationship with a size-limited group of patients for the purpose of using their interaction as a means of removing, modifying, or retarding existing symptoms; of attenuating or reversing disturbed patterns of behavior; and of promoting positive personality growth and development in the participants who have been specifically selected for this purpose.

Group resistance. Collective repression; avoidance by individual participants and by the group as a whole of unconscious material, emotions or old patterns of defense.

Group ritual. Tradition or activity that any group establishes as a standard operating procedure or routine way of performing its functions.

Group stimulus. The effect on the group of several members' communicating with each other. Each member has a stimulating effect on every other member of the group, and the total stimulation is studied for therapeutic purposes.

Group tradition. Activity or value established historically by a group. It determines, in part, the group's manifest behavior.

Group value. Relative worth or standard developed by and agreed on by members of a group.

Hallucinatory psychodrama. A type of psychodrama in which the patient portrays the voices he hears and the visions he sees. Auxiliary egos may be called on to enact the different phenomena expressed by the patient and to involve him in interaction with them, so as to put them to a reality test. The intended effect on the patient is called psychodramatic shock.

Hamartic script. In transactional analysis, a self-destructive, tragic life script.

Herd instinct. Desire to belong to a group and to participate in social activities. Wilfred Trotter used the term to indicate the presence of a hypothetical social instinct in humans. Psychoanalysis views the herd instinct as a social phenomenon, rather than a basic drive or instinct.

Here and now. Contemporaneity, characteristic of many group approaches that emphasize current behavior, rather than the historical-genetic origins of attitudes, feelings, etc.

Here-and-now approach. A technique that focuses on understanding the interpersonal and intrapersonal responses and reactions as they occur in the ongoing treatment session. Past history and experiences are de-emphasized.

Heterogeneous group. A group comprising members from both sexes, with a wide age range, differing psychopathologies, and divergent socioeconomic, racial, ethnic, and cultural backgrounds.

Hierarchical vector. The style of relating to people, to other members of a group, or to the therapist as described on a supraordinate-subordinate continuum. It is also known as vertical vector to emphasize the up or down, dominant or submissive aspect and is contrasted with the horizontal vector or peer vector.

Homogeneous group. A group consisting of patients of the same sex and age range, with similar pathologies and socioeconomic, racial, ethnic, and cultural backgrounds.

Hook. In transactional analysis, to switch one's transactions to a new ego state. For example, a person's Adult state is hooked when he goes to the blackboard and draws a diagram.

Horizontal vector. The style of relating to people, to other members of a group, and to the therapist as equals. It is also known as peer vector.

Hot seat. A technique of Gestalt therapy in which the leader works with one member of the group while the other members watch. Fritz Perls kept empty the seat beside him, and members took their turn in sitting in that hot seat for intensive work with the leader. Although participation by other members was minimal in Perls's groups, most Gestalt therapists today encourage wider participation by all members. Group interactions provide participants an opportunity to confront the internal contradictions of their characteristic ways of behaving, and those experiments in relating combine with contactfulness and awareness to form the core principles of Gestalt group therapy.

House encounter. Group meeting of all the persons in a treatment facility in order to deal with problems that have arisen within the therapeutic community, such as poor morale and poor job performances.

Humanistic psychology. An orientation that emphasizes common human needs, and views a human being as uniquely creative and controlled by his own values and choices. People care not only about whether they are sick but also how they can exercise their power to gain a voice in formulating the policies and regulations that affect them. Therapy is not an end in itself, nor is it only preparatory for some future event; it is a valid and relevant experiential moment. The therapist is a participant in the therapeutic process, and he himself changes during the course of therapy. In such a viewpoint, the group experience is more than treatment; it is a growth experience, aimed at finding better forms of living. Through experiential means, each person can develop his greatest potential or self-actualization. Humanistic psychology is related to the human potential movement and its encounter groups, growth centers, etc.

Hypnodrama. Psychodrama with the patient in a hypnotic trance, during which he is encouraged to act out the various experiences that appear to him or to the therapist to be of particular significance.

I-boundary. The limits within which the subject is willing and free to engage and make contact with other people, ideas, settings, values, etc.

Id. In the structural hypothesis of psychoanalytic psychology, one of the three subdivisions of the psyche, the other two being ego and superego. The id is completely unconscious and is governed by the pleasure principle and the primary process. It contains the psychic representation of the drives and of all the phylogenetic acquisitions.

Ideational shield. A type of rationalization in which the person develops attitudes and behavior patterns that protect him from criticism and rejection. Criticizing another person is unacceptable to him, for example, because of his deep fear that he will be rejected. Both group and individual therapy encourage the recognition of such patterns and provide a setting in which the shield may be dropped and the deeper conflicts dealt with directly.

Identification. An unconscious defense mechanism in which the person incorporates another person or object into his ego system and then acts toward the object as if it had originated from within the self, rather than having been taken from without.

I-It. Martin Buber's term for a damaging type of interpersonal relationship in which the self and other people are treated exclusively as objects. Such an approach prevents mutuality, trust, and growth, and in a group it prevents human warmth, destroys cohesiveness, and retards group process.

Illusion of alternatives. A form of compliance-induction procedure used in strategic intervention in which the patient is offered a choice between two actions, but carrying out either one will constitute a change. It is associated with the work of Milton Erickson.

Illustration. In transactional analysis, an anecdote, analogy, or other concrete example used to reinforce a confrontation or make it more acceptable to the subject. Depending on the situation, an illustration may be chosen from something remote in time or in distance from the group, or it may be taken from an immediate or recent experience within the group.

Imitation. Conscious emulation or modeling of one's behavior after that of another.

Improvement scale. A quantitative assessment of positive response to therapy. Various rating scales have been devised to objectify and assess the effectiveness of different treatment methods so that feedback concerning results can be used in the development of better approaches.

Improvisation. In psychodrama, the acting out of problems without prior preparation or rehearsal.

Impulse control disorders. A group of disorders with the following characteristics: (1) The impulse is ego-syntonic; (2) it contains a pleasurable component; (3) there is minimal distortion of the original form of the impulse; and (4) it possesses a quality of irresistibility. In DSM-III, the group comprises pathological gambling, kleptomania, pyromania, and explosive disorders.

Inappropriate affect. A feeling tone that is out of harmony with the ideas of the subject or incongruent with the situation. It is sometimes termed a splitting of affect from intellect.

Inclusion phase. The early dependency stage of group therapy when each member's concern is with belonging and acceptance, especially by the therapist.

Incorporation. An unconscious defense mechanism and primitive form of introjection, consisting of assimilating an object into oneself through symbolic oral ingestion. It is the primary mechanism of identification.

Individual therapy. Dyadic psychotherapy in which one trained person deliberately establishes a professional relationship with one patient for the purpose of removing, modifying, or retarding existing symptoms, attenuating disturbed patterns of behavior, and promoting positive personality growth and development.

Infrareality. Latent content, the things that are going on beneath the surface. According to J. L. Moreno, who coined the term, the contact between doctor and patient is not the dialogue it seems to be, but is instead, an interview, projective test, or investigative study.

Injunction. In transactional analysis, the directions and instructions given to one ego state by another that become the basis for a person's life script decisions. Usually, it is the Parent ego state that gives injunctions to the Child ego state.

Input overload. In encounter groups, overstimulation of one or more members because of intense pressure to open oneself up to inner feelings or because of negative feedback that the member cannot tolerate. Some patients need reinforcement, rather than dissection or destruction of their defense, and, if not managed appropriately, the intensity of the encounter situation may precipitate a psychotic episode in such patients.

Insight. Understanding or awareness. In psychiatry, insight refers to the conscious awareness that one has some kind of problem or illness and also to some degree of understanding that the problem reflects intrapsychic conflicts and an inability to make a wholly successful adaptation. Intellectual insight is used to indicate a superficial level of awareness that is not adequate to lead to effective changes in behavior. Emotional insight refers to a deeper level of awareness that promotes positive changes in attitudes, behavior, etc.

Inspirational-supportive group psychotherapy. A directive, exhortative type of group therapy, employed often by self-help groups, as well as more traditional therapeutic groups, in which emphasis is on the positive potential of participants and reinforcement for accomplishments or the performance of desired behavior.

Instigator. A member of a therapy group who stimulates others in the group toward action and, in particular, the open expression of their feelings and ideas.

Insulin coma therapy. A form of somatic therapy, developed by Manfred Sakel in the 1930's, consisting of the production of coma by means of the intramuscular injection of insulin. Largely replaced nowadays by psychopharmacological and other somatic treatments, insulin coma therapy was used in certain types of schizophrenia.

Intellectualization. A form of rationalization in which reasoning or logic is used as a way of avoiding awareness of and confrontation with an objectionable impulse. Intellectualization is also used to refer to a brooding or thinking compulsion, a need to worry about insignificant things as a way of avoiding emotions by escaping into a world of intellectual concepts and words.

Intensive group process. High level of personal interaction and involvement within a group, typically manifested in the expression of strong, deep feelings.

Interpretation. In psychoanalytic treatment, the description or formulation of the meaning or significance of a patient's productions and, in particular, the translation into a form meaningful for the patient of the meaning of his resistances, defenses, and symbols.

Intervention laboratory. Human relations laboratory, such as an encounter group or sensitivity training group, designed as an intervention into group conflict or crisis with the aim of resolving it.

Intuitive self. In transactional analysis, the part of the Child ego state that assesses the kind and quality of social operations that will take place with other people.

Isolate. In a therapy group, a member who does not participate in group activities or make contact with others in the group.

I-Thou. Martin Buber's term for a constructive type of relationship based on true sharing and basic trust. In groups, I-Thou relationships promote warmth, cohesiveness, and constructive group process.

Johari Window. A schematic diagram used to conceptualize human behavior. It was developed by Joseph (Jo) Luft and Harry (Hari) Ingham at the University of California at Los Angeles in 1955. The diagram is composed of quadrants—both representing some aspect of a person's behavior, feelings, and motivations—known as (1) blind self; (2) hidden self; (3) public self; and (4) undeveloped potential.

Karate-chop experience. In encounter groups, a semihumorous technique for eliciting aggression from timid or inhibited participants. A more aggressive member faces the timid one, and each makes exaggerated karate-like motions at the other, yelling "Hai!" as loudly as possible after each stroke but making no physical contact with the other. After the exercise, all members of the group discuss the experience.

Kinesiology. The study of body movement and action, particularly as a part of communication; also termed kinesics.

Kinesthetic sense. Perception of muscular movement in one's own body; proprioception.

Latency phase. Stage of psychosexual development, beginning at about 5 years of age with the passing of the Oedipus complex and ending at puberty at about 12 years. Lubidinal energies are only apparently latent during this period, for they remain active but are directed away from the too-dangerous oedipal objects and into the elaboration of more effective defenses, such as the superego, and into increasing mastery in the social sphere. During the latency phase, the energies connected with the aggressive drive are more in evidence than those associated with libidinal strivings.

Lateral transference. In group therapy, transfer to a peer or co-participant of the projections that would ordinarily appear as transference manifestations toward the therapist. Other members of the group are perceived in terms of the subject's experiences within his nuclear family.

Leaderless therapeutic group. In Walter R. Bion's terminology, a group characterized by nonparticipation of the therapist, who remains a silent observer of group interactions, withholding explanations, directions, and support except for rare, nonauthoritarian verbal interactions. Currently, the term is more frequently applied to self-directed groups that have, at least in the beginning, no designated or recognized therapist or leader, although typically a leader ultimately emerges.

Leadership role. The therapy style adopted by the therapist conducting group therapy: the techniques he uses, how he uses them, what he emphasizes in his interactions with the group and its members, etc. One typology subdivides leadership roles into three types: authoritarian, democratic, and laissez-faire.

Libido binding. Used by S. R. Slavson to refer to activity group psychotherapy that engages group members in activities that tie them down to a specific interest or occupation. Immobilizing or libido-binding activities are designed to have the opposite effect from stimulating or libido-activating activities.

Life line. A projective technique in which each member of the group is asked to draw a line representing his life from birth to death. Comparison of the lines drawn and discussion of their differences usually reveal a variety of personally meaningful parameters, such as maturity and academic achievement, that have determined the shape, slope, length, etc., of the individual drawings.

Life review. Reminiscence; the recalling or recollecting of past experiences and, in particular, those deemed by the subject to have been particularly significant. Life review tends to occur in any therapeutic group at times, but it is characteristic of group therapy with the elderly. Erikson's eighth stage of man, integrity versus despair, emphasizes the importance of life review. The older person who can look back on life with satisfaction shows integrity, while the one whose life is a series of missed opportunities or mistakes that cannot be undone is filled with despair.

Maintenance drug therapy. The minimal dosage of a psychopharmacological agent that must continue to be administered without risking relapse. In psychotic states, for instance, very high doses of a drug may be needed for the control of symptoms; once that control is achieved, however, dosage may often be lowered considerably, although it may be necessary to keep the patient on that lower dosage (maintenance dose) for a long time.

Mannerism. A gesture, posture, expression, or other motor activity of short duration that is frequently repeated and thus characteristic of or peculiar to a given person. Sometimes it is used interchangeably with stereotypy, although a mannerism is less insistently and monotonously repeated and is more readily modifiable or controlled if called to the attention of the person. Examples are clearing the throat, tapping the foot, and curling a wisp of hair with the fingers.

Marital counseling. A form of marriage therapy in which a trained counselor helps the couple in resolving problems that trouble them in their relationship by seeing husband and wife both separately and in joint sessions that focus on immediate family problems. This type of intervention was first developed in social agencies as part of family case work.

Marriage therapy. A type of family therapy, based on the systems concept that the marital dyad is a subsystem of the family, involving husband and wife and focusing on the couple's relationship and the effects it has on the individual psychopathology of the partners. Marriage therapy assumes that psychopathology within the family structure, and the social matrix of the marriage perpetuate and engender individual psychopathology which, when fed back into the family unit, aggravates the disturbances in the marriage.

Mattress pounding. A technique used most often in encounter groups that mobilizes a member's suppressed or repressed anger by having him yell and beat a mattress with his fists. In many cases, the mattress soon becomes in fantasy a hated parent or sibling. After the exercise, all members of the group discuss their feelings about it.

Maximal expression. Greatest degree of communication possible. In psychodrama, it results from involved sharing by the group of the three portions of the session: warm-up, action, and post-action. During the action period, the actor patient is enjoined to express anything and everything to the limit, including delusions, hallucinations, fantasies, and soliloquies.

Mechanical group therapy. A didactic approach to treatment employing various mechanical devices to deliver a message with some therapeutic intent. The method requires neither an organized group nor a therapist and has been used mainly in mental hospitals to inform residents about and secure general acceptance of some elementary principles of mental health. One technique is to broadcast brief recordings over the hospital's loudspeaker system; another is to print messages on cards that are placed on breakfast trays.

Mediator. In behavior therapy, anyone who can provide data needed for analysis of the patient's behavior and his response to treatment, such as a parent, teacher, or spouse.

Methadone maintenance treatment. Long-term use of methadone in persons formerly addicted to other opiates, such as heroin. Repeated intravenous or subcutaneous injections of heroin produce peaks of elation; methadone maintenance replaces those peaks with sustained and uniform drug action without notable elation, abstinence symptoms, or demand for an escalation of the dose.

Milieu therapy. Socio-environmental therapy, usually in a hospital or residential setting, utilizing techniques that are specifically designed to promote behavior modification within a stable social organization so that every social experience and treatment experience of the patient will be synergistically applied toward realistic and specific therapeutic goals. The treatments used may include somatic therapies, behavior therapies, individual psychotherapy, sensitivity training, family therapy, psychodrama, other group process approaches, hypnosis and suggestion, communications analysis, and role playing. Milieu therapy is a means of providing an integrated, stable, and coherent context in which the optimal combination of specific treatments can be provided to the patient.

Million-dollar game. A group technique used to explore the meaning of money to the players and to encourage free, creative thinking. The group is told it has a million dollars to be used productively in any way they want, so long as every member of the group is involved.

Mirror. In psychodrama, a person who copies the behavior of another patient and tries to express the latter's feeling in words and movement in order to demonstrate how he is perceived by other people. The mirror often exaggerates and deliberately distorts the patient's behavior in order to rouse him from a passive spectator role into one of active involvement and participation. The mirror is also called the double.

Mirroring. A group process in which the group's response to one member is used to show him how he presents himself to others. The image may be true or distorted, depending on the level of truth at which the group is functioning at the time. Mirroring is used as an exercise in encounter groups and as a laboratory procedure during the warming-up period of psychodrama.

Modeling. A form of behavior therapy based on the principles of imitative learning; it obviates the need for the patient to discover effective responses through trial and error by observing the behavior of the therapist or other members of a group. Outside therapy, the behavior of others may constitute a powerful antecedent in determining or maintaining the problem behavior of which the patient complains.

Modular strategy. A technique used in treatment planning to refer to the different levels of intervention available, with therapist and patient deciding jointly to proceed to a different level of intervention if the current one is not having the desired effect. The assumption in such planning is that less treatment is better than more treatment, and the emphasis is on continuing evaluation and feedback of the results of each treatment approach.

Mother Superior complex. A therapist's tendency to play a maternal role in his relationship with his patients, a tendency that usually interferes with the therapeutic process.

Multibody situation. Interaction between several people, as in a group session. The term emphasizes the evolution of social interaction from narcissism through the dyadic mother-child relationship and the triad of the oedipal period to the complexities of group relationships.

Multidirectional partiality. A technique used by Boszormenyi-Nagy in family therapy in which the therapist sides openly with one family member and then in turn, with another, until every member has been favored. The aim is to heighten the therapist's empathic understanding of each member of the group at the same time that it is made explicit that the therapist has become a part of the system that he is treating.

Multiple double. In psychodrama, presentation in sequence of different parts of the patient's life, each played by a different actor. The first actor, for example, may portray him as he was in adolescence, the second as he was when his mother died several years ago, the third as he is now, the fourth as he may be 20 years from now.

Multiple interaction. Group behavior in which many members participate and interact, both verbally and nonverbally, at the same time.

Multiple reactivity. The behavioral effects on different group members of the provocative or otherwise stimulating behavior of another member of the group.

Multiple transferences. Projection simultaneously onto the therapist and other members of the group of feelings, attitudes, and ideas that were originally held toward members of one's family.

Multipolarity. Slavson's term for the many objects of transference projections within a therapy group, where interpatient transference develops as readily as patient-to-therapist transference.

Munich cooperation model. A type of group therapy, used mainly in hospital and residential settings, in which the group is structured in such a way as to reproduce typical intrafamilial conflicts. Ward personnel observe group sessions and apply interpretations from them to patient-personnel interactions on the ward. Patients support one another in autonomous groups that form after the treatment sessions.

National Training Laboratories. Now called NTL Institute for Applied Behavioral Science, a program introduced in 1947 at Bethel, Maine, to train professionals in group work. Interest in personal development and growth potential led eventually to sensitivity training and encounter groups.

Natural Child. In transactional analysis, the autonomous, expressive archaic Child ego state, free from parental influence, uncensored, affectionate, impulsive, curious, sensuous, and aggressive.

Negative practice. K. Dunlap's term for one of the earliest forms of strategic intervention to be described (in 1928); the subject is directed to practice repetitively the very habit he hopes to overcome.

Negative therapeutic reaction. Worsening of the clinical condition during treatment; often used more loosely to refer to slow, difficult, or less than optimal progress in treatment. Group therapy may afford the major entry point into the defenses that interfere with therapeutic progress.

Network. Those many different people who have an on-going significance in a specific person's or a nuclear family's life in terms of meeting human needs, including the extended family, more distant relatives, friends, and work and recreational contacts. It is also called the supportive social network to emphasize its relevance to the goals of treatment and rehabilitation. The social network is a largely invisible system that is rarely together at any one time.

Neurosis. An ego-dystonic mental disorder, not based on known or demonstrable organic pathology (and, therefore, assumed to be psychological or emotional in origin), that tends to be relatively enduring or recurrent if untreated, and to interfere with the quality or ease of functioning; although in its most severe forms it may be markedly disabling or incapacitating, it does not lead to gross violation of social norms or to loss of reality testing, such as are observed in psychosis or psychotic disorder. Most schools of psychology have a particular theory of its causes, called the neurotic process in DSM-III and consisting of the following sequence: (1) unconscious conflicts between opposing wishes, prohibitions, etc., lead to (2) unconscious perception of potential danger, with accompanying anxiety or dysphoria, which calls forth (3) defense mechanisms, whose variety and intensity mount to constitute (4) symptoms or personality disturbance. Neurosis is also called neurotic disorder and psychoneurosis. Most systems include all or some of the following as types of neurosis: anxiety neurosis, neurasthenia, hypochondriasis, phobia or anxiety-hysteria, conversion hysteria, dissociative disorders, depersonalization neurosis, obsessive-compulsive or anancastic neurosis, and depressive neurosis.

Neutrality. The role of the therapist in group or individual therapy when he is passive, permissive, nonjudgmental, and allows each patient to use him according to the patient's particular needs. Neutrality is also used in group and family therapy to refer to maintaining an even distribution of attention (or other behavior that might be interpreted as showing favoritism) among all members of the group.

Neutralizer. Member of a therapy group who counteracts or otherwise controls the aggressivity, impulsiveness, and destructiveness of other members of the group.

Nonclinical group. Group organized around increasing self-awareness, growth potential, and effectiveness of coping maneuvers in day-to-day living, rather than for treatment of specified disorders or the uncovering and investigation of the psychopathology of participants. Included are problem-solving, experiential, and sensitivity training groups.

Nondirective approach. Technique in both individual and group therapy in which the therapist follows the patient's lead, rather than imposing his own theories or directions on the course of the session.

Nontruster. Person with strong dependency needs whose early negative experiences have sensitized him to rejection or overprotection, the possibility of whose repetition he avoids by developing a facade of independence. In group sessions he may repeatedly reject all offers of support and avoid any attempt by other participants to draw close to him.

Nude marathon. Encounter group session of long duration (from not less than 8 hours to several days), during which participants are unclothed, based on the theory that clothes are a defense against openness and facing conflicts over one's body, that they connote limiting roles and thus program others to respond in stereotypical ways.

Observer. Person who sits with the group but does not participate actively; instead, he discusses his observations with the staff or supervisor in post-therapy meetings.

Ogre. In structural analysis, the child ego state in the father that supersedes the nurturing Parent and becomes a pseudo-Parent.

Open group. Group to which new members can be added at any time during the course of treatment. Most long-term groups that aim for attainment of insight are open. They are sometimes termed continuous groups.

Outsider. Member of a therapy group who feels alienated and isolated from the group, often because he is a nontruster who needs a great deal of extra effort by the therapist and other group members before he can begin to trust someone.

Pairing. Walter R. Bion's term for mutual support between two or more group members who want to avoid facing their problems; it is sometimes used to refer to any attraction between the two group members.

Palo Alto model. A brief therapy approach, generally limited to a maximum of 10 sessions, that is symptom oriented and applicable to families, as well as individuals; its basic assumption is that problems are maintained by the current behavior of the subject and those with whom he interacts and that such problem-maintaining solutions must be eliminated or prohibited.

Paradoxical therapy. Strategic intervention; influencing techniques that employ tactics that appear contrary to the goals of therapy but are, in fact, designed to overcome resistance, foster change, and hasten improvement. In paradoxical prescribing strategy, for example, the therapist directs the patient to perform the very symptom of which the patient complains, such as to practice an obsessional thought or a compulsive action. In paradoxical retraining therapy, the therapist discourages the patient from attempts to change; the therapist may suggest that it may not be possible for the patient to change, or he may adopt a paradoxical position that is an exaggeration of the patient's pathological attitude.

Passive. In group and individual therapy, describing a therapist who is inactive or nondirective but whose presence serves as a stimulus to the patient(s).

Pastime. In transactional analysis, a semistereotyped set of transactions dealing with a particular topic. In contrast with the game of Berne's terminology, pastime has no ulterior motive and no psychological payoff.

Patty-cake exercise. Use of palm-to-palm contact, similar to children's behavior in playing patty-cake, as a way of bypassing verbal defenses in a group. The game usually arouses minimal anxiety, and yet it encourages a dropping of reserve between people who can then get to know each other more easily. Also called hand-dance.

Peer co-therapist. Therapist who is equal in status to the other therapist treating a group; the two therapists are on a par and relate to each other as equals.

Peer-group phenomenon. Interaction of one person in a group on an equal footing with all the other members of the group, with special emphasis on behavior and activities he performs within the group but would not ordinarily perform outside it. The term is also used to refer to the power that a united group can wield in influencing one of its members to adhere to its code and thereby achieve the status of equal to everyone else in the group.

Peer identification. An unconscious process wherein one member incorporates qualities and attributes of another member; it is seen most frequently in a subject with low self-esteem, who identifies with a group member he perceives as having made great improvement in order to feel more at ease within the group and also to participate magically in the improvement he perceives.

Perception. Mental process by which intellectual, sensory, and emotional data are organized meaningfully, and the organism is thereby enabled to make sense out of all the stimuli with which it is bombarded. Perception is a complex ego function and includes at least four aspects: reception, registration, processing (i.e., reorganization in accord with memory, affects, needs, intentions, etc.), and feedback (proprioceptive and autonomic processes that allow the subject to determine if the object sensed is the object sought). Therapy groups, nonclinical groups, encounter groups, and the like have in common the aim to expand and alter perception in ways conducive to the development of each participant's potential.

Permission. In transactional analysis, a therapeutic transaction that aims to neutralize permanently the parental injunctions.

Personal growth laboratory. Sensitivity training laboratory in which primary emphasis is on each participant's potential for creativity, empathy, and leadership. The facilitator encourages use of the widest possible range of experience and modalities of expression, including art, sensory stimulation, and intellectual, emotional, written, oral, verbal, and nonverbal expression.

Personality. Behavior response patterns that are characteristic of and to some extent predictable in each person, who has both consciously and unconsciously evolved a style of living and being that is a compromise between inner needs and the controls that limit or regulate their expression. The personality functions to maintain a stable, reciprocal relationship between the person and his environment and is a composite of ego defenses that are used in coping with the demands of day-to-day living.

Personality disorder. Pattern of relating to the environment so rigid, fixed, and immutable as to limit severely the likelihood of effective functioning or satisfying interpersonal relationships. The pattern is deeply ingrained, chronic, and habitual; it is maladaptive in that it is relatively inflexible; it limits the optimal use of potentialities and often provokes the very counterreactions from the environment that the subject seeks to avoid. It is not always easy to draw the line between normal personality and personality disorder, and often the label is more a social diagnosis of nonconformity than a designation of disease process in the usual sense. DSM-III recognizes the following personality disorders: paranoid, schizoid, schizotypal, histrionic, narcissistic, antisocial, borderline, avoidant, dependent, compulsive, and passive-aggressive.

Personality syndrome. One of the organic brain syndromes in which the predominant clinical feature is either a pathological exaggeration of pre-existing personality traits (obsessiveness, suspiciousness, niggardliness, etc.) or an appearance of personality features that are inconsistent with or contradictory to premorbid character traits (e.g., the previously hostile and irascible spouse becomes a generous, warm, and self-effacing wife, or a previously straitlaced bulwark of the community loses control over sexual, aggressive, or acquisitive impulses.

Pervasive developmental disorders. A group of abnormalities in psychological development characterized by severe distortions in the timing, rate, or sequence of functions that are basic to the development of communication and social skills. Included are: (1) early infantile autism—characterized by withdrawal, self-absorption, aloneness, inability to relate, obsessive need to maintain the status quo, repetitive play, language disturbances, and motility disturbances such as rolling, rocking, or whirling; (2) atypical childhood psychosis—characterized by impaired emotional relationships, flat or inappropriate affect, catastrophic reactions to stress, motility disturbances, and self-mutilation; it has also been called symbiotic psychosis and childhood schizophrenia.

Perversion. An abnormality, deviation from the norm, or dysfunction; but the term is commonly used to refer to sexual deviations, classified as paraphilias and other psychosexual disorders in DSM-III and including: ego-dystonic homosexuality, fetishism, pedophilia, transvestitism, exhibitionism, voyeurism, sadism, masochism, necrophilia, coprophilia, and urolagnia.

Phobic disorder. Phobic neurosis; anxiety hysteria; an anxiety disorder characterized by a persistent, irrational, and intense fear that is a significant source of stress to the subject and interferes with daily functioning because of the need to avoid the feared object. DSM-III distinguishes three subtypes: (1) agoraphobia, with or without associated panic attacks—fear of being alone or of being in public places from which escape might be difficult or help not readily available in time of need; (2) social phobia—avoidance of situations in which the subject might be humiliated, embarrassed, or exposed to scrutiny (e.g., speaking in public, eating in public, using a public lavatory); and (3) simple or specific phobias that are not elaborated into agoraphobia or social phobia.

Phyloanalysis. Trigant Burrow's later term for his conceptualization of group analysis, by which he emphasized the social participation of many persons in their common analysis, which investigated the impaired tensional processes affecting each organism's internal reaction as a whole. He changed the term because the original one was so often confused with group psychotherapy of the analytic type.

Pillow beating. A technique used most often in encounter groups that mobilizes a member's pent-up rage by beating the pillow and yelling angrily until he gets tired. Acceptance of his demonstrated anger by the group as they discuss his behavior is considered therapeutic.

Play therapy. Techniques used with children in which their play activity is used, instead of verbal associations; first used in psychoanalytic treatment of children by Melanie Klein. The child patient reveals his conflicts on a fantasy level with dolls, clay, and other toys, and the therapist intervenes with explanations or interpretations about the child's responses and behavior geared to his level of comprehension.

Political therapist. A therapist whose professional activities are strongly influenced by the personalities of his superiors and by the personal and historical aspects of authority.

Popular mind. The psychology of the mob or leaderless crowd—primitive, fickle, suggestible, impulsive, and uncritical in their perception of reality. LeBon introduced the phrase.

Power phase. Second stage in group treatment, when participants begin to express anger—usually toward the leader, sometimes toward other members—in an attempt to achieve individuation and autonomy.

Pratt, Joseph H. Boston physician who pioneered in the development of group psychotherapy in the United States. During the period 1900–1906 he worked with tuberculous patients, forming discussion groups that first focused on information about the physical aspects of their disease and its treatment, but later moved to discussions of the emotional problems engendered by their illness.

Preconscious. In psychoanalysis, one of the divisions of the mental apparatus in Freud's topographic scheme. The preconscious includes all those parts of the mind (ideas, thoughts, past experiences, other memories) that can be brought into consciousness when willed by the subject.

Premeeting. Group meeting of a group immediately before they join or are joined by the therapist; it is also known as warming-up session and presession.

Pressure cooker. Slang expression for the high degree of involvement and emotional pitch sought by some of the intensive groups, such as marathon groups.

Primal therapy. A type of psychotherapy, developed by Arthur Janov in California, that begins with a 24-hour period of total isolation before a 2- or 3-week period of intensive individual therapy, which is followed by a few months of group therapy with other postprimal patients. During therapy, the patient is expected to experience primals, reliving the prototypical traumas that originally crystallized his suffering and thereby created his neurosis. It is also called primal scream therapy because of the screaming that is usually a prominent part of reliving past trauma.

Primary gain. Reduction of anxiety achieved through defense mechanisms or neurotic symptoms.

Procedural therapist. A therapist who relies too heavily on the written word, formal rules and regulations, and the hierarchical system.

Procedures. In transactional analysis, ulterior transactions that are done with full Adult awareness, as contrasted with games, whose payoff is not clearly understood by the Adult of the acting person.

Process-centered group. Group whose focus is on its own group dynamics—how it operates and through what stages it progresses. Such groups often ask the question, "What's going on here?" rather than the encounter group question, "What are you experiencing or feeling?"

Program. In transactional analysis, the teaching by one of the Parents of how best to comply with the script injunction.

Project Assist. A self-help group for family members of persons with senile or presenile degenerative dementia.

Projection. Unconscious defense mechanism in which one attributes to another the ideas or impulses that he abhors or is blind to within himself. Among the many forms it takes are blaming others for one's own mistakes, scapegoating, ideas of reference and persecution, delusions of infidelity, pathological jealousy, and transference.

Psychoanalytic group psychotherapy. A method of group therapy, pioneered by Alexander Wolf, based on the theory and techniques of individual psychoanalytic therapy. Analysis and interpretation of transference, resistances, and defenses have the same central importance as in individual analysis, but their use is adapted to the group setting. Like individual psychoanalysis, group psychoanalysis has been modified or applied to purposes other than the original one of effecting significant character change, and its principles have formed the basis for many techniques of group therapies that are not considered psychoanalytic.

Psychodrama. Psychotherapy method, developed by J. L. Moreno, in which personality make-up, interpersonal relationships, conflicts, and emotional prooblems are explored through the medium of dramatic methods, such as self-presentation, in which the player/actor/patient duplicates situations he is involved in, and soliloquy, in which the patient duplicates feelings he has had in real situations but did not express, and spontaneous improvisation, in which the patient acts out fictitious or symbolic roles that have been selected by the therapist. Involved in the psychodrama are: (1) protagonist or patient; (2) auxiliary egos, trained persons who will act out different aspects of the patient in order to help him express his feelings; and (3) director, leader, or therapist, who guides those involved in the drama. Psychodrama or role playing is used as an auxiliary technique in many therapeutic and encounter groups.

Psychodramatic director. Leader of a psychodrama session who functions as producer, therapist, and analyst. As producer, he turns every clue the patient offers into dramatic action. As therapist, he attacks the patient at times or supports him or laughs with him or is passive and indirect or is dominating and interfering, depending on the patient's needs. As analyst, he interprets and elicits responses from the audience.

Psychosis. Loosely, any mental disorder; more specifically, one of a particular class or group of mental disorders characterized by impairment of cognitive capacities, affective responses, reality testing, communication, and relations to others of such degree as to interfere with the ability to meet the ordinary demands of daily living. The definition of the term is even more restrictive in DSM-III, where psychotic denotes the existence of one or more of the following: delusions, hallucinations, incoherence, repeated derailment or loosening of associations, marked poverty of thought, marked illogicality, and grossly disorganized or catatonic behavior. Classically, the psychoses were differentiated from less severe disorders, such as neurosis, sociopathy or psychopathy, character or personality disorder, psychosomatic or psychophysiological disorder, and mental retardation; they were subdivided into organic mental disorders and functional psychoses. The latter included the schizophrenic disorders, affective psychoses, and paranoid states.

Psychosocial stressor. A life event judged to be of significance in the development, precipitation, recurrence, or maintenance of a psychiatric disorder, such as the birth of a child, death of a parent, marriage, illness, or natural disaster.

Psychotherapy. Treatment for mental illness or behavior disturbance in which a trained person deliberately establishes a professional relationship with a patient for the purpose of removing, modifying, or retarding existing symptoms, attenuating or reversing disturbed patterns of behavior, and promoting positive personality growth and development. It is assumed that the process and the changes it provokes involve learning mechanisms and that the therapeutic relationship serves as a microcosm in which the patient can subject past behavior patterns to trained scrutiny and assessment and try out, in collaboration with the therapist, different ways of dealing with reality. Psychotherapy is differentiated from other forms of psychiatric treatment, such as treatment with insulin coma, electric shock, psychosurgery, and psychopharmacological agents.

Psychotropic drug. Drug that affects psychic function, behavior, or experience. This large group includes: neuroleptics (antipsychotics or major tranquilizers), antianxiety agents (minor tranquilizers, anxiolytic sedatives), antimanic agents, antidepressants, psychostimulants, and psychodysleptics (hallucinogens).

Public self. The behavior, feelings, and motivations of a person known both to himself and to others. It is a quadrant of the Johari Window.

Quadrangular therapy. A type of marital therapy involving four people: the married pair and the therapist of each spouse.

Rationalization. An unconscious defense mechanism in which irrational behavior or feelings are made to appear reasonable and logical. Ernest Jones introduced the term.

Reactance. Avoidance of any directive or influence that threatens to eliminate one's ability to choose, select, and determine one's own freedom of behavior. Direct suggestions from a therapist always run the risk of arousing reactance.

Reaction formation. An unconscious defense mechanism in which an unacceptable urge is denied through a constantly maintained opposite attitude. Unlike sublimation, where the energy of the original impulse is diverted into acceptable channels, the original energy in reaction formation or reversal formation continues in force and is controlled only because a counterforce of equal intensity must be maintained to keep it from breaking through.

Reaction formation thus limits the subject's potential for expansion, growth, and creativity, but sublimation enhances it.

Reality. The environment as it is and as agreed upon by other people; the whole of the objective world, embracing everything that can be perceived by the five senses.

Reality testing. A fundamental ego function consisting of objective evaluations and judgment of the world outside the ego or self. Reality depends upon perception, memory, and ability to differentiate between ego and non-ego. Reality testing provides the ego with a mechanism for handling both the external world and its own excitation, for it makes it possible for the ego to anticipate the future in imagination and to plan its actions accordingly. How a person evaluates reality and his attitudes toward it are determined by early experiences with the significant people in his life.

Recall. Process of bringing material that has been registered and stored into consciousness at will. Recall is a function of memory and is known also as remembering and retrieval.

Reciprocal inhibition and desensitization. A form of behavior therapy, developed by J. Wolpe in the 1950's, consisting of pairing anxiety-provoking stimuli with responses antagonistic to anxiety (such as relaxation responses) to weaken and finally eliminate completely the anxiety responses. Recurrent exposure of the phobic patient, for example, to increasing doses of the feared object while the patient maintains relaxation, was used to build up a tolerance to the object until the patient was completely desensitized to it, and the object could be tolerated without anxiety. A patient with a fear of heights, for example, would be given relaxation exercises, and, once a suitably relaxed state was reached, the patient was asked to think just for a minute of stepping only as high as from the street up to the curb. As time went on, the height of the imagined climb was increased—first to one stair, then two, then a whole flight, etc., until, finally, the patient could imagine himself going to the top of a tall building. Then he was directed to begin putting his imaginings into reality and to try out his ability to tolerate heights.

Reconstructive psychotherapy. A therapy aimed at producing alteration in basic character structure and behavior patterns to promote better levels of adaptation in the future, as contrasted with forms of psychotherapy that deal only with symptoms, current conflicts, and here-and-now elements of behavior. Reconstructive psychotherapy attempts to uncover unconscious infantile determinants of conflicts and their derivatives.

Recorder. Person who takes notes or minutes of individual or group therapy sessions. Also called observer, he usually is not a member of the group and does not participate actively in it.

Re-enactment. In psychodrama, acting out a past experience as if it were happening again, so that the subject can feel, perceive, and act as he did the first time.

Regression. Unconscious defense mechanism in which the subject retreats to an earlier level of adaptation; the level to which he returns is typically one upon which he had been fixated during psychosexual development. Regression may occur in any type of disorder, but it is particularly frequent and extensive in schizophrenia.

Rehabilitation. Restoration of a handicapped person to a level of maximal function and adjustment; preparation of the patient physically, mentally, socially, and vocationally for the fullest possible life compatible with his abilities and disabilities. Rehabilitation involves the use of all forms of physical medicine in conjunction with psychosocial adjustment and vocational retraining. It is concerned both with primary handicaps, the chronic symptoms that are in an inherent part of illness and the accumulated losses of skills through illness, and with secondary handicaps, including unhealthy personal reactions to illness and unfavorable, inappropriate attitudes toward the handicapped person that develop in his relatives, employers, hospital staff, etc.

Remotivation. Planned group activity whose aim is to tap dormant areas of functioning and help the patient find parts of himself that can be recovered and used despite his illness. Originally evolved to deal with severely regressed senile or schizophrenic patients, remotivation currently refers to a family of rehabilitation techniques to meet a variety of needs. Included are reality orientation, remotivation activities, and primary and advanced remotivation.

Reparenting. In transactional analysis, a technique used in treating schizophrenics. The patient is regressed to a Child ego state, and missing Parent transactions are then supplied and contaminations corrected.

Repeater. Group member who has had experience in another group.

Repression. Unconscious defense mechanism in which ideas, impulses, or affects that are unacceptable are banished or ejected from consciousness. Repression acts only one time, through the anticathexis or energy required for expulsion of the unacceptable material; nonetheless, it is one of the most limiting of all defenses because it requires that whole tracts of mental life be withdrawn from the ego. Repression of material that was once in consciousness is also termed after-expulsion; maintaining repression of material that has never entered consciousness in the first place is known as primal repression.

Repressive-inspirational group psychotherapy. A type of group treatment aimed at bolstering patients' morale and helping them to avoid undesired feelings. Its chief use is with large groups of seriously regressed patients in institutional settings.

Residential treatment facility. A form of domiciliary care in which the patient receives the treatments appropriate to his needs within the dwelling he shares with other patients with similar needs. A children's residential treatment facility, for instance, provides both educational and specific treatment experiences for the emotionally disturbed child.

Resistance. Conscious or unconscious opposition to exposure of repressed material, often manifest as an exaggeration of the defenses already in operation against threatening material.

Resonance. An unconscious sounding board constructed on the basis of experiences in the first 5 years of life that predisposes the person to respond to specific kinds of stimulation in a characteristic way for the rest of his life. Group therapy often elicits such resonance, as when one patient who begins to function regressively at one particular level of psychosexual development provokes another to resonate with fantasies that express his own conflicts concerning that same level of development.

Response cost contingency. In behavior therapy, a punisher. Maladaptive behavior costs the patient something of value, as when a teenager's allowance is docked when he persists in breaking his agreement to come home by a certain time each night.

Review session. Meeting in which each member of the group re-examines his goals and progress in treatment; a technique used in structured interactional group psychotherapy.

Role-divided therapy. In co-therapy, the assumption of different functions by each of the therapists as part of the planned strategy of treatment. One therapist, for instance, may be the provocateur, while the other always remains the passive observer and interpreter.

Role limit. Definition of the functions of the actors or participants in a group situation. In group therapy, for instance, the patient is the patient, and the therapist is the therapist, and there is no reversal of roles.

Role model. Significant other whom the subject imitates in developing a repertoire of coping behaviors. In a therapeutic community or methadone program, for example, a former addict who has been successful in giving up his habit and gaining status in the community will become a positive role model for the recent entrant into the program.

Role playing. Psychodrama technique in which a patient learns through repetition and practice under controlled conditions how to function better in his real-life tasks. In the therapeutic setting of psychodrama, the protagonist can try out his real-life role as student, for example, but, if he fails, he is readily granted the opportunity to try again and again, until finally he learns new approaches to the situations that had always defeated him in the past. He can then apply those improved methods to real life.

Role reversal. In psychodrama, assigning the role of the patient to an auxiliary ego, with the patient playing the other person, rather than himself. The technique elicits distortions of interpersonal expression that can then be explored and corrected.

Roll and rock. An encounter group technique used to develop trust in a participant. The member stands with eyes closed in a tight circle of group members; he is passed around (rolled) from member to member and then placed on his back on the floor. Next, he is gently lifted by the group and rocked back and forth and finally put back on the floor. After the exercise, the group members discuss their reactions.

Schedule of reinforcement. A program, set in advance, for rewarding desired behavior on an intermittent basis, rather than every time it occurs. A fixed-ratio schedule reinforces after a set number of responses has occurred; a variable-ratio schedule sets an over-all average number of responses that are rewarded, but the actual number of desired responses that occurs between each reinforcement varies widely. There are also fixed-interval and variable-interval schedules in which the average time between reinforcement opportunities is the significant factor, rather than the number of responses.

Schilder, Paul (1886–1940). Vienna-born neuropsychiatrist who introduced group psychotherapy at Bellevue Hospital in New York City. His approach combined social and psychoanalytic principles.

Schizophrenia. A group of mental disorders involving disorganization of a previous level of functioning and a tendency to progressive deterioration of the entire personality, with disturbances of multiple psychological processes, such as language and communication, thought content, perception, affect, sense of self, relationship to the external world, volition, and motor behavior. During the active phase of the illness, such psychotic features as hallucinations and delusions appear. The term was introduced by Eugen Bleuler to replace "dementia praecox." The causes of this group of disorders are unknown, although there is strong evidence that heredogenetic factors are involved in many cases. Various subtypes are differentiated on symptomatic grounds: paranoid, catatonic, hebephrenic or disorganized, simple, childhood, schizoaffective, residual, latent, undifferentiated.

Screening. Initial patient evaluation—including medical and psychiatric history, mental status evaluation, and diagnostic formulation—used to determine the patient's suitability for a particular treatment modality.

Script. In transactional analysis, the life pattern of the person based on childhood decisions, a complex set of transactions that are adaptations of infantile responses and experiences. The script operates on an unconscious level as a mold on which a person's adaptation is based.

Script analysis. Analysis of a person's life adaptation—his injunctions, decisions, and life scripts—and the therapeutic process that helps reverse maladaptive behavior. It is the last phase in transactional analysis.

Script antithesis. In transactional analysis, therapeutic intervention designed to avert, at least temporarily, a tragic event in a script.

Script matrix. Diagram used in transactional analysis that depicts two parents and their offspring. It is used in tracing the development of life scripts.

Secondary gain. Advantages gained from an illness over and above the primary gain of reduction or control of anxiety, such as attention, gifts, or other rewards. It is also called epinosic gain.

Secondary process. In psychoanalysis, the mechanisms that govern the functioning of the ego and consciousness, including: judgment, intellect, logic, reality testing, control of the instincts that press for immediate discharge and gratification, and regulation of the drives.

Self-help group. Special-interest group formed to provide mutual help to its members; a formalized mutual help network whose members share a specific problem, such as alcoholism, widowhood, divorce, parental abuse of children, colostomy, cancer, or loss of a child through sudden infant death syndrome.

Self-preservation. Psychodrama technique in which the protagonist plays the role of himself and of related persons (parent, sibling, etc.) as he perceives them, completely subjectively.

Self-realization. Psychodrama technique in which the protagonist enacts, with the aid of auxiliary egos, the plan of his life, no matter how remote it may be from his present situation. For instance, a computer programmer who has been taking acting lessons and would like to try out for summer stock as his first move into a theatrical career can explore what he might have to do to be successful in the theatre and what he would do if he failed.

Sensitivity training group. Educational-experiential technique in which a group of people meet regularly, usually with a specified leader, to learn about themselves, about interpersonal relationships, about group process, and about larger social systems. The aim is not treatment of recognized emotional disturbance; emphasis, instead, is on increasing relatedness and opening communication channels between a person and others in his social system. It is also known as a human relations group or T-group.

Sensory-experiential group. An encounter group with primary emphasis on emotional and physical interaction of participants. The experience itself, rather than examinations of group process, is the reason for the group's existence.

Shaping. An operant conditioning technique consisting of reinforcing small steps or approximations to the desired level of functioning in each of the subject's social and behavioral deficits.

Shifting attention. A characteristic of group therapy in which the focus moves from one participant to another so that no one patient remains continuously in the spotlight. It is also known as alternating scrutiny.

Shock treatment. A form of somatic treatment in which a chemical substance or electric current is used to produce an epileptic-like seizure and unconsciousness. The treatment has proved to be markedly beneficial in mood disorders and certain types of schizophrenia, even though its mechanism of action is only poorly understood. The electrical form of treatment is called electroconvulsive treatment (ECT).

Skills training. Exposure of a patient to situations that provide supervised experience and positive role models in areas where he has demonstrated deficits or conflicts in the past. In social skills training, for example, the patient might be given practice in groups meetings and in joining activities that are appropriate to his age, education, and background.

Slavson, S. R. (1890–1981). American pioneer in group psychotherapy based on psychoanalytic principles. He introduced activity group therapy and was a founder of the American Group Psychotherapy Association.

Social network therapy. A form of group therapy involving not only family members but also other relatives, neighbors, friends, employers, and all who make up the patient's social network and provide a potential source of support, encouragement, employment, etc., that may protect against later relapse.

Social therapy. Rehabilitative therapy whose aim is to improve social functioning. Included are occupational therapy, therapeutic community, recreational therapy, milieu therapy, and attitude therapy.

Socialization. Process of learning interpersonal and interactional skills according to and in conformity with one's society; a person's way of participating both mentally and physically in the group.

Somatic treatment. Physical interventions, such as electric convulsive therapy, psychosurgery, and psychopharmacological agents, as contrasted with psychotherapy.

Splitting situation. In co-therapy groups, the opportunity a patient has to express contradictory or ambivalent feelings that he could not ordinarily express to one therapist by having him express one set of feelings (hostility, for example) to one therapist and their opposite to the second therapist.

Splitting transference. Breaking transference feelings or attitudes into their component parts and having one part directed to one member of the group, another part to a second member, etc.

Square interview. Occasional session in marriage therapy in which both spouses and the therapist of each spouse are present. The two therapists, and sometimes the marital couple as well, are able to observe, experience, and respond to the transactional dynamics among the four of them, thus encouraging a sharing of the same viewpoint by all four people involved.

Squeaky wheel. A person who is forever calling attention to himself but, because of his interactional style, is likely to get an unduly large share of a group's effort and energy.

Strokes. In transactional analysis, the basic motivation for action. People do things in order to get strokes, and all social strokes or interactions convey one or more of the basic dynamics through which one influences another person. Those dynamics are: (1) "I'm okay with myself." (2) "You're okay with me." (3) "I'm not okay with myself." (4) "You're not okay with me." A get-on-with-it event is the experience of "I'm okay" with "You're okay."

A combination of "I'm okay" with "You're not okay" engenders a get-rid-of social operation. A combination of "I'm not okay" with "You're not okay" is experienced as a get-nowhere-with event. The combination of "You're okay with me" with "I'm not okay with myself" is experienced as wanting to get away from the situation at hand.

Structural analysis. Analysis of the personality into its constituent ego states, so that the person knows what his own Parent, Adult, and Child are saying. The goal of structural analysis is to establish and maintain the predominance of reality-testing ego states, free from contamination. It is the first phase of transactional analysis.

Structured interactional group psychotherapy. A type of group psychotherapy developed by Harold Kaplan and Benjamin Sadock, in which the therapist provides a structural matrix for the group's interactions. The significant element in the structure is that a different member of the group is the focus of the interaction in each session.

Subject session. A group technique, often used in structured interactional group psychotherapy, in which a therapist or member introduces a topic for discussion by the whole group.

Substituting. Providing a nonverbal alternate for something that was missed in early life, such as crossing the room to sit beside a group member who needs support.

Substitution. An unconscious defense mechanism in which a person replaces an unacceptable drive with one that is more acceptable. Substitute formation refers to symptom formation, since the symptom itself stands for the unacceptable impulse.

Summer session. In structured interactional group psychotherapy, a regularly scheduled group session during the therapist's vacation.

Superego. In psychoanalytic psychology, one of the three functional divisions of the psyche (the others are the id and the ego) and the last of the three to develop. It is the representative of society with the psyche (conscience or morality) and includes the ego ideal or ideal aspirations. It arises from the internalization of the ethical standards of society and develops by identification with the attitudes of the parents. It is mainly unconscious and has a protective-rewarding function, as well as a critical-punishing one. The conflicts of the oedipal period are particularly significant in its development in that they require changes in the organization of the ego, one of which is the superego.

Surplus reality. Moreno's term for the intangible, invisible dimension of intrapsychic and extrapsychic life.

Survival. For use in a professionally homogeneous group, a game designed to make participants aware of each other's talents. In the game, members are not permitted to continue in their professions but, as a group, must find some other activity in which to work together meaningfully and profitably.

Symbolization. An unconscious defense mechanism in which one idea or object comes to stand for another because of some element or quality they share. The symbol protects the person from the anxiety that the original idea or object would provoke.

Target multiplicity. Slavson's term for the multiple possibilities existing in a group for projecting or displacing hostility onto other patients, who replace the therapist as target.

Target patient. Group member who is analyzed by another group member, the object of the go-around technique in psychoanalytically oriented groups.

Task-oriented group. A group whose conscious focus is on a specified goal, such as finding a solution to a problem or building a product. An experiential group, in contrast, focuses on sharing whatever happens in the group, rather than trying to move it toward any particular goal.

Termination. Planned, orderly conclusion of treatment with the concurrence of patient(s) and therapist, in contrast to dropping out.

T-group (training group). Experience-based learning group that emphasizes self-awareness and group dynamics.

Theatre of Spontaneity (Stegreiftheater). Theatre in Vienna that improvised group processes, developed by J. L. Moreno.

Therapeutic agent. Any device, mechanism, procedure, substance, etc., whether animate or inanimate, that promotes healing in a person with a disorder, disease, or maladaptation. It may be a drug or other somatic modality, it may be a therapist, or it may be people in a group who help their peers.

Therapeutic alliance. Conscious collaborative relationship between therapist and patient in which each implicitly agrees that they should work together to achieve the insight and control that will help the patient with his conflicts. It involves a therapeutic splitting of the patient's ego into observing and experiencing parts and is as important in group therapy as in dyadic psychotherapy. A good therapeutic alliance is needed particularly during phases of strong negative transference in order to keep the treatment going.

Therapeutic atmosphere. All the maturational and growth-supporting elements—cultural, social, medical, etc.—that operate within the therapy setting.

Therapeutic community. Psychiatric or mental hospital that emphasizes socio-environmental and interpersonal influences in the therapy, management, resocialization, and rehabilitation of patients. It helps the patient identify himself with a social group and thereby modify his social behavior because of increased awareness of his role in relationship to other people. The term is also used to refer more specifically to a residential setting for the rehabilitation of drug abusers, consisting usually of a drug-free program combined with provocative encounter group sessions with peers and drug counselors.

Therapeutic crisis. A turning point in treatment, such as a burst of acting out in a patient, the adequate handling of which by the therapist may make the difference between reaching therapeutic goals and withdrawing from the treatment situation.

Therapeutic group. Assemblage of patients under the leadership of a therapist for the purpose of working together for psychotherapeutic ends—specifically, for the treatment of each person's emotional disorders.

Therapeutic impasse. Deadlock in the treatment process, when the patient is inactive and seems unable to gain insight or awareness, no matter how extensive or intensive the interpretations of the analyst are. Therapy sessions become nothing more than scheduled meetings between therapist and patient, and therapy is in danger of collapse. Unresolved resistances and transference and countertransference conflicts are often the basis of the impasse.

Therapeutic role. The position of or the identity of one who aims to treat, improve, or alleviate a distressing condition or state.

Therapeutic soliloquy. Psychodrama technique in which a patient portrays, through side dialogues and side actions, his hidden thoughts and feelings that parallel his overt thoughts and action.

Therapeutic transaction. Interplay between therapist and patient or among group members that is intended to improve the patient.

Therapist surrogate. Substitute for the leader; a group member whose experience, intuition, or training enables him to be an effective group leader in the absence of or in concert with the group therapist. He is also known as a nuclear group member.

There and then. Past experience, rather than immediate experience.

Third ear. Ability to use intuition, sensitivity, and awareness of subliminal cues to gain understanding of and make interpretations about the behavior, attitudes, and feelings expressed in the clinical situation by individual and group patients. First introduced by the German philosopher Friedrich Nietzsche, it was later used in analytic psychotherapy by Theodor Reik.

Tolerance. In group therapy, willingness to endure or allow disordered behavior by co-members. In the area of drug treatment and drug abuse, tolerance refers to increasing resistance to the effects of a drug and the ability to endure its effects without harm. Tolerance is an outstanding characteristic of the opiates, amphetamine, barbiturates, and many other drugs of abuse, including alcohol.

Trading of dissociations. Phenomenon observed in family therapy, when each family member insists that the trouble lies in another member of the family and that the solution would be individual treatment of that member. Each person denies or dissociates his own contribution to the family problem.

Traditional group therapy. Conventional group approach in which the role of therapist is clearly delineated and the other participants are understood to be patients who attend meetings to overcome or resolve some definite emotional problems. This is in contrast to the more recent development of nonclinical groups, whose emphasis is on self-actualization, growth, and the fulfillment of one's potential and not on individual pathology.

Trainer. Professional leader or facilitator of a sensitivity training or T-group; teacher or supervisor of a person learning the theory and techniques of group therapy.

Transaction. Interaction that occurs when two or more persons have an encounter. In transactional analysis, it is the unit of social interaction.

Transactional analysis. Introduced as a form of group therapy by Eric Berne in 1957 and since applied to both groups and individuals, a teaching or learning device with a teleologic emphasis that seeks awareness of what goes on between people socially. It centers on the study of interactions occurring during treatment sessions and includes four components: (1) structural analysis of intrapsychic phenomena; (2) transactional analysis proper, the determination of the currently dominant ego state (Parent, Child, or Adult) of each participant; (3) game analysis, identification of the games played in interactions and of the gratifications or payoff provided; and (4) script analysis, uncovering the causes of the person's life pattern and the childhood decisions that produced it.

Transactional group psychotherapy. System of therapy founded by Eric Berne.

Transference. Projection of feelings, thoughts, and wishes onto the therapist or analyst, who has come to represent an object from the patient's past. The analyst is reacted to as though he were that person; such reactions, while perhaps appropriate to the conditions prevailing in the patient's earlier life, are inappropriate and anachronistic when applied to the therapist in the present.

Transference neurosis. Artificial neurosis that is an outcome of the psychoanalytic situation in which the patient's development, leading up to his infantile neurosis, is re-enacted in the analytic room. The early infantile Oedipus situation reappears, and the analyst comes to represent one or both parents as a love object, as if he were really the original parent in the original infantile setting of the patient. During the period of the transference neurosis, the patient lives out all his old ego attitudes and incest prohibitions.

Transference regression. The psychoanalytic patient's reenactment of his preoedipal and Oedipus complex development that is expressed in the form of a transference neurosis.

Undeveloped potential. The unknown quadrant of the Johari Window, comprising the behavior, feelings, and motivations of a person that neither he nor others recognize but that could, under appropriate conditions, be enlisted to further emotional growth and personality development.

Universality. Total effect of all group members sharing specific symptoms or problems.

VCIA. A label—standing for value, congruence, influence, and activity—for participants in a group whose behavior is viewed as harmonious with group values and including such elements as willingness to take risks, spontaneity, warmth, empathy, openness, expressiveness, and helpfulness.

Vector. A force felt by the therapy group to be operating within it. Originally used in Lewin's field theory of human behavior, it has been applied to various group situations.

Verbal-deep approach. Procedure used in small groups in which communication is conducted exclusively through verbal means and oriented to major goals, as in analytic group psychotherapy.

Verbal-superficial approach. Group therapy procedure in which language is the sole medium of communication and the therapeutic process is structured to attain limited objectives. It is used primarily in the treatment of large groups.

Verbal technique. Any method of group or individual therapy in which words and language are the medium of expression. The major part of most psychotherapy is verbal.

West Coast-style T-group. Sensitivity training or encounter group oriented toward the experience of union, intimacy, and personal awareness, with relative disregard of the study of group process. It is popular in California.

Wild therapy. Group therapy conducted by a leader whose background may not be professional or whose theoretical formulations espouse procedures that deviate markedly from conventional techniques.

Withdrawal. Act of retreating, leaving, or dropping out. It is used to refer to pathological retreat from interpersonal contact and social involvement, as observed in schizophrenia and depression. In a group setting, such behavior creates a barrier to therapeutic progress. The term is also used to refer to abstinence from a drug on which the subject has become psychologically or physically dependent.

Wolf-pack phenomenon. Group process in which a member of the group or the therapist becomes the scapegoat for the other members.

Working alliance. Collaboration between each member and the therapy group as a whole in a shared striving for health, growth, and maturation with the help of the therapist.

Working out.   Stage in the treatment process in which the personal development history and psychodynamics of a patient are discovered.

Working through.   Process of obtaining more insight and changes in personality and behavior by repeated and varied examination of a conflict or problem. Interactions between free association, resistance, interpretation, and working through, constitute the fundamental elements of the analytic process.

Index